HOSPICE AND PALLIATIVE CARE IN AFRICA

A review of developments
and challenges

HOSPICE AND PALLIATIVE CARE IN AFRICA

A review of developments and challenges

Michael Wright
and
David Clark
With
Jennifer Hunt and Thomas Lynch

International Observatory on End of Life Care
Institute for Health Research
Lancaster University, UK
Supported by The Diana, Princess of Wales Memorial Fund
and the Elton John AIDS Foundation

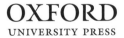

OXFORD
UNIVERSITY PRESS

OXFORD
UNIVERSITY PRESS

Great Clarendon Street, Oxford OX2 6DP

Oxford University Press is a department of the University of Oxford.
It furthers the University's objective of excellence in research, scholarship,
and education by publishing worldwide in

Oxford New York

Auckland Cape Town Dar es Salaam Hong Kong Karachi
Kuala Lumpur Madrid Melbourne Mexico City Nairobi
New Delhi Shanghai Taipei Toronto

With offices in

Argentina Austria Brazil Chile Czech Republic France Greece
Guatemala Hungary Italy Japan Poland Portugal Singapore
South Korea Switzerland Thailand Turkey Ukraine Vietnam

Oxford is a registered trade mark of Oxford University Press
in the UK and in certain other countries

Published in the United States
by Oxford University Press Inc., New York

© Oxford University Press, 2006

British Library Cataloguing in Publication Data

Data available

Library of Congress Cataloging in Publication Data

Wright, Michael, 1944–
    Hospice and palliative care in Africa : a review of developments and
challenges / Michael Wright, David Clark ; with Jennifer Hunt and
Thomas Lynch. — 1st ed.
        p. ; cm.
    Includes bibliographical references and index.
    1. Hospice care—Africa.   2. Palliative treatment—Africa.   I. Clark,
David 1953–   II. Title.
    [DNLM: 1. Hospice Care—Africa.   2. HIV Infections–therapy—
Africa.   3. Palliative Care—Africa. WB 310 W952h 2006]
    R726.8.W75 2006
    362.17′56096—dc22

                                                        2006015480

Typeset by Newgen Imaging Systems (P) Ltd., Chennai, India
Printed in Great Britain
on acid-free paper by Biddles Ltd., King's Lynn

ISBN 0–19–920680–5 (Pbk.:alk.paper)   978–0–19–920680–3 (Pbk.)

10 9 8 7 6 5 4 3 2

Contents

Part 5 **Hospice–palliative care service development in Africa: countries with capacity building activity**

Foreword to Hospice and Palliative Care in Africa

By Sir Elton John

This book is a landmark document for anyone concerned about HIV/AIDS in Africa and the role of palliative care in supporting those affected by the epidemic that is occurring there. It lays down a solid platform of evidence about how hospice and palliative care services are developing across the continent and it provides a baseline against which to measure progress in the future. It is packed full of useful information that will assist those involved in policy and service development. But it is also a powerful testimony to the many individuals who make up the African palliative care workforce and to their shared desire to achieve their goals, often in the face of tremendous adversity. It is both a handbook and a history – a guide to palliative care services in Africa and an analysis of the factors that are shaping their development.

The Elton John AIDS Foundation was born out of the frustration and sadness of watching people that I loved succumb to this disease. Since its inception in 1993, we have disbursed over $100 million to thousands of programmes around the world, including food programmes, counselling, training, prevention education, condom promotion, needle exchanges, fostering and adoption for AIDS orphans, microcredit and much more. Always, a core element of our grant-making is to fund programmes providing essential care to those who have no other support to turn to. Home based and palliative care has been the backbone of the compassionate response to the AIDS epidemic – from San Francisco to Soweto. Now my Foundation is championing the expansion of anti-retroviral medication in the developing world which can have a 'Lazarus effect' for millions. Yet even 'ARVs' are not a cure, and until one is found, palliative care will occupy a central role in the response to this terrible disease.

With the death of Princess Diana in 1997 I lost a dear friend and the world lost a great champion, particularly for the sick. It was my privilege to record a special version of 'Candle in the Wind', which provided some of the first funds for the Diana, Princess of Wales Memorial Fund. Since then, my Foundation has collaborated with the Fund on a number of important projects. In 2001 the Fund launched a Palliative Care Initiative to champion palliative care development in sub-Saharan Africa. It recognized at the time that there were very few major donors interested in this area of work. The overall aim of the initiative was therefore to ensure accessibility and sustainability of palliative care in order to improve quality of life for people with life limiting illness. It also sought to mobilise public awareness as well as policy initiatives and funding programmes in support of palliative care in areas of Africa significantly affected by HIV/AIDS. Many of those with cancer or HIV/AIDS have little or no access to pain relief or drugs for managing troubling symptoms, yet through the support of palliative care teams they can be cared for in their homes. For their families, palliative care can ease the burden of supporting a very sick relative and bring comfort as relatives prepare for bereavement. The Fund's palliative care initiative works in two ways – it gives grants to practical projects as well as advocating for palliative care internationally.

Together, the Elton John AIDS Foundation and the Diana, Princess of Wales Memorial Fund have sponsored the work that led to this wide-ranging and important book. Michael Wright and David Clark, along with their many associates working under the umbrella of the International Observatory on End of Life Care at Lancaster University, have produced a study of hospice and palliative care in Africa that is remarkable in its breadth and depth. I commend this book to anyone interested in the fight against AIDS and in the struggle to promote palliative care across Africa. This is a book with much to teach us all. It captures some of the unique dimensions of the African palliative care experience, but also contains many messages that will be relevant elsewhere. *Hospice and Palliative Care in Africa* deserves to be widely read. I am delighted that the Elton John AIDS Foundation and the Diana, Princess of Wales Memorial Fund have been able to support the research that led up to the book's production and also to make available large numbers of copies to those who will most want to read it – clinicians, policy makers, fund raisers and researchers seeking to promote palliative care across the spectrum of disease to people affected by HIV/AIDS in the African context.

Sir Elton John

Acknowledgements

This project began in September 2003 and throughout our work we have been grateful for the interest and support of Olivia Dix and Andrew Purkis from The Diana, Princess of Wales Memorial Fund and Anne Aslett from the Elton John AIDS Foundation—and also for the funding support from both these organisations. We hope that our efforts have matched their expectations.

Many other colleagues and organisations have helped us along the way. These include Faith Mwangi-Powell and members of the African Palliative Care Association; Anne Merriman and staff at Hospice Africa Uganda; and JP van Niekerk and board members of the Hospice Association of South Africa. We are also grateful for the continuing support of Mary Callaway and Kathleen Foley from the Open Society Institute, New York, as well as Avril Jackson from Hospice Information, Nick Pahl and colleagues at the UK Forum for Hospice and Palliative Care Worldwide (part of Help the Hospices, UK) and Abigail Fowlkes Gutierrez from the Foundation for Hospices in Sub-Saharan Africa. Francoise Porchet was kind enough to assist with some help in translation.

Exceptionally, several individuals have given crucial help in a variety of ways, particularly during visits to African countries: drawing up a programme, gathering together reports and statistical data, assisting with transport arrangements, arranging visits to services and so on. These include Liz Gwyther, Lesley van Zyl, Mandla Mtatembi, Barbara Campbell-Ker, Sibongile Mafata and Davina Bishop in South Africa; Eki Kikule and Immaculate Mukasa in Uganda; Bactrin Killingo, Brigid Sirengo, Zipporah Ali in Kenya; Kristopher Hartwig, Susan Simonson, Karilyn Collins, Mary Ash and Hussein Mtiro in Tanzania; Cromwell Shalunga, John Imbwae, Mary Chidgey and Alison Hill in Zambia; Vicky Lavy, Lameck Thambo, Sam Phiri and Sue Makin in Malawi; Eleanor Warr and Christa Kiebelstein in Botswana; and Sam Mkwananzi, Eunice Garanganga and Val Maasdorp in Zimbabwe.

We also thank all of the people—around one hundred of them—who gave interviews for this study, together with the large number of individuals who kindly completed questionnaires, sent emails, provided documents and materials, and generally steered us along.

Our colleagues at the Institute for Health Research at Lancaster University, as always, have kept our spirits up and provided timely advice. We are particularly grateful to Anthony Greenwood, our Information Officer for many pieces of work and, in particular, the uploading of country reports to our website; and to Justin Wood, who assisted with the maps of Africa. Thanks also go to our programme secretary, Lynne Hargreaves, and to our transcribers—Margaret Jane, Erja Nikander, Karen Mackay and Julie Buttrick. We also appreciate the extended support given by Tracey Sillito, both as a transcriber and in drawing together the final manuscript. And we are grateful to our Norway-based colleague, Lars Johan Materstvedt, for his contribution to the ethical issues section of the Uganda report. Amanda Bingley contributed significantly with our report on the situation in Egypt.

We have enjoyed every moment of our collaboration on this study. We hope it will have a positive impact on the development of hospice and palliative care in the countries of Africa. It has been a privilege to gain some insight into this important work and to meet many of those who are engaged in it. We thank them all for their help, generosity of spirit and, above all, what they have taught us. Any inaccuracies, omissions or mis-representations are ours alone.

Michael Wright, David Clark, Jennifer Hunt, Thomas Lynch
January 2006

Part 1

Summary

Chapter 1

Overview of the study

The African context

The continent of Africa encompasses an estimated population of around 826 million[1] people spread across a vast expanse of land. The second largest of the continents, Africa contains 22 per cent of the Earth's land surface. The USA, China, India and New Zealand could all fit within the African coastline, together with Europe from the Atlantic to Moscow, and much of South America (Fig. 1.1).[2]

John Reader comments:

> Distances within the continent are vast—7,000 kilometres from the Cape of Good Hope in the south to Cairo in the north, and approximately the same distance again from Dakar in the west to the tip of the Horn of Africa in the east. The Nile is the world's longest river—6,695 kilometres from source to estuary; both the Zaire and the Niger rivers are more than 4,000 kilometres long and the Zaire alone drains a basin covering 3.7 million square kilometres, which is larger than all of India (3.2 million square kilometres); on the world scale, only the Amazon basin is larger—7.05 million square kilometres[2] (p. 2).

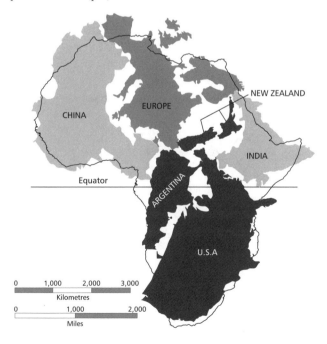

Fig. 1.1 The size of Africa in relation to other portions of the world.

Source: Published with permission from Reader J. (1998), Africa: A Biography of the continent. Penguin.

The countries of Africa can be divided into five regions: North Africa, West Africa, Central Africa, East Africa and Southern Africa. Any division of Africa is arbitrary since some countries could easily fit into more than one region. For example, Burundi and Rwanda are sometimes considered part of East Africa rather than Central Africa. Also, Tanzania may be grouped with the countries of East Africa; here it is placed in Southern Africa due to its membership of the Southern African Development Community[3] (Table 1.1).

Among the countries of Africa, the sovereignty of Western Sahara has remained unresolved since Morocco claimed the northern part in 1976 and the remainder in 1979. After more than a decade of hostilities, a United Nations (UN)-administered cease-fire has remained in effect since September 1991, yet all attempts to hold a referendum have failed. Since the World Health Organization (WHO) provide no data on Western Sahara and the United Nations Development Programme has no human development information, we acknowledge the territory of Western Sahara but have not included it in our study as a sovereign country. Neither do we include islands—such as Madagascar—that are located in the African region. Consequently, this review focuses on the 47 countries on the continent of Africa that are recognized by WHO.

Table 1.1 Countries of Africa by region

North Africa (6)	West Africa (15)	Central Africa (9)	East Africa (7)	Southern Africa (11)
Algeria	Benin	Burundi	Djibouti	Angola
Egypt	Burkina Faso	Cameroon	Eritrea	Botswana
Libya	Cote d'Ivoire	Central African Republic	Ethiopia	Lesotho
Morocco	Ghana	Chad	Kenya	Malawi
Tunisia	Guinea	Congo (Congo-Brazzaville)	Sudan	Mozambique
Western Sahara	Guinea-Bissau	DR Congo (Congo-Kinshasa)	Somalia	Namibia
	Liberia	Equatorial Guinea	Uganda	South Africa
	Mali	Gabon		Swaziland
	Mauritania	Rwanda		Tanzania
	Niger			Zambia
	Nigeria			Zimbabwe
	Senegal			
	Sierra Leone			
	The Gambia			
	Togo			

As we began this review, the complex difficulties currently faced in Africa continued to unfold. In her paper *Tradition and Change*, Grace Wamue summarizes them thus:

> Africa is undergoing serious problems of hunger, malnutrition, bad governance and AIDS. All these are issues that have affected the lives of those living in the continent. For a continent still struggling to free itself from the untold legacies of external domination through slavery, colonization and neo-colonialism, the latest devastation by AIDS and other scourges brings a double tragedy . . . In the face of these challenges, the indigenous African values that held the communities together have come under stress. The sages of African cultural values have either succumbed to old age or to the numerous problems facing our continent. African scholars on the other hand have at times had to rely on views by foreigners on their cultural values.[4]

For Reader, this situation is exacerbated by the twentieth century challenges which faced newly independent states:

> While the effects of poverty, civil war and cultural challenge are plain to see, the causes are neither simple nor easy to eradicate. Crucially, the dream of Africa becoming a continent of peaceful democratic states evaporated in the latter half of the twentieth century when >70 coups occurred in the aftermath of independence. By the 1990s one-party states, presidents-for-life and military rule had become the norm as resources were squandered, the privileged accumulated wealth and the majority suffered[2] (p. 657).

There are dangers, however, in oversimplification, and a more penetrating view highlights differences on the ground that relate to both internal and external influences. For example, Paul Nugent[5] suggests that decolonization during the 1960s varied according to the European decolonizing power. Experiences therefore were not uniform, but varied from region to region. Although military regimes were often repressive, they were not all the same: some were designed as caretaker governments or reforming movements— though there may have been problems sustaining such intentions in the longer term. What is clear, however, is that African debt remains deeply problematic and the question arises as to why sub-Saharan Africa was not part of the worldwide rise in prosperity over the last 50 years. Addressing this issue, Roel van der Veen[6] points to two factors inherent in African society that pre-date colonialism and seem to inhibit progress: patronage and presidentialism. Through patronage, a leader distributes favours to family, friends and a chosen few, whereas presidentialism includes the tendency towards authoritarianism among political and community leaders; in effect, both practices undermine democracy.

Against this backdrop, the UK Prime Minister Tony Blair announced a *Commission for Africa* in February 2004. The accompanying press release was unequivocal about the need for action: Africa is the only continent to become poorer in the last 25 years; its share of world trade has halved in the generation; and it receives less than 1 per cent of direct foreign investment. Five objectives were set:

1. To generate new ideas and action for a strong and prosperous Africa, using the 2005 British presidencies of the G8 and the European Union as a platform.

2. To support the best of existing work on Africa, in particular the New Partnership for African Development and the African Union, and help ensure this work achieves its goals.

3. To help deliver implementation of existing international commitments towards Africa.

4. To offer a fresh and positive perspective for Africa and its diverse culture in the twenty-first century, which challenges perceptions and helps deliver changes.

5. To understand and help fulfil African aspirations for the future by listening to Africans.

The Commission reported on 11 February 2005[7] and proposed a 'coherent package' which addressed the 'interlocking' problems which affect Africa—the 'vicious circles which reinforce one another'. Activity is targeted in key areas. Governance and capacity building focus on the building of systems and staff in national and local governments, where confidence would be improved by more transparency and accountability. Violence is to be tackled with the support of the UN and regional organizations, with stronger agencies for mediation and funding for post-conflict peace building. A skilled workforce would be built by investing in people through the rebuilding of education and health systems, together with a scaling up of the services to deal with human immunodeficiency virus (HIV)/acquired immune deficiency syndrome (AIDS). The economy would be strengthened by an improved climate for investment, doubling the expenditure on infrastructure and placing an emphasis on agriculture and small enterprises—with a particular focus on women and young people. Improvements must also be made to Africa's capacity to trade by removing unfair barriers and facilitating the movement of goods within the country. To implement these changes by 2010 would require an additional US$25 billion and involve the building of a new type of partnership.

Paul Vallely, co-author of the report of the *Commission for Africa*, makes a plea for a broader understanding of the challenges being faced in Africa and for out-dated myths—often perpetuated in the media—to be dispelled. He writes:

> What the critics neglect to say is that things are changing. When I first began to report on Africa two decades ago, there were more than 20 major wars; today, there are just four or five. Then, half the countries were run by dictators; today, two thirds have had democratic elections (some more free and fair than others). For the past 30 years, Africa has stagnated economically; in 2003, growth exceeded five per cent in 24 African countries. The flow of cash to Africa from relatives abroad has increased dramatically in recent years. A new entrepreneurial class is emerging across the continent, as is a new generation of politicians.[8]

Against this background of hope for Africa, it is important to remember that hospice pioneers emerged in Africa just a little over 25 years ago. So the history of palliative care should be seen in the context of social and political change, ideological conflict, civil war, economic fragility and an inadequate infrastructure. When coupled with the effects of famine, poverty, a rampaging AIDS pandemic and, in many areas, a hostile climate, it is little wonder these obstacles appear formidable.

Palliative care in Africa

We are currently witnessing a worldwide growth in concerted efforts to improve the quality of end-of-life care. These efforts focus on the relief of suffering in the face of terminal disease; they address physical, social, psychological and spiritual issues; they are based on multidisciplinary team work; they employ partnership strategies to bring together public health planners, clinicians, non-governmental organizations (NGOs), business and academia; and their efforts are supported by an evidence base grounded in rigorous research. Since the modern hospice movement began during the 1950s and 1960s, it has been estimated that hospice and palliative care services have become established in >120 countries of the world.

In 2002 the WHO defined palliative care as follows:

> Palliative care is an approach which improves quality of life of patients and their families facing the problem associated with life-threatening illness, through the prevention and relief of suffering by means of early identification and impeccable assessment and treatment of pain and other problems, physical, psychosocial and spiritual. Palliative care:
>
> ◆ Provides relief from pain and other distressing symptoms
>
> ◆ Affirms life and regards dying as a normal process
>
> ◆ Intends neither to hasten or postpone death
>
> ◆ Integrates the psychological and spiritual aspects of patient care
>
> ◆ Offers a support system to help patients live as actively as possible until death
>
> ◆ Offers a support system to help the family cope during the patient's illness and in their own bereavement
>
> ◆ Uses a team approach to address the needs of patients and their families, including bereavement counselling, if indicated
>
> ◆ Will enhance quality of life, and may also positively influence the course of illness
>
> ◆ Is applicable early in the course of illness, in conjunction with other therapies that are intended to prolong life, such as chemotherapy or radiation therapy, and includes those investigations needed to better understand and manage distressing clinical complications.[9]

The HIV/AIDS pandemic has become a huge burden for Africa, the world's most affected region; >20 million African deaths have so far been linked to the disease. In 2003, among an estimated 34–46 million people living with HIV infection worldwide, some 26.6 million were in sub-Saharan Africa—an area which also has the highest estimated adult prevalence rate of 7.5–8.5 per cent.[10] The scale and character of these problems create particular difficulties in offering palliative care for people with HIV infection: during critical opportunistic infections, often in deeply impoverished circumstances, and up to the end of life. There are also major issues involved in the care of those bereaved and orphaned.

Several initiatives are underway to promote the development of hospice and palliative care in Africa (Appendix 2). The WHO is involved in a joint palliative care project for cancer and HIV/AIDS patients in Botswana, Ethiopia, Tanzania, Uganda and Zimbabwe.[11] The Diana, Princess of Wales Memorial Fund has supported palliative care initiatives in the nine countries of Ethiopia, Kenya, Malawi, Rwanda, South Africa, Tanzania, Uganda, Zambia and Zimbabwe.[12] The Foundation for Hospices in Sub-Saharan Africa,[13] now a part of the National Hospice and Palliative Care Organisation in the USA,[14] has a growing programme of twinning schemes. The Open Society Institute has a grant support programme for South Africa.[15] An evidence base for the African palliative care context is also beginning to emerge, with an analysis of models of service delivery[16] and an appraisal of the literature relating to services in sub-Saharan Africa.[17]

Since 2004, the effects of a major global policy initiative are also being felt, through the US Government's President's Emergency Programme for AIDS Relief (PEPFAR).[18] This endeavour covers 15 countries in total, 12 of which are in sub-Saharan Africa. PEPFAR is being used to provide antiretroviral (ARV) drugs for 2 million HIV-infected people and to prevent 7 million new infections. It also seeks to provide care for 10 million individuals and orphans infected and affected by the disease, and to build health system capacity in Africa. Fifteen per cent of its US$15 billion dollar budget is earmarked for palliative care.

The first annual report of the PEPFAR programme provides considerable detail on investment in palliative care capacity building and service development.[19] The figures are impressive. Among 5400 US Government-funded outlets and programmes providing palliative care in the 15 PEPFAR countries, 5350 are listed in sub-Saharan Africa. Furthermore, of 36 700 individuals trained to provide palliative care, about 35 400 are in sub-Saharan Africa. Regarding patients: a total of 854 800 HIV-infected individuals have received palliative care (824 100 in sub-Saharan Africa); whereas 241 100 individuals have received palliative care in the form of tuberculosis (TB) care and treatment (~240 500 in sub-Saharan Africa).

The remarkable point about these data is not just the high numbers said to be receiving palliative care but the spread of patients and programmes across the region of sub-Saharan Africa—especially in countries where palliative care services have previously been unknown to the international community. For example, it is claimed that palliative care was received by a total of 15 500 individuals in Ethiopia from a total of 200 palliative care outlets/programmes. In Mozambique, 27 700 individuals received palliative care from 71 outlets; in Namibia, 19 800 individuals received palliative care from 200 outlets; and in Rwanda, 17 600 individuals received palliative care from 300 outlets. The question arises: how have 5350 outlets/programmes in sub-Saharan Africa been scaled up to provide palliative care services in such a short space of time?

Unfortunately, details of methodology, training and client accounting procedures are not provided in the PEPFAR report. Yet perhaps we can gain some clues from the PEPFAR definition of palliative care and inclusion criteria[19] (p. 49):

Palliative care

For HIV positive people, care covers a continuum from diagnosis with HIV infection until death. While the vast majority of HIV positive people do not meet critical criteria for antiretroviral treatment (ART), they nonetheless need basic health care, symptom management, social and emotional support, and compassionate end of life care. Basic health care and support includes routine monitoring of disease progression and prophylaxis and treatment of opportunistic infections, cancers and other complications of immune suppression, such as water-borne diseases and tuberculosis. This holistic approach to the full spectrum of care services from the time of a diagnosis of HIV infection until death is considered to be palliative care. Building upon definitions of palliative care developed by the US Department of Health and the World Health Organisation, President Bush's Emergency Plan supports an interdisciplinary holistic approach and interventions to relieve physical, emotional, and practical suffering.

Palliative care includes all clinic-based and home/community-based activities aimed at optimizing quality of life of HIV-infected (diagnosed or presumed) clients and their families throughout the continuum of their illness . . . ; social and material support such as nutritional support, legal aid and housing, and training and support for caregivers.

Inclusion criteria
Number receiving upstream system strengthening (palliative care) support

Number of individuals . . . includes those supported through contributions to national, regional, and local activities such as training, laboratory support, monitoring and evaluation, logistics and distribution systems, and protocol and curriculum development.

Number receiving downstream site specific (palliative care) support
Number of individuals . . . includes those receiving services at US Government-funded service sites.

These statements seem to suggest a PEPFAR definition of palliative care that, by 'building upon' the US Department of Health and WHO definitions, has broadened the parameters of palliative care. In fact, it appears that every HIV-infected person receiving any form of treatment from US Government-supported outlets is designated as being in receipt of palliative care. These parameters are further widened by a notion of upstream support that includes items such as curriculum development. In the absence of information to the contrary, it may be assumed that these factors have a bearing on patient numbers.

Significantly, the US-based AIDS Healthcare Foundation (AHF)—the largest AIDS organization which operates free AIDS treatment clinics in the USA, Africa, Central America and Asia—has raised serious questions about the figures published by PEPFAR. A news item published on 24 March 2005 states:

AIDS Healthcare Foundation . . . today expressed concern over treatment number claims made by officials from the Presidential Emergency Plan for AIDS Relief (PEPFAR), President Bush's ambitious $15 billion dollar, five-year global AIDS treatment plan. In a letter accompanying the first Annual Report of the Emergency Plan, U.S. Global AIDS Coordinator Randall L. Tobias stated that, 'The Emergency Plan reached 155,000 people with treatment support in just eight months—152,000 of them in sub-Saharan Africa'.

'Even if this number of people on treatment via PEPFAR were accurate, it still represents a mere eight per cent of PEPFAR's stated—and Congressionally mandated—goal of getting two million people on treatment worldwide with less than three years to go in the five year emergency plan,' said Michael Weinstein, President of AIDS Healthcare Foundation. 'A closer examination of PEPFAR's report to Congress today reveals that the program is actually providing direct, downstream site-specific support for treatment with life-saving anti-retroviral therapy and care to just over 67,000 individuals—only three percent of the overall program target—far, far below Congressional intent'.

'We and other AIDS advocates and organizations have made formal requests to try and get an accounting of the how these PEPFAR funds have actually been spent', said AHF's Weinstein. 'We did this in order to examine how the money—$865 million released by June 2004—had been spent and to clarify repeated inconsistencies in the treatment numbers administration officials were claiming. In mid-September 2004, PEPFAR officials claimed 25,000 people on treatment, yet this current report now states that 155,000 were on treatment by the end of September, a 130,000 increase in just a two-week period. Many of us are simply seeking more accountability and transparency in this crucial program. In response to our own formal request, however, we were largely directed to the websites—and press releases—of the CDC, the Department of State and the White House'.[20]

While the PEPFAR initiative has the potential to improve quality of life in Africa, more transparency in its reporting procedures would clearly be beneficial, and debate about the scale and character of its impact will doubtless continue.

In November 2002, with the support of The Diana, Princess of Wales Memorial Fund, 28 African palliative care trainers from five countries met in Cape Town and began to evolve a strategy for more systematic development. They produced the 'Cape Town

Declaration'.[21] It stated that palliative care is the right of every adult and child with life-limiting illness; that the control of pain and other symptoms is a human right, making access to key drugs imperative; that all health care providers need appropriate training in palliative care; and that such care should be delivered at all levels—primary, secondary and tertiary. The Declaration further galvanized those present to take forward the creation of the first all-African palliative care association. So a steering group was formed, and work began in earnest to forge the aims, objectives and structures of the new venture. Just 18 months later, The African Palliative Care Association (APCA) held its first annual general meeting in Arusha, Tanzania, and its first board was elected with representatives from Ghana, Zimbabwe, Nigeria, South Africa, Kenya, Tanzania and Uganda. Over 150 delegates from 22 African countries gathered for the first Pan African Conference of the newly created APCA. The association aims to: promote study, knowledge, training and research in palliative care; foster networks and links at all levels of palliative care; address ethical issues; establish an international communication network; sponsor publications; disseminate achievements; and promote access to resources. Its objectives include: the promotion of standards; advocating for palliative care at governmental level; securing the availability of drugs; encouraging the development of national associations within Africa; promotion of training programmes; devising standard guidelines; and advocacy.

It has been in this context of growing interest and support that our review of hospice and palliative care development across Africa has taken place.

The study

Purpose

Growing interest in hospice and palliative care in Africa has created the need for an informed overview of the state of development across the continent. We have set out to provide a fuller evidence base concerning what palliative care provision presently exists in the countries of Africa and to generate intelligence on barriers to development and how they may be overcome. We also wish to stimulate a more informed debate and improved policy making among intergovernmental and governmental organizations on the problems facing end-of-life care in the region. Our work is intended as a focus for the efforts of existing researchers and palliative care workers and to stimulate research capacity building through the involvement of new colleagues. We also seek to promote heightened awareness among international funders and donors, with the potential for increased involvement in and additional resources for new and existing programmes.

Methods

This study was undertaken as part of the global development programme of the International Observatory on End of Life Care (IOELC) at Lancaster University, UK.[22,23] Within the programme, we are building a systematic overview of palliative care development across the regions of the world, focusing in particular on hospice- and resource-poor, and transition economies. A key feature of our approach is the production of in-depth 'country reports' that analyse the current state of hospice and palliative care at the national level, against key parameters, and which are published for open access on the IOELC website. Our study was carried out between September 2003 and July 2005; data presented as 'current' therefore relate to that entire time period, though on occasions more specific times are given.

Building on earlier studies,[24,25] a review methodology has been developed to include the following dimensions. First, we collate and compare relevant epidemiological, demographic and health system data gathered from governmental, public health and NGO sources, both within and outside the country. Secondly, we record non-anonymized 'on the record' in-depth qualitative interviews with key personnel, both by telephone and face to face; these explore the narrative of hospice–palliative care in the lived experience of in-country 'palliateurs' and seek to uncover the story of why and how individuals became involved in hospice–palliative care developments, their achievements and frustrations, the perceived opportunities and barriers and their visions for the future. Thirdly, we undertake a systematic analysis of published hospice, palliative care and related sources, including the 'grey' literature (newsletters, reports and technical documents), as well as information from web-based sources. The approach makes extensive use of web-based information and e-mail communication, as well as site visits and ethnographic fieldwork methods. It involves the development of a network of collaborating colleagues within each country to facilitate data collection and to validate findings.

This work leads to the production of individual country reports, against an agreed template. Country reports include a homepage with geo-political information and a map. They provide a narrative history of hospice and palliative care and give details of current services, describing how these are funded and reimbursed, together with estimates of workforce capacity and coverage, and details of educational programmes. Case studies of individual 'success stories' are reported together with oral histories of key individuals and activists. Data on opioid availability are presented along with information on the public health context, population, epidemiology, health care system and political economy. Key ethical issues in the delivery of hospice and palliative care are described. A strategy for the validation of findings has been developed. Draft country reports are circulated in-country for checking and validation. At this stage, inaccuracies are removed, omissions identified and the text revised. When this process is completed, the finished report is published on the worldwide web within the global development section of the IOELC website.[26]

We describe in this report data collated through the production of 26 African country reports using the above methods and which can be viewed at www.eolc-observatory.net . The present study involved 107 interviews with 97 participants in 14 African countries, as well as field visits to Uganda, South Africa, Zimbabwe, Tanzania, Kenya, Malawi and Botswana. It was made possible by close working relationships with very many hospice–palliative care colleagues across the region and in particular through links with the newly formed APCA and involvement in its inaugural conference in Tanzania in June 2004.[27]

As we have seen, the WHO defines palliative care as 'an approach that improves the quality of life of patients and their families facing the problems associated with life-threatening illness, through the prevention and relief of suffering by means of early identification and impeccable assessment and treatment of pain and other problems, physical, psychosocial and spiritual'.[9] In Africa, many of the organizations delivering such care adopt the term 'hospice' in their title. It is also the case that in the African context, the scope of palliative care is being expanded to include programmes where ARV treatments are delivered alongside psycho-social and symptom-oriented care, thereby extending quality of life to the poorest people. This requires thinking about hospice and palliative care within a preventative and public health model in which care can be delivered across the complete trajectory of the disease and in which well constructed home-based palliative care services can serve as an important platform for education, primary disease prevention and also the support of patients receiving active treatment. HIV/AIDS exacerbates the already great need for palliative care that exists in developing and resource-poor countries where health care is limited and where late presentation is common, even for conditions that could be prevented or cured, and where poverty and gender inequality further compound the seemingly insurmountable challenges of living a meaningful and satisfying life.[28] To commentators in developed countries, some of the services provided by palliative care organizations in Africa may seem unfamiliar:

> Although the definition of palliative care is globally relevant, what constitutes palliative care needs and services in sub-Saharan Africa is continent-specific, particularly in the light of poverty and HIV disease. Necessary components include practical care, pain and symptom control, counselling/emotional/psychological support, income generation, financial support for food, shelter, funeral costs and school fees, respite, spiritual care and orphan care[17] (p. 4).

Given this process of evolution in definition, organizational culture and scope of activity, we adopt the inclusive term 'hospice–palliative care' to capture the range of specialized activities relating to the holistic care of persons with life-threatening illness and the care of those bereaved.

Results

History and current levels of organizational development

The history of hospice development in Africa stretches back to the late 1970s, when services first appeared in Zimbabwe and in South Africa. Island Hospice was founded in Harare in May 1979 and had developed 17 regional branches by 1997.[29] In an anniversary speech in 2004, social worker Rona Martin recalled the impact of the AIDS epidemic upon the service:

> Twenty five years ago who could have known how the spread of HIV/AIDS would change the face of hospice care in Africa? Our first AIDS patient was in 1986 and we continued to take patients with HIV referred in the usual way. However, as with the rest of the country, we were slow to realize and respond to the full impact of the pandemic. It became clear, however, that in order to reach our increasing numbers of families in need, we would have to change the way we work . . . Island had always worked in the community with its home based care, but now with the increased need it became necessary to partner with other groups committed to home care . . . Training, always a part of our work with medical students, nurses and caregivers, became increasingly important. Our separate training department was formed in 1996 to respond to demand. Spreading skills in palliative and home based care through training and mentoring continues to be seen as the way forward.[30]

Also in the late 1970s, hospice initiatives were developing in South Africa—in Johannesburg, Port Elizabeth, Cape Town and Durban. The visit of Cicely Saunders to South Africa in 1979 added impetus to these developments, and within a year or two hospice organizations were operating in a variety of settings throughout the country. The approach to care, as noted by Thembi Nyuswa, at Highway Hospice, in Durban, was new and unfamiliar:

> When I first came to work for the hospice, it was on a part-time basis and I became the first black sister. It was quite different, you know, from the usual kind of nursing that I'd always been involved in. And I discovered that the hospice concept was also a very new thing to the average black patient. At that time, all the patients were referred to us from the provincial hospitals. They would get admitted in the hospice inpatient unit and when they went home there was no follow-up system to see how they were doing until they were re-admitted. So, I worked here on and off because I had to finish my studies; and when I left to do my psychiatric medicine the matron said, 'Thembi, go and finish your studies and come back and start an African home care service', which I was excited about. So I went and finished my studies, got my drivers' licence and there I was: I came back and I started this service.[31]

After the start made in these two countries, it was another decade before hospice and palliative care developments began to occur elsewhere in Africa: in Kenya and Swaziland (1990); Botswana, Tanzania and Zambia (1992); Uganda (1993); Sierra Leone (1994); Morocco (1995); Congo-Brazzaville and Nigeria (1996); Malawi (1997); Egypt (2001); and the Gambia (2004).

Our review identified 136 hospice and palliative care organizations in 15 countries—an area with a population of 407 million people. The vast majority of these are non-government, charitable and faith-based organizations. Over half (76) were found in South Africa, which has more such organizations than all of the other African countries combined (Table 1.2). Several organizations have developed additional branches, which we define as a service that has local 'ownership', a discernible local structure, local pro-activity and a local focal point; sometimes, these branches are referred to as 'satellites' of the 'primary' or 'mother' organization—a tendency that is most marked in South Africa and Uganda.

Although in South Africa there are 37 organizations that have free-standing hospice inpatient facilities, eight out of 15 countries with hospice–palliative care in Africa have no such facility and in general there is an emphasis on the development of home care services. These are found in 14 out of 15 countries and are provided by 111 of the 136 organizations identified. Forty-nine organizations have hospital-based services, found in 11 out of 15 countries. Day care services and clinics are run by 87 organizations in 14 out of 15 countries.

Opioid availability issues

This limited development of hospice–palliative care organizations is also reflected in the low level of opioid use across the continent: 29 countries reporting no morphine use at all in 2000–2002 (Appendix 1). Also, whilst a clear match exists between the country with the most reported defined daily doses of morphine[32] and that with the most hospice and palliative care services (South Africa), elsewhere it is difficult to explain why Namibia, the

Table 1.2 Hospice and palliative care: organizational provision in Africa (15 countries)

Country	No. of organizations	No. of known branches	Organizations making inpatient provision		Organizations making outpatient provision	
			Hospice	Hospital	Home care	Day care/clinic
Botswana	3	0	0	1	3	3
Congo	1	0	0	1	1	0
Egypt	3	0	2	1	1	1
Kenya	8	3	0	6	8	6
Malawi	5	0	0	4	2	3
Morocco	1	0	0	1	0	1
Nigeria	2	0	0	1	1	1
Sierra Leone	1	0	1	0	1	1
South Africa	76	42	37	19	61	49
Swaziland	4	0	1	0	3	2
Tanzania	4	0	0	3	3	3
The Gambia	1	0	0	0	1	1
Uganda	8	124	2	6	7	6
Zambia	6	0	6	0	6	6
Zimbabwe	13	6	2	6	13	4
Total	136	175	51	49	111	87

Central African Republic and Tunisia report higher morphine use than other countries when this review could identify no hospice or palliative care services in those countries. There were also many reported problems of morphine availability, and these were exacerbated by fears of using the drug, on the part of both practitioners and patients. We cite here a small number of many examples identified, and note that the use of opioids is a prominent issue of on-going importance.

In Cote d'Ivoire, whilst it is reported that limited supplies of opioids are available in the main cities, they are not accessible to rural communities.[33] In Tanzania, all morphine is distributed by the Ocean Road Cancer Institute in Dar es Salaam, following approval by the regulatory pharmaceutical board in 2001. The Medical Stores Department of the Institute is responsible for importing the raw powder, mixing it into an oral solution and distributing the different strength solutions to other health care providers throughout the country. In recent years, the palliative care team has been using the drug with great success, and has led training sessions for doctors. Outside of the hospital, however, resistance continues. Dr Hussein Mtiro, Acting Head of the Palliative Care Team at the Institute explains: 'They still think that they prefer pethidine than morphine, and pethidine is not very good for chronic pain. Sometimes they go for tramadol, this is an expensive drug and mostly they get it injected'.[34]

Current in-country information suggests there is no injectable morphine in Malawi, although the Ministry of Health distributes morphine tablets (MST). Morphine solution for oral use has recently been introduced as a result of a close relationship between the Ministry of Health and the Lighthouse hospice programme in Lilongwe, which has lobbied for its introduction. Lighthouse orders the parabene powder from the UK; it is then mixed with the preservative propylene glycol by the government Central Medical Stores pharmacists. Supplies of the oral morphine are distributed by this department to hospitals and clinics around Malawi where palliative care is practised. Supplies have been uninterrupted since the introduction of this system, and indicate the benefit of co-operation between government and the private sector. Yet in Nigeria, a country of 120 million people where in 2003, 490 000 adults and children are thought to have died from HIV/AIDS, no oral morphine is available.[35]

Nevertheless, there are some examples of outstanding success in tackling the problem of morphine availability. Uganda is a particular example; here morphine for cancer and HIV/AIDS patients is provided free of charge by the government, and in a ground-breaking innovation of March 2004 a Statutory Instrument[36] was signed by the Minister of Health authorizing palliative care nurses and clinical officers to prescribe morphine as part of their clinical practice. At Hospice Africa Uganda, pharmacist Peter Mikajjo comments:

> We prepare [liquid morphine] in a very simple way whereby it cannot take a lot of time and cannot be costly. Morphine is prepared out of morphine powder: there are actually two types—either morphine sulphate or morphine hydrochloride—but basically we are using morphine sulphate and we prepare enough that can be used in a week.[37]

If morphine is required by patients in the Kitovu Mobile Home Care programme, one of Uganda's eight palliative care organizations, a referral is made to the programme doctor. Once the doctor prescribes the morphine, the patient or a family member can collect the medicine from nurses at a nearby centre. Kitovu palliative care physician and medical consultant Mary Simmons explains the impact morphine has made on both patients and health workers:

> Pain and symptom relief not only benefits the patients, but the family and even our staff. The suffering of caregivers is intensified when they see their patient suffering. Their relief is obvious when the patient no longer suffers. As for our staff, they repeatedly tell me how grateful they are for palliative care. Before we had morphine, they felt helpless in the face of the suffering of their patients. Now they know something can be done.[8]

A key contributor to the campaign for morphine availability in Uganda has been Dr Jack Jagwe, who describes his role as follows:

> My role in Hospice Africa Uganda is that of the senior advisor on policy, drugs and advocacy. Policy concerns how palliative care relates to Government health policies so that we don't have any conflict. The second one is about drugs, how to access palliative care drugs and most specifically the availability of morphine to patients in palliative care. And the third one is advocacy—to try and convince Government and top health policy makers about the value of having palliative care for so many patients in our country who are dying from HIV/AIDS and cancer. First of all: I'm a physician by training, and I've been in the Government services for 30 years 'til my retirement—and I got interested when Dr Anne Merriman came to Uganda in 1993. By then I was the Deputy

Director of Medical Services in charge of clinical services and also in charge of essential grants in the country. That's when she came and mentioned that we should have drugs like morphine available for these people. And after that, when I retired officially from the Government, I became Chairman of the National Drug Regulatory Body in Uganda. Since then I've been interested in palliative care, and in 1998 when she organized a national workshop I was appointed Chairman of a task force which worked out a national policy on palliative care. That draft was thoroughly discussed and eventually submitted to the Ministry of Health and it was incorporated into the Health Strategic Plan of 2001–2005.[39]

Problems of opioid availability were a recurring theme throughout the review, even in the countries better endowed with hospice–palliative services.

Categorizing development

Taking into account the overall development of hospice–palliative care in Africa, we are able to group the continent's 47 countries into four categories: (1) no known hospice–palliative care activity; (2) countries with hospice and palliative care capacity building activity; (3) countries with localized provision of hospice and palliative care; and (4) countries where hospice and palliative care activities are approaching integration with the wider public health system. In this typology, characteristic activity within each category is shown in Table 1.3.

Table 1.3 Typology of hospice–palliative care service development in Africa

1 No known activity	2 Capacity building	3 Localized provision	4 Approaching integration
	Presence of sensitized personnel Expressions of interest with key organizations (eg APCA, HAU, AHPC, Hospice IInformation) Links established (international) with service providers Conference participation Visits to hospice–palliative care organizations Education and training (visiting teams) External training courses undertaken Preparation of a strategy for service development Lobbying of policymakers/health ministries	*A range of capacity building activities but also:* Critical mass of activists in one or more locations Service established—often linked to home care Local awareness/support Sources of funding established, though may be heavily donor dependent and relatively isolated from one another, with little impact on wider health policy Morphine available Some training undertaken by hospice organization	*Capacity building and localized activities but also:* Critical mass of activists countrywide Range of providers and service types Broad awareness of palliative care Measure of integration with mainstream service providers Impact on policy Established education centres Academic links Research undertaken National Association

The location of countries in each of the four categories is shown in Fig. 1.2.

In Table 1.4, we show the ratio of hospice palliative care services to population in each of the four categories.

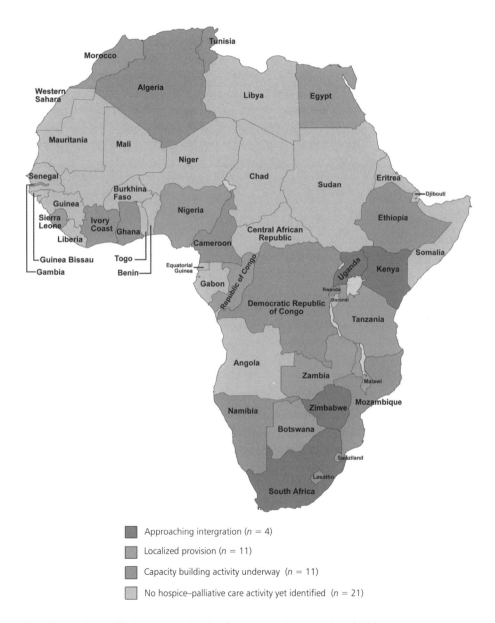

Fig. 1.2 Hospice–palliative care service development in the countries of Africa.

Table 1.4 Ratio of hospice–palliative care (PC) services to the population within Africa (47 countries)

Country	Population (millions)	Total PC services	Ratio (1:millions)
No developed services identified			
Angola	13.184		
Benin	6.558		
Burkina Faso	12.624		
Burundi	6.602		
Central African Republic	3.819		
Chad	8.348		
Djibouti	0.693		
Equatorial Guinea	0.481		
Eritrea	3.991		
Gabon	1.306		
Guinea	8.359		
Guinea-Bissau	1.449		
Liberia	3.239		
Libya	5.445		
Mali	12.623		
Mauritania	2.807		
Niger	11.544		
Senegal	9.855		
Somalia	9.480		
Sudan	32.878		
Togo	4.801		
Total population (21 countries) = 160.09 million			
Capacity building			
Algeria	31.266		
Cameroon	15.729		
Cote d'Ivoire	16.365		
Democratic Republic of the Congo (Congo-Kinshasa)	51.201		
Ethiopia	67.850		
Ghana	20.471		
Lesotho	18.000		
Mozambique	18.537		

Table 1.4 (Contd.)

Country	Population (millions)	Total PC services	Ratio (1:millions)
Namibia	1.961		
Rwanda	8.272		
Tunisia	9.728		
Total population (11 countries) = 259.38 million			
Localized provision			
Botswana	1.770	10	0.177
Congo (Congo-Brazzaville)	3.633	2	1.817
Egypt	70.507	6	11.751
Malawi	11.871	12	0.989
Morocco	30.072	2	15.036
Nigeria	120.911	3	40.304
Sierra Leone	4.764	3	1.588
Swaziland	1.069	6	0.178
The Gambia	1.388	2	0.694
Tanzania	36.276	11	3.298
Zambia	10.698	20	0.535
Total population (11 countries)	292.959	77	3.805
Approaching integration			
Kenya	31.540	25	1.262
Uganda	25.004	155	0.161
Zimbabwe	12.835	34	0.378
Total population (three countries)	69.379	214	0.324
South Africa	44.759		

Population source: WHO World Health Report 2004.

Group 1: countries with no known hospice palliative care activity (*n* = 21)

The review may have failed to identify palliative care activity in some countries where such activity does exist. It is considered, however, that there is currently no tangible activity in some 21 countries: Angola; Benin, Burkina Faso; Burundi; Central African Republic; Chad; Djibouti; Equatorial Guinea; Eritrea; Gabon; Guinea; Guinea Bissau; Liberia;

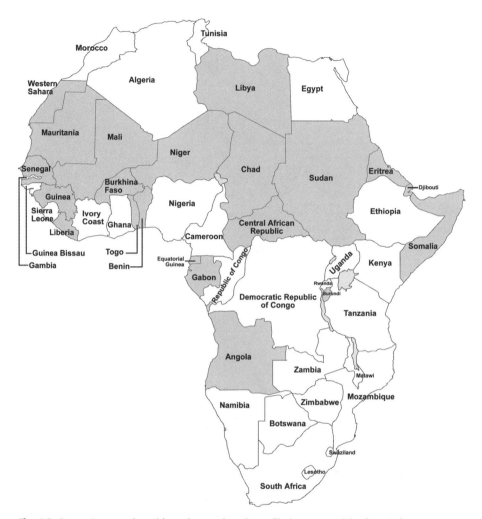

Fig. 1.3 Group 1: countries with no known hospice palliative care activity (*n* = 21).

Libya; Mali; Mauritania; Niger; Senegal; Somalia; Sudan; and Togo. This represents a region of 160 million people, mainly concentrated in western, central and northern areas of the continent.

Group 2: countries with capacity building activity (*n* = 11)

In 11 countries (Algeria; Cameroon; Cote d' Ivoire; Democratic Republic of Congo; Ethiopia; Ghana; Lesotho; Mozambique; Namibia; Rwanda; and Tunisia), there is evidence that steps are being taken to create the organizational, workforce and policy

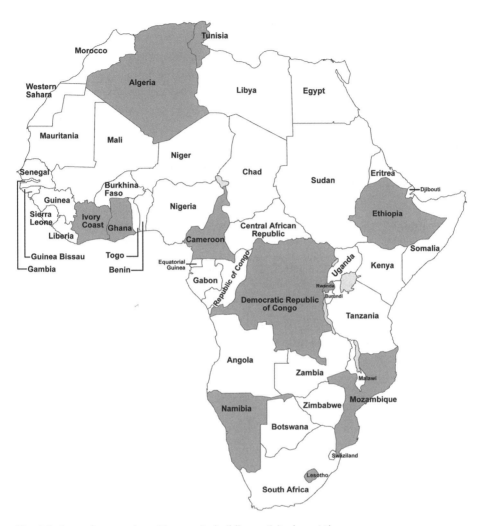

Fig. 1.4 Group 2: countries with capacity building activity (*n* = 11).

capacity for hospice–palliative care services to develop, though currently no operational services exist. In five of these (Cote d' Ivoire; Ethiopia; Mozambique; Namibia; and Rwanda), the country is part of the PEPFAR programme, which is proving a key driver of palliative care innovation. There is evidence in all 11 countries of various developmental activities: attendance at or organization of key conferences, personnel undertaking external training in palliative care; lobbying of policy makers and health ministries, and incipient service development, usually building on existing home care programmes. We cite selected examples.

In Cameroon, an oncology nurse working in a Prevention of Mother to Child Transmission programme administered by the Ministry of Health is studying for a palliative care diploma with Hospice Africa Uganda and has become a member of APCA in order to strengthen the ability of his organization to lobby government to develop palliative care support for those living with cancer and AIDS. He identifies the need for further training and for funds to be sourced to support this work and highlights the importance of collaborating with other African countries.[40] In the Democratic Republic of Congo, a nurse supported by an organization called International Youth Association for Development describes the beginnings of a palliative care service in Kinshasa, despite the difficulties experienced in the country. The service is linked to two European NGOs and relies heavily on volunteer support, particularly from young people:

> Some patients are cared for in the hospital but the condition is not good. Our organization provides student nurses and doctors to help volunteers in Kinshasa; about 80 patients are being cared for at home. We would like a clinic. If we have a clinic it would be easier for the patient. We would like to have autos for transport for the nurse volunteers; we want to have computers; and also education. We would like to give medicine for the patient at home, but we would like to have more experience with palliative care. There is a need for education for nurses and for doctors.[41]

A conference on the theme of *Pain and Supportive Care for the Maghreb* (Tunisia, Morocco and Algeria) was held in Tabarka, Tunisia, in September 2004, but it is reported that no home care provision exists for people with cancer, opioid prescriptions are restricted to a period of 1 week and morphine is expensive and only available in sustained release form.[42] There are no established palliative care services in Ghana; in the absence of formal structures, individuals in Ghana have begun to incorporate palliative care principles into home-based care projects with AIDS and cancer patients.[43] Terry Magee, director of education at Myland Hall Education Centre (St Helena Hospice, UK), has been involved in education initiatives in Ghana for the last 2 years. She notes:

> There are a number of initiatives that are a mixture of outreach and social and health support for people who are living in communities—rural communities mostly—who have HIV and AIDS, and there are services developing within the hospitals in Kumasi and Accra, to try to produce more information and more awareness for patients about issues like pain and symptom control and family support. As yet, there isn't a hospice as such, but the idea of hospice is very much alive in the practice . . . we did a series of story telling workshops with the students where we talked to them about what holistic care was all about, and we outlined the principles of hospice care, and we asked them to tell us stories of where they felt that was happening in their own practice, and how they were making that happen, and we heard some wonderful examples—it's not got a label 'hospice' over it, but it's hospice care nonetheless. Some lovely stories of where the care was delivered to a person, or the actions taken by health care professional, or a social care professional had resulted in some very, very fine holistic care and good quality of life in dying people, and some very fine examples of very appropriate after death care and support.[44]

A draft US Government Rapid Appraisal for HIV/AIDS Program Expansion in Lesotho[45] identifies palliative care as a critical important component of an integrated health plan to combat the effects of HIV/AIDS in the country. However, palliative care is, in reality, not at all developed.

Clinical and medical comprehensive palliative care and palliative care for children are nearly non-existent. Given the lack of progress in palliative care, service delivery in this regard primarily consists of fragmented social, spiritual and psychological support (with limited bereavement support)[45] (p. 36).

The National AIDS Strategic Plan 2002/2003–2004/2005 for Lesotho makes no reference to palliative care and there are no palliative care policies or guidelines for pain control, and these have not been integrated into general health policies for dealing with cancer and other illnesses. Advocacy for palliative care is minimal, and it appears only on a limited basis in the nurses' training curriculum. Despite this, some plans have been developed at the local level for the creation of the Tsepong Community Hospice, to serve the areas of Tebellong, Qabane, Linakeng and Thabana-Tsooana. The objectives of the project are: to alleviate the effects of the HIV/AIDS crisis; to facilitate the development of a culture of community; to involve home-based care; and to develop an effective network of stake-holders such as churches, traditional healers and medical centres.[46] This initiative is being promoted by Sister Virginia Moorosi of the Machaberg Hospital at Qacha's Nek and would seek to raise funds through agricultural and horticultural projects. A needs assessment for HIV/AIDS was conducted in the district in 2003.[47] The report states that the hospice committee involves a large number of local people from several villages as well as a number of key individuals in the District of Qacha. A field has been donated for a building plot; rocks have been gathered and some fruit trees planted; there is potential for further land to be used for agricultural purposes. The vision in the community is to build a facility for respite care, and to offer training courses to the long-term sick. However, plans for the building will require significant capital investment beyond those available in the district. Sister Virginia Moorosi describes the situation:

I'm a social worker, so my work is to see the welfare of people, to see that people are having the higher standard of living, understanding how they can be infected or affected by HIV and AIDS and other terminal diseases, so while I was doing the research going on making the assemblies in the societies, I realized that there was a need to build a hospice where people can get counselling, where people, when they are neglected by their families, maybe two to three days they can come to the hospice to get counselling, even to get moral support, spiritual support, counselling, and other things, maybe washing, this can maybe raise their spirits up and go back to their families . . . After the research, I got 3000 orphans in that place, it's where I was thinking that I can build a hospice for alleviation of those people living there, to give them education and to see how they can come to a better knowledge of how to understand how to take care of themselves, even these affected orphans. Up to now, I have made a training of support groups, these are volunteers, people in the villages, and I did ask the government but the government also it's helping very little by supporting as well the workshops, to support the sick people and to those orphans by distributing the kits, and the paracetamols and small medicines to take care of the sick people . . . Because out of the research I made I have realized that many are dying alone in their families because of the neglect they get, because of the poverty, they don't get food nutrition and their cleanliness hygienically, they are not given by the carers because financially people in Lesotho are very poor and many are not working so they cannot tolerate with the sick people for a long time.[48]

Concerned individuals committed to establishing palliative care services in Rwanda have sourced initial funding for specific projects. Financial support was found to send two Rwandan nurses to Nairobi Hospice for training; the British government paid for the same nurses to attend the APCA conference in Tanzania in June 2004. A US-based hospice linked with a Tanzanian hospice has also shown interest in financially supporting palliative care development in Rwanda.

We came across repeated examples of these small-scale initiatives in each of the 11 countries categorized as 'capacity building'.

Group 3: countries with localized provision (*n* = 11)

A further 11 countries [Botswana; Congo (Congo-Brazzaville); Egypt; Malawi; Morocco; Nigeria; Sierra Leone; Swaziland; Tanzania; The Gambia; and Zambia] demonstrate

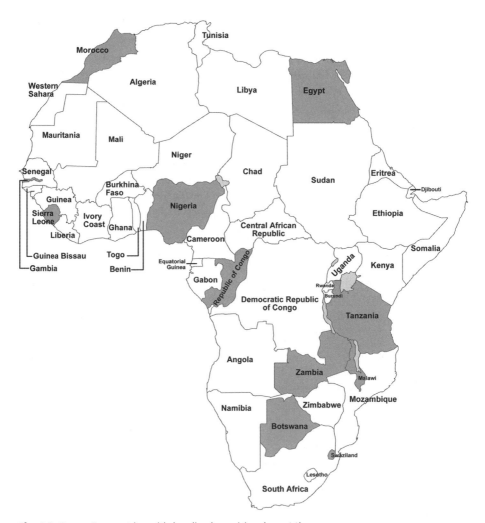

Fig. 1.5 Group 3: countries with localized provision (*n* = 11).

evidence of the localized provision of hospice–palliative care in a context where small numbers of isolated services have gained a toehold (Table 1.4). Four of these countries (Botswana, Nigeria, Tanzania and Zambia) form part of the PEPFAR initiative; three have support from the Diana, Princess of Wales Memorial Fund (Malawi, Tanzania and Zambia); and two form part of the WHO community health initiative for palliative care (Botswana and Tanzania). Table 1.4 shows that in small countries such as Botswana, the ratios of hospice–palliative care services to the population can be as high as 1:177 000; whereas in countries with a large population such as Nigeria, the ratio is as low as 1:40 million. In total, across these countries, 77 services exist for a population of 292 million.

In Botswana, there is some optimism that the government is committed to providing quality health care services to its entire population and has established a suitable base for strengthening palliative care services by its primary health care delivery system, community home-based care programme, national HIV/AIDS activities, National Drug Act, cancer management protocols and strong partnership among the government, civil society and private sector.[11] In Congo, L'Association Congolese Accompagner (ACA) was founded in 1996 by Soeur Eliane Julienne Boukaka, of the Congregation Occiliatrise. ACA cares for incurably ill persons, particularly those with AIDS and cancer, and offers support in the hospital and in the home; about 50 people are in the care of ACA on a given day. It is the only service of its type in a country of 3.6 million.

Palliative care is being introduced to Nigeria through the Palliative Care Initiative (PCIN), Nigeria based at the College of Medicine, University of Ibadan. PCIN is a multidisciplinary group of medical specialists formed in January 2003 and, in addition to sensitizing the public to the importance of palliative care, it has sponsored some of its members to attend palliative care courses and conferences in other countries. It operates a pain and palliative care clinic at the University College Hospital, Ibadan. This was commissioned in February 2005 to provide support for patients with chronic pain and cancer patients.[49] In its current form as a chapter of the International Association for the Study of Pain, the group is working towards including palliative care in the curriculum of medical and nursing students, based upon guidelines developed by Hospice Africa Uganda. Funding has been obtained to develop home-based palliative care services. A 'train the trainers' programme is expected to produce locally trained palliative care practitioners.

Hospice developments began in Sierra Leone in 1994. Gabriel Madiye, founder of The Shepherd's Hospice, contacted St Christopher's Hospice, London, and subsequently made contact with hospices in the USA. However, at the same time, Sierra Leone was engulfed by a civil war and, during the hostilities, the hospice premises were destroyed twice.[50] The vision survived, however; Gabriel Madiye recalls:

> It all started with the recognition of the problem in a very genuine way and it continued with organizing community effort; sensitizing people around the problem to see how they can rally around . . . My own role in the hospice has been management, planning and research; making sure that services are appropriate to the needs of the local community. And I try to make sure that our programmes are based on sound research. Because of that, we have always maintained good donor relations—with donor confidence and donor interest in our work. We initially started from

nowhere and today, over the last four years, we have been able to work with 11 international donors, including the World Bank, WHO, Bread for the World, Help the Hospices, and now we are doing some work with Comic Relief . . . The Shepherd's Hospice itself is a facilitating institution: we have patients referred to us; we train their family care givers; we train volunteers; the volunteers pay visits to the home once every week, and the family caregiver is almost always there in the home. The professional team is multidisciplinary consisting of the social worker, a medical officer and the nurses; they stay at the hospice and they have a routine schedule to visit those patients . . . we are mobile; we can go in.[51]

Swaziland is another small country that has stimulated several hospice–palliative care initiatives: Hope House; Swaziland Hospice at Home; Parish Nursing; and the Salvation Army; in addition, several community-based church organizations provide supportive care to terminally ill patients.[52] Future Care Hospice was officially registered as a charitable organization in October 2004 and is The Gambia's first service of this kind.[53] The hospice provides home care and day care services and the programme includes symptom control, domiciliary care and prevention advice.[53]

In Zambia, inpatient units have featured heavily in the way the country's six hospice organizations have developed their services. A visiting expert commented:

[There was] the presumption throughout all we met in hospices in Zambia that for everyone there came a time when they were too sick to stay at home. We found this rather sad, when we have witnessed dying at home to bring so much more peace for patient and family in other parts of Africa.[54]

In Tanzania, palliative care is delivered by four organizations: Selian Hospital, Muheza Hospice Care, PASADA and Ocean Road Cancer Institute. Faith-based organizations, particularly the church-related hospitals, provide 50 per cent of the health care in the country,[55] and plans are in place to extend palliative care coverage into the Christian hospitals (~82) throughout Tanzania. The Evangelical Lutheran Church, which has its national headquarters in Arusha, is introducing palliative care into its 20 hospitals. The Diana, Princess of Wales Memorial Fund has supported palliative care development in Tanzania through the award of grants, including: a one year project to set up palliative care training and referral facilities for Muheza district at Teule Hospital, and to establish home-based care in the area; and a three year grant for PASADA to move from clinic-based to community-based health services and to strengthen the palliative care component of its work. PEPFAR support has also been made available to some of the country's hospice–palliative care services.

Group 4: countries approaching integration (n = 4)

The review identified four countries in which hospice–palliative care services are achieving some measure of integration with wider mainstream service providers and gaining greater policy recognition (Kenya, South Africa, Uganda and Zimbabwe).

Kenya

In Kenya (Table 1.5), there are six established hospices: Nairobi, Meru, Kisumu, Nyeri, Eldoret and Coast (Mombassa). A further service is developing in Nyaharuru. There are

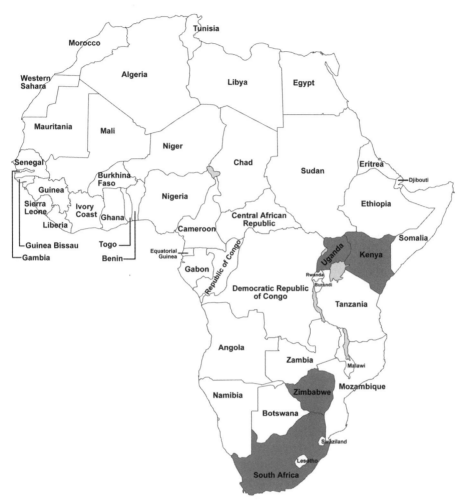

Fig. 1.6 Group 4: countries approaching integration (*n* = 4).

palliative care teams in two mission hospitals, Chogoria Hospital and Maua Methodist Hospital, both in Meru district. A total of 25 services is being provided. The government of Kenya does not yet have an official palliative care policy although it is supportive of palliative care in the country. The Ministry of Health is working on a 5-year Health Sector Strategic Plan and has invited Nairobi Hospice to sit on that committee. Nairobi Hospice is also consulting with the Ministry of Health on the development of a manual guiding palliative care for cancer of the cervix. The Government of Kenya supports the hospice in kind by paying for the salaries of three nurses seconded to the hospice by the Ministry of Health. It has also donated a plot of land on which the hospice can build its own offices. The training programmes offered by Nairobi Hospice are aimed at alleviating the continuing resistance to the use of morphine in Kenya amongst some doctors and nurses. The difficulties in accessing morphine are being addressed by the national hospice association. Nairobi Hospice Chief Executive Brigid Sirengo comments:

> It's very difficult to get some of the senior doctors to change their minds to prescribe morphine, particularly if the patient is experiencing a lot of pain and needs higher doses of morphine. They are very, very apprehensive about that: they are quite reluctant. But with the training we hope that things will change.[56]

Important networking with the Ministry of Health was undertaken when the hospice was established to ensure a supply of morphine for patients. The hospice imports morphine powder from the UK for reconstitution as liquid morphine for hospice distribution within Kenya. Injectable morphine is also available. Other drugs prescribed by Nairobi Hospice are guided by the WHO analgesic ladder: ibuprofen, dihydrocodeine, paracetamol, aspirin and laxatives are available, and amitriptyline and diazepam are used for depression and anxiety. Antibiotics, mystatin and antifungal drugs are prescribed for people living with HIV. ARVs are not prescribed. There is no palliative care formulary to date. Most drug costs for all Kenyan hospices are covered by a Dutch donor: Nairobi Hospice-The Netherlands.

The Kenya Hospice and Palliative Care Association was formed in October 2004 to promote palliative care countrywide by developing more hospices with a standard quality of care. A second objective is to supply smaller hospices with drugs that can be bought in bulk in Nairobi. It is anticipated that all existing hospices will be members, as well as other organizations providing elements of palliative care in related fields. Hospice Care Kenya (UK)[57] is a UK-based charity that supports hospices in Kenya by providing funds for various projects. Significantly, Hospice Care Kenya (UK) sponsors a doctor rotation programme by paying the salaries of local doctors who work at Kenyan Hospices for 3 months. After this placement, doctors should be able to provide palliative care and train others in palliative care in whichever part of the country they are working. Four doctors successfully completed this rotation in the year 2002–2003.

Kenya is a country within the PEPFAR programme. The Diana, Princess of Wales Memorial Fund has supported palliative care development in Kenya by awarding grants to Maua Methodist hospital and the Nairobi Hospice. Through the Foundation for Hospices in sub-Saharan Africa, Nairobi Hospice has a twinning arrangement with VITAS-San Antonio, Texas, USA. This partnership was the first between hospices in Kenya and America. The VITAS-San Antonio programme is part of the VITAS Innovative Healthcare Corporation. One of San Antonio's nurses is a native of Kenya, and was instrumental in spearheading the twinning efforts with Hospice Nairobi.[58] Meru Hospice is twinned with Hospice Care Incorporated in Wisconsin, USA.

In June 2001, Nairobi Hospice, in collaboration with Oxford Brookes University, UK, launched a 14 month Diploma in Higher Education; Palliative Care. This part distance learning and part block system enables health care professionals from around Africa to undertake the diploma while continuing to work. The first class of students graduated in September 2002. In another scheme, students from colleges and other hospices are offered 4 week clinical placements at Nairobi Hospice for palliative care experience. The hospice offers two separate training courses each lasting 1 week for health care professionals and community volunteers. During the year 2002–2003, 52 health care professionals and 68 volunteers completed these courses. Consultation is taking place with the Ministry of Health to include palliative care in the curriculum for nurse training. The hospice provides introductory palliative care training to third year medical students at the teaching hospital. In January 2004, 25 medical personnel (clinical officers and nurses) from the District Hospitals in the Coast Province were trained by this hospice in a 5 day palliative care course. The intention was to enable the trainees to set up small palliative care units in their respective stations with support provided by the hospice. Plans are in place for similar workshops in 2005 for health workers and volunteers.

The training programme offered by Nairobi Hospice has equipped other hospices around the country with trained staff and so expanded national coverage: 'The people that we have trained are the ones that have gone out and started those hospices so that other people who cannot reach us at least they will have palliative care accessible and available for them'.[59] The positive attitude towards Nairobi Hospice by the Kenya Government has significant implications for palliative care in this country. Senior Medical Officer, Zipporah Ali observes:

> . . . the Ministry acknowledges and appreciates palliative care, and for us that is very, very important, and we are at an early stage working with the Ministry so that palliative care can eventually be part and parcel of the main health care delivery system.[60]

Uganda

Overall in Uganda, eight organizations are delivering 155 hospice–palliative care services (Table 1.5). Hospice Africa Uganda (HAU) is an NGO founded in 1993 to promote hospice developments in the countries of Africa which lack palliative medicine. Its objectives are: (1) to provide a palliative care service to patients and families within a 20 km radius of the Makindye premises and to promote this care throughout Uganda; (2) to carry out education programmes in palliative medicine to health professionals at undergraduate and post-graduate levels; and (3) to encourage the initiation/consolidation of palliative care in other African countries by providing a training facility.

Its services began in a two-bedroom house loaned by Nsambya Hospital and subsequently moved to alternative accommodation, donated free of charge by Henry Mary Kateregga, before the current premises at Makindye were secured with the help of the organization Ireland AID[61] in 1994. In January 1998, the service was extended with the founding of Mobile Hospice Mbarara. An outreach clinic was established and supplemented by the inception of roadside clinics for those outside of the 20 km catchment area. In June 1998, a third service was founded—Little Hospice Hoima—to demonstrate how a simple service could be introduced using existing health facilities and personnel. As a result, an affordable service reached out to the villages, supported by community volunteers who helped to identify those in need.[62]

From the outset, the gains made in Uganda were recognized by WHO:

> In the last ten years, thanks to NGO initiatives, progressive government involvement and the support of the WHO country office, Uganda has been able to include palliative care in the government health agenda which has resulted in the allocation of resources, improved morphine availability, and the provision of training at all levels of care and to undergraduate and post graduate health professionals. It has integrated palliative care into the existing health system at a district level and is planning to extend the programme to other districts and eventually to the rest of the country.[63]

The WHO has also recognized the value of research undertaken in Uganda by Ekiria Kikule:[64]

> A needs assessment study recently undertaken in Uganda . . . showed that the distribution of terminally ill patients was 73% HIV/AIDS, 22% cancer, 3% both and 2% other diseases. The majority of patients preferred to be cared for at home and, in fact, 87% of the caregivers were family members who were very supportive. Among the various needs shared by patients and their caregivers, the major ones were food and welfare. Poverty and sickness combined to put families in a critical situation. Patients experienced pain and other symptoms quite often and 65% declared them a problem. The main fears expressed by the patients were fear of death and abandonment. The study concluded that the home is the best place to care for the terminally ill.[11]

The key person behind Hospice Africa Uganda has been Anne Merriman, a doctor from Liverpool who had previously worked in Singapore and Kenya. She recalls her motivation:

> . . . what I wanted to do was to set up a hospice somewhere that would be a model from which other countries could say, 'Look it works in our situation' . . . So what I wanted to do was set up a model that was affordable and to show . . . that it could work in the African situation . . . and we really felt Uganda was the best place. [Firstly] the Government was trusted and we would be able to get funding from outside. Secondly, they had a huge AIDS epidemic, you could see the people suffering even driving along the road, it was so big at that stage, you know, it's gone right down now but it was very big then. And also the Ministry of Health were really fully behind us and promised to get in the morphine . . . it was a big struggle . . . but we got it in and I made a lot of enemies trying to get it in because, although the Minister was behind me, people like the pharmacists were very against what I was doing and we had a lot of trouble getting the Ministry of Health on board. In fact we didn't get it on board 'til five years later, '98. So it was a very difficult time and it was only in '98 when we held the big conference for the stakeholders in palliative care and we got the finance from SCIAF, the Scottish Catholic International Aid Fund. . . . And we were the first country in Africa to do that . . . and it's been taken up seriously and they have moved forward on it.[65]

Hospice Africa Uganda received a pledge of 50 million shillings from the Ministry of Health for the financial year 2003–4;[66] but continues to rely on the support of many donors, including: Hospice Africa (UK), the British High Commission, the Government of Ireland, the States of Jersey, Singapore and Canada, CORDAID (The Netherlands), CAFOD (England), SCIAF (Scotland), the Nuffield Foundation, the Diana, Princess of Wales Memorial Fund and the RAF (UK). Rotarians worldwide have contributed; DANIDA and USAID are committed during 2004. The Diana Fund has supported a Uganda-based training programme for other African countries (2001) and APSO, VMM (Ireland) and VSO have supported expert volunteers. In future, the hospice aims to raise 10 per cent of its running costs in Uganda.[67]

Another significant contributor to palliative care development in Uganda is the UK-based Christian organization Mildmay International which, after a study tour to Africa in 1991, developed training programmes in East Africa, funded by the British Council. This in turn led to an invitation from the Uganda AIDS Commission to set up a care and training programme in Uganda. The Centre opened in 1998 and Mildmay has an agreement with the Ministry of Health to manage the Centre and its activities until 2008. Director of the study centre, Julia Downing explains:

> The Mildmay Centre was developed in order to provide and demonstrate good-quality holistic, comprehensive, outpatient care for patients with HIV/AIDS-related health problems, and to teach and train health workers throughout Uganda and the region in such care.[68]

The Palliative Care Association of Uganda (PCAU) was founded in 1998. It is chaired by Dr Lydia Mpanga; Julia Downing is co-editor of the PCAU journal with Anne Merriman, and the organization has >180 members. The association's aims include: introducing and maintaining standards; bringing together key players and stake-holders; establishing a journal; quarterly continuing medical education (CME) update; publications; advocacy; and co-ordination of education and CME. Throughout the 56 Districts of Uganda, there are eight hospice–palliative care organizations delivering 155 services.

Uganda is the first and only country in Africa that has made palliative care for people with AIDS and cancer a priority in its National Health Plan, where it is classed as 'essential clinical care'.[69]

Zimbabwe

In Zimbabwe, 13 organizations provide 34 palliative care services (Table 1.5). A crowded public meeting in May 1979 resulted in the establishment of Island Hospice Service—among the first of its kind in Africa. In a country which became independent from Britain in 1980, the developing service operated in a receding colonial framework where whites still held social and financial power. Yet over the next 24 years, the organization changed from 'a charitable institution, relying on volunteers, initially with patients who were elderly, middle class and mostly white'[28] to something more attuned to the wider population of Zimbabwe. David McElvaine, a former Senior Administrator of Island Hospice writes:

> Zimbabwe's pre-independence history also had a marked effect on public opinion regarding death and bereavement. The bloody and protracted struggle for independence had personally affected hundreds of thousands of people. The need for skilled bereavement care was at its zenith when Island Hospice was formed. These large-scale events, coupled with our early focus on public relations and education were strong contributory factors to our successful establishment and have remained crucial to our continued functioning.[29]

At the outset, Island Hospice was a specialized unit with qualified and experienced staff who delivered care to a relatively small number of people. As the reputation of the service spread, 'the patient profile changed. There were more black patients and they tended to be younger (conforming to the pattern of cancer in Africa), they lived in small, overcrowded houses and spoke Shona'.[70]

Table 1.5 Hospice–palliative care services in three African countries approaching integration

	Free-standing unit	Inpatient unit	Paediatric inpatient unit	Hospital unit	Hospital support service	Home care	Day care	Paediatric day care	Paediatric clinic	Clinic/Drop-in center	Mobile clinic	Total
Kenya												
Nairobi Hospice					1	1	1			1		4
Meru						1	1			1		3
Eldoret					1	1				1		3
Nyeri					1	1	1			1		3
Coast					1	1				1		3
Kisumu						1	1					2
Maua Methodist Hospital					1							1
Maua Methodist Hospital Home care projects (branches)						3						3
Chogoria Mission Hospital					1	1						2
Total services					6	10	4			5		25
Uganda												
Association François-Xavier Bagnoud						1						1
Hospice Africa Uganda					2	1	1			1		5
Mobile Hospice Mbarara					2	1	1				2	6
Little Hospice Hoima		8			2	1					2	6
Mildmay International		1			1	1		1	1			5

								Total
Joy Hospice, Mbale	1		1	1			1	4
Kitovu Mobile Home Care				1				1
Branches of Kitovu Mobile							124	124
Home care								
PC Unit: Lira Regional Referral Hospital		1		1		1		3
Total services	1	1	9	7	3	1	127	155
Zimbabwe								
Bekezela Home Based Care				1				1
Dananai Home Based Care (Murambinda)			1	1				2
FACT Mutare				1				1
Island Hospice, Bulawayo			1	1				2
Island Hospice, Harare			1	1			2	4
Island Hospice, Mutare			1	1				2
Island Hospice branches				6				6
Lubancho House, Hwange				1				1
Mashambanzou	1	1		1			1	4
Methodist Church of Zimbabwe (Epworth Project)				1		1		2
The Mildmay Centre			1	1	1		1	4
Morgenster Mission Hospital			1	1				2
Seke Rural Home Based Care				1				1
Thembelihle Halfway Home	1			1				2
Total services	2	2	6	19	2		5	34

Island Hospice has centres in Harare (established 1979), Bulawayo (1981) and Mutare (1985), and incorporates six autonomous branches throughout the country.[71] Services range from a full palliative home care service—including palliative nursing support, counselling and volunteer services—to simple nursing care. Island Hospice, Harare is twinned with three hospices: two in America and one in Wales. Whilst celebrating 25 years of hospice care in Zimbabwe, there have also been many challenges in recent times. A commentator in 2004:

> . . . in the past three years Island has had to deal with challenges above and beyond the call of normal hospice duty. In 2000 the country began experiencing increasing political instability and polarization. When certain areas of the city become impassable due to strikes, stayaways and turmoil, staff safety becomes a concern . . . Economic hardships have increased the brain drain, and many professionals are leaving the country. Medication is expensive, if available, and medical bills are above the reach of many of the population. This strains already weakened health and welfare systems and adds to the pressure on an established and well-respected organisation like Island . . . All of this inevitably affects service delivery. There are clinical supervision meetings in fuel queues; nutritional supplements have to be sourced in order to safely implement certain medication regimes; administration and accounting functions have become extremely challenging . . . foreign donors have to be patient with the massive changes in budget items.[72]

There are ongoing issues in Zimbabwe concerning the availability of appropriate analgesics. Island Hospice Harare uses the WHO pain ladder and keeps a supply of morphine for patients who are unable to collect the drug from the government hospitals of Pariryanetwa and Harare. A local firm produces morphine whenever powder can be imported, although availability is erratic. The hospice doctor writes a prescription after discussion with a nurse. The Ministry of Health and the Drug Control Council have given permission for a hospice nurse to prescribe drugs falling within the Dangerous Drugs Act providing the prescription is validated by a hospice doctor. Island Hospice Bulawayo does not prescribe morphine; the service liaises with the patient's doctor who prescribes the necessary morphine. Island Hospice Mutare does not prescribe morphine. Bekezela Community Home Based Care has access to doctors at Inyati District Hospital. These doctors prescribe morphine in injectable and MST forms; volunteers administer paracetamol and aspirin. Dananai Home Based Care (Murambinda) has access to three doctors at Murambinda Mission Hospital, who may prescribe liquid morphine. Family AIDS Caring Trust (FACT) has three qualified nurses who have responsibility for morphine prescription, supervised by a volunteer doctor.[73] Lubancho House is limited to the administration of paracetamol; morphine is difficult to access and the hospital supply is frequently exhausted. Morgenster Mission Hospital does not prescribe morphine to home care patients, though where a patient is taking morphine on discharge from hospital, relatives are able to collect repeat prescriptions (tablets and syrup) as required.

The Hospice Association of Zimbabwe (HOSPAZ)[74] is a registered public voluntary organization (PVO) whose mission is to provide national co-ordination, training and advocacy to support organizations in their provision of hospice and palliative care. All organizations describing themselves either as palliative care providers or home-based care groups in Zimbabwe have been invited to register with HOSPAZ, and a database of members is currently being constructed. Palliative care standards have been devised by HOSPAZ and approved by the Ministry of Health, although there is no implementation policy as yet. HOSPAZ is twinned with the Ohio Hospice and Palliative Care Organization, Arlington, Ohio, USA.

WHO notes that in Zimbabwe, palliative care still has some way to go at the level of policy:

> Zimbabwe has a long tradition in palliative care provided by the hospice movement, however this is still not widely integrated into the health system. There is no exclusive national policy concerning palliative care although palliative care policies are included in the following documents: the Home Based Care Policy, the Discharge Policy and the Ten Year Plan produced by the Committee for Prevention and Control of Cancer in Zimbabwe (PCCZ). Like Hospice Uganda, Island Hospice in Zimbabwe provides training at various levels in palliative care within the community, within the country and to neighbouring countries.[11]

Eunice Garanganga, clinical and technical adviser to HOSPAZ, sums up the success of hospice care in Zimbabwe:

> We have lots of successes . . . Zimbabwe was the first country to bring hospice into Africa, and that has grown; it has given us strength to go on, just knowing that we are Mother Hospice . . . And we have grown in the sense that training started in 1983 when doctors at the medical school came to say, 'We don't know how to break bad news, can you come and do some lectures with final medical students on breaking bad news?' So that was our opportunity to sell everything in hospice, sell everything in palliative care. So we started training even in pain control, breaking bad news, communications skills, symptom management, in 1983 . . . We've realized the numbers are huge in home-based care, and we are grafting palliative care onto home-based care groups so that the quality remains very good. So again, in Africa, we were the first to come up with standards for home-based care, and we are proud of that . . . We have also embarked on a rural model: this was initiated by WHO. The WHO chose five countries in Africa, and Zimbabwe's one of them, to initiate palliative care and see how to go about it through the Ministry of Health. At some stage the funds were not there and HOSPAZ sought the funds so that this project can go on, and we can see how to graft palliative care onto a district hospital. The training—the hospital, the health professionals—is going on at the moment. We are going to evaluate and see if it can be taken to another area. We are going to learn a lot, so even through difficult circumstances we are taking strides to try and maintain our palliative care standards in Zimbabwe.[75]

South Africa

In South Africa, around 60 organizations linked to the national association—the Hospice and Palliative Care Association of South Africa (HPCA)—provide a range of services for patients and their families (Table 1.6). Many of these organizations have branches which provide palliative care services in local settings. Service types include: inpatient care; home care; day care; clinics/drop-in centres; hospital support teams; education and training; patient support groups; bereavement care; foster parent support groups; orphan support groups; and hospice care for the homeless.[76] Between 2003 and 2004, data returned to HPCA indicate that 24 613 patients were cared for, of whom 12 413 had an AIDS diagnosis and 9233 had cancer. Most referrals originated from family, friends or state hospitals.

Table 1.6 Palliative care provision in South Africa: Hospice and Palliative Care Association members/affiliated members, 2000

Date opened	Organization
Pre 1984	Grahamstown Hospice
	Highway Hospice, Durban
	Hospice Association of Witwatersrand, Johannesburg
	St Francis Hospice, Port Elizabeth
	St Luke's Hospice, Cape Town
	South Coast Hospice, Port Shepstone
	Msunduzi Hospice, Pietermaritzburg
1985–1989	Franschoek Hospice, Franschoek
	Goldfields Hospice Association, Welkom
	Helderberg Hospice, Somerset West
	Hospice East Rand
	Howick Hospice
	Khanya (Lighthouse Hospice/ Amamzimtoti), Umkomaas
	Knysna/ Sedgefield Hospice
	Naledi Hospice, Blomfontein
	Pretoria Sungardens Hospice
	Vryheid Hospice
	Wide Horizon Hospice, Vereeniging
1990–1994	Chatsworth Hospice
	Estcourt Hospice
	Golden Gateway Hospice, Bethlehem
	Good Shepherd Hospice, Middelburg
	Hospice Association of Transkei
	Hospice in the West, Krugersdorp
	Hospice North West, Klerksdorp
	Kimberley Hospice
	Newcastle Hospice
	Parys Hospice
	Drakenstein Hospice, Paarl
	St Bernard's Hospice, East London
	Stellenbosch Hospice
	Viljoenskroon Hospice
	Worcester Hospice
	Zululand Hospice Association, Empangeni

Table 1.6 (*Contd.*)

Date opened	Organization
1995–1999	Breede River Hospice, Robertson
	Cotlands Hospice, Johannesburg
	Impilo (Zazile Hope for Life Care Centre) Johannesburg
	Ladysmith Hospice Association
	Moretela Sunrise Hospice, North West
	Nightingale Hospice, De Aar
	Rustenburg Hospice
	St Nicholas Children's Hospice, Bloemfontein
	Sparrow Ministries, Roodepoort
	Tygerberg Hospice, Bellville
	Verulam Hospice
2000–2004	AIDS Care Training and Support, White River
	Arebaokeng Hospice, Tembisa
	Beautiful Gates Ministries, Muizenberg
	Brits Hospice, Brits
	Centurion Hospice, Lyttleton
	Comfi Care, Hartswater
	FWC HIV/AIDS Hospice Shelter, Melville
	Good Samaritan Hospice, Bethulie
	Holy Cross Hospice, Gingindlovu/ Emoyeni
	Hospice of White River, Witbank
	Ladybrand Hospice
	Morningstar Hospice, Welkom
	Potchefstroom Hospice
	Philanjalo Hospice, Tugela Ferry
	St Joseph's Care and Support Trust, Sizanani
	Tapologo Hospice, Rustenburg
	Themba Care, Century City
	White Rose Hospice, Witbank

In South Africa—unlike most other African countries—palliative care services can be found in hospital settings countrywide. Examples include: Cape Town (2 Military Hospital, Wynberg); Durban (Addington Hospital, McCord Hospital, Parklands Hospital, St Mary's Hospital); Johannesburg (Chris Hani Baragwanath Hospital); Soweto (Johannesburg General Hospital); Port Shepstone (Murchison Hospital; Port Shepstone

Hospital); and Pretoria (Pretoria Academic Hospital). In Cape Town, palliative care provision at the 2 Military Hospital is described as follows:

> Situated within a general hospital, the patient has access to palliative care and all its facets from the time of diagnosis of curable and incurable cancer. A major advantage is the availability and affordability of a full multidisciplinary team, which can provide services and support to other departments, e.g. dietician. Additionally, this particular hospice is combined with a rehabilitation unit, which allows cost effective use of staff as well as space. The issues of loss/grieving/disability and impact on psycho/social functioning are similar. Because of this system, by the time a new symptom develops or some serious event occurs, the patient and family are familiar with palliative care, the ward and the system.[77]

At South Coast Hospice, Port Shepstone, in collaboration with a range of partners, an innovative form of care has been developed, known as *Integrated Community-based Home Care* (ICHC). The approach includes several elements. *Clinical management*—providing early diagnosis, including HIV testing, appropriate prophylaxis and treatment of opportunistic infections as well as effective management of pain and symptom control. *Nursing care*—promoting and maintaining hygiene and nutrition, teaching the family and microcommunity basic nursing skills and comfort as well as emergency measures, supervising the taking of medication. *Psycho-spiritual support*—providing counselling and spiritual support, including stress and risk reduction as well as planning, promoting and supporting the acceptance and disclosure of serostatus and enabling coping and planning for the future of the family, in particular placement of children. *Social support*—providing welfare services and legal advice; providing information and referrals between the partners who make up the care network, including poverty alleviation and pastoral and bereavement care; and facilitating peer support.

The ICHC model was piloted at seven hospice sites across South Africa in 1999–2000 on behalf of the South African national Department of Health HIV/AIDS Directorate. Research conducted by HASA (now HPCA) and the University of Natal demonstrated the replicability and cost-effectiveness of ICHC and recommended the model be rolled out countrywide. South Coast Hospice was subsequently awarded a research tender by the South African Department of Health to develop Port Shepstone as an HIV/AIDS TB/sexually transmitted infection (STI) demonstration site.[78] In 2002, a review of the model was undertaken by the Centre for AIDS Development, Research and Evaluation (CADRE) on behalf of the POLICY Futures Group.[79,80] Their report concludes that hospices are being transformed and expanded as a direct result of the emerging needs of the HIV/AIDS epidemic. However, the underlying ethos of care provision combined with an understanding of the community contexts is maintained within the ICHC model.[81]

Despite the numbers of organizations and services in existence, hospices in South Africa are usually registered as not-for profit organizations. A small amount of money is available from government but, in the main, the hospice has to source its own funds. Barbara Campbell-Ker, executive director, Hospice Association of the Witwatersrand:

> The spirit can be extremely willing but we are as good as the resources that we have, and we have to find all our money. The Department of Health gives us about 2 per cent or 3 per cent of what we require— if we're lucky—and that isn't done just by handing it out, but after completing funding proposals.[82]

This can place a considerable burden on hospice organisations; Lesley van Zyl, general manager of Highway Hospice (Durban), describes the impact of dwindling funds:

> The challenge for me is always to balance the books. We've gone through some fairly tough periods where we had to retrench staff [make staff redundant] and we moved from being predominantly in-care units—correctly I believe—to care for patients in the community by opening various day centres. So we've opened day centres in Chesterville, in Umlazi, in Phoenix and in Inanda, and difficult as it was and as painful as it was, I personally believe it was the right thing to do. We had two years where we were battling to raise funds and we had to down-size. So, you know, we make a loss year—it's not good; but if you make it in two years, it's worse. By the time we get to the third year you really have to do something. So we reduced our beds from 16 to eight. It was a particularly difficult thing to do; and also I think whenever you are facing the staff and you have to tell them that some of them are going to be without work, that's really tough.[83]

The Hospice Association of Southern Africa was formed in 1987 'to represent, facilitate and co-ordinate development and growth of hospice in the region'.[84] By 2002, the Association was made up of around 50 member hospices, although large areas of the country were without a palliative care service.[85] Today, the Association has changed its name and geared up for the challenges brought about by the AIDS pandemic and the urgent need for expansion.[86,87] Josef Lazarus, strategic adviser to the board of HPCA identifies the significance of these issues:

> In 1997 I was asked to do a strategic planning exercise for the national organization, in terms of its future direction . . . Instead of having a CEO who couldn't possibly fulfil all the functions as required in development, because they're so varied, we identified five key portfolios that are required for hospice development; they being patient care, education and training, organizational development, advocacy and public relations and fundraising.
>
> That has pretty much revolutionized the Hospice Association in South Africa. The people that you've seen here like Liz Gwyther and André Wagner and Joan Marston, they are conveners of those development subcommittees and they've taken full ownership and responsibility for their portfolio with the expertise of their subcommittee. The Hospice Association was asked to do three major tenders for the national Department of Health—done by these development subcommittees. These development subcommittees now sit on a newly formed steering committee of the Department of Health for palliative care in South Africa and that steering committee is now forming similar subcommittees for operationalizing palliative care throughout South Africa—so that model is now beginning to be replicated by the national Department of Health. It's been a very exciting journey the last five years.[88]

As yet, palliative care coverage in South Africa is quite comprehensive in some areas but non-existent in others. Services are particularly sparse in the Northern Cape, Mpumalanga and Limpopo. HPCA intends to have a hospice service in each of South Africa's 170 health authorities by 2009. Kath Defilippi, HPCA board member and manager, South Coast Hospice, Port Shepstone outlines the significance of a new association with the Council of Health Services Accreditation for Southern Africa (COHASA)

> Our aim is to move hospices along as fast as possible to the place of full accreditation, but to do it in a non-threatening, supportive way. And then, in order to be a mentor . . . to other organizations, and very importantly to Department of Health organizations. We believe that to fulfil that function effectively a hospice should have full accreditation. And so, so that's what we're really very excited

about at the moment. HPCA have partnered with COHSASA who are a very professional outfit—COHSASA stands for the Council of Health Services Accreditation for Southern Africa—and they are internationally recognized. And so HPCA have signed a formal Memorandum of Understanding with COHSASA and together we've developed hospice standards of care, which is wonderful for us, but it's also very good for them because in fact they have acknowledged that in some ways we have improved their standards.[89]

South Africa is a country within the PEFAR programme and in 2004 became one of the first beneficiaries of its palliative care funding stream. HPCA's mentorship programme is the basis of the PEPFAR-funded work. The mentorship programme was supported for the two and a half years up to June 2004 by Open Society Institute, and is being used as the vehicle for the PEPFAR funding, of which the first year's grant is US$2 million. The aim of the programme is to deliver quality palliative care to patients and families, by taking organizations that have a component of clinical palliative care but that also have good management, good governance and financial accountability. The idea is to develop those organizations, starting with standards of clinical care, to which are added standards of management and good governance. There are different levels of accreditation: pre-entry level, entry level, intermediate level and those that get full accreditation. This covers the range of services that hospices offer: home-based care services, inpatient services, day hospice, spiritual counselling, bereavement counselling, education and training. There are six objectives for the programme of PEPFAR-funded work: (1) to build capacity in the national office; (2) to strengthen services; (3) to develop new hospices; (4) advocacy; (5) palliative care research and training; and (6) monitoring and evaluation.

Concluding comments

This review of hospice–palliative care developments in Africa highlights the impact of individual, charismatically led service initiatives, but also reveals some of their limitations. If the enormous needs are to be met, it will be necessary to harmonize hospice–palliative care into a variety of other structures and to reduce the risk that well organized small-scale services remain islands of excellence in an ocean of unrelieved suffering. This requires engagement with the institutionalized health care system, as well as systems of family and community support. Cultural, spiritual and socio-economic support systems must also be engaged, together with the efforts of both governmental and non-governmental agencies. Public engagement and consumer involvement are likewise vital. In particular, palliative care should be integrated with, and not separated from, the mainstream of medical practice and health and social care.

Guidelines on policies and strategies for the effective implementation of palliative care development are extremely important. The establishment of public health programmes in palliative care has now been described extensively.[28] The principles have been outlined in detail in a series of WHO documents, and good examples exist concerning the establishment of public health programmes in palliative care. Establishing a national policy offers the best way to ensure, in a cost-effective manner, adequate palliative care for the greatest number of patients and families. WHO recommends three foundation measures based on: governmental policy, education and drug availability. These are important for establishing sustainable palliative care and achieving meaningful coverage. Yet, on their own, they are insufficient to achieve the necessary changes. The examples cited here, especially for the four countries we define as achieving some measure of integration of their hospice–palliative care services, show how foundation measures, NGOs, faith-based organizations and inspired individuals make up a highly complex mosaic of activity. At present, we remain remarkably ignorant of how to guide hospice–palliative care developments in a country in order to capitalize on this rich synergy, whilst avoiding the pitfalls of insufficient resources, burn-out of personnel, policy inertia and governmental indifference.

Palliative care has different characteristics in different regions. Within Africa, there are diverse attitudes towards death and dying informed by multiple meanings and traditions. This has important implications for the identification of appropriate models and places for hospice–palliative care. The cultural beliefs that underpin health, sickness and the societal responses to them need to be identified in order to ground palliative care in the African context.[17] Policy makers commonly extrapolate Western biomedical approaches to African nations,[90] yet effective hospice–palliative care requires integration into the existing continuum of care.[91] Unique, culturally specific community systems and rituals have helped individuals and communities to cope with dying and suffering; old cultural traditions exist for curbing total pain that could be empowered rationally in hospice-palliative care infrastructures.[92] Those who ignore culture are doomed to failure in Africa. Outside prescriptions only succeed where they work with the grain of African ways of doing things. They fail where they ignore, or do not understand, the cultural suppositions of the people they seek to address. Alongside medical or biological explanations for disease, many Africans will also look for explanations that are spiritually or culturally related (as in the case of traditional healing). In reducing the transmission of HIV and AIDS, the importance of cultural attitudes is paramount, indeed, where cultural norms have not been taken into account in HIV and AIDS prevention strategies, prevalence rates have continued to rise.[93] The changing face of hospice–palliative care on the continent entails the integration of African home-based care programmes with a Westernized model of palliation—this will require a sensitive recognition of the complex cultural synthesis that will undoubtedly be involved. In the face of such overwhelming needs and problems, the results it might produce must surely make the attempt worthwhile.

Our purpose in this volume is to map out in detail what has so far been achieved and also to form a picture of the developments that have occurred—as well as the obstacles that remain—through the words of those most actively involved. We move next to a series of oral history accounts of hospice–palliative care development in Africa. We then turn to in-depth country analysis, grouped by the three stages of development we have formalized here; 'approaching integration', 'localized provision' and 'capacity building'. We hope the book will be used as a ready source of information about hospice–palliative care development in Africa in the early part of the twenty-first century. We hope in due course to extend our studies in Africa further with more in-depth analysis of the factors that promote and inhibit such development.

References

1 WHO: The World Health Report 2004.

2 Reader J. *Africa: A Biography of the Continent*. London: Penguin, 1998.

3 See: *Thinking Regionally*. African Policy Information Centre. Available at: www.africaaction.org/bp/regmap.htm

4 Wamue GN. Tradition and change: oral history, belief systems, AIDS, and the challenges of modernity among the Agikuyu people of central Kenya. Paper presented at the 12th conference of the International Oral History Association, University of Natal, South Africa, 24–27 June 2002.

5 Nugent P. *Africa Since Independence*. London: Palgrave, 2005.

6 Van der Veen R. *What Went Wrong With Africa?* Amsterdam: KIT, 2004.

7 Available to download at: http://www.commissionforafrica.org/english/report/introduction.html

8 Valley P. Will they never learn about Africa? *Church Times* 17 June 2005.

9 Sepulveda C, Marlin A, Yoshida T, Ullrich A. Palliative care: WHO global perspective. *Journal of Pain and Symptom Management* 2002; **24**(2): 91–96.

10 UNAIDS/World Health Organization: *AIDS Epidemic Update* 2003.

11 WHO. *Community Health Approach to Palliative Care for HIV/AIDS and Cancer Patients in Sub-Saharan Africa* 2004:8. Available to download at: http://whqlibdoc.who.int/publications/2004/9241591498.pdf

12 See: www.theworkcontinues.org

13 See: www.fhssa.org

14 See: www.nhpco.org

15 See: www.soros.org

16 Harding R, Stewart K, Marconi K, O'Neill JF, Higginson IJ. Current HIV/AIDS end-of-life care in sub-Saharan Africa: a survey of models, services, challenges and priorities. *BMC Public Health* 2003; **3**: 33.

17 Harding R, Higginson I. *Palliative Care in Sub-Saharan Africa. An Appraisal*. London: King's College and Diana, Princess of Wales Memorial Fund, 2004. See: www.theworkcontinues.org/causes/pall_library.asp

18 See: http://www.usaid.gov/our_work/global_health/aids/pepfarfact.html

19 *Engendering Bold Leadership*. The President's Emergency Plan for AIDS Relief. First Annual Report to Congress, 2005. http://www.state.gov/documents/organization/43885.pdf

20 See: www.aegis.com/news/pr/2005/PRO50339.html

21 The Palliative Care Trainers' Declaration of Cape Town, November 13 2002. *Journal of Palliative Medicine* 2003; **6**(3): 339–340.

22 www.eolc-observatory.net

23 Clark D, Wright M, Bath P, Gatrell A. The International Observatory on End of Life Care: a new research and development initiative in end of life care. *Progress in Palliative Care* 2003; **11**(3): 137–138.

24 ten Have H, Clark D. (eds). *The Ethics of Palliative Care: European Perspectives*. Buckingham: Open University Press, 2002.

25 Clark D, Wright M. *Transitions in End of Life Care: Hospice and Related Developments in Eastern Europe and Central Asia*. Buckingham: Open University Press, 2003.

26 See: http://www.eolc-observatory.net/global_analysis/regions_main.htm

27 Defilippi K, Downing J, Merriman A, Clark D. Editorial: a palliative care association for the whole of Africa. *Palliative Medicine* 2004; **18**: 583–584.

28 Stjernswärd J, Clark D. Palliative medicine—a global perspective. In: Doyle, D, Hanks GWC, Cherny N, Calman KC (ed.), *Oxford Textbook of Palliative Medicine*, 3rd edn. Oxford: Oxford University Press, 2003: 1199–1224.

29 **McElvaine D.** Zimbabwe: the Island Hospice experience. In: Saunders, C, Kastenbaum R. *Hospice Care on the International Scene.* New York: Springer, 1997: 52.

30 **Martin R.** Speech delivered at the celebrations marking the 25th anniversary of Island Hospice— 22 January 2004.

31 IOELC interview: Thembi Nyuswa—8 August 2004.

32 'The term *defined daily doses for statistical purposes* (S-DDD) replaces the term *defined daily doses* previously used by the Board. The S-DDDs are technical units of measurement for the purposes of statistical analysis and are not recommended prescription doses. Certain narcotic drugs may be used in certain countries for different treatments or in accordance with different medical practices, and therefore a different daily dose could be more appropriate.' International Narcotics Control Board. *Narcotic Drugs: Estimated World Requirements for 2004. Statistics for 2002.*

33 IOELC interview: Beugre Kouassi—4 June 2004.

34 IOELC interview: Hussein Mtiro—10 November 2004.

35 IOELC interview: Professor Olaitan Soyannwo—4 June 2004.

36 Ministry of Health, Republic of Uganda. *Statutory Instruments 2004:24 The National Drug Authority (Prescription and Supply of Certain Narcotic Analgesic Drugs) Regulations, 2004.* Ministry of Health, 2004.

37 IOELC interview: Peter Mikajjo—10 March 2004.

38 **Simmons M.** The integration of palliative care using oral morphine into an existing home care programme. *PCAU Journal of Palliative Care* 2003; **6**(3): 28.

39 IOELC interview: Jack Jagwe—10 March 2004.

40 IOELC interview: George Mbeng—4 June 2004.

41 IOELC interview: Anselme Kananga—8 April 2005.

42 **Porchet F, Schaerer G, Larkin P, Leruth S.** Intercultural experiences of training in the Maghreb. *European Journal of Palliat Care* 2005; **12**(1): 35–37.

43 IOELC interview: Mary Opare—4 June 2004.

44 IOELC interview: Terry Magee—25 March 2005.

45 USAID and CDC. Rapid Appraisal for HIV/AIDS Program Expansion, Lesotho. September 5–13. Draft report, 2004.

46 Information provided by Sr Virginia Moorosi.

47 Graham Thomas, Wales Lesotho Link. HIV Health Needs Assessment 2003: Tebelong Community, Qacha's District, Lesotho.

48 IOELC interview: Sr Virginia Moorosi—2 June 2004.

49 Personal communication: Olaitan Soyannwo—25 March 2005.

50 **Hurton S.** The Shepherd's Hospice—Sierra Leone. *Hospice Information Service* 1999; **7**: 1.

51 IOELC interview: Gabriel Madiye—4 June 2004.

52 Personal communication: Sibusiso Dlamini—5 June 2003.

53 IAHPC news online: 2005, **6**(3). See: http://www.hospicecare.com/newsletter2005/mar05/editor.html

54 **Merriman A.** *Report of Visit to Zambia to Assess, Share and Assist with Advice re Palliative Care Provision.* 21 February–1 March; 2004: 9.

55 IOELC interview: Mark Jacobson—4 June 2004.

56 IOELC interview: Brigid Sirengo—2 June 2004.

57 Kate Jones, Hospice Care Kenya. hospice.care.kenya@virgin.net

58 FHSSA newsletter 17 December 2003.

59 IOELC interview: Brigid Sirengo—1 November 2004.

60 IOELC interview: Zipporah Ali—2 June 2004.

61 See: http://www.fias.net/Donor%20Page/Ireland-Donor.htm

62 **Wheatley S.** Little Hospice Hoima celebrates five years. *Hospice Information Service* 2003; **12**(3): 9.

63 WHO: *Community Health Approach to Palliative Care for HIV/AIDS and Cancer Patients in Sub-Saharan Africa*. Progress Report. August 2002.

64 **Kikule E.** A good death in Uganda: survey of needs for palliative care for terminally ill people in urban areas. *British Medical Journal* 2003; **327**(7408): 192–194.

65 IOELC interview: Anne Merriman—9 March 2004.

66 **Kikule E.** A word from the executive director. In: *Hospice Uganda Eleventh Annual Report: 1 April 2003 to 31 March 2004*: 17.

67 Hospice Uganda. *Some Facts about Hospice Uganda: January 2004*.

68 **Downing J.** Welcome from the Mildmay Centre, Uganda. In: *Conference proceedings—Palliative Care: Completing the Circle of Care*, 16–17 September 2003.

69 Ministry of Health, Republic of Uganda. *National Sector Strategic Plan 2000/01–2004/05*. Kampala: Ministry of Health, 2000.

70 **Williams S.** Global perspective: Zimbabwe. *Palliative Medicine* 2000; **14**: 225.

71 See: http://site.mweb.co.zw/islandhospice/

72 Anon. International Perspective. Island hospice and Bereavement Service (Island) hits a quarter century 'not out' in 2004. *Progress in Palliative Care* 2004; **12**(1): 30–31.

73 Personal communication: Pardon Myambo—19 March 2004.

74 Personal communication: Carla Lamadora—13 November 2003.

75 IOELC interview: Eunice Garanganga—20 September 2004.

76 **Wright M.** A survey of delegates at the HPCA annual general meeting, Rustenburg, South Africa. Unpublished, 2004.

77 IAHPC newsletter, October 2003. See:
http://www.hospicecare.com/newsletter2003/october2003/page7.html

78 **Defilippi K.** South Coast Hospice: integrated community-based home care. *South Coast Hospice Information Leaflet*, April 2002.

79 Part of the Washington-based Futures Group International, the POLICY Project aims to facilitate the development of policies and plans that promote and sustain access to high-quality family planning and reproductive health (FP/RH) services. The project also addresses HIV/AIDS and maternal health policy issues. See: http://www.policyproject.com/index.cfm

80 Centre for AIDS Development, Research and Evaluation (Cadre) on behalf of the POLICY Project. *Integrated Community Home-based Care in South Africa: A Review of the Model Implemented by the Hospice Association of South Africa*. National department of health Government of South Africa, 2002. Report available in full at: http://www.policyproject.com/pubs/countryreports/SA_Hospice.pdf

81 See: http://www.eldis.org/cf/search/disp/docdisplay.cfm?doc=DOC12596&resource=f1

82 IOELC interview: Barbara Campbell-Ker—11 August 2004.

83 IOELC interview: Lesley van Zyl—8 August 2004.

84 **Buckland P.** Hospice in Southern Africa. In: Saunders C, Kastenbaum R (ed.). *Hospice Care on the International Scene*. New York: Springer, 1997: 48.

85 **Gwyther E.** South Africa: the status of palliative care. *Journal of Pain and Symptom Management* 2002; **24**(2): 236–238.

86 **Defilippi K.** Palliative care issues in sub-Saharan Africa. *International Journal of Palliative Nursing* 2000; **6**(3): 108.

87 Foundation for Hospices in sub-Saharan Africa. *Challenging Times*. Liverpool: New York, 2000.

88 IOELC interview: Josef Lazarus—13 August 2004.

89 IOELC interview: Kathleen Defilippi—12 August 2004.

90 **Lau C, Muula AS.** HIV/AIDS in sub-Saharan Africa. *Croatian Medical Journal* 2004; **45**(4): 402–414.

91 African Palliative Care Association. The Palliative Care Trainers Declaration of Cape Town. *Journal of Palliative Medicine* 2003; **6**(3): 339.

92 **Stjernswärd J.** Uganda: initiating a government public health approach to pain relief and palliative care. *Journal of Pain and Symptom Management* 2002; **24**: 257–264.

93 http://www.commissionforafrica.org/

Part 2

A narrative history of hospice–palliative care in Africa

Chapter 2

Oral history in Africa

In this second part of the book, we focus on the history of hospice and palliative care in Africa, as seen through the medium of storytelling.

Language is a defining feature of human beings and, in Africa, a land of over a thousand different peoples,[1] storytelling may be categorized in a variety of ways.

First of all, stories are integrally related to what is termed *tradition*. For Africans, tradition is grounded in the collective experience of the whole community. In effect, it 'constitutes the totality of all that successive generations have accumulated since the dawn of time, in both spiritual and practical life. It is the sum total of the wisdom held by a society at a given moment of its existence'.[2] In the absence of written records and sacred writings, this wisdom is transmitted through cultural and linguistic structures, encapsulated in what is known specifically as the *oral tradition*. The oral historian Grace Wamue comments:

> Oral tradition becomes crucial as sages [storytellers] of African philosophy strive to pass on the core teachings of the people's religious and cultural history. As custodians of traditions and repositories of oral history, elders and sages have with time exercised considerable power and influence among the peoples of Africa.[3]

Secondly, these stories may be viewed as *oral testimonies* or *histories*. Unlike the oral tradition, regarded as the word of mouth transmission of information over a period longer than the current generation, oral histories relate to the lifetime of the storyteller. In the absence of documentary information in many African countries, these oral histories are invaluable sources of information provided by individuals who have been directly involved in any given historical events or circumstances.

The Centre for Popular Memory (CPM)—part of the Department of Historical Studies at the University of Cape Town—has been established to record people's stories. The Centre acknowledges that:

> People have the right to be seen, heard and remembered. For marginalised individuals and groups who have felt the pain and the joys of the past these needs tend to be acute. Storytelling through various media can play a small but significant part in meeting these needs.[4]

The Centre is one of numerous organizations in South Africa and beyond that preserves and disseminates oral history. CPM mostly undertakes research in the Western Cape, but intends to extend its work to other African countries. Stories are recorded in several languages and focus on a broad range of topics, including:

- Migrancy and refugee experiences
- Forced removals in Cape Town and beyond

- Trauma and violence
- Social impact of HIV/AIDS
- South African life stories
- Heritage and cultural practice.

Outcomes include: *Testimonies of passage: Congolese and Nigerian migration and identity in Cape Town* (2004)—which is based on interviews with >120 refugees; *Imini Zakudala: Gugeletu elders remember* (2003)—a study that explores social trauma experienced by residents during the unrest in 1980s South Africa; and *Umqomboti, utywala and lucky stars: stories of liquor in Langa between 1930 and 1980* (2002)—a project that drew on 40 interviews with Langa residents involved with the underground liquor trade to explore the histories of people living under apartheid.

Oral histories have also been utilized to determine critical issues identified by social groups. One study concerned leaders of black Christian women's organizations in Sobantu, on the outskirts of Pietermaritzburg and Umlazi, Durban's biggest black township.[5] This research was initiated by the Sinomlando Project (formerly known as the Oral History Project) of the School of Theology, University of Natal in 1999. Twenty women were interviewed (in Zulu) in Pietermaritzburg, and 14 in Umlazi. These interviews highlight issues that concern leaders of black women's organizations in their homes, the church and the community. They include: cultural oppression of women; concerns about the rape of girls by family members; the impact of segregated worship; discrimination against women in leadership roles; and the relationship between Christianity and traditional African religion.

Alongside insights gained into social and political development, oral histories also have a role to play in health care—not least by illuminating the nature and occurrence of disease. Study of the history of disease and related phenomena is difficult in Africa due to the problem of sources, in particular the lack of: medical archives; data relating to hospital admissions; and patient charts and reports. In this scenario, oral histories assume a special significance. In a paper presented at the International Oral History Association conference in South Africa (2002), César Nkuku Khonde comments on this issue:

> The maintenance of medical archives, a long-standing tradition in developed countries, still poses a problem in Third World countries in general and in Congo-Kinshasa in particular. Nonetheless, Africa offers other possibilities for retaining significant facts: for example, memory to which one has access by the spoken word. These sources, called oral sources, supply less polished but more particular information on most diseases. They permit completing and confirming the limited written data available, but more especially they become the only source of information on diseases and on the effects of the diseases within the family, the neighbourhood, the city, the country, or the society.[6]

Importantly, Khonde demonstrates how, in the case of Congo-Kinshasa, oral sources are able to contribute to public health history in four distinct categories. *Oral tradition* may encapsulate the case of an individual—a prince, for example—whose incapacity prompts a modification to the royal line. *Oral histories* provide information from people who have contracted a disease or who lived at a critical moment. *Material and immaterial sources* rely on accompanying narratives for explanation. For example, the use of medicinal plants can only be understood through the explanations of those who used them, with details of the mode of preparation, means of consumption, target disease and modalities of treatment. *Retrospective epidemiological studies* may detect disease within a family or region through research into life histories.

In sub-Saharan Africa, the AIDS pandemic has assumed disastrous proportions, and there is a strong argument for the disease to be seen essentially as a public health issue.[7] Yet Wamue maintains that in combating the disease, oral tradition also has a role to play. Interventions such as peer counselling and the oral transmission of information resonate with the African cultural heritage, where ancient wisdom reflected in myths, proverbs and songs links the traditions of the past to issues of the present. She concludes:

> Oral traditions in the African context have the role and the power to uphold and creatively adapt moral values and principles . . . The role of the sages in teaching the youth on prevailing taboos on sexual matters and moral conduct must be re-examined. Notwithstanding the socio-economic and political challenges of modern times, oral transmission has a role in Africa . . . African renaissance can only be achieved through a dynamic reclaiming and incorporation of those values that have escaped documentation and may eventually be lost with time.[8]

Turning to end-of-life care, Elizabeth Grant and her colleagues worked in this way by collecting oral histories from Meru patients and their families in rural Kenya. The study aimed to construct accounts of patients who were facing death, detailing their experiences and their physical, psychological, social, spiritual and other expressed needs. Thirty two-patients—and their carers—were listened to. The authors conclude:

> Many patients felt they were dying in a way that neither they, nor their families, would have wished. They cited overwhelming pain, lack of money, a sense of burden, guilt about not providing adequately for others, and a need for the very basics of life. By outlining their needs, this study draws attention to gaps in service provision and allows the voices of patients and their carers to be heard and incorporated into the planning process.[9]

In the context of widespread stigmatization of people with HIV/AIDS, silence around diagnosis and the early death of parents are having a detrimental effect upon children who eventually become orphans. As social structures change, memories of dead parents fade and a state of confusion ensues. To combat this confusion, an innovative project based on memory boxes was initiated in Kampala (Uganda) that relies heavily on oral history to collect memories that relate to a family. Though the concept was developed by the National Community of Women Living with HIV/AIDS in Kampala, the programme has a cross-cultural and international relevance.

According to Philippe Denis and Nokhaya Makiwane,[10] the purpose of the memory boxes is to promote *resilience*.[11] This goal is achieved by using an oral history methodology. Parents are encouraged to share stories as a way of keeping family memories alive and to facilitate the process of bereavement. Reporting on the Memory Box programme located within the School of Theology at the University of Natal (South Africa), Denis and Makiwane state:

> The memories of the families are kept in a 'memory box'. Memory box is a metaphor. But the term also designates a physical object: a box which can be decorated with photos or drawings and which contains the stories of the deceased person as well as various objects pertaining to the history of the family.
>
> Creating memory boxes is a process. The fact of sharing the memories of the sick person or of the deceased, of recording those memories and of storing them in a memory box, helps the family members to break the silence about disease and death. The unknown becomes a little less unfamiliar. The memory boxes create the space to talk about sickness and death and in this way to cope with the loss of the loved person[10] (p. 67).

In this study, we wish to reflect the richness of oral history in the African context through the voices of health workers and other individuals caught up in the development of hospice–palliative care across the continent. Our research methods—especially designed for resource-poor settings—are grounded in a social science approach. In sociological research, the study of a phenomenon through the personal recollections of events, their causes and their effects forms part of the biographical tradition of qualitative enquiry.[12–14] The International Observatory on End of Life Care (IOELC) values this tradition and makes use of it alongside other research methods. In 2005, the Observatory published an oral history of the hospice movement in the UK, drawing on an extensive archive that has been developed systematically since 1995.[15] Reports of our study in Central/Eastern Europe and Central Asia have also drawn on an extensive oral history archive, mostly developed since 2001.[16]

As part of this review, we conducted 107 recorded interviews with 97 key personnel who described their work in 14 African countries. These interviews explore the development of hospice–palliative care through the lived experience of in-country activists. They seek to discover why and how individuals became involved in hospice–palliative care developments; their achievements and frustrations, the perceived opportunities and barriers within the field, and visions for the future.

It is from this oral history archive that extracts have been drawn for inclusion in the country reports and, also, in the following three chapters of this part of the book. In each case, the participant has given permission for such extracts to be reproduced and attributed. In the interests of clarity, these extracts were lightly edited to remove any repetition, but care was taken to maintain the sequence of ideas and the rhythm of the speech. Eventually, the draft manuscript was available to the interviewees before being passed for publication. Many of those interviewed reviewed their extracts and sent encouraging comments by way of endorsement, and in some cases requested minor modifications to the text.

Collectively, these interview extracts give a remarkable insight into the undocumented history of palliative care development in Africa. In the following chapter called 'Personal motivations', there are moving accounts of the huge impact made by the illness, or death, of a friend or family member. Some participants speak of their religious conviction, others about a desire for better patient care, or a heightened sense of fulfilment in their professional role. In the chapter entitled 'Confronting the issues', interviewees tell of the changes brought about by questioning the culture. Advocacy is seen as an essential pre-requisite to policy development, supported by comprehensive programmes of education, training and, increasingly, research. Other issues relate to the widespread poverty of patients and their families; the delivery of spiritual care in the African context; and to staff support through a 'caring for the carers' programme. In the chapter, 'New models, new care', attention is paid to the relationship between palliative care and existing health systems; to the development of strategies for reaching the poorest of the poor, particularly in remote rural areas; and to the development of a team approach.

The extracts presented here provide valuable perspectives on many of the issues contained in the country reports and constitute a first attempt at setting out an unfolding history of hospice–palliative care in Africa.

References

1 Mbiti JS. *African Religions and Philosophy*. London: Heineman, 1969: I.

2 Zahan D. *The Religion, Spirituality, and Thought of Traditional Africa*. London: The University of Chicago Press, 1979: 47.

3 Wamue GN. Tradition and change: oral history, belief systems AIDS, and the challenges of modernity among the Agikuyu people of central Kenya. Paper presented at the 12th conference of the International Oral History Association, University of Natal, South Africa, 24–27 June 2002.

4 CPM. See: http://web.uct.ac.za/depts/cfpm/home.htm

5 Phiri I, Worthington J. The leaders of black women's organisations in the Natal Midlands and in Umlazi from oral evidence. Paper presented at the 12th conference of the International Oral History Association, University of Natal, South Africa, 24–27 June 2002.

6 Khonde CN. The potential of oral sources for the history of disease in Congo-Kinshasa. Paper presented at the 12th conference of the International Oral History Association, University of Natal, South Africa, 24–27 June 2002.

7 De Cock KM, Mbori-Nagacha D, Marum E. Shadow in the continent: public health and HIV/AIDS in Africa in the 21st Century. *Lancet* 2002; **360**(9283): 734.

8 Wamue GN Tradition and change: oral history, belief systems AIDS, and the challenges of modernity among the Agikuyu people of central Kenya. Paper presented at the 12th conference of the International Oral History Association, University of Natal, South Africa, 24–27 June 2002.

9 Grant E, Murray A, Grant A, Brown J. A good death in rural Kenya? Listening to Meru patients and their families talk about care needs at the end of life. *Journal of Palliative Care* 2003; **19**(3): 159–167.

10 Denis P, Makiwane N. Stories of love, pain and courage: AIDS orphans and memory boxes. *Oral History* Autumn 2003: 66–74.

11 Philippe Denis and Nokjaya Makiwane follow the International Resilience Project's definition of resilience: 'a universal capacity which allows a person, a group or a community to prevent, minimise or overcome the damaging effects of adversity'. See: Grotberg E. A guide to promoting resilience in children: strengthening the human spirit. *Early Childhood Development: Practice and Reflections, No. 8*. The Hague: Bernard Van Leer Foundation, 1995: 7.

12 Bertaux D. *Biography and Society: The Life History Approach in the Social Sciences*. Beverley Hills: Sage Publications, 1981.

13 Denzin NK. *Interpretive Biography*. London: Sage Publications, 1989.

14 **Wengraf T.** *Qualitative Research Interviewing: Biographic Narrative and Semi-structured Method.* London: Sage Publications, 2000.

15 **Clark D, Small N, Wright M, Winslow M, Hughes N.** *A Bit of Heaven for the Few? An Oral History of the Hospice Movement in the United Kingdom.* Lancaster: Observatory Publications, 2005.

16 For example: **Clark D, Wright M.** *Transitions in End of Life Care: Hospice and Related Developments in Eastern Europe and Central Asia.* Buckingham: Open University Press, 2003.

Chapter 3

Personal motivations

I said to my husband, 'One day I want to pay back to this
organization. I want to make a difference. I want to go out to
the community and tell the people that there is something
which can be done for somebody until the person stops
breathing'. So it happened that I joined the hospice.
Zodwe Sithole

The history of hospice–palliative care development in Africa began in the late 1970s
when services appeared in Zimbabwe and South Africa. In Zimbabwe, Island Hospice
was founded in Harare, and in South Africa, hospice initiatives began around the
same time in Johannesburg, Port Elizabeth, Cape Town and Durban. Hospice and
palliative care developments appeared in other African countries in around 1990 and, by
2005, our study had identified 136 hospice–palliative care organizations operating in
15 countries across the continent, with capacity building evident in 11 other countries.

In many instances, this activity has occurred in difficult circumstances—political
repression, civil war, widespread poverty and an AIDS pandemic. Yet visionary pioneers
and activists have emerged across the continent to bring about better care for the dying
person and family members. The question arises: why have these 'palliateurs' committed
themselves to a marginalized—frequently stigmatized—group such as the dying? Some
of the answers are found in the following extracts that cluster around the activist's
experience of illness or death, religious conviction, raised awareness of palliative care or
simply a desire to provide better care for dying people. The dates given are those upon
which the interview took place.

Impact of illness and death

Personal experience of illness and death is often reported as a strong motivation for
hospice activity.

> When the hospice was being introduced in our hospital—we are a group of more than 15 nurses—
> we received the induction. By that time, my mother-in-law was suffering from cancer; so I was
> anxious to know, 'How can I take care of her?' That's why I remained after all of the nurses said the
> programme was not very important; for me, it's very important because I was in need.
> Dr Kristopher [Hartwig] is the one who introduced hospice here. So at that time I was very happy
> to work with Kristopher, also [for him] to visit my mother-in-law and tell me how I can take care

of her. And they took care of her, and she died peacefully, without pain. So I'm happy to know about hospice and what hospice does in the community. And that's why I am happy also working in hospice, yes. **Paulina Natema, hospice nurse and spiritual counsellor, Selian Hospital, Tanzania; 5 November 2004**.

It's a long time ago now, its 25 years. The year after [our daughter] Frances died, which of course was my motive, I did a course in communication with UNISA, and then I went over to England; and being there I went to see St Christopher's; so that was the first time I had visited St Christopher's. And then I had all these wonderful ideas about starting here. So I went to see my psychologist friend, John McMaster, who was very interested and I said to him, 'What shall we do with all this? And he said, 'Why don't *we* have a symposium?' because I had just come back from a symposium in Johannesburg, which was about the Compassionate Friends, I think; and that's how we went ahead. He got permission from the head of his department, with use of all the facilities, and he and I got on with drawing up a sheet of queries for whoever came, and we sat there biting our nails. We had one of the big lecture halls at the University, which would have been awful if we had only 12 people turn up, but in fact the hall was packed. It's a wonderful thing to work for, hospice. And for me it was very important at the time, after Frances, because it was a very great loss; and for her to die that way from cancer, without any of the concepts of hospice—there was nothing at all—it was dreadful. **Maureen Butterfield—founder, Island Hospice and Bereavement Service, Harare, Zimbabwe; 7 June 2003**.

I was working at the psychiatry department at the main Grotte Schuur hospital in Observatory [Cape Town] and I left to have a baby, my second child. The day before my baby was born, my Mom died suddenly, and I experienced grief like—I'm not sure I can explain what the grief felt like; but I knew when I'd gotten through that I wanted to do something more for people that experience grief. And I—being a very spiritual person—I prayed about it and I asked God to show me what's in line for me. And lo and behold, the next morning one of our newspapers had an advert for ten sisters needed in the St Luke's Hospice community [service]. I applied; and I got a part-time post in the ward at St Luke's Hospice. It was great working with people as they came in. I could see the difference St Luke's made in their lives. I could see the difference St Luke's made in the lives of the families as well, and I think the satisfaction was of knowing that you were part of the team that was doing the good work. I then got tired after two and a half years with just being in the ward; and I was about to leave the St Luke's family when a post became available in the community. I had no driver's licence, I had no experience of community, but within two months, I managed to get my driver's licence and I was taken on orientation, and I've been on the community now for 12 years. **Jeanette Daniels—community palliative care nurse, St Luke's Hospice, Cape Town, South Africa; 6 August 2004**.

I live alone with my Mom, so I have all the time to give to these patients. I had a very painful experience. My husband died very tragically; it was a sudden death. He wasn't ill or anything and five years ago he just went to do a job and he—in his car—he died of a massive heart attack. He was quite young, 48 at that time. And then my Dad: I clung to my Dad and he got cancer; he ended up with leukaemia at the age of 74. But he was still fit, he was still working and he just died suddenly; and that's what made me decide to come to do this work for terminally ill patients. It's a calling I think, so that's when I moved into hospice. **Jennifer Padayachee—nursing sister and manager of Phoenix day centre, Highway Hospice, Durban, South Africa; 9 August 2004**.

My sister died of cancer of the breast. At that time I was staying in Johannesburg and she was in Durban. So this Friday, I 'phoned her. I could hear that she wasn't OK, she couldn't even speak to me. Then I took the earliest flight to Durban. That was on Friday. When I arrived at home it was very late in the evening. She wasn't on medical aid, so she was attending one of the public hospitals, the Oncology Department. So the only hope we had as a family was the oncology clinic; so we waited for Monday to go to the clinic. The first thing [in the morning] we went to the oncology clinic. I remember my sister was sitting on the wheelchair. I was pushing her, and her son was with me and my cousin. We went to the doctor's room. The doctor checked her side, look at her, and he said to her, 'Elizabeth, I'm sorry, there is nothing I can do for you; the cancer's just spread throughout your body'.

You know, for us, as a family, we didn't know what to do, where to go; we didn't know. By profession I'm a nursing sister, but I didn't know much about hospice. So we wheeled Elizabeth out of that doctor's room, trying to be strong for her now, you know. We wanted to cry. The doctor said, 'There's nothing I can do for you'. So what were we supposed to say to her, or do to her? We went home. So her son said, 'Auntie, listen, I think there's a place called hospice who helps the patient who's got cancer'. So we said, 'Let's not even telephone, let's try to see them'. So we left her at home.

We went to Highway Hospice. We found the sister and we explained to her, and she said, 'OK, this is what we'll do'. That was now on Monday. She said she is going to try and get the sister who was working in that area; she would come and visit my sister at home. The following day, early in the morning, round about nine o'clock, that sister was there to assess my sister, yes. I mean, for us just to see her coming in, it was such a relief. *Oh God; here is someone who is going to help us!* So she said, 'She does need admission' and she was going to contact the hospice doctor to check whether there was a bed available for her. So Wednesday, she 'phoned us early in the morning to say that we can bring her in; so we took her to hospice. I must say, as a family we were really struggling through a threat that she was going. I mean, she was really terminal at that time, and you know, there was no counselling, nothing.

So we arrived at hospice. They admitted her; but at that time she was semi-unconscious. So they put her in a room and immediately organized counselling for us, because to me she was my mum, my sister, my friend. Then the very same day hospice said to us, to me and my sister's son, 'If you want you can spend the night with her'. So we spent the night with her in her room and she died the following morning. Then, I said to my husband, 'One day I want to pay back this organization. I want to make a difference. I want to go out to the community and tell the people that there is something which can be done for somebody until the person stops breathing'. So it happened that I joined the hospice, yes. **Zodwe Sithole—palliative care nurse, Highway Hospice, Durban, South Africa; 12 August 2004.**

Religious conviction

We also found considerable evidence of the place of the spiritual domain in the personal motivations of palliateurs. In the following extracts, some identify a sense of calling; others speak of divine intervention, the humanitarian implications of faith or the outcome of prayer.

I was thinking of how I became involved and it's quite strange. I had just finished a degree in Psychology and English and two of my children had started school and the third one had just started nursery school, and a friend of mine 'phoned me and she said, 'They are going to be starting a hospice, do you want to go along to the first meeting?' And I said, 'No I certainly don't. I don't know anything about hospice and I've never worked with dying patients and this isn't for me at all'. And I asked my husband's advice—he's a medical doctor—and he said, 'Why don't you go along, you can't lose anything', and so along I went. And another thing: looking back, I don't really know why I went. I am a committed Christian. I really believe that it was God putting me there and that's really all I can say. I didn't go with any great and wonderful skills that I could offer them. My background is in education. When I went they said to me 'Are you a nurse?' and I said, 'No I am not'. But I said I was just willing to help in any way. I could perhaps just answer the 'phone and do anything. And so I started. We were all new and I don't think any of us knew too much about what a hospice was—but we learnt; and we did all sorts of things. We did the cooking and we did the answering the 'phone and I actually eventually went out with the nurses to help with patients; and

I enjoyed it very much; and I found that I could relate to them; and when we later started getting AIDS patients, I found that I enjoyed working with them and perhaps I had something to offer. **Sue Cameron—HPCA board member and manager of the Centre for Palliative Learning, Pretoria Sungardens Hospice, South Africa; 26 April 2005.**

I had nothing to go back to [in Britain] and I went to do some STI clinics because I knew that was needed out here; and I went to the local hospice because I'd always been interested in palliative care, and I thought this is a field that is really, really needed in the Third World. And so the hospice took me on and said, 'OK, you can run the day hospice three days a week', and I just loved it: I've never felt so happy. I'd loved general practice, but this was a completely different part of medicine, and I just then realized that this was what I wanted to do. We came out again for a very short locum at the end of 1998 and I was landed with running the whole Obstetric Department here at that stage: I wanted to do palliative care—within my bones there was palliative care—but there was nobody doing obstetrics, so I ended up doing 44 caesarean sections, two ruptured uteruses, and being absolutely frightened to death by not knowing as much as I ought to have known about what I was doing. And I came back and I thought, 'I'm never going back there to do obstetrics again but I do want to go back and do palliative care'. And I applied to Cardiff at that stage to do the Diploma in Palliative Medicine; the hospice at home took me on on a full-time job; my mother had recently died and so I had a very elderly father to look after. In '99 we came out again for a short-term. Again I was doing a lot of obstetrics, some palliative care, and—that's right, we came back for the millennium and my father died very soon after that; and I just felt that this was the Lord saying, 'OK. You're OK. You can go to Africa'. I completed the Diploma and we came out here in September 2001, which was when the palliative care here started.

I'm not a preachy-preachy missionary. I'm a missionary who believes that God is working through me in this place. I do believe in the power of prayer and I believe the power of prayer has perhaps got us here in the first place and has then given me a wonderful team of workers; and they are a very committed team. We have Muslims on our team in the hospice as well as Christians of all denominations. I don't believe that people must be preached at at the end of life to go to heaven: I strongly disbelieve this. I think that our faith should be shown through our works and if people ask questions we answer them, and we pray with them if that is what they want. **Dr Karilyn Collins—medical director, Muheza Hospice Care, Teule Hospital, Muheza, Tanzania; 7 November 2004.**

I started at the hospice in 1986, having in my fifties had cancer, was very ill, recovered, and an opportunity came along. I needed to regain my self-confidence because I had lost my job as a result of having cancer and being so ill, and our church had said that hospice was looking for a volunteer to do their books; and I prayed about it for a week, went and spoke to the administrator and said I'd prayed about it and I'd heard that he needed someone, and he looked at me and said, 'But I've found somebody'. And I thought, 'Gosh, as a new Christian it seemed quite strange that here I was so sure that I belonged at hospice and he didn't want me'; so I shrugged my shoulders and thought, 'Well I've got it wrong'—turned away, and he ran after me and said, 'but give me your name anyway', which I did, and 'phone number. And the very next morning—I remember, five to eight—he 'phoned me and he said, funnily enough, the man—that chartered accountant that he had got—found that the job was too big and he would need to have someone else with him, and could I come now for an interview, which I did. I was interviewed by a panel of five men and that's where it started.

I started as a volunteer, was invited onto the board virtually straight away, and worked more and more and more—eventually was working three mornings a week, taking work home, working on the board, and after two years was asked on the staff as a half-day worker. I resigned from the board because I felt it was inappropriate to be a board member and a staff member, and in 1992 became a full-time member in charge of finance and admin—and well, five years ago became the executive director.

To be blunt: nobody joins hospice to get rich! So you certainly have to have a calling. There are a couple of people that are perhaps a little off-beam as far as why they're at hospice, but certainly there are a lot of people who believe that it is their calling; it is where God wants them to be; it is their mission field, and we take it from there. So yes, there are a lot of people who are extremely dedicated, and if, like myself, it became a job, it became a job incidentally. One's circumstances can change, but the original idea was because of it was your calling. **Barbara Campbell-Ker— executive director, Hospice Association of the Witwatersrand, South Africa; 11 August 2004**.

I really loved doing family medicine and became invited to begin hospice work when a director of our county-wide programme retired; so I did the necessary initial education. I eventually worked for seven years as medical director for a hospice, and that connection was one of those doors that open that you only look back and you go, 'Oh, my goodness! If I'd only known, I might not have gone in that door', because of all the changes that would come about in our feelings, our understanding of life and the faith, and who we are; you can't turn away.

So my friend, Mark Jacobson, who works in Tanzania at Selian Hospital, when he heard I was doing hospice work, invited me—and I was able to come for a period of two months and help to begin a very small, humble programme at that hospital, and that has grown in five years. I had continued my work in family medicine, and our family came at that time: Rebecca and I have five children. At that time we came with three of our children, and when I left in '99 Mark was asking me, 'Won't you come back and do this?' and I couldn't imagine it. I just said no.

But when I was here for that seminar teaching, it was my first time to see the Selian Hospice, to meet with staff who were doing it, and to listen to them. I know I heard a lot from patients, which authenticated what I heard from the staff, but to hear how these people were brought in and the amount of compassion that would draw someone in who was living in the village life; these are not people going home to a nice garden and porch like I'm doing now—they're going back to the people who they've just finished seeing, and they know that people had been dying all around them, literally, without any knowledge. They would die and nobody would know, and that was all that the people knew how to do in that time in the 80s and 90s, and I think even now, in most of the country. I've tried to write about this: but the evangelist was telling me over and over, 'May God forgive us for all those people who died before'. So I didn't get over that, and I don't.

It was two years before we actually came, but it took two years to do the logistics. How can we live here? Who can support us? Is there a church who will do it? Is there someone else? Actually, everybody thought it was a great idea but, well, families aren't cheap; but we found out eventually we had support from the Lutheran Church in the USA and some support from another church. So we feel very fortunate to have a chance to be a part of such a—I don't know how to talk about it, but it's such a privilege. **Dr Kristopher Hartwig—physician, Selian Hospital, Arusha, Tanzania; 4 November 2004**.

I was married with a number of children, six children, and I was working as a clinical tutor running the midwifery ward and doing all the clinical teaching, and it was, you know, very unsociable hours, and the children were growing up, and we had bought a holiday house on the South Coast of KwaZulu Natal; and we sent my husband down to see if he thought he could make a living there, because we felt we were at a crossroads and that, you know, either the rat race was going to consume us or we were going to have to make a move. So the plan was: we'd go down to the South Coast and I would be like a full-time wife and mother, make a beautiful garden and play a bit of golf and bridge. But that's not the way things turned out because—I mentioned the spiritual maturity that was kind of setting in, I joined a prayer group and, quite out of character, found myself one day asking my friends in the group to pray for me to be open to, and to know, whether God had anything specific he'd like me to do, because I actually had some time on my hands, which I wasn't used to having. And the very next week, the local newspaper, the *South Coast Herald*, had an article about a woman trying to start a hospice movement, and so, you know, it felt like real divine intervention—and it still does 22 years later. **Kath Defilippi—chairperson of APCA; HPCA board member and chief executive officer, South Coast Hospice, Port Shepstone, South Africa; 5 June 2004.**

I was actually living in Mozambique for quite a while and then we moved to Lesotho and in that time my children were quite small, but they had to go back to school, so we had to move back to Pretoria; and then one morning I was sitting there and thought to myself, 'I can't stay at home for the rest of my life, I'd better get myself going and if the children are going back to school, that's a good place to start'. So I picked up the 'phone and for some reason I just felt that I need to 'phone the hospice: I saw this place with the board outside the building that said Hospice Centurion, and I thought to myself, 'I wonder if something's happening there'. So I actually 'phoned the sister and Sister Jackie said to me, 'You would not believe it, but you know I just prayed this week that the Lord will send someone to come and help me to do the home based care'. And she was crying and I was crying because I just had this confirmation in my spirit that that's exactly where the Lord wanted us to be. So, it was just being obedient to what he actually said that I felt in my spirit that I need to get involved in the hospice. **Elna van der Merwe—nursing services manager, Centurion Hospice, Pretoria, South Africa; 13 August 2004.**

Raised awareness

Among the range of ways in which people were drawn towards hospice and palliative care in Africa was a sensitization to the nature of such care. The next set of interview extracts show that for some, this awareness came through contact with a hospice organization: a chance occurrence in some cases. Others heard of hospice care at seminars or conferences, by word of mouth or through the publications which explored issues around care at the end of life.

Hospice experience

I'm a trained nurse and I'd been hearing about hospices for several years. The opportunity came in 1991, when I went to the Sixth International Conference at St Christopher's Hospice and that gave me a wide knowledge of what it is all about. From that moment, I felt like flying home to start everything, and that was where Anne Merriman and I got to know each other. She decided to visit me in 1993 and I was so happy to receive her in Nigeria. Unfortunately what would have been in Nigeria is what is in Uganda now. We went to the Ministry, we went to all the people that need to know about this health care system to help the needy—they all gave me promises—and after she left, she left on April 1st '93, I went back to St Christopher's again for some other courses in various areas, multidisciplinary courses, and I told them there: 'I am ready to start single-handedly whether I get anybody's support or not'. **Olusola Fatunmbi—nurse, founder of Hospice Nigeria; 4 June 2004.**

Well I'm a medical practitioner by profession but got involved in palliative care issues in the year 2000 when I went for the doctor rotation at the Nairobi Hospice. It is there that I got to interact with lots of patients, and palliative care made a lot of sense to me, because it is first of all something that I didn't have the opportunity to learn in medical school; it wasn't in the curriculum. But over and above that I got to interact with patients who came from my village. Quite a number of them needed that; and they came from far away, almost 300 kilometres, sometimes for two-weekly reviews or monthly reviews, or to get two weeks' supply of morphine, which at the end of the day didn't make sense to me. So what I did was: after my doctor rotation programme, I decided that palliative care is what I want to do. So I went back to my village and decided to carry out a small study to find out whether palliative care was necessary; whether cancer was a big problem. I knew AIDS was but I wasn't too sure about cancer. But what came out from the small survey I did was that cancer care was very essential. So after that I decided, 'well, this place certainly needs a hospice'. **Dr Bactrin Killingo—founder, chief executive, and physician, Meru Hospice, Kenya; 2 June 2004.**

My background is very interesting because I came from an accident and emergency department where the work was purely resuscitation and passing on the patients to other people to look after. And I had an urge to follow up and know what was happening to these patients we were passing on; so I needed to do some community work. But during that time if you trained as a community nurse you were posted away from your family to other parts of Zimbabwe, which I did not want to do; and this opportunity arose for me to go and relieve a nurse who was going for maternity leave from a hospice. And before I knew it, I only worked there for two months, they told me they wanted me to continue working. So I wrote back and gave my resignation and joined hospice in 1986. At that time, there were very few patients who had cancer, and especially among the black people; the majority were white patients who suffered from cancer diseases; and I found that hospice was more than just a job because of our interactions with the patients, knowing them more, and their families and so on. So I really got to like it and I thought, 'Well, I think I would like to pursue palliative care for life'. And that's what I'm doing. **Eunice Garanganga—clinical and technical adviser, Hospice Association of Zimbabwe (HOSPAZ); 20 September 2004.**

Personal influences

I was at University in 1979, doing nursing education at university in Johannesburg, when Dame Cicely did a tour of South Africa. The professor in the department asked us, a small group of us (there were seven of us actually) whether any of us had heard of her or *hospice*, and none of us had. And she said, 'Well it was a revolutionary way of caring for the dying', and she thought that, as future nurse teachers, we ought to go to a two-day symposium on death and dying, and that the department were going, but that if we all decided we didn't want to go we could spend the time in the sociology department. So we actually got into a huddle over tea and sort of tried to figure out which was the lesser of these two evils. And my friends still tease me because I was the one who said, 'Two days of death and dying, how morbid can you get? Let's get the sociology over and done with'. However, it wasn't meant to be that way, and four voted to go to the symposium and three to stay. So we went. And then, you know, Dame Cicely had such an impact on me; and I realized how I'd been lying to patients when they had made attempts to talk about not getting better and I had cheerfully brushed it off and said, 'Oh, rubbish, you're looking great today; we'll have you out of here in no time', and how unaware I had been of the incredible suffering that the family were going through; so busy rushing around doing my tasks perfectly and feeling I was a wonderful nurse. And I just thought, 'I really have to make amends'. **Kath Defilippi—HPCA board member and manager, South Coast Hospice, Port Shepstone, South Africa; 5 June 2004.**

I became involved in hospice through a senior medical student at the time that I was deputy dean at the Medical Faculty at the University of Cape Town: her name was Chris Dare; she was a friend of Cicely Saunders, now Dame Cicely Saunders, who was the founder—or regarded as the founder—of the modern hospice movement, at least in the UK. And Chris Dare, who'd been a physiotherapist, had decided to do medicine in order to commence hospice activities in South Africa. When she approached me I had no idea what hospice was about, and she said it was about care of the dying and I said, 'Well, so care of the dying, what does that mean, and why is it different? Everyone does that anyhow'. And I assisted her to bring Cicely Saunders out. We had a week's wonderful programme at which she presented the key elements, which are still important in hospice. And from that meeting, which was in the early '80s, the hospice movement in South Africa developed and Chris Dare has, by many including myself, been regarded as the founder of the hospice movement in South Africa. So that was the start. **Professor J. P. van Niekerk—chair of HPCA and manager of PEPFAR project, South Africa; 13 August 2004.**

I first joined the hospice in 1996 as a locum doctor. Previously I had been working here on and off as a volunteer doctor out of my own interest, and I had a friend who was also working here so she actually introduced the hospice to me. I worked for about one and a half years as a locum doctor and then moved on to complete my Masters at the University of Nairobi . . . the hospice asked me to come and work for them again, so since I had a lot of interest in palliative care I said I'd come back and work for the hospice, and I've been at the hospice since then as the senior medical officer.

Being a doctor at the hospice is not easy. Many times I've felt isolated from my colleagues, class mates and doctor friends—who constantly ask me what I'm doing in a place like the hospice. Most feel it is a place for nurses and that I'm wasting my knowledge in a doomed place. There are very few doctors who are in palliative care full time; in fact, I think there's just we two. When I decided to do a diploma course in palliative care, there was disbelief and many asked me why I just would-n't stick to my Public Health, which would ensure I got a better job, better pay and status. I tried to explain to them the passion I felt for those in need of this special kind of care, and that the dying still needed a doctor's care. My social life may not amount to much, but the smiles on my patients' faces, the grateful looks from their families, the simple card saying 'thank you' makes my day. I feel privileged to work in a hospice. I have learned a lot and I'm still learning, especially learning to give and love—and learning to live. **Dr Zipporah Ali—senior medical officer: Nairobi Hospice, Kenya; 1 November 2004.**

I was at home. I'm a professional nurse and I had two young children and I heard about Greta Schoeman at the church we both attend. I had some time previous to this nursed my 23-year-old sister-in-law with a brain tumour and I just said to Greta, 'Look, I'm missing people and nursing. I'd love to volunteer and help you a couple of hours a week'. So I started with Greta when she started the Highway Hospice. I was with Lesley [van Zyl], and Lesley was pregnant when she came forward as a volunteer; and Greta opened her little guest cottage in her home for those patients that otherwise would have gone—had to have gone—into hospital. And Lesley used to come and sit with the patients so that those of us who were mobile could go out and do the home care. And then Lesley became, after the baby was born, our first home care sister. **Karen Hinton—chairperson, Hospice Association of KwaZulu Natal and quality assurance adviser, Highway Hospice, Durban, South Africa; 8 August 2004.**

The group that started the hospice was inspired by Dr Elizabeth Kübler-Ross and because of her the centre is called Shanti Nilaya, which means 'final home of peace'. Then in '94 we heard that Dr Ross was coming to South Africa to present one of her workshops. I wrote to her and I said 'there's no way she's coming to South Africa without blessing Shanti Nilaya'—and I gave her some background history. And we were very blessed. She came to our hospice and sort of blessed it and opened it for us; and I then attended one of her Life, Death and Transition workshops that she presented. That really got us started, you know, and we've been going ever since. **Marisa Wolheim—executive director, Shanti Nilaya, Hospice in the West, South Africa; 13 August 2004.**

Better patient care

This group of extracts focuses on the desire to provide better care for patients, and what this means in the African context.

My background is as a nurse and midwife. I worked in the UK as a health visitor. I moved to Zimbabwe in 1994 and during that time the Ministry of Health had placed an advert for someone with a background in nursing who was willing to work on the cancer programme and perhaps do some basic training in palliative care. There were training modules prepared, and I thought, 'This sounds interesting'. With my community background I thought it would give me an opportunity to meet more people and I agreed to apply. Training of health professionals went on for over one year covering the whole country until April 1996.

I started in the Ministry of Health in October 1994, with the contract seconded by WHO. This was the time when the Cancer Prevention Committee had set up the Cancer Control Programme and decided to work on a 10-year plan; and in it was palliative care. So they agreed they would employ a programme officer who'd be a nurse, to help in introducing it. Really this was a palliative care awareness programme, working closely with Island Hospice, and this was a challenge—but we trained in April in Zimbabwe and the health professionals, both nurses and doctors, had a week's awareness workshop on palliative care. When that was over, it was by now the end of the year, and the Ministry of Health was supposed to take over the funding of my post. The money was unfortunately not found, although they expressed an interest in keeping me. Island Hospice was at the time setting up a training department and I was approached and agreed to apply for a post with hospice. And really I have not looked back since. I've continued to grow and realize how much I didn't know about caring for the terminally ill and the bereaved. However it's challenging but enjoyable work. **Sambulo Mkwananzi—training manager, Island Hospice and Bereavement Service, Harare, Zimbabwe and board member APCA; 20 September 2004.**

Originally I trained as a registered nurse and then a registered midwife, a community health nurse. I had further training in nurse education and administration and did a continuing education programme in the care of the terminally ill—and that really interested me. And then an opportunity lent itself. As part and parcel of being a professional nurse, we are expected to update our skills and when there was an advertisement for a training programme for care of the dying, I was very, very interested. At that time, HIV/AIDS was coming on the scene and cancer, as I knew, was a problem; so it appealed to me. After I had finished the course, there was an advertisement in the press: they wanted to start a hospice and they were looking for either a doctor or a senior nurse, and they said training in the care of the dying would be an added advantage. I was working in Nairobi, in the Nursing Council, which is a statutory body in Kenya that governs the education, training and practice of nursing in the country. So when I looked at that advert, it was just me. So I applied and I got that job with the Nairobi Hospice. It was during its formative years and they [wanted] a professional who would help to set up the service. **Brigid Sirengo—chief executive officer, Nairobi Hospice, Kenya; 2 June 2004.**

I must say that our work with palliative care here in Arusha has been some of the most exciting work that I've been involved with in my career. I've been in Tanzania as a doctor for almost 20 years now, and about five years ago we had our first opportunity where we had a patient who actually asked us to come and care for him at home. He was dying from a lymphoma and he didn't want to be in hospital and he asked if, as his caregivers, we could provide him with some care at home, and some pain relief for his disease, and he wanted to go through this process of dying. And this really triggered for us a kind of eureka moment.

Of course, this is an important part of what we're trying to do in Tanzania in terms of the continuum of care that we want to give our patients. And there was in that an assumption that because there were centuries of tradition of dying at home, that there was also a tradition of knowing how to care for people at home, and sadly, that turned out to be an incorrect assumption. People were wanting to die at home, but most of the people were going home to die in a place where no-one knew how to care for them, where there was no-one to relieve their symptoms. There were great difficulties for families being able to talk to somebody who was dying, about their dying—about what that would mean for the family. There was lot of secrecy around it.

So we were struck by that realization when we started to be asked to care for people at home. From that realization we began to explore. We were aware of hospice and palliative care in the global sense, but we hadn't really been involved with it here, in Arusha, and really not in Tanzania, that we were aware of. I think as we discuss further how Tanzania has developed, there's three or four programmes that have made a serious effort to move into palliative care; and we kind of debate amongst ourselves which of us actually stumbled on it first. But we began to explore actively at that point and invited in some people with more expertise to talk with us about it and explore how we might move in that direction. **Dr Mark Jacobson—medical director, Selian Hospital, Arusha, Tanzania; 4 June 2004.**

I'm a qualified nurse. I worked at the Baragwaneth Hospital for 23 years, but just before I left there, I left in 1995, the standards of nursing were really deteriorating. Things were no longer as they used to be. I felt that this is not the nursing I had been taught, this is not what I can give to the people. I resigned at the Bara in 1995 and then I went into a first aid organization. For three years I was a first aid instructor, but I found the job to be monotonous, repeating the same thing, and then I felt that I needed some nursing. And then there was a post for a hospice coordinator and I applied for that post. And here I am, where now I can see that the nursing care that I was taught, I'm able to provide. **Sibongile Mafata—co-ordinator, Soweto Hospice, South Africa; 10 August 2004.**

I'm the medical doctor here at the Soweto Hospice. I've been here for seven months. Before this I was doing GP work at my private practice and I was reaching people with HIV/AIDS. As you are aware, we've got this AIDS pandemic and it's a challenge to everyone. So I thought that maybe it would be better for me to come to hospice where I could render services to more people. Since I have been here I've realized that AIDS is not just a physical illness, it goes beyond that. It's important that people are taken care of in total, that is: emotionally, socially, psychologically, and spiritually. So for me I do get a lot of fulfilment as a medical doctor and also caring for people in these other spheres that I've talked about. **Dr Thobi Segabi—palliative care physician, Soweto Hospice, South Africa; 10 August 2004.**

My background is basically public health. I studied public health and served the government of Sierra Leone, Ministry of Health and Sanitation, for some time; and I served as Public Health Superintendent in charge of [one of the] districts until 1995, where I noticed that there was a need to provide some care for people with terminal conditions, whose needs were not catered for by the health care service at that time. And that interest drove me into dialogue with health care service providers like the National Health Service Ministry and other community health services to see how we can look for a service that caters for terminal cases—at that time more HIV and few cancer cases. **Dr Gabriel Madiye—founder and executive director, The Shepherd's Hospice, Freetown, Sierra Leone; 4 June 2004.**

Sense of fulfilment

Finally in this chapter, we present some extracts that highlight a sense of fulfilment found in hospice care, despite the many challenges.

I'm a child care manager. I started work at Cotlands [Johannesburg] in June 2001. Before that I was working in a government hospital, and I left there because I wasn't getting any job satisfaction, due to the government policy of having free treatment for all patients. A lot of patients were coming to hospital; I'm primary health care trained and we were not allowed to use the facilities to the full. So none of us were getting job satisfaction and I had to leave the government service. From there I began working for general practitioners where I liked nursing the patients who were HIV positive. I decided to look for a full-time job and needed a place that was a sort of healing place; and I wanted to work with children. So fortunately for me, I saw the advert in one of the newspapers; it said *Cotlands*, and I thought, 'Cotlands? Cotlands was a place where there are babies', but I wasn't sure which type of babies. So I made an application and I came to Cotlands.

To my surprise, when I saw these children, I just fell in love with them. I knew that this was the place I wanted to work in. Initially, I started working as a hospice sister; and I noticed that these children were so sick when they came in. A child really needs just love, and I had a passion for that. I also trained for palliative care, which has increased my influence on the way things are done. So when hospitals say, 'There's nothing we can do', we come in and say, 'There's a lot that can be done for this child'. **Stella Dubazana—child care manager, Cotlands Hospice, Johannesburg, South Africa; 11 August 2004.**

Five years ago, when I joined hospice, I had no idea what hospice was all about. I, as a single parent, came to hospice because I would have weekends off with my children; but surprisingly, when I got to hospice, that is all what I wanted to do, the work was so fulfilling. As a professional nurse who has been working in theatre for a long time, not knowing that you can look at a patient as a whole, holistic patient, it was quite a challenge for me. But it was fulfilling for me as well. So, that's why I'm still at hospice, yes. I have a Diploma in Palliative Care, and that made me more confident facing the problems that I had to, because most problems we encounter are social problems rather than the disease itself. So it was quite a challenge, you know. **Angie Sehoke— palliative care nurse, Hospice North West, Klerksdorp, South Africa; 12 August 2004.**

Palliative care for me has been a discovery by accident actually. I've done some palliative care as a medical student, Robert Twycross was one of my teachers, but then in my time in Newcastle I'd finished doing my membership exams and I was registered to go home to Uganda. But I decided to do some locums before going home, to earn a bit of money to get back; and a friend of mine who I'd gone to college with had been working in a hospice in Sunderland and she had an accident. So she was looking around for somebody who could do her locum while she was off, and she asked me if I wanted to do the job. I said 'fine'. So I went along. It was a month's locum during which I really fell in love with palliative care, because it's very much a holistic approach. You not only deal with the whole of the patient and their family, but I've found that palliative medicine uses the whole of me. It's taken up my music, taken up my faith and my spirituality, and all the other things. My family's involved and my medicine is involved and I really find it satisfies many different parts of who I am and is very absorbing. **Dr Lydia Mpanga Sebuyira—director, clinical services, Hospice Africa Uganda; 21 September 2004.**

Chapter 4

Confronting the issues

Long time ago in our ancestral ages, people dying of incurable illnesses used to be thrown into the forest to be fed to hyenas . . . Now we have modern day hyenas and forests, which are the public hospitals.
Bactrin Killingo

This chapter focuses on challenges faced by hospice and palliative care activists in Africa. These include a questioning of the culture inherent in health care institutions, community groups and the wider society; they also highlight issues that relate to governments, education, policy, patients and palliative care services.

Questioning the culture

Eduardo Bruera suggests that the success or failure of a palliative care programme is directly related to its ability to change the culture of the host environment.[1] In the African context, this necessitates an overt challenge to the culture of societies as well as some constituent organizations. The following extracts illuminate the magnitude of the task, while demonstrating how palliateurs have questioned the legitimacy of patient abandonment and stigmatization, of myths around HIV and AIDS, the withholding of information by physicians, and the reticence of medical practitioners to prescribe morphine.

> This place, Africa, has a way of doing things; it has a culture. It is uncommon to talk about death and dying. Traditionally, people who are dying of a terminal illness are abandoned, they are cast away. Long time ago in our ancestral ages, people dying of incurable diseases used to be thrown into the forest to be fed to hyenas. Anybody who had a terminal illness that a traditional healer couldn't handle was thrown away into the forest. Now we have modern day hyenas in forests which are the public hospitals. Where someone has a terminal illness the family says, 'OK, fine, let's take you to the hospital' and then they—they abandon you. You die there and thereafter taken to a congested mortuary and after that you are basically buried in a public cemetery. So, because of the cultural background—there are a lot of connotations, just like any African setting where, if you have a terminal illness and the traditional healer can't handle it, then most likely you have a curse and the village doesn't want to have anything to do with you; but in modern-day times, stigma surrounding terminal illnesses still persists. Families don't know how to take care of their dying patients at all. They get, you know, emotional turmoil, frustration, suffering—and the only way out is through an escapist kind of strategy, of just dumping you somewhere. They know you won't walk back home, so they just dump you and run away.

Against this background we have an entry point where we say 'something can be done'. We tell families: 'something can be done'. We tell the health care professionals in the public institutions and private institutions who know nothing about palliative care: something can be done. And over time, through our interaction with the various people we have taken care of, slowly but surely the community have started understanding that, yes, something can be done, even for a dying person. A lot of care can be provided, and that is how we have been able to succeed in interacting with the government through the district hospital, who are our hosts, and for whom we take care of their patients, and from where we have had an entry into the community as we follow up these people who haven't had care before; to tell people it is OK to care for a dying person. And this is how we do it, but we tell them that we can't provide this care alone, we need your participation and your involvement on the same. **Dr Bactrin Killingo—Founder, Chief Executive and physician, Meru Hospice, Kenya; 2 June 2004.**

The social circumstances that the vast majority of our patients live in are really very, very difficult and traumatic; some, many, households have no piped water or electricity, and have to walk four kilometres to the nearest river to fetch water. And we often get to places where starvation is an enormous problem: there's been nothing in the home but water for two days. I think you've heard me say that in the African context holistic care has got to be looking at emergency food relief, empowerment in terms of trying to break the whole poverty cycle. Nutrition is so important, so that the little bit of money there is doesn't get wasted on junk food, but something relatively substantial. And, we found that it was no good controlling people's pain and leaving them with hunger pains, or teaching families how to do nursing care and then not having the strength to even turn an emaciated patient because they had no energy, because they really were starving., I often wonder how many of the so-called AIDS deaths are actually starvation deaths. So poverty is very traumatic. There's also a lot of violence associated with it, a lot of desperation and substance abuse, and things that people do to try and escape the horrific reality. In a rural area, many of the cultural norms are extremely beneficial and wonderful; there are some tremendous rituals in respect to dealing with grief, that are so constructive and good; but there are also horrific myths—such as having sex with a virgin can revert HIV status—and so we have a terrible problem of even babies and little girls being raped; it's just heart-breaking. **Kath Defilippi—chairperson of APCA; HPCA board member and chief executive officer, South Coast Hospice, Port Shepstone, South Africa; 5 June 2004.**

At that time, the culture of medicine was that when you were diagnosed with a terminal disease, then nothing could be provided for you and you had to be asked to go home and die—because the stigma about HIV was so intense, even amongst health caregivers and medical officers. So as somebody who was in charge of public health, I believed in the rights of patients to care, no matter what their background. You should not be discriminated against in the health care delivery system because of your status, being terminal or otherwise. I thought there was a need for some research, to come up with a system whereby people with terminal conditions could be cared for. Initially I never knew there was any option like that. I never knew there was a way forward called palliative care, except that I recognized the need and I said that we must go in search of something. **Dr Gabriel Madiye—founder and executive director, The Shepherd's Hospice, Freetown, Sierra Leone; 4 June 2004.**

Perhaps I could start before I was involved with hospice. I was privileged to be a medical student at the University of Cape Town and we had a world-famous surgeon who taught us that, when somebody was diagnosed with cancer, it was inappropriate to tell them that, because they behaved inappropriately. They blamed the surgeon, they denied the presence of the disease, they became angry—and all of those things which today we understand are natural, normal human responses to such a situation. So that was part of our training. **Professor J. P. van Niekerk—chair of HPCA and manager of PEPFAR project, South Africa; 13 August 2004.**

To get the doctors to actually accept hospice was quite difficult. I came back with a lot of literature from Robert [Twycross], from Sobell House [Oxford], and I got it all photostatted and handed it out to the GPs and the oncologists. I very well remember a case that we were doing. Karen [Hinton] and I used to do most of the home care work in the early days, and I remember going out and arguing with the oncologist about the use of oral morphine. In those days, they were using that dreadful drug, Brompton's cocktail, and of course, to get their pain controlled with that, you needed to give massive doses. So I was going out and finding that these patients were hallucinating. They were having a terrible time and still not pain-controlled. So I finally talked this oncologist into just giving us plain morphine. And the next day, I went to visit this patient. There were two new bottles from the pharmacy: one plain morphine and one of Brompton's cocktail. So I rang him up and said, 'What are you doing?' He said, 'Well, OK, you can do what you like with your morphine but I still want him to have the Brompton's cocktail.' And, you know, it took years for these doctors to really accept morphine. Now, you'd think they'd never been without it. In those days they didn't want to know, a lot of them; not all of them, there were a few around. **Greta Schoeman—founder, Highway Hospice, Durban, South Africa; 9 August 2004.**

The vast majority of our patients [at Chatsworth Hospice] are cancer patients, not more than five per cent are HIV/AIDS sufferers. So our involvement with HIV/AIDS is mainly preventive, and the promotion of behavioural change. We have regular workshops for the community. Community organizations, women's groups, and even schools are targeted. Schools are invited over a period of a week per year to spend a day with us and the whole programme is gone through with them, so much so that lots of our fundraising is, has been, initiated by schoolchildren, so it is extremely useful. They grow up knowing that it's their responsibility as well. Taking care of the elderly and the sick is part of their social structure; so hospice is playing a very useful role in the community, not just providing patient care, but also stimulating this culture of service and social responsibility. **Dr C. N. Pillay—president, Chatsworth Hospice, Durban, South Africa; 12 August 2004.**

I think everybody in palliative care has experienced the association of hospice and palliative care with death. So there's been that attitudinal barrier to making people understand that hospice is about quality of life, about living. Hospice started in apartheid South Africa as a multiracial, multifaith [service]; you could have your treatment no matter what your race was, what your religion was and whether you could pay or not; but my colleagues who started hospice had their initial requests for Department of Health funding turned down because we didn't segregate our wards or our beds, notwithstanding that most of our care happened in the home. And it seemed that when the democratic government took over, they weren't looking to put funds elsewhere so they continued the trend of not funding hospices. From the HIV point of view, there's been a concept that palliative care is for people who die, mainly because hospices provide end-of-life care. So the concept of palliative care being available throughout the course of the illness hasn't yet been taken on board. The HIV physicians, who are really striving for their patients' survival, don't want their patients to go into a palliative care service because it feels to them like giving up; they haven't yet learned how much can be done for patients in that kind of setting. **Dr Liz Gwyther—HPCA board member, education and research co-ordinator, South Africa; 4 June 2004.**

Relationships with government

In this section, we first include extracts that relate to the development of palliative care in the context of apartheid South Africa.

Because of apartheid, South Africa was the polecat of the international society. We were South Africans, and we were in South Africa, so we didn't have access to all the wonderful developments in palliative care that were happening internationally, and we had to develop anything we needed ourselves. So we probably wasted a lot of energy reinventing wheels. In fact, I can remember how relieved I was when I did once get a glimpse of a nursing course that had been developed—I think it's the ENB 931 or whatever it is—and wow! Ours was just about the same, which was wonderful. But at the same time we were an embarrassment to the South African government because we said it was against hospice philosophy to be having any kind of different care for people because of different colour, and that everybody had to have access to care; that the care we gave was based on need, not ability to pay or colour of the skin, or creed, or anything else, and that that was the way we were operating. Of course, the other thing was the segregation in South Africa: we actually were breaking the law going into black areas to care for patients, and it was because of that that we also knew we had to develop the skills of people who were allowed to be there, who lived there, like the primary health care nurses, and we were there in a consultancy availability. **Kath Defilippi— chairperson of APCA; HPCA board member and chief executive officer, South Coast Hospice, Port Shepstone, South Africa; 5 June 2004.**

One of the remarkable things is that hospice, right from its early days in the '80s in South Africa, has always been totally open and non-racialistic, at a time when in this country it was extremely difficult to do. I think that that influence has been quite important in our country—that in fact people are all valuable in their own right, no matter who and what they are. Interestingly enough, one of the demands that Dame Cicely Saunders made before coming to South Africa, was that the Radiotherapy Department at Grotte Schuur [Hospital] was racially integrated; and I could satisfy her on that one. The reason for that was that, as a Medical School, the University of Cape Town was at the forefront, going against government policies, and such services as Radiotherapy were integrated; you couldn't divide them and double them. So that was one of her demands and we were able to meet it. **Professor J. P. van Niekerk—chair of HPCA and manager of PEPFAR project, South Africa; 13 August 2004.**

Yes, we did start in apartheid South Africa but I think in those early hospices there was no apartheid. We just went in and ignored the apartheid. We went into black, Indian, white, coloured, wherever; and I can actually remember, in the original little house here [in Durban], which was in '85 to 86, we had a three-bedded room with a black person, a Hindu person and a coloured person—three patients all together in one room—and that was in the apartheid days. I think our hospices just over-rode apartheid. So I think we were probably one of the organizations that didn't have a hospice for whites and a hospice for blacks. Our hospice was open and—we acknowledged it in our pamphlets and in our first talks—it was for all people of all races with no religious or other discrimination. **Karen Hinton—chairperson: Hospice Association of KwaZulu Natal and quality assurance adviser, Highway Hospice, Durban: South Africa; 8 August 2004.**

I think lots of exciting things were happening at the end of the 1970s; at the individual level things were breaking down. One of the difficulties in retrospect—at the time, too, I suppose—was that there were some people who felt we shouldn't be party to those things because they actually allowed the regime to be shored up in a way, because they could point to them and say, 'Well look, we're not clamping down on that bit of inspiration', so it wasn't a clear cut, easy argument. But indeed, yes, there were initiatives occurring and the hospice initiatives were by and large done on non-religious and non-racial lines and that was very exciting; but it wasn't done without problems. **Dr Richard Scheffer—medical director, Rowcroft Hospice, UK; 24 March 2005.**

Two of the nurses who worked very closely with me were married to doctors who worked in the hospital. So we got them signed up quite quickly prescribing morphine properly. But when a patient went home, there was nowhere they could get it again; they were sometimes over 60 kilometres away and there's no public transport infrastructure in place, and it's expensive to try and get a taxi to come back. So, you know, we sort of gave them a taste of proper pain control and then they went home. When that supply of morphine was finished and the pain returned, probably with greater intensity because of disease progression, they had the terrible choice of having to use money to come back and be admitted. Also, they could come in three days in a row, sitting at outpatients, before a doctor saw them—and they couldn't afford that. I was horrified when I realized that we'd actually done them a disfavour.

So we worked about trying to get ourselves out there. This was in the height of the apartheid era, but we actually got permission the first time from the police to go to a primary health care clinic to talk and that was fine. And then we discovered—and in those days, white people didn't know black people in South Africa—we discovered these amazing women who were kindred spirits; and there were nurses in the primary health care clinics who were nurses just like us. So I told them all about hospice philosophy and what-have-you, and they liked what they heard. They were so committed to caring for people, and they had hardly anything to do it with in those days. Then I said, if they were interested we could have a small team to do a symptom control workshop to teach them how to really do it; you could even prevent pain in most patients. In those days they were patients with an advanced malignancy, as common cancers were cervix and oesophagus. And, they were open to it; it was like a wonderful revolutionary discovery for both the black primary health care services and ourselves. We've been working together in a close partnership since then. **Kath Defilippi—chairperson of APCA; HPCA board member and chief executive officer, South Coast Hospice, Port Shepstone, South Africa; 5 June 2004**.

With me being part of the [black] community and knowing their culture, they were amazed this was actually happening. I had both Western medicine and an understanding of their traditional values and where they were coming from, so it was quite an eye-opener for me and I found it very challenging. Of course, working at hospice, you don't actually look after people of your own race, which was also quite interesting, especially during the apartheid era. I used to go and relieve in other areas and, for some people, it came as a shock, seeing me knocking at their door, on the doorstep, coming as a nurse; and you could sense they were not at ease until they proved to them-selves you knew what you were doing. They were asking those kinds of questions. Of course, having gone through the course and with experience I knew just about as much as everyone else knew. But I must say, with the hospice, it's a place where you find you're part of the family. I haven't found any place as supportive as the hospice is for their staff. **Thembi Nyuswa—palliative care nurse, Highway Hospice, Durban, South Africa; 8 August 2004**.

I'm pleased you raised the racial issues, with which we still grapple with difficulty in this coun-try. Organizations that are charities, NGOs, were often started by people who had reasonable means themselves, which would free them up to do such work. And those typically came from church groups, but also from white people who had the financial means which black people in this country did not have. That is still reflected in some of our structures at the national and regional levels, to the extent that when we looked at our board, the national board [HPCA], we identified that our demographic mix was not appropriate; and so, hopefully as a temporary measure, we did not change our constitution, but we got the annual general meeting of the board to agree that the regions would supply not one board member but two, at least one of whom would not be white.

So we still grapple with those questions, and those are some of the realities that we have to deal with. We don't move as quickly as some would wish. The Department of Health in particular believes that we should look completely different to what we are; but we have our own realities to face and we believe that we are very conscious of those needs. At the same time we have to provide the developmental expertise that ensures that we put all the appropriate structures and standards in place to go forward in strength rather than in weakness. **Professor J. P. van Niekerk—chair of HPCA and manager of PEPFAR project, South Africa; 13 August 2004**.

Turning to other African countries, the following extracts highlight relationships with government in Swaziland, Uganda, Tanzania and Kenya.

[In Swaziland], the steering committee came to the conclusion that the first thing that we needed was permission from the Ministry of Health, and we needed to register as a non-government organization. This was not easy; it was *not* easy at all. I thought my first port of call must be the Minister of Health. I got there, and actually was introduced to the principal secretary to the Minister of Health. His name was Chris Mkonta. I got very friendly with him and we ended up on Christian name terms, so you can understand how long this took. The first thing he said was that he couldn't give me permission, after I'd given him the outline of what we were trying to do, but I must go down and register as an NGO and then, once I'd got the registration for an NGO, I could go back and he was sure the Minister of Health would give me permission.

This was a journey of an hour between the two cities. The Ministry of Health was in Mbabane and the NGO headquarters were in Manzini, and in between was a hill that's in the *Guinness Book of Records* as being one of the most dangerous in the world. So I was going up and down this hill. I went back to the NGO and the lady who was in charge, Sarah Dlamini, said, 'Oh, it sounds very good and I'm sure I *could* help you, but you have to have permission from the Ministry of Health'. I obviously told her, 'Well, you know, this is where I'd just been'. I think I had probably six journeys and in the end I thought, 'This is not on; this is absolutely ridiculous, I'm going to do a sit-in', and I went up, saw Chris, said to him, 'I've just about have enough. I just can't do this any longer, and I'm not leaving this place until I get some sort of permission'. So I said, 'All I need is a letter stating that it's all OK for me to do this'. Anyway he sort of turned around and said, 'Will you follow me?' I followed him thinking, 'Oh I'm going to get my letter', and he opened a door and there was the biggest desk I've ever seen, with the largest lady I've ever seen sat behind it, and this was the Minister of Health, Dr Fanny Freidman. And she then questioned me, and I gave her my story, and I left and went back down that hill, clutching my letter—and we were registered as an NGO on 4 July 1990. It was no mean feat! **Stephanie Wyer—founder Swaziland Hospice at Home; 1 July 2003.**

[In Uganda] we learnt of the epidemic of HIV/AIDS in 1982 and officially the diagnosis of this disease was made. There was no doubt about the diagnosis; but because of political turmoil, and also the primitive idea that if we mention this disease tourists will not visit our country, the politicians of that time kept quiet about it. But we knew the disease was around. So from when the National Resistance Movement came into power in 1986, the government—and His Excellency, the President of Uganda, Mr Yoweri Kaguta Museveni—was very open about this disease and he said, 'There are people dying, why should we keep quiet? If you have an enemy, you raise an alarm and say, 'Here's an enemy'; so that openness and the political will caused people to be aware. People talked about this disease, and people got information, people got to know how the disease spreads. So I think that awareness, and knowing the routes of infection of this disease, helped this country—for many people know how to avoid this disease. I think that attitude has helped: the awareness, the communication, the education, has helped people to avoid being infected. And eventually, of course, condoms came; but at the beginning, only about 5 per cent of the people were using condoms. Now about 15 per cent are using condoms. So I don't think [the reduced incidence] is mainly due to condoms, but the background of openness, education, information and taking other precautions—like the screening of blood transfusion and education about use of syringes. All these have contributed to lowering the incidence of HIV/AIDS. **Dr Jack Jagwe—senior adviser, national policy, drugs and advocacy, Hospice Africa Uganda; 10 March 2004.**

[In Tanzania], the Orphans' Department has changed a lot over the last two years. A lot of our staff have been trained in Zimbabwe and in Uganda on bereavement, and they've brought that into the work they're doing now. They're also doing a lot of work with memory books, or memory boxes, whatever you want to call them. We've done a lot of lobbying within the legal system because of the huge problem concerning the abuse of these children—and in particular sexual abuse. During the past two years, the numbers of kids who are now talking about it has become huge. So we've done a lot of lobbying and actually the Global Fund has given us the money within the grant to do a write-up of the psychosocial support that we are giving. According to them, there is no other organization doing it in Tanzania and it would be helpful for everybody else. So once we do get the money we will do that. **Mary Ash—executive director, PASADA, Dar es Salaam, Tanzania; 9 November 2004.**

Nairobi Hospice is situated on government land, because the government recognizes the value of the service we provide, so they have accommodated us in the grounds of the National Hospital. In 2001, the government gave us an acre of land, very near to where we are at the moment. That was an important development because in Nairobi city, buying land is very, very expensive. So we are very grateful that the Kenya Government acknowledges and appreciates what we are doing, and that they have donated land to us. So the task now is to raise money to be able to put up our own structure.

The government do not give us hard cash as such, but they support us in kind, which is equally as significant. At the moment, I have got three nurses on my staff who are government employees, and you would appreciate that manpower is quite expensive—a burden on the hospice budget—so the fact that three out of the six nurses are sponsored by the government: that is really very good support. Of course their goodwill and recognition is also a big contribution; and the land, it has been valued very much. **Brigid Sirengo—chief executive officer, Nairobi Hospice, Kenya; 2 June 2004.**

Education, training and research

Education and training is one of three foundation measures identified by WHO as being crucial to the development of palliative care. These extracts demonstrate how, in Africa, initiatives in palliative care education range from basic courses for community groups to university-based post-graduate degrees. Alongside these education programmes is a growing interest in research.

I think they do deal with palliative care, maybe not 100 per cent adequately, but there's a lot of support from the families. The idea of still being a family is important; I don't know if it will still be there with the next generation—they're different from the rest of us—but usually family support is there for patients who are dying; and even if it's not family, the neighbours. If you go to a slum area where people have come from different parts of the country to live and work in Nairobi, we find it's the neighbours who are cooking for patients, who are washing their clothes and who are supporting them. These are neighbours, they're not their relatives, sometimes because their relatives live very far away. So I think that kind of care at home has been there throughout. Probably now, they are facing different challenges, like HIV/AIDS, and they don't know how to deal with it. Usually what we do is to give them some training, when we go out there, on how to take care of these patients.

We hold a one week training course twice a year at the hospice for health care professionals, and also for non-health care volunteers; this is just an introductory course for those who want to get to know something about palliative care. We've had funding from the Diana Memorial Fund to train in all the provinces in Kenya. This is on going and has made a big difference in care for those with life-limiting illnesses. The Ford Foundation has also funded training—for both health care professionals and community-based workers—in the two largest slums in Nairobi. Slowly, we are spreading the work of Dame Cicely Saunders and we hope, and pray, that palliative care will become available to all in the near future. **Zipporah Ali—senior medical officer, Nairobi Hospice, Kenya; 1 November 2004.**

Our latest milestone in our development is that in June 2001, Nairobi Hospice, in collaboration with Oxford Brookes University, has developed a Diploma in Higher Education: Palliative Care. This is a programme that is partly distance learning and partly the block system. It is very convenient to our health care professionals because they can do this Higher Diploma while they continue working, and it's also convenient because not everybody can manage to go to the UK or anywhere else for long periods of time because of cost and other constraints. So this is a programme that we are running and that's why tomorrow I have to leave because on Saturday we have a class graduating, so I will have to be there at the graduation ceremony. **Brigid Sirengo—chief executive officer, Nairobi Hospice, Kenya; 2 June 2004.**

We're training hospital staff, usually nurses, although it's been a mix and some of them clinical officers; I'm not sure what the equivalent would be outside of East Africa, but you could call them physician assistants in the USA. Then there has been a lot of training of church-related people— lots, lots and lots—and a lot of what we call volunteer training. Mark [Jacobson] is fond of saying that he had never heard of volunteers and he remembers learning Swahili in the 1980s: there wasn't a word ['volunteer'], there just wasn't. People helped but the idea of this kind of helping, was not within the framework that we had. What Selian has done with their training of volunteers has been to take church parish workers: lay people who are visiting folks who are sick, and maybe bringing them something from the church, or praying, or doing just the basic things. That link has been very special because it's a very motivated group, and a group that doesn't seem to require the usual incentives that a lot of volunteer groups do require, at least in this context. **Dr Kristopher Hartwig—physician, Selian Hospital, Arusha, Tanzania; 4 November 2004.**

There's such a wealth of work that's happening in our hospices at the moment that needs to be documented. I have had a growing interest in research since doing my own research project which was around the need for palliative care education for South African doctors, and because I'm teaching a research-based degree. We have about 23 research projects that have come out of the University of Cape Town programmes since 2001, which really inform us so much about what's happening in palliative care in Africa. A lot of my teaching is based on articles from peer-reviewed journals. Those articles are published overseas and we need a body of evidence-based medicine in Africa that's relevant to African conditions. So the research in palliative care is at an early stage now, and it's really exciting to be in at that early stage and to be encouraging research skills—which doesn't have to be the high-powered, academic, university-based research; it can happen in the community. We're doing a small research project at St Luke's Hospice where our community caregivers are collecting the information around symptom control for their patients over just a single, one-month period. It's really important because we've said to the Department of Health, 'We make a difference in our patients' lives' but where do we have the evidence to back that up? So we're looking at what the intervention over a month does for three specific symptoms of pain, diarrhoea and shortness of breath. For the community caregiver, who often doesn't have any school-leaving training, we've provided a three-month training course in basic nursing care, HIV/AIDS awareness and some palliative care concepts and principles. So they're going in and they're asking their clients on a mild–moderate–severe scale: what are these three symptoms like? what are they like a week later? and what are they like at the end of the month. So we're hoping to be able to show the Department of Health that we really are making the difference that we claim. **Dr Liz Gwyther— HPCA board member; education and research co-ordinator, South Africa; 4 June 2004.**

The course—a two-year Masters degree in palliative care—runs through the Family Medicine and Primary Care Department of the University of Cape Town, so palliative care falls into the Family Medicine fold. It is not widely accepted yet in the undergraduate teaching, although I think the advent of HIV is going to change that in due course; perhaps it has already and I'm not aware of it yet. I do some undergraduate teaching, but in Family Medicine not in Palliative Medicine, and I've done a little bit of postgraduate teaching—also in Family Medicine. So that's another area of interest, teaching, and now latterly research.

The course involved three components. We had course work which covered the range of palliative care and 13 assignments that ranged from ethics, to clinical issues, to teamwork that were written over two years. There was a portfolio where we took cases from our own practice. There were 11 or 12 of us on the course and each person brought their own cases and the portfolio was a learning process. My two cases were both GP-based because I am a GP, I'm a family physician: the one was mismanagement and the other based on the fragmentation of care—because GPs and family physicians are marginalized in the treatment of cancer; both patients were cancer patients. Those were my two portfolios. Then the third component was the research component. My hypothesis was that outcomes would be better if general practitioners or family physicians were involved in the patient's [palliative] care. **Dr Alan Barnard—GP and hospice physician, St Luke's Hospice, Cape Town, South Africa; 12 August 2004.**

Until this year, I was predominantly with education and I think had a hand in developing the education [in South Africa]. I was very fortunate to be on the National Sub-Committee for Patient Care and Education, and I think very privileged to have been on the team of nurses to develop the curriculum for our Certificate course for professional nurses, which has been accredited with the Nursing Council. So for me the greatest success I can always talk about is that specific Certificate course because I never dreamed that we would now have a Diploma course for nurses. I think also the education centre here is another success for Highway, and provincially and nationally we are fortunate that we do have a very good reputation for the training given here, and I think Highway can be quite pleased about that. **Karen Hinton—chairperson: Hospice Association of KwaZulu Natal; quality assurance adviser, Highway Hospice, Durban: South Africa; 8 August 2004.**

[At Mildmay International] we run an 18-month Diploma course with the University of Manchester on HIV/AIDS Care and Management, which is a multidisciplinary programme. We're just re-writing that to upgrade to a degree course; in fact we had our first graduation last Friday. Then we have a year-long programme with two mobile training teams. Each team has a nurse, a doctor or a clinical officer, a counsellor and a driver, and they work in the districts in Uganda. So they're working in six districts over a year-long period. It's a module programme, trying to strengthen HIV/AIDS/palliative care in the rural setting—not bringing people from the rural setting to Kampala, but us going there and trying to encourage the development of palliative care services, HIV/AIDS services, networking and referral, and strengthening care in the rural setting.

This is quite an unusual idea, yes. I've been asked by WHO to share the model and so we've been trying to develop that and share it. We also run short courses on all aspects of palliative care: paediatric clinical care, paediatric HIV/AIDS palliative care, communicating with children, psychosocial and spiritual care, use of ARVs in resource-limited settings, introductory courses on palliative care, courses on palliative care for religious leaders, teachers—so a wide variety of short programmes and clinical placements.

I'm currently doing my PhD, looking at the impact of palliative care training on care in the rural setting in Uganda. **Julia Downing—director, Mildmay International Study Centre, Kampala, Uganda; 2 June 2004.**

Part of the challenge is the resistance from senior health professionals. It is now improving because we have the junior health professionals coming on these courses and we expect them to go back, train others and introduce palliative care to their work settings. But then their seniors, the senior health professionals, sometimes don't support them. So we've done a lot of advocacy among the senior health professionals. We've organized sensitizations for them and we are involving them in our whole range of activities; some of them have presented sessions on our courses. We've invited them for updates for the Palliative Care Association of Uganda. We've interested them in referring patients. So that has been a challenge, but we are managing it and so far the results have been positive—especially now palliative care is part of the five-year national strategy plan. The Ministry of Health is at the forefront of the initiative, and of course the Ministry of Health is their boss. So really it is much more positive than before. **Fatia Kiyange—education administrator, Hospice Africa Uganda; 10 March 2004.**

I studied medicine here at Makerere and after my medical degree I got married and I went and lived in Kenya for eight years. We have three daughters and when they were attending school the whole day, I went back and did a Masters degree in public health; and it was during that time that I stumbled on palliative care—really stumbled on palliative care—I didn't even know the words *palliative care*. But as I thought of what to do for my thesis I thought of the quality of life of people who are terminally ill with HIV/AIDS and I wanted to do something there, and that is when my lecturers introduced me to Dr Merriman with another doctor, I know him as Dr Jan [Stjernswärd]. So I talked with them about what I was trying to do during my research into quality of life, comparing those who were in home care programmes and those who were not and they said, 'Quality of life is going to be difficult because there are no instruments applicable to Africa'. And then they said, 'Why don't you look into their needs?' so I said, 'Fine, I may do that'.

So what I did was to write a concept paper and then a proposal and then Dr Merriman read it with one of my lecturers in public health, and they said, 'Oh, this is a good one, go ahead'. So the contact I got with the people who were in their homes suffering from HIV/AIDS and their families gave me a lot of results and really opened my eyes to that phase in a patient's life where the doctor says 'There's nothing I can do, please go home now'. And that has, you know, always bothered me when I was doing medicine, because a person would come in—usually our people come in late—and we go through all the tests and diagnose their disease from an academic point of view, and then sit the family down and say, 'Yes, this is cancer but there's nothing we can do. Please go home, don't go the witch doctor'. And I was curious to know what happened next. How do they handle that period between 'there's nothing the doctor can do' and death. So, going around collecting data really opened my eyes to that period and I was hooked to palliative care after that.

So when I finished my thesis I really enjoyed it and the people opened up. They were not afraid of talking about death. The families were very receptive, they came up with recommendations of how we can help. The home care programmes managers welcomed the study.[2] They said, 'We've always wanted somebody to do a study for us so that we know that what we are doing is helpful'. And after my degree Dr Merriman invited me and said, 'Look, we've always wanted to do a study like this one in another district, a rural district, can you come and do it for us?' I said, 'Fine, no problem.' So I came in and joined the hospice in February 2001, mainly to do that research for them. **Dr Ekiria Kikule—executive director and research co-ordinator, Hospice Africa Uganda; 10 March 2004.**

I'm looking at pre-service training, so I'm going to incorporate this into our curriculum for the graduates, as well as those at the diploma level, and also look at those already in service. We are going to organize in-service education to incorporate palliative care into practice. As we said, you can see that our major need is education, and education needs funding. **Mary Opare—acting dean of the School of Nursing, University of Ghana, Legon, Accra, Ghana; 4 June 2004.**

Traditional healers are in the community, living with the people and seeing them through their suffering. Fortunately, some of us are now double trained. I am a medical doctor and I'm a traditional healer. We have come a long way in educating the biomedics, because we understand their language. We can talk to them in their language. We have gone a long way in educating the traditional healers, because we understand their language. We can tell them to realize the gaps. Traditional medicine has a lot missing; Western medicine has some things missing. They can both play a complementary role. And in any case, the target is the patient and we cannot claim dominance over the patient. The patient claims the right to see whichever person is of value to him and in that respect, patients have opted for traditional healers. So they see value. **Dr Yahaya Hills Sekagya– general secretary, National Integrated Forum for Traditional Health Practitioners, Uganda and president PROMETRA Uganda; 9 September 2004.**

When we started [in Pretoria] we needed to train volunteers and because my background was in education, I became involved in training programmes to support the work of the hospice; and from very humble beginnings training a few volunteers we now have probably the largest centre for palliative learning in the country. [Initially], we drew up a whole programme for training volunteers and that was going along quite well; and then I was involved in the work in one of the former settlement areas. When I worked there trying to establish a hospice, I would get repeated requests from a young woman in the area saying, 'Can't you train me to be a nurse?' This was impossible, but I thought, 'What about caring skills?'

So I went back and spoke to a nursing colleague and we put together a training course and we had our first group of six of these women and we learnt as we went along. We gave them the theory and we gave them the practice and then we employed them at hospice as carers in that area—and four of them are still doing that, from the very first course. Over the years we've probably trained about 200 women from both those communities in the basics of home care skills, and I think that's has been one of my greatest rewards: we've been able to provide the skills to make people marketable. A lot of these women have now gone into nursing. They are qualified nurses themselves or they are able to give drugs in retroviral centres. So it's been a wonderful way of empowering women who had very few skills to be able to get work and support their families and to make a difference. That's been a great reward for me. The Department of Health then asked me to develop that programme and it's actually become the national training programme for home-based care. So I think that has made a difference and has, you know, been a great sense of pleasure for me. **Sue Cameron—HPCA board member and manager of the Centre for Palliative Learning, Pretoria Sungardens Hospice, South Africa; 26 April 2005.**

In the rest of this chapter, we focus on issues concerning patients, staff and the palliative care service. Patient issues include: the implications of poverty, the late presentation of patients, African perspectives of spirituality and HIV denial. Staff issues relate to salaries, personal safety and professional support; whereas service issues highlight the cultural context of palliative care, the challenges posed by rural areas, the need to include special care for family members, and breaking down resistance to the use of morphine.

Patient issues

In the rural areas there is always a cousin to help us with the care; so there is, to that extent, a relative. With those that are living in the rural areas, at least the poverty is not as severe as it is in the informal settlements—because there they've got land; they plant something. Here, there's no land. Even if you tell them about the importance of famine, there's no land for them [to grow things] because one house is crowded in on another. Sanitation problems arise and, because they've erected these houses themselves, it's a challenge to put sewerage systems in. So we always have problems: tummy problems. We are always having skin problems—they're the majority. Maybe in some areas you find that there's just one trench and then everyone will have a bath and wash his clothes in that trench, and then the trench runs past the other families. **Mandla Mtatambi— palliative care nurse and manager of Inanda day centre, Highway Hospice, Durban, South Africa; 9 August 2004.**

Most of our patients are very poor; some live in slum areas. So say you go into the homes and you want to give them morphine: if they've not had any food for some days, sometimes you have to dig into your pockets and buy them a packet of milk and a loaf of bread so they can eat this and then take their drugs. We encourage patients to be in their homes and not in hospitals. We sensitize the family and talk to them and prepare the families for death at home; because these patients, if they go to the hospitals—particularly if they're HIV/AIDS positive or are at the end of life with advanced cancer—nobody's going to provide the care they need. People actually keep away from them, including the medical staff. So we prefer them to be in their homes. They're happier in their homes; and even the family finds it easier to be in the home with the patients and not visiting them in hospitals hence avoiding travelling long distances. **Dr Bactrin Killingo—founder, chief executive and physician, Meru Hospice, Kenya; 1 November 2004.**

I think one of the real challenges is that when people's cancer is so advanced you're looking at palliative treatment anyway, and that's a really difficult thing for people who have suddenly been told that they have got cancer and it's incurable. It's like a double whammy. Women don't have smears, they don't have mammograms, they don't know to look for breast lumps, they don't know about signs of early bleeding in post-menopausal women—or any of the signs that could alert them to thinking, ' I think this might be cancer'. It's really difficult.

And I guess the other thing is that, come the wet season, it's really awful to try and get out to people. You've said, 'Right, I'll call on Wednesday', and then there's a flooded river and you can't get there, or your car breaks down, or the person's gone up country to do the planting and so they're not there. So to just chat or even find the person is an achievement. **Ruth Wooldridge—co-founder, the Nairobi Hospice, Kenya; 23 January 2005.**

I do think the African way of looking at spiritual issues is different because of the ancestral spirit issues. No matter how people are educated or religious, in the context of formal religion, I find that when there's difficulty in the family, or someone who's being sick, there's always an urge to work through the ancestral spirit and then carry out the appropriate ritual. I think this can really bring a lot of peace to the dying person. They can feel they've made peace with their God. They've prepared the way for those who are ahead to welcome them, and sometimes this links with the fact that when people are dying they'll sometimes mention the name of a person who died—perhaps years before them—an adult or a great-grandparent, and this is all seen as positive. The ancestors are welcoming them and it helps those left behind feel our loved one has gone the right way. **Sambulo Mkwananzi—training manager, Island Hospice and Bereavement Service, Harare, Zimbabwe and board member APCA; 20 September 2004.**

What I find in the communities I work in, like the Indian area of Phoenix, is the whole myth that HIV and AIDS does not affect the Indian person. The families are now in a crisis because the disease is actually attacking them. I'm working with the patients, the families, there's a lot of work there. One's got to counsel them and make sure the neighbours are not rejecting them. Family members are also keeping away. Whereas previously, when there's death, it's the culture, the rituals, which bring families together. But now it's tearing that family apart from the rest of the community. Another challenge they are facing is that the Hindu women especially—and the Moslem women—are not allowed to come out of their homes for a period of time around the time of a death. So while they may need counselling because verily the husband's dying, and death may be very sudden, they are not allowed to come out to see the social workers. **Goonam Jacob—social worker, Highway Hospice, Durban, South Africa; 8 August 2004.**

Staff issues

Unfortunately, I have been running the service with serious hardships, serious problems, especially with respect to funding, because up until March this year, for the last perhaps one and a half years, our staff, who are six, have been doing that without pay. This is something I usually don't talk about. I only talk about it when I'm asked, because we started with a, kind of, sacrificial approach because the apathy to death and dying in Meru was too much. People don't talk about death and dying in Meru, and I'm sure that is common everywhere else. People don't talk about their sexuality and that is why we have problems with HIV/AIDS containment. So we started small, started quietly but effectively. We've reached a stage now where we couldn't do without, for example, support for staff in terms of salaries. But we didn't know how to go about it, because all the proposals we sent to various donors, basically brought the answer that they don't fund salaries. They didn't see the need for supporting someone who was going to die anyway. But fortunately, in March, we got twinned by Hospice Care Incorporated in Wisconsin [USA], who are able to send us some small little monies for support of staff and for support of other things like communication that we had a problem with; but we are still a long way off providing for staff. At least staff can now get a loaf of bread and survive. **Dr Bactrin Killingo—founder, chief executive and physician, Meru Hospice, Kenya; 1 November 2004.**

Phoenix has got a major problem with drug and alcohol abuse, woman abuse. In the area it's very rife and I am in danger quite a bit. But with the grace of God, you just risk your life to go and see your terminally ill patients. For our patients that have got cancer, the family background from where they come is absolutely devastating. I have one patient and she's got cancer of the breast. Her husband's an alcoholic, her son is a drug addict, and they just break all the bottles if there's no money to buy more alcohol. Quite a number of times when I've got there they were violent with the wife. The husband was going over with this broken bottle, almost wanting to rip her open and saying, 'Why don't you die?' And quite a number of times I've transported her to her relative's home nearby. **Jennifer Padayachee—nursing sister and manager of Phoenix day centre, Highway Hospice, Durban, South Africa; 9 August 2004.**

Much as we take care of these children, the morale of the caregivers goes down when we lose a child. So I do a lot of counselling, especially with the caregivers. We've realized that with most children it's in the small hours of the morning—that is 4.00 a.m., 5.00 a.m., when their immune system is at its lowest—when they die. So I come in in the morning and counsel the staff members that were on nights, because they work a shift and they have to come in again in the evening, yes. And apart from counselling the night staff, I do a lot of counselling with staff members during the day because, once a child dies, much as we say we take care of terminally ill children and we know they are going to die, we always feel we have lost a child. So we do a lot of 'care of the caregivers' work. **Stella Dubazana—child care manager, Cotlands Hospice, Johannesburg, South Africa; 11 August 2004.**

One of the major stresses of our staff is the poverty, witnessing the poverty. Going into a home: yes, OK, we can come with our expertise, do something about the pain, and the vomiting, and all of those things. But to have to walk away from that home—where you know when you walk away there is no bread on that table—is hard. The medication that you've brought: you're saying you must take this with something to eat; and there's nothing to eat.

Now our staff, where they can, leave some money for a loaf of bread. And that's for today. But until we've been able to access, for instance, a disability grant for them—which is something positive we can do, but it's going to take about three months, and you can't put bread on the table every day for three months for a family we know are hungry—it's that feeling of helplessness, I think, in the face of great poverty which is difficult. As carers, we always feel there's something we can do; but it's having to come to a place where sometimes there's nothing you can do, particularly in the area of poverty. Also, we have a child whose mother is dying and we're really searching for a family member that's going to be able to take care of this child when mum dies, and sometimes that's impossible to find. So I think it's the feelings of helplessness; that's the kind of stress I would say that our sisters and our care workers find the hardest. **Lesley Lawson—co-founder, St Francis Hospice, Port Elizabeth, South Africa; 26 April 2004.**

Service issues

I think to talk about the challenges, we have to consider the overall context of the African countries, their culture, their past history, their economic state at the moment, whether there was war, poverty, hunger. All these things influence palliative care and its provision. However, the palliative care necessity has arisen really from HIV/AIDS. Cancer has been there, but in the African countries that I'm linked with, the highest cause of death has been infections—and cancer is outside the top ten causes of death. But HIV/AIDS is very much there with all the infectious diseases, so governments are beginning to take notice.

The HIV/AIDS epidemic is increasing in most of the African countries and the highest level we have seen is 38 to 40 per cent in Botswana. These countries where it's going up have a huge problem caring for these people, both within hospitals and at home; and all the research that's been done in Africa shows that people want to die in their own homes, but there are cultural and governmental issues which prevent people dying in their own homes. In fact, a lot of research needs to be done on that, to see if we can change things so that people could die comfortably in their own homes. So it's often the legal issues, the cultural issues, and the poverty issues that decide where a patient will die. **Dr Anne Merriman—founder and director—medical services and education, Hospice Africa Uganda; 20 July 2004.**

I was thinking before the interview about the different challenges to palliative care in the region. One of those, I think, is the language issue, in that [in West Africa] the majority of the countries are Francophone countries, French-speaking countries. We have some Anglophone countries and then one country that speaks Portuguese, Guinea-Bissau. And so in terms of what I've seen, it's easier to have involvement from outside agencies, particularly the USA and the UK, with Anglophone countries. So since some of the leading agencies for palliative care are UK and US based, it makes sense that it would be an Anglophone country that would be more advanced in that. **Caroline Bishop—technical adviser of HIV/AIDS, Catholic Relief Services, West Africa; 4 June 2004.**

At that time I was writing to Help the Aged, UK, to see if they could come in with funding so that we could construct a centre whereby medical care could be provided for the terminally ill. Help the Aged directed me to an appropriate institution. In their own words at that time, if I was looking to provide care for terminal patients, like cancer and AIDS patients, then I needed to approach St Christopher's Hospice. That was how I knew that an institution specializing in palliative care existed in the UK. I contacted St Christopher's Hospice and it came back to me with a lot of information about hospice and palliative care and even gave me addresses of hospices in the USA and in Canada. I contacted hospice and palliative care training groups in the USA and I received some information, and that information was able to build my library, which I used to set up the first hospice in Sierra Leone—Shepherd's Hospice. **Dr Gabriel Madiye—founder and executive director, The Shepherd's Hospice, Freetown, Sierra Leone; 4 June 2004.**

The only thing I haven't said is the difficulty to get something established in our rural areas. I'm covering four provinces, which is a huge area: Gauteng, Limpopo, Mpumalanga and the North-West Province. By next month, we're hoping to have another team in place, which is going to make it a little bit easier. If you look at Mpumalanga and Limpopo, we have nothing in place, so I'm busy trying. There's only one established programme, which is a rural programme, and we're needing to set something up within the urban and semi-urban areas, because there's just nothing. It's also the distances: these areas are vast. We have to travel a lot to get to the places and that is the difficulty. We're trying to prioritize what we need to do. Even if we just have one or two established hospices in Mpumalanga and Limpopo, we can start from there and develop further; that is our priority at the moment. We're talking to a hospital—it's actually a government hospital, called St Rita's—and we're doing a presentation to them on the 27th [August 2004] to ask them to give back-up beds for the inpatient unit. This is so we can have our patients from the home-based care programme going into the hospital when they need to—just for pain and symptom control, or acute things that you can't treat at home. That's the difficulty of the job: setting things in place in the provinces where the infrastructure's a little bit shaky. **Brenda Dass—provincial (PEPFAR) co-ordinator Limpopo, Gauteng and Mpumalanga, South Africa; 12 August 2004.**

The hospice looks at the care of one with life-limiting illnesses, in totality, and their families. That gives rise to the two programmes that we have. One is an end-of-life programme for cancer and AIDS patients. But in the era of HIV, we were faced with the challenge of responding to the plight of people who are HIV positive, for the following reasons: there are those who presented to us with cancers who are HIV positive, and these individuals had spouses and children who were HIV positive. When they passed on we found there was no way we were going to abandon the spouses and families, because they too started entering into non-cancer-related chronic illnesses. So we felt we needed to come up with a formal support for people living with HIV/AIDS. That is where we got involved with other service providers in treating the opportunistic infections, offering prophylactic measures, and providing antiretrovirals. **Dr Bactrin Killingo—founder, chief executive and physician, Meru Hospice, Kenya; 1 November 2004.**

We just have to battle with these fears that people have. There is a very, very strong fear around the use of morphine. It's very difficult to get some of the senior doctors to change their minds and prescribe morphine, even if the patient is experiencing a lot of pain and needs higher doses. They are very apprehensive about that; they are quite reluctant. But with training, we hope that things will change. Part of our training programme involves the medical students, so we hope that as the doctors come out of the training school, some of them will have had some orientation in palliative care, so they will be much more comfortable prescribing morphine. But it is a problem for most doctors, and of course, nurses too. **Brigid Sirengo—chief executive officer, Nairobi Hospice, Kenya; 2 June 2004.**

I think perhaps one of the biggest challenges that we've faced—and to a certain degree we're still facing, but it is decreasing—is to change the perception of hospices: from the kind of a relatively insular organization that provides services just for its immediate locality, in isolation from other services, not linking up with the local not-for- profit and governmental health services—to shift from that traditional kind of insular hospice, to the hospice becoming more of a broker for palliative care within a particular region, and this is where we have been trying to move hospices towards.

The AIDS situation in South Africa is so great that hospices cannot possibly provide the support that's required for AIDS patients. The skill of hospices in South Africa—its particular niche—is 2-fold in a way. One, it provides exemplar services, high quality exemplar services, which is captured in the quality of care; and building on that particular niche, it has developed quite a strong education and training capability and capacity. And so more and more the direction that hospices in South Africa are moving towards, is to retain its exemplar quality services, but to use those exemplar quality services as a spring board for capacity building, through education and training. So a hospice in a given region will provide education and training for other health service organizations around palliative care; will become the facilitator and catalyst for more teamwork around palliative care within a particular area. **Josef Lazarus—strategic adviser to the HPCA board, South Africa; 13 August 2004.**

References

1 **Bruera E.** The development of a palliative care culture. *Journal of Palliative Care* 2004 **20**(4): 306–319.

2 See: **Kikule E.** A good death in Uganda: survey of needs for palliative care for terminally ill people in urban areas. *British Medical Journal* 2003 **327**(7408): 192–194.

Chapter 5

New models, new care

> What I think is always most important is respect for the person as an individual; respect for who they are and what has brought them through their lives to the place where they're at in terms of their culture, their faith, their environment.
> *Lesley Lawson*

In this chapter, we focus on the broad range of hospice and palliative care initiatives in Africa. The role of advocacy is acknowledged and attention is paid to developing services at the national level and in specific localities. A team approach is considered a central feature of palliative care, and this is explored in the African setting; so too is spiritual care—an important component that is grounded in the richness of African culture. Finally, we turn to paediatric care and the measures taken to deal with the rising number of HIV-infected children, orphans and child-headed families.

Advocacy

I joined the Diana Fund in May 2002 as an international advocacy officer for palliative care. My job was to persuade donors, in the UK and overseas, to support palliative care, because palliative care is very poorly funded. Now things are improving. When I joined, there were very few donors supporting palliative care and we thought it was good to have an advocacy officer to talk to donors, to encourage them to talk and to support palliative care. Then beyond that, to talk to government so that palliative care can be included in government policies, regulations and national health strategies, so that palliative care drugs can become available. Of course, that ties in with talking to health professionals' training institutions, so they can put palliative care in the curriculum. Also, trying to talk to NGOs who are not palliative care providers but doing HIV/AIDS work, to integrate palliative care into their work. **Faith Mwangi Powell—executive director, APCA; 14 November 2004**.

Back in November 2002, there was a meeting held in Cape Town for trainers involved in palliative care in Africa. It was convened and funded by the donor, The Princess of Wales Memorial Fund, and they got together palliative care trainers from South Africa, Zimbabwe, Kenya, Uganda and Tanzania. We met and we discussed issues around palliative care, particularly palliative care training in the respective countries, and we shared with each other what we were doing. That was an eye-opener for some of us—to see what other people were doing—but we were also looking at the wider impact and the wider provision of palliative care within Africa. As a group, we put together what we called the Cape Town Declaration, which was a declaration on our vision—and beliefs as well—for palliative care in Africa. We believed: that palliative care is a right to all people with an illness that's not responsive to curative treatment; that it was a right to everybody in

Africa; and that we were committed to trying to ensure drugs were accessible, including morphine, which isn't accessible in many countries; around training. Just around our commitment to palliative care. We felt very strongly that we wanted to put this in writing; that we wanted to sign our names to it so that we were committed to it; so that it wasn't just a paper exercise; so that, if nothing happened, we could come back to each other and say, 'Look, we were committed to this three years ago. Where have we got to? What's going on?' But also as an advocacy tool—so that countries where palliative care is just beginning could use it as an advocacy tool, saying that people are committed to the development of palliative care in the African region. Out of that meeting, and part of that Cape Town Declaration, was that we felt there was a role for a Pan-African Palliative Care Association where we could all work together to promote palliative care within the region. **Julia Downing— director, Mildmay International Study Centre, Kampala, Uganda; 2 June 2004.**

I'm a palliative nurse working with the Cameroon Baptist Convention. I work as a supervisor of the Prevention of Mother to Child Transmission Programme, which is part of the HIV/AIDS programme. In our service, we have an AIDS control programme, which looks at ways of prevention and support. We've come a long way with the prevention of mother to child transmission, and we now have support groups focusing on awareness. To talk about the country generally, I would say we have raised a lot of awareness, with a lot of NGOs and all private organizations taking part under the control of the Ministry of Health. The Minister of Health has been very supportive and receptive to our activities. Looking at where we are now and where we should be next, I would say that awareness has mostly been raised; now we realize that there is more need for care. We realize there is a need to start antiretroviral therapy, which the government strongly supports, and we also realize that palliative care will bring holistic care for all patients. As we see an increasing incidence of cancers and HIV, we feel this is the right time to get into palliative care. **Ndikintum George Mbeng—nurse, HIV/AIDS counsellor/trainer, Cameroon Baptist Convention Health Board; 4 June 2004.**

It took us some time to package the Cancer Society in Ghana and, God willing, on the 23rd of this month, the Head of District will formally inaugurate it. We've already got the registration certificate and the deputy executive director and I came to this conference [in Arusha, 2004] as the Ghanaian champions, to learn, and go back home and champion the cause of palliative care. Last month, we had our first sensitization and training of trainers programme. We had three Ugandan specialists in palliative care and two from the UK. They came and they did a wonderful job and the news spread about the nation; they are asking questions on palliative care. Then you come to HIV: we have a comprehensive HIV programme in Ghana, but minus palliative care. It is sad. We have morphine on prescription, but we need to engage in advocacy, we need to go and talk to our government and address all the health needs in an HIV programme. Fortunately we have a dynamic director of the Ghana AIDS Commission and we know he will listen to us. In the near future, we will initiate training, proper training of trainers, and then we'll spread it at three levels. We want to train the professional; we want to train the community staff, though at the roots level we have the community's health centres; and then we want to train the Red Cross and volunteers, and go into full-scale palliative care. We believe, and I strongly believe, there's a place for palliative care in Ghana, because we are going on the National Health Insurance Programme and this will reduce the funding of the National Health Programme. **Dr Vinolia Tonugble—physician and trustee of the Cancer Society of Ghana; 4 June 2004.**

My position in the association [HPCA] is really to promote palliative care throughout South Africa. One of the problems is that people don't really understand the concept of palliative care; they tend to think of it as either home-based care or it's care of the dying—and they don't see the big picture of what palliative care is. So it's really informing people of what this is, of getting the government on board. We've been very lucky. We've had somebody in government whose been a great promoter of the concept of palliative care—and HPCA—for a few years. He's not one of the really top-level guys, he's in a deputy director post, but he's just caught on to this idea of palliative care and we've worked very much with him. Of course we've worked with the Ministry, but we've had a lot of problems. A lot of it is the concept. They see HPCA as a very white, wealthy, middle-class organization and of course, if we look at our stats, the leaders of HPCA still tend to be from the white community; it's a historical fact. But actually the staff of HPCA, the volunteers, are predominantly from the previously disadvantaged groups in South Africa—and it's trying to get this picture across to people, and to try and get the government to not only put resources into palliative care but to include it in the continuum of care, and this they have done, which is very exciting; it's been included now from community, from prevention, through the clinics into the hospitals; it is baby steps, it's still right at the beginning. But we've also been able to set up a national task team to get together other role players in palliative care with the Department of Health. We called that meeting in Pretoria and now we have a working group which consists of about twenty people; but within that working group there is a steering committee of five chairs of task teams, and three of those chairs come from HPCA. One is Liz Gwyther, who is doing research and education; the other is Mpho Seboyane from Moretele Sunrise Hospice—who is looking at issues around caregivers because most of our care is provided by community care workers; and then of course, I'm doing paediatrics, no surprise. But then we have another task team looking at clinical care. We're meeting next month for two days—we've all got our basic plans and we've got our basic subcommittees together—to really look at how we're moving this forward. **Joan Marston—HPCA board member and founder of St Nicholas Children's Hospice Bloemfontein, South Africa; 21 September 2004.**

I think all I can say is: it is very difficult to describe in words hospice activities in resource-limited settings—very, very difficult. I can only encourage people to come and visit our programme. See it for themselves and capture it in their minds and hearts, and go and describe what they see for themselves. That is the best way I think I can describe what would be most useful to others. I invite as many people as possible to come and see what we are doing; it's easier for them to get to see that, than for me to go over there [abroad] and describe it. **Dr Bactrin Killingo—founder, chief executive and physician, Meru Hospice, Kenya; 2 June 2004.**

In terms of palliative care and AIDS: seropositivity and AIDS is a problem in our country as almost 10 per cent of our population is infected. This is why, for some years, we have been mobilizing our resources to try to fight against this infection. There is even one Ministry completely dedicated to this cause; so it shows how much of a problem it is. Concerning treating and caring for patients with AIDS, palliative care has not been well enough developed in my opinion and we, as neurologists, deal with many patients suffering from neuro-AIDS. Our wish would be that in the incoming programmes and future health developments, palliative care could be integrated as a complete part of care offered to persons living with AIDS. This is why we hope that in the three years to come, a maximum of professionals taking care of those persons will be sensitized; then we think that professionals should be educated and trained in palliative care in order to implement it. For sure there will be a need for many people to advocate in this direction towards governments, NGOs and other associations. But I do think that within the three next years we can at least sensitize and educate and begin to get things structured. **Professor Beugre Kouassi—neurologist, University of Abidjan-Cocody/Ministry of Health Cote d'Ivoire; 4 June 2004.**

Service developments

A macro view

I went to the World Pain Congress in 1996, following which I came back [to Nigeria] and got a group together in the University Teaching Hospital to start a palliative care team. That group metamorphosed into the Society for the Study of Pain in Nigeria, which is now a chapter of the

International Association for the Study of Pain, and I'm on the Council of the International Association for the Study of Pain. I also teach post-graduates, because we have a West African College of Surgeons and I'm on the Council of that and also I belong to the Faculty of Anaesthesia. So I am trying to use my expertise to spread the word round, to train and introduce palliative care. Right now, at Ibadan, we have a new group in the College of Medicine and we've introduced palliative care into the curriculum of medical students and nursing students. The proposal has been sent from the Faculty, it's now awaiting confirmation at the College level, so that once that is passed it can go into the curriculum. I visited Hospice Uganda, and with some assistance from the Diana Fund, my College, and individual funding, three of us from my group have now visited Hospice Uganda. We are working towards more capacity building in terms of training, and we're working towards having a training of trainers course, because we found that a lot of people—even the senior ones—have a lot of problem using opiates, and also with the concept of a multidisciplinary team approach to the management of medical problems.

So in terms of palliative care: right now we have a lot of individuals, oncologists, surgeons, physicians, just managing patients as best as they can. But regarding the holistic approach: we've just introduced that using a small clinic in the radiotherapy clinic and a group of us, two anaesthetists, one oncologist, one nurse and a psycho-oncologist who does counselling, we run a clinic there once a week. Patients on the ward are also referred to us, patients with terminal illness. **Professor Olaitan Soyannwo—dean of clinical sciences, College of Medicine, University of Ibadan, Nigeria; 4 June 2004.**

Island Hospice made a decision in the late '90s to move into the community instead of having hospice based in a place in town, in Harare. We moved to where the communities are, where hospice care could be provided to different communities. We started in one suburb in Harare then we moved on to two other areas. In one area, hospice is based at a hospital outpatients department about 27 kilometres outside of Harare. Hospice nurses there work alongside nurses and doctors advising patients at diagnosis. In Africa, we don't talk of end-of-life care because there's no adequate care before the end. You need to help professionals break bad news, to talk to patients about their condition, diagnosis and prognosis. They support staff and see patients at outpatient clinics; they provide home visits; they train community groups in that area—the community home-based care groups. We work very closely with the Red Cross, who provide good training for their volunteers—but again, we're grafting palliative care onto home-based care groups. So Island Hospice staff train Red Cross nurses in dealing with the terminally ill, and there's such a good partnership.

We had the project evaluation earlier this year, in February 2004, and it was encouraging to see that although there were challenges, we are moving in the right direction. Island continues to work with what is already in the community because we realize we can't do it all. We have to move into communities, see what's there, try and give the skills that we identify are missing, to improve the quality of care. In another suburb—where a group of people living with HIV and AIDS has been providing home-based care to that community—we were approached to provide training. Our nurses give support to these volunteers and train them before they go and see patients.

The other thing we are doing is to work closely with faith-based centres, whether they be the hospital or the health care communities of different faiths, because they are also responding to HIV and AIDS by developing their own home-based care groups. Again, we try and bring in the palliative care element, and the same issues arise: basic symptom control; communication; spiritual matters; factors that cause emotional pain; how to deal with children of parents who are dying, or children who are sick. **Sambulo Mkananzi– training manager, Island Hospice and Bereavement Service, Harare, Zimbabwe and board member APCA; 20 September 2004.**

My own belief is that for sustainability of hospices we have to become part of the formal health care system. It is true that at first, care of the dying was left to the NGOs and the communities, and hasn't been part of formal health care; and care of HIV patients in South Africa started just with the response of communities: the families of people who were suffering—and the neighbours of people who were suffering—were doing the initial work. The hospices have supported them in that and have trained them; and we've come up with this really effective model for palliative care and HIV/AIDS which is a standard not only to care for HIV patients, but has expanded the scope of practice.

Whereas we would go in to do the symptom control and the psychosocial and spiritual support, now we're also talking prevention. Now we're also doing treatment support, because our caregivers are the best treatment buddies—or what are being called in the formal health care system, *patient advocates*, because they've formed that relationship. We're also identifying the potential orphans. There are some wonderful bereavement programmes for children. The pre-bereavement work that is being done around the memory box concept that came out of Uganda is important—and the scope of practice in hospice has expanded to include food security and poverty alleviation. There is a wonderful programme that St Luke's Hospice instituted in conjunction with the UCT Institute of Ageing. It was a programme to empower grandparents. Firstly, doing home-based care for their children who are dying of AIDS, and then looking after the orphans, their grandchildren. Nobody was bringing in any income because the income-earning generation was the generation that was sick—and that was dying. So it was business skills, it was money management, it was home industry-type things that were done in this course, as well as AIDS awareness and care of people who are ill. At the end of that programme—I was at the certificate ceremony for the first group of grandparents who were trained—there was singing, and a wonderful rhythm and tradition that people have. Then one grandfather said, 'Please, let me translate this hymn because this is what you've done for us. The song is about the light of Jesus bringing love into our world, and what you have done is bring love and light into the dark world of HIV'. It was just such a moving experience. This group of grandparents have now formed their own NGO that they called 'Grandmothers Against Poverty and AIDS'—GAPA—and they've got their own shop and they're doing their income generation in their homes whilst caring for their grandchildren. And they have had this kind of economic empowerment, which is not anything that would have been a hospice function in the traditional model, but has become so in the new model. **Dr Liz Gwyther—HPCA board member; education and research co-ordinator, South Africa; 4 June 2004.**

I refused to go to Kenya without them getting in palliative morphine. I refused to go to Uganda without them bringing it in; they've got it in. Now these other countries need to make sure that would be the minimal thing that they would require before they really start palliative care, because the biggest fear of patients and even of health professionals, when we ask them, is severe pain coming towards death. That's the thing people fear the most and it's the thing that carers and families fear the most: to be dealing with pain which they can't control. It disrupts not only the patient, but the whole family. So this is the first essential I would see to bring palliative care into a country and after that, the rest will follow. **Dr Anne Merriman—founder and director, medical services and education, Hospice Africa Uganda; 9 March 2004.**

[The essence of hospice care?] What I think is always most important is respect for the person as an individual; respect for who they are and what has brought them through their lives to the place where they're at in terms of their culture, their faith, their environment—because we have in our care, people who have never known family in the way that we know it. We see people, women particularly, suffering what we would see as abuse; but for them it's the norm. We see people that have come from poor rural areas. At the other end of the spectrum we have people of great wealth, who are very sophisticated. We try and be to people in whatever situation they are in—whatever their background, whatever their journey has been, whatever their needs are—I think with a real acknowledgement of the fact that each and every one of us is an individual, is treasured in the image of God. And we need to seek what it is that's important to them rather than what is important for us.

If we want to serve—and we want to be the best we can be—we want to equip ourselves with all the knowledge that we need to be able to do the best in terms of the pain and symptom control; all of those things. But we fail if we lose sight of the fact that people will come to us with many different things in terms of education, in terms of ability, or how they—even culturally— deal with their emotions. How they think and feel is something we need to understand and we can't know it all in a classroom. It comes with experience. But the starting point, I think, is absolute respect for the human-ness of each one of us, and to let the people that we meet teach us what it is they need in order to cope in the situation in which they find themselves, whatever that is; and for us to know we have our limitations. For instance: the resource may well be a traditional healer if that's the persons need. Where do we direct them for that? We have our bag of knowledge, but we're not just dictating how we think they should be coping with this journey at this time; it's very much a discovery of what their need is. **Lesley Lawson—co-founder, St Francis Hospice, Port Elizabeth, South Africa; 26 April 2004.**

The local level

I came out to Muheza long-term in September 2001 because my husband was going to be the medical superintendent of Teule Hospital. He was going to take over from Dr Elizabeth Hills, who was still here at that stage, and I had recently finished a Diploma in Palliative Medicine from Cardiff. I was very fired up with a great love of palliative medicine, but I came to Teule without a job description, with ideas of my own about setting up palliative care. Teule is a district designated hospital which means it's half mission: the mission is the United Society for the Propagation of the Gospel—which is an Anglican Mission—and a government hospital, a district hospital. Here, Dr Hills had had the foresight to start a small team of palliative care: there was one nurse and one nursing auxiliary, and that nurse had already been to England to have six weeks' training through the Hereford–Muheza link; this was Mary, and she had been out and worked with me at St Michael's Hospice in Hereford, so she already knew what palliative care was. And this little team was going through the wards with a bucketful of equipment, looking at patients who were referred to them who were on the point of dying, and they were very much looking at the very terminally ill patients. There was also a Department of HIV that were running from a converted container. It was dreadful. The temperature went up to goodness knows what. There were just two rooms in this container: one where people sat and waited, and one where people had their counselling. There were two counsellors and the District AIDS Co-ordinator and they'd been doing that since 1992. So this little HIV team were running in the hospital with very little space.

So, I think it was the first week of October, I called a meeting and I said, 'OK, we're going to form a hospice here that's going to be for terminal patients—for cancer, for HIV—who's interested? Let's have the whole of the HIV team, let's have the whole of the palliative care team and other representatives who might be interested'. The hospital physio came along, the hospital chaplain came along, one of the auxiliaries from the TB Department came along, and we had our first meeting—and we discussed what we should be called. I wanted to be called 'St Thomas's Hospice'—because I thought there were lots of doubts about what we were doing, and also I trained at St Thomas's—that was voted out. Everything was done very democratically. They said, 'We want to be Muheza Hospice Care'. So that was where the name came from. The District AIDS Co-ordinator, who is a very far-thinking person and was Chairman of Tanga AIDS Working Group, could see that this could be an NGO and could attract outside funding, and he said 'We need to be recognized outside the hospital, therefore we need a proper constitution'. He was the one who really made us set up as an independent NGO. So at that meeting we set our constitution, we set our chairman, our officers, and we decided that we would apply for independent status as an NGO within the country. So that was done very, very early on. **Dr Karilyn Collins—medical director, Muheza Hospice Care, Teule Hospital, Muheza, Tanzania; 7 November 2004.**

We didn't have any funds initially at all, and I would never advise anybody to go about it the way we did, because we rushed in where angels fear to tread; but our husbands were very generous because they were letting us use their cars and paying for the petrol. I remember the first time a patient died and her husband said in lieu of flowers he'd give us a donation. There was incredible excitement, and we bought a firm mattress with it. Then as donations came in we bought equipment and, yeah, it was just amazing, you know. When I think we're sitting now with this massive budget of close to five million rand a year that it costs us to run our show, how it happened. Of course, we were working out of each other's homes, and I mentioned the need for a place for storing our equipment. How thrilled we were that we were acquiring so much, but it was difficult. I remember I actually had a commode that had a nice wooden lid. When it wasn't in use it had been in my lounge with a thing of flowers on it as if it was a coffee table!

I didn't know any doctors here [in Port Shepstone], but my husband happened to play golf with one of the clinic sisters' husbands. So she introduced me to the first doctor—well to some-body who really knew the sort of medical professionals in the area. Then, when P. had a bout of nausea and vomiting, I 'phoned her GP who I'd never heard of, and he came around. I felt a bit embarrassed because he didn't know me or anything; and here I was almost like an impostor with his patient. I said, 'If I'm not mistaken, the nausea is likely to recur. I am a professional nurse and if it is OK with you, if you'd like to leave me a repeat prescription for the anti-emetic, I could get here perhaps before you next time she needs medication?' He was amazingly receptive. He actu-ally ended up being our first medical director, and he also was a very respected, senior kind of general practitioner in a small-town area—and we needed an advocate like him to get other doctors on board.

Perhaps an important thing to say is: like all the hospices in South Africa, we had inherited the British model and that was the hallmark. Very soon I realized that the people in our part of the world who had the greatest need for pain and symptom control, and holistic care, lived in the outly-ing areas. And they were black people. We were a group of middle-class white women at that stage, you know—all volunteers—and it just didn't make sense to have this wonderful little, comfortable, service for people—who certainly needed it—but not nearly as badly as others who had virtually no access to health care at all. **Kath Defilippi—chairperson of APCA; HPCA board member and chief executive officer, South Coast Hospice, Port Shepstone, South Africa; 5 June 2004.**

I'm a retired surgeon. I was head of the department of surgery at the large hospital in Chatsworth since its inception in 1969. It was as a result of my experience that we felt the need to establish a hospice. Having done an audit of the hospital records, we found there were a large number of cancer patients who would have been deemed to be incurable but who were lost to the hospital. So they, obviously, were left alone, and isolated and possibly neglected. There was tremendous community support for hospice in Chatsworth. This hospice was established in 1991, and it has grown considerably since. We now have a very busy domiciliary unit with an average of over 250 patients—almost all cancer patients—in the service. We have a day care centre which is very popular. An average of 30 patients visit—these are ambulant patients—and we have an inpa-tient unit of 10 beds. I might mention that we take into our programme patients who are not necessarily terminally ill, but they are deemed to be incurably ill. We find that very, very useful, because patients become very familiar with the hospice environment. So eventually when they do become terminally ill, they come into a familiar environment, and this is extremely useful. They're with friends. Here again, traditionally—I might mention the large majority are patients of Indian origin—it's traditional for patients to want to die at home. And this can happen with our hospice: to be at home for the final few days. We encourage this. **Dr C. N. Pillay—president, Chatsworth Hospice, Durban, South Africa; 12 August 2004.**

I went to Swaziland to support my husband and I thought, 'Well what on earth am I going to do here? I'm not used to this sort of life'. So I thought, 'OK, I've got some background in palliative care, why don't I offer? So I rang round the hospitals asking did they have any knowledge of palliative care and people said, 'What's palliative care? What's terminal care? They just had no idea whatsoever, so I just thought, 'Oh well, I suppose I'd better go on with my first hobby which is reading'; and that's what I was prepared to do—and have a nice holiday in Swaziland. Then as soon as I got to the library, as people do in Swaziland, there were questions being asked. It was a lady called Kay Knowles who was doing a stint in the library, and she said, 'What's your background?' and I told her, and she said, 'Well, let's set up a hospice'. I said, 'I'm sorry, I don't think this is quite me'. And she said, 'Oh when things don't happen in Swaziland, we make them happen and I'll help you'. **Stephanie Wyer—founder, Swaziland Hospice at Home, Swaziland; 1 July 2003.**

In Nairobi, we started providing the service and training in 1990. In 1994, it was a milestone for us because we started to provide a day care service; that is something that we had to plan for. By day care service, I mean on a Thursday; it is specifically on a Thursday. Those patients who are not too ill and are able to come to the hospice spend the whole day with us. It is a very good experience for them because the patients share and interact with one another. They don't feel isolated in their suffering. It gives them the opportunity to be seen, to be reviewed by the clinical team, and it is a respite for the main carers. It is also a good opportunity for the volunteers to do something for the patients. They like it. They do the shopping, the cooking, the serving of the meals and they interact with them. So it's a rich experience not only for the patients and families but also for the carers as well. For us that is a milestone. **Brigid Sirengo—chief executive officer, Nairobi Hospice, Kenya; 2 June 2004.**

St Luke's [Cape Town] at that time was growing. I started having 30 to 40 patients from the Constantia area going into the poorer areas. And they started a new hospice, a community hospice, in a totally new area which St Luke's hadn't been involved with. I immediately asked for a transfer to start this new hospice in the Grassy Park Area. That was eight years ago and I'm still in that area. It's the area that I live in. It's the area that I'm familiar with; people I'm familiar with—people's habits, people's culture—and I actually feel less stress working in the area that I know. St Luke's is not well known in the area. We've had to do a lot of fieldwork, educating the public; had to have a lot of public relations talks—at meetings, at church groups, at mosques; and I think St Luke's is always welcome in the homes. I get a great satisfaction at seeing what a difference we make.

The patient must be told the prognosis. But by the time we get to the patient, they've either forgotten, or they've not heard, or they need clarification. That takes up a lot of our first assessment meeting—telling patients about the disease. I spend quite a bit of time sitting with the patient, drawing the body, showing the part that's been affected, and giving the information I have. I actually try and draw it for them. **Jeanette Daniels—community palliative care nurse, Grassy Park (St Luke's Hospice), Cape Town, South Africa; 6 August 2004.**

A team approach

International perspective

We can see hospice [Africa Uganda] now expanding into our third objective which is to help other African countries start their own hospice. We're actually seeing more and more of that now. We're looking at having a team that's dedicated to going and training in other countries and perhaps that same team doing the follow-up. So that would be a mobile and travelling team. We're seeing more responsibility put on us by the Government and other groups to train and to go out. So I think we're ambassadors; but we still have to make sure that we have a well run, exemplary service, so that's why I want to remain small in terms of the service we're providing. That service is also a place where we welcome more and more people to come and be with us and learn by apprentice-ship, as it were—then go back and do the same. So I think in the next five years or so we see ourselves remaining very much as we are, consolidating what we have, but then reaching out to more and more people. **Dr Lydia Mpanga Sebuyira—director, clinical services, Hospice Africa Uganda; 21 September 2004.**

Community focus

It's always something that's amazed me: that women from communities which are often so poor themselves come forward. We give them the training and empower them to do the caring, and they are willing to serve their community. It's a humbling experience to talk to some of these care-givers—many who earn very little, some earn nothing at all—who work completely as volunteers; and the fact that they are willing to get out there and do what is a very difficult job: to confront illness and death and sadness and poverty day after day. I can think of fewer things that are more difficult to do. I am just humbled by their willingness to get involved. **Sue Cameron—HPCA board member and manager of the Centre for Palliative Learning, Pretoria Sungardens Hospice, South Africa; 26 April 2005.**

The devastating economy and the high numbers of our patients infected by HIV and AIDS forced our country to embark on home-based care. On one hand it's a challenge; but it was a good thing because the communities responded very well to this overwhelming challenge which we are facing. Hospitals could not accommodate all the patients and what it meant was that there was diversity in the care which was being given by different groups. Some will just go in and pray—and they call themselves a home-based care group; some are relieving the patient groaning in pain; some will go and sweep the home or do some gardening—and call themselves home-based care. Because of this diversity, it has forced us to look at the standards of care which is being given. So we developed standards of care through a multidisciplinary team from different organizations who were experienced in palliative care and home-based care, and so that document is completed. What we are doing now is creating awareness of these home-based standards. We hope it will be a tool, an advocacy tool for best practices; to identify the gaps. Then training will come in, mentor-ing will come in, follow-up visits will come in—and it will also advocate for resources. So although it is a challenge, I think we have grown, because we are trying to get quality care right through to the community. **Eunice Garanganga—clinical and technical adviser, Hospice Association of Zimbabwe (HOSPAZ); 20 September 2004.**

Our programme consists of a team, based at the hospital, which is giving the leadership as well as the medical back-up for the care that we're providing at home. This team meets and trains vol-unteers in the communities around us. Those volunteers then become the weekly visitors to the patients that we're following as a hospice/palliative care programme. Right now, at any given time, we're carrying a group of about 300-plus patients in this programme. So a small team of medical/nursing staff support about 120 volunteers out in our surrounding communities and work with them to provide the ongoing care in the home. What that consists of in the home is: in addition to simply a ministry of presence, of being with people and being in prayer with them, it's also a caring where we have symptom relief. We also have in Tanzania—and in our programme, for about a year and a half now—the availability of oral morphine. So increasingly we're able to provide that for patients who are in pain. It really is a holistic outreach in palliative care. It's completely community based, in that all of our work is done in the homes of our patients. Some patients in hospital are introduced to and acquainted with the programme in hospital, but we don't have an inpatient component of our programme. **Dr Mark Jacobson—medical director, Selian Hospital, Arusha, Tanzania; 4 June 2004.**

Interdisciplinary approach

I think perhaps I should say that the fundamentals of hospice and palliative care, in terms of an interdisciplinary approach, remain essential, whatever the context we're working in is. It's just how it's arranged. So in some areas, it's not possible for one non-profit organization to employ the whole range of interdisciplinary professionals. Then they've got to access them from somewhere else—and we are thrilled that we've been able to do that, and that we've now got doctors with a qualification in palliative medicine. We've actually employed one part-time medical officer for the last couple of years, thanks to the Elton John's AIDS Foundation, but most of our doctors are really working in the formal health care sector and they do give our patients a great deal of care.

We run a very small back-up inpatient unit. Every day a doctor does a ward round there and is available on call for that day; only one doctor is employed part-time. So I think to emphasize the need for proper, effective medical coverage, you've got to have proper diagnosis, everything's still got to be treated. Taking the medical implications seriously is very important. Also, the psychosocial issues are enormous, and the need for support and counselling; and I think one of the things that I will be saying tomorrow in my presentation [at the AGM, 2004] is the challenge of the transference of skills.

At South Coast Hospice and in South Africa generally, we've transferred a lot of skills that are traditionally done in the First World by professionals, to professionally supervised non-professionals who are highly trained and supervised. We now, I believe, have to go another step: we've got to transfer skills from trained, employed, community caregivers to the community at large in terms of reaching the coverage that's required. One of the areas where we've started doing that is with memory work for children. So I think we're back to balancing quality and coverage. It's applying the principles of good palliative care, but somehow working out a way of doing it in a viable fashion. **Kath Defilippi—chairperson of APCA; HPCA board member and chief executive officer, South Coast Hospice, Port Shepstone, South Africa; 5 June 2004.**

Although there's line managers, supervisors and directors—there's very little hierarchical emphasis. We work as a team. So if there's a failed bus service and staff can't get in to work on time, then it doesn't matter who you are, we all go down and either feed babies, change them or do whatever it takes. For us, the children are our clients and their well-being comes first. Once in a while, we have what we call a clean-up day. Everybody comes dressed casually and it means scrubbing down fridges, scrubbing walls or whatever; and again, that for us is the team working together in practice. **Bonnie Haack—director, Human Resources and Training, Cotlands, Johannesburg, South Africa; 11 August 2004.**

Social work perspective

Coming from a non-medical background, I have appreciated here at [Highway] Hospice the fact that we have interdisciplinary team meetings four days a week. I feel I've learnt a lot from these meetings because you can ask questions you don't understand. It's a learning process. It's also finding out what's happening with the patient. It's also support for each other. We have a meeting once a week with all our home care sisters as well, when referrals are made to the social workers. Also, when new staff start at Highway Hospice—and volunteers—they are able to attend a course through our Education Department which runs over a period of 12 weeks. I've found that was beneficial because you could deal with your own feelings about death and dying, and you also had people from the community. You had volunteers, and you had staff in that course. So you learnt what their experiences were—and that's helped me in terms of assisting the Education Department and being able to give back in that way.

Challenges for me as a social worker: often I've found it difficult because sometimes my work is so short term. I'm dealing with pre-bereavements, so often I'm seeing families for a short time. Sometimes there's a high turnover of patients so I find that difficult sometimes. It's also, I think, difficult in terms of the breakdown of family life, particularly now with AIDS. The family structure is such that children don't know the normalities of the family unit; we're dealing with the mother, the father and the child who have AIDS.

I can remember a little boy of 10 being in our unit. He was just 10 and he had experienced the death of eight family members at that age. He was the saddest child I have ever met. I almost felt, could we even get through to him? The only living relative he had was his grandfather, and he was obviously not being well looked after; there were problems. We were eventually able to arrange a foster care placement because we noticed the only time this child ever showed any expression was when we talked about a person that was in his church, a lady that he had obviously identified with, and she was screened for foster care placement. She agreed, and they actually looked after this little boy. For me it was wonderful when he left here. He left in a wheelchair—he couldn't walk—and he came back literally bouncing in here to say 'hello' to us. It was about emotional love and care and just being part of a normal family. That family also learned so much through him, through his illness, and, after his death, they have become very involved talking about AIDS, forming support groups. That was good.

Another highlight for me was when a man was admitted to our unit. He had been a day centre patient for many years. He was a good ambassador for hospice. He used to tell people not to fear hospice and tell them about his experiences. When he was admitted to our unit, he was terminal and he expressed his sadness that he wouldn't live long enough to see his daughter graduating. I 'phoned the university and explained the position. Although they couldn't actually do a graduation outside of the university, the Vice-Chancellor agreed to come to hospice with her robes on and take pictures with this man's daughter. Within a short time, the whole family was hearing about it. The son suddenly said he's coming from Johannesburg. It really was a very moving experience. The father actually insisted on getting dressed in a suit. He was very weak but he insisted on it. He had to stay in the bed—he was too weak to even stand—but it's something I'll never forget. It was won-derful. And yes, there've been difficult situations. But I can say we have made a difference in the lives of some of the people. The journey is sometimes difficult but we feel we do make a difference. **Rosemary Schütler, social worker, Highway Hospice, Durban, South Africa; 8 August 2004.**

Counsellor

Unfortunately the term 'counselling' has many, many connotations and in Uganda there is actually no recognized role of the counsellor. So there's no governing body around counselling. But what we're talking about generally is not counselling perhaps as we know it in the UK—when we're looking at big theories—it's more round communication skills. It's more communicating in an appropriate way, not being afraid to communicate with somebody who's dying, not being afraid to talk about whatever is culturally appropriate for them in their setting.

So we have to work within the tribal traditions and the tribal cultures. In Uganda, as in many of the African countries, there's many different tribes and each tribe has their own beliefs about death. In one tribe, they will talk about death, in another tribe they won't. In some tribes, the moment somebody dies you don't talk about them ever again, because you don't talk about the dead; in another tribe it's OK to. So we get people, when we're doing our training, to explore what is culturally appropriate in their particular community and to work with that. We're not saying, 'Well you must talk to everybody about the fact that they're dying' if that isn't done in that culture. **Julia Downing—director, Mildmay International Study Centre, Kampala, Uganda; 2 June 2004.**

Home care sister

I found such a change in the home care because, starting off as the co-ordinator, things were just really basic to start with: answering the 'phone, passing on the contact. But as the years have passed, families have brought difficulties, social problems have increased, our way of medicating has changed. Palliative care taking off has definitely changed the home visit for the sister. Before, it was a case virtually of just going to hold your hand and doing some counselling; but now, the sisters are very well trained and they do a lot of work as far as counselling, education and anything to go with palliative care is concerned.

I find today a lot of calls that come through on the telephone are for other resources. Everybody seems to 'phone hospice if they have a problem. So we have to build up quite a big resource base in order to give the person the right contact, who to 'phone. We never send them away without an alternative. AIDS has definitely made an impact on the home nursing care. When we started off with the cancers, it was basic medicines, basic nursing. As our AIDS patients increased, the symptoms were different, the counselling was different. We had a problem as far as culture goes in the acceptance of the disease, the disclosure of the disease. So with the advent of AIDS, it really has changed the nursing for the home sister. We are very lucky to have a proficient palliative care doctor because we really go beyond the call of duty as far as looking after the patients. Dr Sarah [Fakroodeen] did mention a couple of success stories, and this is happening all the time. Doctors are beginning to accept our care. We find they are 'phoning for information as far as pain control goes, or they are referring patients to hospice for specific symptoms. **Rosemary de Jager—home care co-ordinator, Highway Hospice, Durban, South Africa; 8 August 2004.**

Physician

Getting palliative medicine recognized as an essential part of medicine is important, particularly where we are dealing with oncologists and specialists in other fields. Over this weekend, a patient of mine—I've been his GP for many years and he's got cancer of the lung—had a chest pain and they rang the physician. He was immediately admitted into intensive care and given oxygen and the whole works, with a cardiac monitor and all that. When I saw him, I had to explain to the physician who was treating him that the chest pains were due to his cancer; he needed palliative care and some painkillers rather than keeping him in intensive care and monitoring him.

Another challenge is patient care: symptom relief—bringing comfort and relief to that patient. But I think the biggest challenge is the transition you have to get the patient to make: from fighting death to literally accepting death, finding peace in it. And also, getting the patient's family to come to terms and let go. To realize they have had some very good times with the patient but now the time is coming where they must make the best of what they have and not expect cure any more. **Dr Sarah Fakroodeen—palliative care physician, Highway Hospice, Durban, South Africa; 8 August 2004.**

Caring for staff

One of the things that we are passionate about is the care of our staff. We call it 'supervision'. We have a professional person, not on our staff, who has a doctorate in social science. She's an excellent counsellor and facilitator, and our staff are compelled to meet her on a monthly basis in a group situation. They also have access to her in between if they need support on something that might have happened within the month. That session is to be used, not so much for personal therapy, but for the kind of stuff that comes up in their day-to-day work with patients. As they look back over the month, was it a death that was difficult? What was it that drained them emotionally?

In between, of course, we have regular daily ward rounds. For instance, in our unit, we have weekly meetings with our home care team where patients are discussed in terms of their symptoms and their needs. It's also an opportunity to say: how was I feeling as I left this family? To have an opportunity to weep if they need to; to be angry; just let it out—and there would be support from within the team. Then there is professional support from somebody who can be really objective with them—to challenge them, empathize with them.

We also have what we call stress days once a month. It's not a holiday. It's not a sick day. There's just a day off to take. You have to take it within the month, but take it you must. Also, through our in-service training we are continually looking at ways to help people balance lives. We talk a lot about balancing our lives. For example, holidays. Staff are not allowed to accumulate their holidays, they must be taken regularly. And we have parties. We party together sometimes and we pray together. If we're not caring for our staff then we're nowhere. We're caring for the people—but if we're not caring for the people that care for the people, then I don't believe we're doing what we should be doing and want to do. **Lesley Lawson—co-founder, St Francis Hospice, Port Elizabeth, South Africa; 26 April 2004.**

Spiritual care

Speaking from my own background as an African person, and also from what I see and from what I hear in our own countries or communities: spirituality is there but it's not like the Western culture when you talk about spirituality. The body's there, the soul is there, but there is another component which is connected to our ancestors, connected to our background, really. For me, doing palliative care and trying to realize that people are different, I think it is just taking people where they are and acknowledging our differences. Just trying to accommodate that and have open communication whatever the poor believe. It's their beliefs and their values. I try and say that a person is valuable no matter where they come from, no matter what their beliefs, and not to impose our own. So being health care providers we try and accommodate that. We might not do it as effectively as in other countries, because in other countries I see a spiritual person is employed to do that. In Africa, our nurses and social workers do the work at home, and if we need help we might then go out and find other people who are more experienced in that kind of field.

In the African context people bring their own rituals and beliefs. You might find somebody who will say, 'Well I think I need to go and appease the spirits and go and brew beer'. Brewing beer is a ritual which is done to appease the spirits. You can give beer for thanksgiving; just to thank your spirits, or to find out what is it you have done wrong and why you've got this ailment. Then you can brew when somebody's died. It's as if you are just saying, 'Well, take your child'; sending the soul to where it belongs, which is the ancestors. People might go and brew beer and come back—because they have had that dialogue. Otherwise, if you don't have that dialogue, normally they disappear and they don't come back. So that dialogue is crucial, yes. It is very important in our care, these spiritual issues. **Eunice Garanganga—clinical and technical adviser, Hospice Association of Zimbabwe (HOSPAZ); 20 September 2004.**

Spiritual care plays a large and very important part in our programme. We believe it's possible—certainly with our Hindu patients—to anticipate the dying process and prepare the patient for this with the mantras and the prayers. The patients are taken through this—it's extremely useful—and this is presented to the patient when they reach the stage of acceptance. When the terminal stage eventually arrives, the patient is reminded of the prayers he needs to think about. Eventually, he ideally will die with the thought of his deity in his mind, and this promises him salvation—as in the Christian faith. In Hinduism, it's getting towards moksha and liberation, and we are promoting this because of our interest in spiritual care. We have recently completed a series of workshops on the perspectives of the various mainstream faiths on spirituality in hospice; in particular—dying and death and preparing the patient for this, and we've found it extremely useful. There appears to be a common thread running through all the faiths, and hopefully we'll have this compiled into a small booklet. **Dr C.N. Pillay—president, Chatsworth Hospice, Durban, South Africa; 12 August 2004.**

[Scott Peck] puts people into four spiritual stages.[1] Stage one: being like a child who actually knows nothing at all about God. Stage two—which a lot of children are still in—is where everything is quite concrete. You approach God through structures and the structures have to be in place for you to worship God. So it's all about going to church. If you don't go to church, or the mosque, or whatever is your form of religion, you can't talk to God. Stage three is where people start questioning—and that's where a lot of teenagers are. They start questioning what they've been taught as children, they start finding out about other religions and wondering, 'Does God really exist?' perhaps adults, too, who move from one religion to another or change faith. Stage three and stage four are where somebody becomes more and more mature, at peace in their relationship with God. God does not necessarily have to be found through a structure. There is a personal relationship and for lots of people that comes—we've seen this happen—as they come closer to death. They might have come through the struggles of stage three but as they come to peace with their diagnosis and the fact that their life is shorter, patients might also come to terms with their relationship with God. Where they come to a stage of acceptance and peace: that's stage four.

We try and make a [spiritual] assessment by asking people, 'What does God mean to you? How do you relate to God? Somebody might say to you, 'I relate to God through church and prayer'. 'Do you talk to God on your own?' that sort of thing. You hope at the end you'll have an understanding of where they are. It's a very difficult assessment and we are still going through discussions about how we can assess spirituality. Quite often you can't assess it in one sitting. As you get to know your patient they open up and they're able to talk to you more about their faith. Some people are very open and they'll say, 'God is real to me'. They might be able to relate to you some religious experiences. Some people tell you they've had visions of God, or a conversion experience, or a healing experience, different things like this; those statements help you.

We also noticed that people change. There's a spiritual journey that people go along, even as we are looking after them. Sometimes we have people for several months, or even years, and you can see them going through different stages. You can see them going back and forth; it's never a static thing. So even as health professionals, we try and keep our minds open; to see where a person is; to recognize how is this going to help me to help them on their spiritual journey. And part of that is to see the interaction between the patient's insight into their disease, diagnosis and prognosis, and their spiritual stage and awareness. For example, we might find that someone who hasn't accepted they have cancer, or that the cancer is very advanced and they may die soon, may not actually be doing the spiritual work that goes along with, 'Am I dying', and 'am I dying soon? Am I ready to meet my maker? They might not do that if they don't know where they are in terms of their disease. But, as they come to terms with that, they might go through the stages of 'God doesn't love me. How could he let me go through this? and all of that. So we try and help them. We ask, 'Do you want to speak to somebody else about this?' And if they want to we can contact a priest or an Imam. Sometimes they want to pray with us so we pray with them; it's very much an individual thing. **Dr Lydia Mpanga Sebuyira—director, clinical services, Hospice Africa Uganda; 21 September 2004.**

Paediatric care

I'd always had a great deal of interest in caring for the dying in the wards that I'd worked in and read a lot of the works of Cicely Saunders. But I lived in Bloemfontein. There was no hospice movement there and when the hospice started, it was started by a Methodist Minister. I went along as a volunteer and I worked as a volunteer relief nurse and as a caregiver and I did that for about 18 months. When they needed a full-time hospice nurse they asked me if I would take on that position. So I went in as a hospice nurse, which is still my favourite role. I still say 'I'm going back to it after all this is over'. Then I went on to become the director of the hospice; and then founded the Children's Hospice when we started seeing so many children with HIV being referred to the children's programmes.

I just felt there needed to be a special programme for children. They tended to get tacked on to the end of the adult programmes and although they always receive beautiful care, there was nothing that was specifically child focused. I was fortunate enough to have a very, very responsive Department of Health. I went to the Head of Health and I said to him 'Prof, we really need a place where we can care for children; it could be the centre of a children's hospice programme' and I really actually thought he'd say, 'Nice try Joan, good luck'. But he didn't. He said to me 'Joan, you're right. You actually do need that'. So the Department of Health provided a house for the children's hospice which is now an inpatient treatment unit and is much too small. We have 18 beds there, six day care centres and a programme that reaches 750 children in home care; so it's a very big programme. But I was just very lucky living in a very supportive community and having a Department of Health that actually caught the vision and came along with us. So that's really how I got involved. **Joan Marston—HPCA board member and founder of St Nicholas Children's Hospice Bloemfontein, South Africa; 21 September 2004.**

We started children's day care because the children of the patients—call them orphans and vulnerable children, or infected and affected children—were roaming the streets because there's no care. One little one even ran in front of a motor vehicle and got killed. So we thought, 'Well, we have to do something'. So we sent 10 of our community care workers for an early development training course so that they were equipped to help care for these little ones. We do ask that the children that come are at least potty trained. So we don't contend with the very little ones and that makes caring a little easier. **Barbara Campbell-Ker—executive director, Hospice Association of the Witwatersrand, South Africa; 11 August 2004.**

I started the hospice in 1999 and renovated the old stables as rooms for the HIV/AIDS patients. The hospice is 40-bedded; I take 20 adults and 20 children. The ward for the children is empty most of the time due to the fact that children don't want to separate from each other, even if they're sick. We will only take a child in when the child is fast dying, just to separate the child from the others.

We've got about ten projects. One of them takes the orphan children as well as those who are underprivileged. We have just finished building a day care centre crèche for 200 children. Why did we do that? Because we have about 468 child-headed households. These homes are run by children. So we take the little ones into the crèche and give a chance for those who are looking after them to go to school. We fetch the children in the morning and bring them back home in the afternoon.

At present I'm building them houses. I've got houses from Holland. These are pre-fabricated houses—it's a two-room house—for those children who haven't got houses, where their parents left them without a house. The container brings 15 at a time, and I'm going to get 215 of these houses. We've already started putting them up. **Sr Priscilla Dlamini—founder, Holy Cross Hospice, Gingindlovu, South Africa; 12 August 2004.**

The care continues around the child and then it continues at home. What we have realized is that, once we go into the home of an HIV-positive child, we sort of adopt the family because they are destitute. You can't see a child that is [HIV] positive and say, 'I'll give you food, clothing and treatment', and leave the family. So we adopt that family as a whole. We have support groups for them; they meet twice a month when they share their problems and advise each other, and then our social worker will help arrange different types of grants, or apply for a grant for the child. **Stella Dubazana—child care manager, Cotlands Hospice, Johannesburg, South Africa; 11 August 2004.**

The memory box concept is being accepted fully by the social workers. The volunteers are having lots of training delivered by the hospice and we are using it quite successfully with children. But what is behind it is a very specialized therapy. South Coast Hospice is having a three-day work-shop next week. There are representatives from the hospice that are going in order to get more training, then they'll train the other caregivers here. We find there are hundreds of children that have been orphaned through the HIV/AIDS crisis, and we have to see them in groups.

The aim of the memory box is to help the child cope with the death of the loved one—and through painting and the collection of valuable little items that belonged to the loved one, to come to terms with the grief. I think with a lot of families, unless they are assisted at the correct time, they carry these problems into other areas of their life. We find it affects their schoolwork, their relationships with their siblings and with the community. There's a lot of aggression and inner sadness that seems to be perpetuated and it comes out in other forms which may not be acceptable to society. **Goonam Jacob—social worker, Highway Hospice, Durban, South Africa; 8 August 2004.**

Another aim of the memory box is that it gives the child a sense of identity because, as they grow up—or even as an AIDS orphan—the child will obviously ask the question: Who am I? Where did I come from? So, ideally, the memory box is started to enable the living parents or grandparents to give the child something—so that in future they can look at a photograph or at a little item (like we have our memories and want to look back) so they feel that they weren't just fostered or sent to a home without any recognition of 'who I am'. Even in the most rural poverty areas, where perhaps there isn't anything materialistic for the mother to put into the memory box (sometimes it's just a stone that she has held in her hand), the caregiver will write a little note and say, 'This stone, when you hold it in your hand, remember your mummy has also held it'. In some of the areas, the community caregivers will take a photograph. If the mother wants a photograph taken, that will be done and put in the memory box—and the granny, and the children, and also the little house, no matter how humble it is, so that child, as they grow older will think, 'Well, I am. I was someone. I'm not just an AIDS orphan. I had a mother, and my mother did remember me before she died'. I think that's what so special about the memory box. **Karen Hinton—chairperson, Hospice Association of KwaZulu Natal and quality assurance adviser, Highway Hospice, Durban: South Africa; 8 August 2004.**

I think one of the great problems is that we're scared of talking of a life beyond this life to children. We're scared about talking about it to other people as well, it's not just to children—but we don't want children to know about death because we think death is frightening. We fear it and we have all the guilt and everything that goes along with being adult. The children have a very sort of straightforward view of the afterlife and they'll talk about it quite easily. I think it's also a matter of love, of bringing a presence of love into their lives and telling them that's what the afterlife is as well; that's what heaven is. It's love; and if they can experience it here it's going to be even greater where they're going to.

It's listening to their stories. Children often in their stories will talk about some fears that they have of death, fears of where their parents have gone to because their parents have died. Will they see them again? Will they be cared for? Looking at their paintings, at their drawings, what are they telling us there? What are they telling us when they're just playing on their own or singing? It's just really being very aware and also bringing the comforting power of prayer into their lives. And we really have cases where the children, when they're dying, the first person they want is Father Keith. They say, 'Please call Father Keith; he must come and pray for me', and they experience that power of prayer. They'll also talk. We've had children talk about dreaming of their parents who've died or feeling their presence, and I think a lot of it then is allowing the child the freedom and the right to speak about this and not saying, 'Oh that was just a dream', or 'You're imagining things', of actually allowing them to express their spiritual feeling. Of course when you get to older children it becomes more difficult because they think like adults and they go through all the emotions that an adult goes through. Then, it's really dealing with those emotions but keeping on assuring them of love. At the bottom of everything that's what it is isn't it? **Joan Marston—HPCA board member, founder of St Nicholas Children's Hospice Bloemfontein, South Africa; 21 September 2004.**

References

1 For an exposition of his views on the stages of spiritual growth see: Scott Peck M. *The Different Drum*. London: Arrow, 1990: 186.

Part 3

Hospice–palliative care service development in Africa: countries approaching integration

In Africa, there are 21 countries in which we were unable to identify any hospice–palliative care development; 11 countries in which capacity building activities are under way; 11 countries with localized service provision; and four countries where hospice palliative care services are approaching a measure of integration with mainstream services providers. We now report on developments in these latter three categories, beginning with the group of countries approaching integration. Individual reports are presented for each country in each category, using the standard template developed by the International Observatory on End of Life Care.

The countries of Kenya, South Africa, Uganda and Zimbabwe are categorized as 'approaching integration' (Fig.1). In these countries, hospice–palliative care services are characterized by: a countrywide critical mass of activists; a range of providers and service types; a broad awareness of palliative care on the part of both health professionals and local communities; a measure of integration of palliative care services with mainstream service providers; the availability of strong, pain-relieving drugs; an impact of palliative care upon policy; the development of recognized education centres; academic links forged with universities; the performance of research; and the existence of a national association.

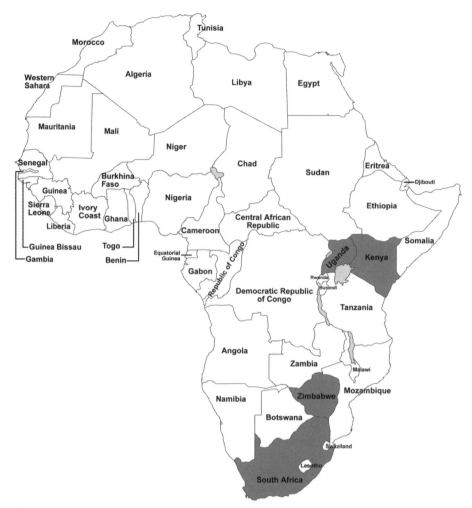

Fig. 1 Countries in Africa where hospice–palliative care services are approaching integration with mainstream service providers.

Chapter 6

Kenya

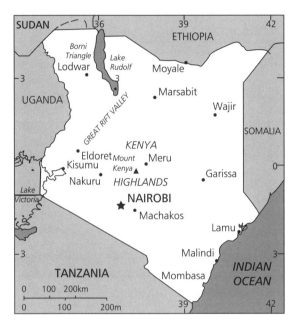

Kenya (population 32.02 million) is a country in Eastern Africa bordering the Indian Ocean that covers an area of 582 650 km^2. Its boundaries border Tanzania, Uganda, Sudan, Ethiopia and Somalia. The capital of Kenya is Nairobi.

According to the UN human development index (HDI), Kenya is ranked 148th out of 177 countries worldwide (value 0.488)[1] and 19th out of 45 in African countries for which an index is available. This places Kenya in the group of countries with low human development.

Palliative care service provision

Current services

Eight organizations in Kenya provide palliative care services (Table 6.1).

The government of Kenya has no official palliative care policy although it is supportive of palliative care in the country. The Ministry of Health is working on a 5-year Health Sector Strategic Plan and has invited Nairobi Hospice to sit on that committee. Nairobi Hospice is also consulting with the Ministry of Health on the development of a manual regarding palliative care for cancer of the cervix.

There are six established hospices in the country: Nairobi, Meru, Kisumu, Nyeri, Eldoret and Coast (Mombassa). A further service is developing in Nyaharuru. There are palliative care teams in two mission hospitals, Chogoria Hospital and Maua Methodist Hospital, both in Meru district.

Table 6.1 Palliative care provision in Kenya

Kenya	Free standing unit	Hospital unit	Hospital support team	Home care	Day care	Clinic/ Drop-in centre	Grand Total
Nairobi Hospice			1	1	1	1	4
Meru				1	1	1	3
Eldoret			1	1		1	3
Nyeri			1	1	1	1	4
Coast			1	1		1	3
Kisumu				1	1		2
Maua Methodist Hospital		1					1
Maua Methodist Hospital home care projects (branches)				3			3
Chogoria Mission Hospital		1		1			2
Total services		6		10	4	5	25

Nairobi Hospice

Nairobi Hospice was founded in 1990. From the outset, the approach of this hospice was two-pronged: to provide a home-based care service and training. The 2003 Annual Report describes this hospice as aiming to provide:

> ... the highest quality of total care possible for people with advanced cancer and AIDS, and to provide counselling and support for their families and other individuals important to their care ... The care is given to terminally ill patients on an outpatient basis, in the hospitals and in the patients' own homes within a radius of 20 kilometres. The service combines patient care, education and training of relatives, community and health care professionals[2] (p. 14).

A day care facility was initiated in 1993 and operates every Thursday for up to 20 patients. Zipporah Ali, a physician from the Nairobi Hospice, describes the service:

> [We] have somebody who has offered us a van, a tour van that goes to pick up the very sick patients from their homes and they'll be dropped here. They usually spend the whole day here. They're able to have breakfast. Lunch is cooked for them by the volunteers—and, of course, they will be reviewed by the medical team for their medical needs. If there's any counselling to be done, it is all done on that day. So the patients spend the day among themselves. They interact and share whatever is going on in their lives, and I think this is a very positive thing for them.[3]

An acre of land was provided by the Kenya government in 2001 in the grounds of the Kenyatta Hospital in recognition of the work of the hospice. Fundraising is underway to generate money to build permanent premises on this land.

Nairobi Hospice has an average caseload of 100 patients per month. Referrals come mainly from Kenyatta National Hospital in whose grounds the hospice is situated. Other referrals come from private doctors and hospitals in Nairobi. Upcountry patients are referred when they receive radiotherapy, chemotherapy and associated hospice support, and swell the hospice numbers to around 1500 patients. Over 90 per cent of patients are from upcountry and only 6 per cent from Nairobi itself.

From July 2002 to June 2003, the total number of home contacts reached 1186, whereas hospital contacts were 1862. Follow-up bereavement visits numbered 116, and related to 132 deaths during that year. Over 60 per cent of these occurred at home[2] (p. 16). There were 601 new cases referred to the hospice during 2002–2003, an increase of nearly 10 per cent compared with the previous year. The gender profile indicates around twice as many female patients as males. The increase is attributed to effective marketing of the service, and a positive reputation in the community. Cancer of the stomach is one of the three most common cancers seen at the hospice. This follows cancer of the breast and cervix[2] (p. 15). An estimated 65 per cent of cancer patients are expected to be HIV positive; approximately 25 per cent of patients are non cancer-related, HIV positive.[3] It is estimated that from inception to the 30 September 2004, about 5690 patients have been registered with Nairobi Hospice.[4]

The service provides symptom control, psycho-social support and bereavement support. Care is mainly home based, although there is an outpatient clinic for patients well enough to attend. The hospice team also makes hospital visits. Those patients who are not too ill to come to the hospice spend the day at the day care centre. This also gives them the opportunity to be examined and reviewed by the clinical team, and provides respite for the main carers. Volunteers do the shopping, cooking and serving of meals, and socialize with patients.

Most Nairobi Hospice patients live in poverty in the slum areas of the city and environs. One of these, Kibera, is the largest slum in sub-Saharan Africa, where close to a million people occupy shanty dwellings with few facilities.[5] Provision of food is often necessary so that patients can take their medications safely. Nairobi Hospice is the main trainer in palliative care in Kenya.

Meru Hospice

Meru is situated at the base of Mount Kenya and is hilly, with plentiful rain and volcanic soils. Meru Hospice provides a multi-faceted programme for those living with terminal cancer and AIDS. This includes:

- Care and support—including physical, psycho-social and material support for the patient and family
- Nutrition—a 2 acre garden provides space where families are taught agricultural methods to produce high yields. Counselling on nutrition and diet is provided
- Care of orphans—including the facilitation of adoptions, enrolling children into school and providing clothing
- Economic empowerment—and rehabilitation of patients well enough to return to work
- Medication—including ARV treatments
- Public awareness
- Providing palliative health care training in the community.

These goals are accomplished through two separate but interlinked services. An outpatient hospice clinic based in the grounds of the district hospital receives referrals for both cancer and HIV-positive patients. This is referred to as the End of Life Care Programme. Home visits are made twice a week to patients in both district and private hospitals as required. An HIV/AIDS care centre in another part of town has been developed specifically for patients living with AIDS. This daily service provides counselling, nutrition education, symptom control and treatment, and ARV support. It also serves as a recreational centre for children affected by AIDS. Partnerships with other HIV/AIDS organizations, such as UNICEF, avoid duplication of services.

Both programmes link families with microfinancing institutions to develop business projects. A local bank provides low interest loans for income-generating activities to people living with AIDS who may have lost jobs through ill health. Bactrin Killingo comments:

> Now we have become involved, we have provided patients with physical support, social support and spiritual support. They are back on their feet. Their children are back on their feet. But they have nothing to do. So we felt that economic rehabilitation [was necessary] in terms of providing them with opportunities for them to go back and use their energies, to go back to life, and also be able to support their children and support themselves.[6]

On average, 8–10 new patients are referred to the hospice each month, accumulating a patient load of between 100 and 150 per month. Up to 10 patients attend the HIV/AIDS day centre each day and spend approximately 3 h receiving medical and emotional attention.

Eldoret Hospice

This palliative care team was established in 1994.[7] The number of patients cared for by the end of 2004 reached 1342. In 2004, a total of 103 visits was made to patients in hospital and 35 home visits were made. The hospice has eight admission beds, but these are not in use at present due to inadequate resources.

> Presently, we visit the patients in hospital following consultations by the ward doctors. We assess the patients and put them on appropriate palliative treatments. We follow up the patients while they are in the ward. On discharge they pass through our clinic before they go home. At our clinic, we review them and give them a new appointment.[8]

The team visits the hospital twice weekly on Mondays and Fridays. Home visits are done on Tuesdays and Thursdays.

Coast Hospice

This hospice was established in 2001 and is hosted by the Coast Provincial General Hospital. Based in Mombassa city, it is the largest government hospital in the province. The disused morgue has been donated to the hospice for renovation and rehabilitation into a clinic. The patient base starts with a visit to those diagnosed with cancer in the hospital. After discharge, follow-up support in the form of symptom management and pain control is provided at the patient's home. In 2004, a total of 1088 contacts with patients was made. Of these, 52 per cent were hospice clinic based, while 42 per cent were seen in the wards; the remainder were home visits. There were 424 new patients registered in 2004.[9]

Nyeri Hospice

Nyeri hospice is a non-profit-making registered charitable organization. Services include home-based care, hospital consultations, day care, outpatient, bereavement services and training. Established in October 1995, originally as a satellite of the Nairobi Hospice, its objective is to extend quality palliative care to rural areas of Kenya.[10] Initially, care for people living with HIV/AIDS was achieved through networking with a home-based centre in Karatina. However, from mid-2005, home-based care for these patients will be provided by the hospice.

The goals of the hospice are stated to be:

◆ Relief of pain and other distressing symptoms

◆ Psychological and spiritual care for patients, so that they may come to terms with, and prepare for, their own death as fully as they can

◆ A support system to help the patient live as actively and creatively as possible until death—thereby promoting autonomy, personal integrity and self-esteem

◆ A support system to help families to cope during a patient's illness and in bereavement

◆ Ongoing emotional support to carefully selected staff.[11]

Palliative care awareness campaigns are considered a priority. These are directed at professionals in the surrounding hospitals as well as monthly hospice awareness campaigns to the lay community (adult classes, churches, primary and secondary schools and chiefs' *barazas*[12]) in the surrounding divisions. These campaigns have been sustained for the last eight years and have covered most catchment areas.

Each month, an average of 130 patients are seen, 30 home visits made and 24 new patients registered.

Maua Methodist Hospital

Since 2002, three home care programmes have become established, with organizational, nursing and medical support based at Maua Hospital. Palliative care co-ordinator Stephen Gitonga comments:

> It's a home based sort of care. We have nurses from the hospital, we have a doctor and we have a clinical officer who is involved in this care. We make visits at a community level every week, one day a week. The hospital is really running on a very tight budget, because of the resources and, as such, when they are available they move with the nurses to the community. The patients know the days that we come and they will come [to see us]. If they are not able to come, the volunteers will come who will give us the report and, depending what the volunteers tell us, we conduct home visits.
>
> So we go and see the patients there. We assess whether we have to adjust the morphine, whether we need to give them more drugs. We are able to do that at that level, and the volunteers are very instrumental. The patients who are now in our programme who are also receiving antiretroviral drugs, they have become changed images, they will come and report those patients who are not taking their ARVs and as such we are really in touch in that way.

The other thing also is that, because we believe this a community-based palliative care programme, we have set up community-based clinics at the community level. And we have equipped these clinics with very basic drugs, that the patients can access from there, so that if they need brufen, if they need paracetamol, the drugs are there and the patients are able to access the drugs.[13]

Chogoria Mission Hospital

In 2001, palliative care physician David Allbrook visited Kenya on an International Association of Hospice and Palliative Care (IAHPC) travel fellowship and later gave some background information about Chogoria Hospital:

> At Chogoria Hospital, in South Meru, HIV/AIDS, malaria, cancer, and cardiac problems account for the majority of deaths. In year 2000, 286 cancer cases were diagnosed, comprising 27 gastric, 19 breast, 16 esophagus, and 17 primary liver cancers. Deaths attributable to HIV/AIDS were 20: 36 per cent of adult deaths. Half of bed occupancy in this hospital is said to be HIV/AIDS related.[14]

Community Health Adviser Elizabeth Grant and her colleagues enquired into the meaning of a good death in rural Kenya. The study was conducted on the eastern slopes of Mount Kenya, the home of the Meru people:

> We listened to 32 people with ongoing cancer or AIDS, and to their carers as they talked about end-of-life experiences and care needs. Patients described how the support of close family relationships, and the care shown by their community and religious fellowships helped meet many of their emotional, social and spiritual needs. But physical needs often went unmet. Patients died in pain. Some suffered in poverty; others were troubled by the guilt of using all available family resources to pay for treatment and care. Accessible pain relief, affordable clinic or inpatient care when required and help to cope with the burden of care were among the key needs of the patients. Until these are available, many will not die well.[15,16]

Kenya is a multifaith country and most Kenyans subscribe to some form of religion. Zipporah Ali:

> I think we are very spiritual people. OK we have got Christians, we've got Muslims, we've got Hindus, we've got Buddhists, whatever . . . but I think people are very conscious of spirituality here, and religion, because actually we don't differentiate between spirituality and religion. Women have fellowship groups, the young folk have youth groups, so these groups are very supportive. And it's very rare that we ask somebody, 'Do you go to Church?' and they say, 'No, I don't go to church'. You find that almost everybody goes to church. The Muslims here are also very supportive to children. The other day we had some people visiting from a Hindu community. They were coming to support our patients—and our patients are not Hindus, most of them are Christians. So I think there's a lot of spirituality going on; it's something of a platform for most of the things that we do in this community.[3]

Reimbursement and funding for services

Nairobi Hospice

The Government of Kenya supports the hospice by paying for the salaries of three nurses seconded to hospice by the Ministry of Health. It has also donated a plot of land on which the hospice can build its own offices. Other funds come from fundraising activities such as golf tournaments, sponsored walks, and Voices for Hospices every 3 years. A support organization, Friends of Hospice, encourages Kenyans to become friends of the hospice at a nominal fee of 1000 Kenyan shillings per year or to take out a corporate membership. Up to 90 per cent of patients cannot pay for hospice services so the majority receive a free service, including drugs. A UK-based charity, Hospice Care Kenya supports a doctor on the doctor rotation programme and covers the costs of the Oxford Brookes training course. A donor from The Netherlands covers many of the drugs costs. The Ford Foundation provided US$36 000 for a 1 year project from late 2004 to train community workers in palliative care. The Diana Fund[17] supported a 3-year palliative care training programme for health professionals at a value of £60 000.

The Nairobi Hospice Annual Report 2003 indicates a much reduced surplus of funds—attributable to several reasons—including a 40 per cent drop in local donations and a 45 per cent drop in Friends of Hospice. This may be related to changes in fundraising staff. Overall expenditure increased significantly due to the need to pay salaries formerly subsidized by a Hospice Care Kenya (UK) grant, and the recalling of seconded staff by Kenyatta National Hospital. In the same year, drug costs rose 145 per cent due to increased purchasing and free issues to poor patients[2] (p. 13).

Nyeri Hospice

The hospice team writes:

> As the hospice is a charity, we must raise funds to support our work. Patients pay what they can but this is usually very little because they have used their resources for drugs, treatment and travel to appointments, often down to Nairobi and there is little left. The hospice team of staff and volunteers work very hard to raise funds to support this work. We have had several fundraising events such as golf competitions, camping safaris, concerts—which have been a hard work, a lot of fun and quite lucrative.[18]

Meru Hospice

Approximately 80 per cent of funds are external donor dependent. Hospice Care Kenya (UK) was instrumental in providing seed money to establish the programme. A twinning arrangement with Hospice Care Incorporated in Madison, Wisconsin (in 2004) resulted in a grant that has contributed towards staff expenses. Local funds are raised through corporate institutions, business people and sale of T-shirts. About 5 per cent of running costs comes from patients who pay for the service. The UK Forum for Hospice and Palliative Care Worldwide provided funds for Bactrin Killingo to study for a diploma in palliative care at a value of £1500.The ARV programme was free in 2004 but will ultimately need to be charged to patients.

Eldoret Hospice

Funds are primarily sourced from local donations. Fundraising activities include charity dinners, raffles, charity walks and a membership campaign.

Coast Hospice

Running costs are sourced from donations from Friends of Hospice. This scheme obtains an annual amount of 1000 Kenya shillings from individuals and 10 000 Kenya shillings from companies. Fundraising activities include charity walks, dinners and golf tournaments. Hospice Care Kenya (UK) considers proposals for funding for training materials and building funds.

Maua Methodist Hospital

The Diana Fund has provided £123 962 to support a 3 year project to establish a system for caring for the very sick, including access to morphine.

President's Emergency Plan for AIDS Relief (PEPFAR)

During the 2004 financial year (FY), funding of around US$75.36 million was enacted for country-managed programmes in Kenya and $21.22 million for central programmes. During FY2005, it is anticipated that a total of US$136.01 million will be enacted: US$115.14 million for country-managed programmes and US$20.87 million for central programmes.[19]

Opioid availability and consumption

The training programmes offered by Nairobi Hospice are aimed at alleviating the continuing resistance to the use of morphine in Kenya amongst some doctors and nurses. The difficulties in accessing morphine are being addressed by the national hospice association.

Nairobi Hospice

Important networking with the Ministry of Health was undertaken when the hospice was established to ensure a supply of morphine for patients. The hospice imports morphine powder from the UK for reconstitution as liquid morphine for hospice distribution within Kenya. Injectable morphine is also available. Other drugs prescribed by Nairobi Hospice are guided by the WHO analgesic ladder. Strong analgesics, other painkillers and adjuvants including ibuprofen, dihydrocodeine, paracetamol, aspirin and laxatives are available. Amitriptyline and diazepam are used for depression and anxiety. Antibiotics, mystatin and antifungal drugs are prescribed as necessary, especially for people living with HIV. ARV treatments are not prescribed. There is no palliative care formulary to date. Most drug costs for all Kenyan hospices are covered by a Dutch donor: Nairobi Hospice-The Netherlands.

Meru Hospice

The WHO analgesic ladder is used as a guideline for pain control although most of the patients are late referrals and consequently are introduced to morphine immediately. The use of generic drugs reduces costs. Most of the patients cannot afford to pay for morphine, and Meru Hospice provides liquid morphine free of charge.

Eldoret Hospice

Morphine syrup is generally used for pain control. In 2004, 12 litres of morphine were used:

> However, sometimes our patients have to make do with dihydrocodeine tablets. When the powder is out of stock, as it happened sometimes last year, the other alternative we would use is morphine sulphate tablets.[20]

Coast Hospice

Coast Hospice gets drug donations from the same Dutch organization as Nairobi Hospice.

Nyeri Hospice

An average of 1 kg of morphine powder is used annually.[21] The following morphine policy is in place as a guideline to nursing staff.

Nyeri hospice: policy on administration of oral morphine

Morphine is a narcotic and is under the DDA, it should therefore be closely monitored, regulated and should be stored in a locked cupboard within a cupboard.

- The prescribing officer should be authorized and knowledgeable on the use of morphine.
- Patients on morphine at home should be regularly monitored and the use of the drug clearly indicated on the 'blue sheet' that patients carry home, yellow record sheet for all medications.
- The patients at home should carry only a 2 weeks supply of morphine unless under very special circumstances, e.g. patients who live very far away.
- The morphine ordered or dispensed out, or received back from patients who are not using it any longer should be clearly entered in the DDA book provided.
- Morphine should be ordered before the stock runs out; a balance of 1000 ml should always be in stock.
- Unless otherwise indicated, morphine syrup should be given every 3–4 h.

The International Narcotics Control Board (2004)[22] has published the following figures for the consumption of narcotic drugs in Kenya: codeine 28 kg; morphine 2 kg; dihydrocodeine 6 kg; pethidine 49 kg.

For the years 2000–2002, the average defined daily dose consumption of morphine for statistical purposes (S-DDD)[23] in Kenya was 1. This compares with other African countries as follows: Swaziland 1; Egypt 2; Uganda 4; Zimbabwe 13; Namibia 73; South Africa 103. Twenty-nine countries reported no morphine consumption during 2000–2002 (Appendix 1).

National and professional organizations

Kenya Hospice and Palliative Care Association

This national association was formed in October 2004 to provide palliative care country-wide by developing more hospices with a standard quality of care. A second objective is to supply smaller hospices with drugs that can be bought in bulk in Nairobi. It is anticipated that all existing hospices will be members, as well as other organizations providing elements of palliative care in related fields.

Hospice Care Kenya (UK)[24]

This UK-based charity supports hospices in Kenya by providing funds for various projects. Significantly, Hospice Care Kenya (UK) sponsors a doctor rotation programme by paying the salaries of local doctors who work at Kenyan Hospices for 3 months. After this placement, doctors should be able to provide palliative care and train others in palliative care in whichever part of the country they are working. Four doctors successfully completed this rotation in the year 2002–2003.

Hospice 'twins'

Through the Foundation for Hospices in Sub-Saharan Africa, (FHSSA)[25] Nairobi Hospice has a twinning arrangement with VITAS San Antonio, Texas, USA. This partnership was the first between hospices in Kenya and America. The VITAS San Antonio programme is part of the VITAS Innovative Healthcare Corporation. One of San Antonio's nurses is a native of Kenya, and was instrumental in spearheading the twinning efforts with Hospice Nairobi.[26] Meru Hospice is twinned with Hospice Care Incorporated in Wisconsin, USA

Palliative care coverage

Nairobi Hospice

The service offers home visits to patients within a radius of 25 km from Nairobi. It is estimated that this serves a population of three million.[4] The majority of referrals are made by Kenyatta National Hospital.

Meru Hospice

The radius covered by this service is up to 100 km, but more realistically the patient catchment is within a radius of about 20–50 km as transport difficulties limit visits. The approximate population is 800 000–1.2 million. Referrals come mainly from the district hospital. Local patients who have received treatments in Nairobi are advised by Nairobi Hospice to contact Meru Hospice once they return home.

Eldoret Hospice

The Hospice receives patients mainly from Moi Teaching and Referral Hospital and the surrounding hospitals. Patients come from a radius of about 150 km.

Coast Hospice

The Coast province has a population of about three million people. Mombassa city has approximately one million people. Coast Hospice is responsible for palliative care patients in the whole province. The attending doctor at the Coast Provincial General Hospital completes the hospice referral form in order that the patient can receive palliative care after discharge. Referral forms are circulated to all hospitals and clinics, and public talks raise awareness of the service.

Nyeri Hospice

The districts of Nyeri, Kerugoya, Murang'a, Laikipia and Nyandarua are covered by this hospice. Satellite hospices in these areas are planned to take palliative care into these communities. A satellite hospice at Nyahururu has been established.

Education and training

Nairobi Hospice

In June 2001, Nairobi Hospice, in collaboration with Oxford Brookes University, launched a 14 month Diploma in Higher Education Palliative Care. This part distance learning and part block system enables health care professionals from around Africa to undertake the diploma while continuing to work. The first class of students graduated in September 2002.

Jane Appleton, programme leader in palliative care at Oxford Brookes University, reflects on the course:

> I first became involved in palliative care education in Kenya in around 1999. Brigid Sirengo, the chief executive officer at Nairobi hospice, had undertaken a course with Oxford Brookes University, and my predecessor, Sue Duke, had kept in touch with Brigid and had visited Kenya. It was around 1999/2000 that we first began to think about the diploma in palliative care being delivered in Kenya, and that approach really came from Brigid Sirengo wanting to develop something more. The Nairobi hospice had already done a considerable amount of education—introductory courses, level 1 courses around the country—and they were interested in having a course at diploma or degree level. So the approach came from Brigid but it took a number of years to really get that going. We had a visit to Kenya to set up the details of the programme and then the first course started in 2000. We're on the third course now and we're planning a fourth to start next year, I think.
>
> The students came on the programme because they wanted to develop their knowledge and skills—and mostly the students we've had have been very experienced practitioners. They were not really new to palliative care. They had a lot of years experience but they were coming on the programme to develop further and to gain the recognized qualification. I think the diploma level was an incentive, and the fact that the programme was very practice focused was another positive factor. And the range of students from different African countries—and disciplines—I think was another attraction.
>
> We feel we have a programme that's very student-centred, and that the programme is not content-driven particularly; it's about working with the students, where they are in their particular practice context. It is a practice-based course, so it wasn't our context that drove it. Some of the key things we were trying to do were around trying to develop practitioners who were able to have a critical debate about palliative care practice—and that debate was very focused on the practice that they were engaged in.[27]

Students from colleges and other hospices are offered 4 week clinical placements at Nairobi Hospice for palliative care experience. The hospice offers two separate training courses each lasting 1 week for health care professionals and community volunteers. During the year 2002–2003, 52 health care professionals and 68 volunteers completed these courses. Consultation is taking place with the Ministry of Health to include palliative care in the curriculum for nurse training.

The hospice provides introductory palliative care training to third year medical students at the teaching hospital.

Meru Hospice

While Meru Hospice does not provide any formal training, there is informal teaching to final year student nurses at the Medical Training College, church groups, women and youth community groups, and health care providers at the district hospital. This covers principles of palliative care, principles of pain management and nursing management.

Eldoret Hospice

This hospice has yet to develop its own training programmes fully. In March 2004, a group of 18 participants including pastors, teachers and health professionals attended an initial training session for hospice volunteers.

Coast Hospice

In January 2004, 25 medical personnel (clinical officers and nurses) from the district hospitals in the Coast Province were trained by this hospice in a 5-day palliative care course. The intention was to enable the trainees to set up small palliative care units in their respective stations with support provided by the hospice. 'As we are charged with the responsibility of providing palliative care to patients in the whole province, we find that not only is this not practical but we would also be spreading our already skeleton staff too thinly, hence the annual training programme'.[28] Plans were in place for similar workshops in 2005 for health workers and volunteers.

Palliative care workforce capacity

Nairobi Hospice

There are posts for six nurses; one social worker co-ordinates volunteers; and two doctors examine patients at the hospice and accompany the team on home visits. The administrative support team consists of a finance administration officer, a secretary, two drivers and two support staff (cleaner/messenger). Approximately 40 volunteers are used for a variety of jobs including patient counselling and fundraising.

Meru Hospice

The service is run by one doctor, two nurses, two social workers and one clinical officer. The workload is shared between the clinic and the day centre, with one nurse and one social worker attending at each.

> There are times I also get to go with the social worker and sometimes we also . . . out-source a physiotherapist from the district hospital because we can't afford to keep her so we get to look for her. When we identify certain spiritual needs that somebody has, say somebody's a Muslim, we identify a certain Muslim spiritual leader who can come over with us to go for home visit so the visits are on a needs basis.[6]

The doctor and one nurse have undergone palliative care training at Nairobi Hospice.

Eldoret Hospice

The health care team comprises three nurses seconded to the hospice from the Moi Teaching and Referral Hospital, and volunteer doctors who act on a consultative basis on the board. The hospice pays salaries for the accounts clerk/secretary, driver, cleaner and a gardener.

Coast Hospice

The service is provided by a team of eight that includes one doctor, a clinical officer, three nurses, a secretary, a manager and public relations/fundraising co-ordinator. The doctor and two nurses are government hospital employees seconded to the hospice. They are given a small allowance. All other employees are paid an allowance. The board of trustees comprises seven volunteers.

Nyeri Hospice

The management of this service is entrusted to a board of directors. The hospice team consists of four nurses, a doctor on rotation, one part-time social worker, a fundraiser, an administrative secretary, a driver and three support staff.

Maua Methodist Hospital

The hospice team consists of: two doctors; three clinical officers; two registered nurses; eight community nurses; administrative and support staff; and 120 volunteers.[29]

History and development of hospice–palliative care in Kenya

Nairobi Hospice

One source of inspiration behind the development of the hospice movement in Kenya came from Ruth Wooldridge, a British nurse working in Nairobi who was deeply moved by the death of Nancy, a young woman who had cancer. Nancy's story features prominently in the history of Nairobi hospice and helped form the mission of the hospice:

> Nancy died of cancer. Her real life story illustrates the many problems experienced by the terminally ill and their families.
>
> Nancy was a 26-year-old woman with two young sons who lived in one room with no running water. By the time her cancer was diagnosed and she went for medical attention the disease was too far advanced to cure. The treatment she had included surgery and radiotherapy, but this did not help and she began to get a lot of pain. When her illness reached this stage she had to give up her job as a teacher and so she no longer had any income to support herself, her children and her mother who came to help.
>
> Nancy's condition deteriorated. She was in pain, unable to sleep, constipated, and having difficulty passing urine. She went back to hospital and was given some tablets but no-one explained to her why she was not improving, why she was having such pain, or what she might expect to happen next. For the last month of her life, she lay on the mud floor of her house, nursed by her mother. She was incontinent and in continuous pain.
>
> Before she died, her mother, who had been unable to get help in any other way, put Nancy on her back and carried her to hospital. By this time, Nancy was semi-conscious; she had bedsores and was in continuous pain.
>
> Nancy died in hospital, four days later, away from her family.[30]

Ruth Wooldridge takes up the story:

> I just thought, 'palliative care is what we need here'. So I spent about a year looking at all the hospitals and oncology departments and speaking to doctors—and realized that there was absolutely nothing for people with advanced cancer. Then a friend of mine, who was also VSO,

sent me an article that Robert Twycross had written—it was in the *Nursing Times*—about the absence of palliative care overseas. I wrote to him outlining the situation in Kenya and he wrote back saying he was going to visit South Africa. So I responded that it would be brilliant if he could just come through Kenya. We could organize a workshop and call a group of people from clergy to social workers—anybody who is interested—as well as oncologists and nurses. We held it at the cathedral; it was a big workshop. Some of the oncologists presented their work and Robert helped them to see what they could do for patients with advanced cancer. So it gave us the green light, really.[31]

Brigid Sirengo continues:

They held a workshop in February 1988 . . . And at that workshop it came out very clearly that cancer was a problem in the community and we did not have the facilities to take care of cancer patients, especially those who were terminally ill. And it was also quite clear that the doctors and the nurses were not trained to take care of the terminal phase. So that is how the hospice was born: from that workshop it was decided that a steering committee should be set up to establish palliative care in the country. So from March 1990 we started taking care of the terminally ill cancer patients. From the outset the objectives were to train people in palliative care and to provide a service.[32]

As the demand for a hospice gathered momentum, crucial support came from Professor Kasilli, a haematologist who worked at Kenyatta Hospital. Having spent time in Glasgow, he understood the importance of palliative care and became an enthusiastic activist. First, he chaired the workshop, then co-wrote a proposal for government and finally took the hospice forward as its chairman, remaining committed to the service until his death in 1996.

Although the concept of hospice had originated in Britain, efforts were made to ensure it was translated into a Kenyan service and accepted as such by patients and health professionals. Writing in 1991, Jane Moore—a contemporary of Ruth Wooldridge and co-founder of Nairobi hospice—tells how the hospice became grounded in Kenyan culture:

Although strong links have been forged with the UK and Zimbabwe, from the beginning the prevailing philosophy of Nairobi Hospice has been 'This is a Kenyan Hospice in Kenya, for the people of Kenya'. Every step has been devised and developed in the context of the Kenyan model of care, and made appropriate to the social, economic, geographical and human situations which are a mosaic of diversity, even within Nairobi itself, let alone elsewhere in the country.[33]

Nyeri Hospice

Nyeri Hospice developed as a satellite of Nairobi Hospice (1995). According to the hospice team at Nyeri:

Right from the start there had been concern about the patients from rural areas who are first seen in Nairobi but are then sent home. These people have even fewer resources available to them and the family is often left to cope alone because the community is suspicious and worried that the illness may be contagious. The establishment of an umbrella of hospices, functioning independently but linked through professional co-operation was envisaged.

Nyeri Hospice was launched on the 1st October 1995. Today, it is a registered Charitable Trust and although it is autonomous in its management and financial provisions, it has the support and guidance on a professional level from the Nairobi Hospice.

The Nyeri Hospice is the first rural project to be established and provides quality palliative care to patients and their families. Through the years, we have become known in the lay and professional communities and the demand for hospice services has grown.

Eldoret Hospice

The idea of having a hospice in this town was mooted in 1992 by a nurse, Mrs Rose Abira. She encouraged other nurses to get involved and together they developed the beginnings of a palliative care approach at Moi Teaching and Referral Hospital.[20] In 1994, a palliative care team was established. A year later, the hospice was approved by the Ministry of Health and awarded a charitable organization number. In 1996, a small plot of land was given to the hospice by the Moi Teaching and Referral Hospital where the construction of premises began in 1997. By 2000, an independent one storey hospice building had been established and services began operating from there in July 2001.

Coast Hospice

The hospice was started in August 2001 by Faustine Mgendi, a physician who is currently chairman of the board of trustees. It is hospital based and has developed to provide continuity of care to the many terminally ill patients who are discharged from the formal health sector.

Maua Methodist Hospital

In his retirement, David Allbrook was on a world tour that took in parts of Africa when an unusual turn of events led him back to Kenya and palliative care:

We did a tour around Uganda and I missed out the Uganda Hospice; and we went to Kenya and did the same thing. We were just leaving the Methodist guest house and my colleague there—one of my ex-students—said 'Oh, I just want to introduce you to my bishop', and 'my bishop' turned out to be an ex-presiding bishop of the Methodist Church of Kenya. I said 'Oh I've come from Meru; I nearly was posted there when I was a young doctor but I never got there, but we did actually travel there in 1954 with my wife and little boy'. He said, 'Oh, yes. I remember you, I was a young teacher'. So we talked a bit. I was getting a bit anxious about the plane and he said, 'Anyway, come back and we will do anything we can for you. You come and visit the Methodist University there and teach there if you want to, or come to the hospital and teach there. And so I said, 'Yeah, OK, OK'.

I communicated and nothing happened. Then I couldn't get this out of my mind. So anyway, I decided as I haven't heard from them I'll see if I can find them on the net. I did—and sent an e-mail off to the medical superintendent. Heard nothing for a month/six weeks, something like that, then suddenly got an e-mail back from Deitmar Zeigler who was the new medical superintendent. It said, 'Come, come now!' Like that. And I got a travelling fellowship from the International Association of Hospice Palliative Care and I went over for four or five weeks.

I used that time to do a feasibility study and I worked with Deitmar. Deitmar was a hugely dynamic thirty-something surgeon. Trained in Scarborough in England with his wife, he was the driving force behind the whole idea of palliative care in Meru district—and he needs to be honoured for that. At the end of the time, I advocated that the person who should be selected for [palliative care] training should go to the Uganda hospice because the Uganda hospice offered hands on, practical, down to earth training, at a grass roots level, and that was what was wanted.[34]

Nurse Stephen Gitonga was selected for training and he takes up the story:

> When we started, we targeted some specific areas. These areas were identified by the community through a church leaders meeting. The leaders of the church went down and mobilized their people and told them they could do something, and the hospital offered to give them technical advice. But starting the programme and raising resources was up to the community, because they had seen the dangers of HIV/AIDS. They were burying members of their community each and every other Saturday and as such they reached a level where they were seriously suffering. That is why they came up and said, 'Yes we are ready; we can mobilize the regional resources that we have'.
>
> We right now have three pilot project areas that we are working in. The first area started operations in February 2002. The second programme, after seeing the good things that were happening with the first programme, started in October of the same year. The programme is managed from the hospital. We are the facilitators. We are really trying to help communities and their health committees who in turn manage the programmes. They go and identify the volunteers so that they can reach out, vet, and give the care that is needed to our people in our villages. So essentially I would say it is the community's project. It does not belong to our Methodist hospital. We are just facilitators.[13]

Hospice success stories

Nairobi Hospice

The training programme offered by this hospice has equipped other hospices around the country with trained staff and so expanded national coverage.

> The people we have trained are the ones that have gone out and started those hospices, so that other people who cannot reach us will have palliative care accessible and available to them.[32]

The positive attitude towards Nairobi Hospice by the Kenya Government has significant implications for palliative care in this country.

> The fact that the Kenya government has given us land means that the Ministry acknowledges and appreciates palliative care, and for us that is very, very important. We are at an early stage, working with the Ministry, so that palliative care can eventually be part and parcel of the main health care system.[35]

An external evaluation in 1996 concluded that Nairobi Hospice was achieving its aims, and this is confirmed by positive comments from patients and families. That many of the medical staff are formally trained in palliative care is seen as another indicator of success.

Meru Hospice

Bactrin Killingo:

> I think we have been able to do what palliative care is meant to achieve: provide quality care to more than 200 people in the last two years. That to me is a success. The other success is seeing other individuals who are interested in participating. I started with me alone; now we have six, seven others. The community has also become aware of the need for these services. Every weekend I have an invitation from a church to go and talk to them about care of the dying. For me that's a success because people are aware of this service.[6]

Coast Hospice

Sound relationships with state health services have succeeded in integrating palliative care into the broader health provision. Lack of funding is all that inhibits plans to expand community palliative care skills by this hospice to health care providers in the district.

Nyeri Hospice

This hospice lists several notable successes in its vision to provide quality palliative care in the rural setting:

+ Operating from its own premises, it has experienced a significant rise in the number of patients seen each month and has set up a satellite centre in Nyahururu

+ Recent developments include a day care centre, bereavement service, and home-based care for HIV/AIDS patients

+ Government supports the service by seconding nurses to the programme

+ Since 2000, the hospice has benefited from the doctor on rotation programme facilitated by Hospice Care Kenya (UK). Public awareness of palliative care has been increased and there are regular training programmes for volunteers, professional health workers and schools.

Maua Methodist Hospital

The successes of this hospice programme are stated to be:

+ Accessibility of palliative care in the rural communities

+ Involvement of churches and local communities

+ A new appreciation that something can be done for people who are terminally ill

+ Availability of antiretroviral drugs

+ The advocacy of patients being treated

+ A broader support base, including the Ministry of Health.[13]

Life/oral histories

Professor David Allbrook—chaplain, Kalamunda Hospital, Perth, Australia; formerly dean of the Medical Faculty, University of East Africa: interviewed by Michael Wright, 11 February 2005. Length of interview: 1 h 7 min.

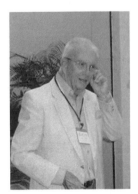 David Allbrook was born in London in 1923. A committed Christian, after he qualified in medicine (University College), his thoughts turned to the mission field—an opportunity which was denied him after he developed TB. Instead, he entered academic life and developed an interest in research—especially muscle regeneration—and subsequently took up a post at Makerere Medical College, Uganda, in 1952. He was offered a Fulbright Scholarship in the USA, where he became interested in electronic microscopy (EM), and later returned to Makerere to set up the first EM Unit in Africa. As the countries of Uganda, Tanzania and Kenya became independent, he became Dean of the Medical Faculty of the University of East Africa. In 1965, he left Africa to become Professor of Anatomy at the University of Western Australia, a position he held until in 1986. During the latter part of his career, David Allbrook developed an

interest in palliative care. He had met Cicely Saunders during the 1940s and spent time at St Christopher's in the early 1980s. He became involved in palliative care development in Australia, in India and in the countries of sub-Saharan Africa. In 2001, he was awarded a travel fellowship by the International Association of Hospice and Palliative Care, and advised on the establishment of a home care service in the Meru district of Uganda. In this wide-ranging interview, David Allbrook tells of his medical career, his research interest, his involvement in hospice development, the impact of his faith upon his life, and the place of medical ethics. He currently serves as chaplain in a hospital near his home in Perth, Western Australia.

Jane Appleton—*programme leader, palliative care; School of Health and Social Care, Oxford Brookes University, (UK)*: interviewed by Michael Wright, 1 February 2005: Length of interview: 20 min.

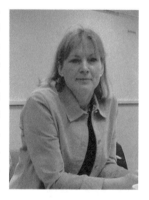

Jane Appleton became involved in palliative care education in Kenya during 1999 amid increasing interest in the establishment of a diploma course for health professionals. Brigid Sirengo had previously undertaken training at Oxford Brookes University and contacts had been maintained. Importantly, she was aware of the benefits that such a course would bring and was an enthusiastic advocate of palliative care education. Eventually, the first course began with nine students in 2000, building up to 15 students by the third year. The course is run jointly by Nairobi Hospice and Oxford Brookes University and has attracted a wide range of participants: doctors, nurses, physiotherapists, social workers and counsellors. In addition to local interest, applications have been received from Ethiopia, Uganda, Malawi, Tanzania and Zimbabwe. Jane Appleton speaks of the challenges associated with the course: of securing funding; the demands of distance learning; access to IT; and the availability of palliative care literature. She speaks also of the nature of a practice-based course in a different cultural setting, of the commitment of the students and teaching staff, and of her future hopes for palliative care education in Kenya.

Dr Zipporah Ali—*senior medical officer, Nairobi Hospice*: interviewed by David Clark, 2 June 2004. Length of interview: 29 min.

Zipporah Ali first became involved in palliative care as a volunteer, in 1994, whilst working as a medical officer at the National Hospital in Nairobi. In 1996, she was employed by Nairobi Hospice and undertook a programme of training in palliative care, at Oxford Brookes University, in the UK. She describes the work of Nairobi Hospice—its inpatient and day care services, home care programme (within a 25 km radius of Nairobi), advocacy work and extensive training programmes, linked to Oxford Brookes University. The work is supported by the Friends of Nairobi Hospice. There are plans for

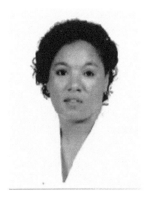

a new hospice building, on land donated by the government. Initially cancer patients only were cared for, but since 2002 the service has also been available to people with HIV/AIDS. She comments:

> We're sensitive about cultural issues, we encourage patients to be in their homes and not in hospitals; encourage that at home. We actually sensitize the family and talk to them and prepare the families for death at home. Because these patients, if they go to the hospitals, because particularly if they're HIV/AIDS positive or they're really terminally ill with cancer, nobody's going to pay them attention now, so, people actually keep away from them, the medical staff and everybody else. So we prefer them to be, we prefer to have them in their homes and they're happier in their homes, and even the family finds it easier that they have to be in the home with the patients and not visiting, travelling distances to be with the patient.

Zipporah Ali goes on to talk about the wider development of hospice services in Kenya and the role of Nairobi Hospice in supporting these. A member of the newly created steering group and then board of the African Palliative Care Association, she describes the origins and early plans of APCA.

Stephen Gitonga—*palliative care co-ordinator, Maua Methodist Hospital*: interviewed by Michael Wright, 22 September 2004. Length of interview: 24 min.

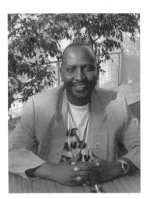

Stephen Gitonga is a trained nurse who responded to a Maua Hospital initiative to establish a palliative care service in eastern Kenya. After visiting Hospice Africa Uganda, he was instrumental in developing a palliative home care service and now holds the position of palliative care co-ordinator. As awareness of palliative care was raised, local communities were mobilized and began to take responsibility for sick people in their localities. Since 2002, three pilot programmes have begun, each training local volunteers to identify those in need of palliative care and to deliver a basic level of service. This home-based care is supported by professional nurses and physicians, to whom referrals are made as appropriate.

Stephen Gitonga speaks of the challenges of establishing a new service; of the way morphine is prescribed and dispensed; of the improvement of patients on ARV therapy; and of the benefits of community involvement and local clinics. There is still much to be done: myths around morphine continue; despite a 60 per cent subsidy from the Diana Fund, patients have to find 40 per cent of the cost of their care; stigmatization and social exclusion are commonplace. Despite these difficulties, support from international donors has helped nurture the service. The Ministry of Health provides HIV testing kits and ARVs for 50 patients free of charge, and the network of faith-based organizations ensures that palliative care services reach the poorest areas of the community.

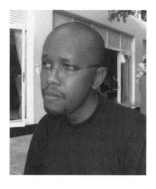

Dr Bactrin Killingo (1)—*founder, chief executive, and physician, Meru Hospice*: interviewed by David Clark, 2 June 2004. Length of interview: 32 min.

Bactrin Killingo trained in medicine in Kenya and became interested in palliative care issues in 2000, when working a rotation at the Nairobi Hospice. Here he saw patients coming from vast distances and resolved to try to set up a service in his own home village of Meru, where— with the assistance of Nairobi hospice—he began to raise awareness of the issues. By 2002, he had set up a community-based NGO, Meru Hospice. A UK-based organization, Hospice Care Kenya also assisted with funding. Initially staff worked without pay. In March 2004, the hospice was twinned with Hospice Care Incorporated in Wisconsin, USA. Meru Hospice seeks to address six issues in a rural context: treatment of symptoms and opportunistic infections; care and support; nutrition; care of orphans and vulnerable children; economic empowerment; and rehabilitation. Approximately 80 per cent of costs are donor dependent, and the balance is raised locally. Bactrin Killingo remarks, 'Now that we've started something, it's like a bush-fire, we just can't put it off'.

Dr Bactrin Killingo (2)—*founder, chief executive, and physician, Meru Hospice*: interviewed by Jenny Hunt, 2 November 2004. Length of interview: 48 min.

Although Bactrin Killingo was brought up in the city of Nairobi, his family originated in Meru district. His parents encouraged their children to maintain strong links with their cultural heritage. They also imparted the virtues of caring and making a difference in the lives of others. Such values affected his decision to study medicine, but he found the field of medicine frustrating in its limitations to spend quality time with a patient and to see beyond the purely physical. A 3-month rotation period at Nairobi Hospice while working at Kenyatta Hospital changed his perception of patient care.

> It is there that I got to interact with lots of patients, and palliative care made a lot of sense to me because it is first of all something that I didn't have the opportunity to learn in medical school, it wasn't in the curriculum. But over and above that I got to interact with patients who came from my village, and quite a number of them needed that and they came from far away, almost 300 kilometres, to sometimes come for two-weekly reviews or monthly reviews, or to get two weeks' supply of morphine, which at the end of the day didn't make sense to me. So after my doctor rotation programme, I decided that palliative care was what I wanted to do, so I went back.[36]

Realizing the value of a doctor–patient relationship, Bactrin Killingo saw the possibility of gathering a fuller picture of the patient's needs, and providing a more comprehensive form of care. With effective pain relief, patients could begin to manage other issues, and he saw in palliative care 'a completeness in the provision of care'. He returned to Meru to undertake a needs assessment and confirmed there was a gap in services for the terminally ill. Knowing the limited professional resources available, his vision has been to encourage the community to help provide good care for the dying. Simple teaching methods and practical experience have begun to achieve this. The model of community involvement is incorporated into the Meru Hospice logo that symbolizes family, community and health care providers surrounding the patient.

Bactrin Killingo shares his dream of providing palliative care for as many as possible in this district that helped send him to medical school. His determination to ensure sustained funding to achieve this is motivated by his belief that human resources are vital to the provision of palliative care and need to be paid for. He concludes that palliative care is not only an important service, it is *essential* in the Kenyan environment of poverty and AIDS.

Brigid Sirengo (1)–*chief executive officer, Nairobi Hospice*: interviewed by David Clark, 2 June 2004. Length of interview: 29 min.

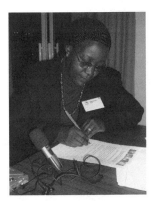

Brigid Sirengo trained as a registered nurse, as a registered midwife and a community health nurse, and then had further training in nurse education and administration. In 1989, whilst working in Nairobi, Kenya, she undertook a continuing education programme which cultivated her interest in the care of terminally ill people. Soon afterwards, she was appointed to the embryonic Nairobi Hospice. She undertook further training in Zimbabwe at Island Hospice, followed by training at several UK hospices and centres. She obtained a BSc in Palliative Care from Oxford Brookes University through distance learning. She is now chief executive of the Nairobi Hospice.

Brigid Sirengo offers some reflections on what involvement in palliative care has meant for her personally, 'Working in palliative care has been a very enriching experience for me . . . It has helped me to grow; it has changed my perception and life. I no longer take my life for granted . . . it has helped me to be much more focused and to really concentrate on things that matter in life, because when you see, more or less daily, people very sick and within a very short time they will have died and gone, then it helps me to really evaluate my values, my perceptions, so that I really try to . . . set my own priorities and concentrate on those things that matter'.

Brigid Sirengo (2)–*chief executive officer, Nairobi Hospice*; Zipporah Ali—*senior medical officer, Nairobi Hospice*; John Njoka—*senior nursing officer, Nairobi Hospice*: interviewed by Jenny Hunt, 1 November 2004. Length of interview: 56 min.

Brigid Sirengo provides a history of the development of Nairobi Hospice in the early 1980s. She tells of a patient dying in pain of cancer of the cervix. This alerted Ruth Wooldridge, who was nursing the patient, to the need for pain control. A workshop in February 1988 identified that palliative care should be available for terminally ill patients, and in 1990 the first patients were seen. Nairobi Hospice was created to provide this service and also palliative care training.

Zipporah Ali explains the referral links between government and private hospitals, and Nairobi Hospice. She describes the extensive training programmes that have been developed for health workers, and the rotation system for doctors to gain experience in the hospice setting.

Focusing on the role of the newly formed Kenya Hospice and Palliative Care Association, Zipporah Ali explains that this national body is well placed to import bulk supplies of drugs that will then be re-distributed to other hospices. It will also concentrate on developing and training further hospices countrywide. Good relationships with the Ministry of Health result in this hospice being consulted on national policies relating to end-of-life care. The donation of a plot of land on which to build their new premises is proof to this team that the hospice concept is accepted by the Kenya government.

John Njoka was trained in community psychiatric nursing. This equips him to help with palliative care training, and to visit patients both at home and at the hospice.

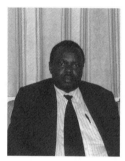

The team provides information on how the hospice serves the three million population of Nairobi and also deal with referrals from upcountry. After explaining that the hospice was developed for cancer patients, Brigid Sirengo highlights the current involvement with patients dying from AIDS. There is discussion around the number of patients seen since inception; a figure of 500 new patients (in the year) confirms the increasing demand for this comprehensive service that now includes a day centre and home-based care.

The interview ends with the team summarizing its successes and difficulties. An external evaluation confirmed that service provision is good, and this is borne out by the feedback received from patients and families. An area of difficulty is funding. Zipporah Ali describes the current trend of increasing community financial support in the face of dwindling external funding.

Ruth Wooldridge—*co-founder, the Nairobi Hospice*: interviewed by Michael Wright 23 January 2005. Length of interview: 1 h 3 min.

Ruth Wooldridge trained as a nurse at St Thomas's Hospital (London) and, in her early career, became concerned about the care of cancer patients and their families. She worked as a volunteer in Uganda (VSO) during the 1970s and returned to Africa in 1982 to take up a nursing post in Kenya. It was during this time that she met Nancy, a young teacher with cancer whose painful death made a deep impression on her. As she advocated for hospice, she persuaded Robert Twycross to visit Kenya on his way to South Africa. The effect was overwhelming and resulted in a grass roots movement towards a hospice service. With Jane Moore, Ruth Wooldridge wrote a proposal for the Kenyan government and, with local support from Professor Kasilli, a piece of land was acquired in the grounds

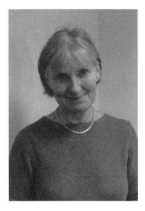

of Kenyatta Hospital (Nairobi); the Tudor Trust funded the erection of premises. An education project began and the hospice opened for patients in 1990. Ruth Wooldridge speaks of the challenges facing hospice development in resource-poor countries, of the need for communication and policy change, and of the place of spirituality and care for family members. She then turns to her work in South Africa, India and, more recently, in Rwanda. Ten years after the genocide in Rwanda, she was shocked to find how much needed to be done to support impoverished communities. She was heartened, however, by the presence of visionary people who, with appropriate training, could help to establish palliative care services.

Public health context

Population

Kenya's population of around 32.02 million people is made up of the following ethnic groups: Kikuyu 22 per cent, Luhya 14 per cent, Luo 13 per cent, Kalenjin 12 per cent, Kamba 11 per cent, Kisii 6 per cent, Meru 6 per cent, other African 15 per cent and non-African (Asian, European and Arab) 1 per cent.

Religious groups include: Christian—Protestant 45 per cent, Roman Catholic 33 per cent; indigenous beliefs 10 per cent; Muslim 10 per cent; other 2 per cent.[37]

Epidemiology

In Kenya, the WHO World Health Report (2004) indicates an adult mortality[38] rate per 1000 population of 509 for males and 448 for females. Life expectancy for males is 49.8; for females 51.9. Healthy life expectancy is 44.1 for males; and 44.8 for females.[39]

HIV/AIDS is a huge burden for sub-Saharan Africa. Throughout the region in 2003, an estimated 23–27 million people were thought to be living with the disease which also caused up to 2.5 million deaths. This represents a huge loss and impacts significantly on health systems and social and family structures.

Kenya is one of the worst HIV/AIDS-affected countries in Eastern Africa. Estimates suggest that in Kenya, between 820 000 and 1.7 million people were living with HIV/AIDS at the end of 2003. In the same year, up to 200 000 adults and children are thought to have died from the disease (Table 6.2).

UNAIDS reports:

> Trends indicate that the annual number of AIDS deaths is still rising steeply and has doubled over the past six years to about 150,000 deaths per year. New infections, however, may be dropping to around 80,000 each year. The majority of new infections occur among youth; especially young women aged 15–24 and young men under the age of 30. HIV infection among adults in urban areas (10%) is almost twice as high as in rural areas (5–6%). The president and his government have demonstrated strong political leadership in the battle against HIV/AIDS, exemplified by the president's personal engagement and his declaration of 'Total War on HIV/AIDS' in March 2003.

Table 6.2 Kenya HIV and AIDS estimates, end 2003

Adult (15–49) HIV prevalence rate	6.7 per cent (range: 4.7–9.6 per cent)
Adults (15–49) living with HIV	1 100 000 (range: 760 000–1 600 000)
Adults and children (0–49) living with HIV	1 200 000 (range: 820 000–1 700 000)
Women (15–49) living with HIV	720 000 (range: 500 000–1 000 000)
AIDS deaths (adults and children) in 2003	150 000 (range: 89 000–200 000)

Source: 2004 Report on the global AIDS epidemic.

President Kibaki has also established a Cabinet Committee on HIV/AIDS, which serves as the highest-level HIV/AIDS policy and leadership body of the government.

The National AIDS Control Council (NACC), established in 1999, provides overall coordination and leadership to the multisectoral response to the epidemic. Its recent Joint Institutional Review brought an enhanced understanding of the roles and relationships of decentralized government structures and how they can contribute more effectively and efficiently to the overall national response. Kenya is the recipient of US$129 million through the Global Fund for HIV/AIDS over five years. It also benefits from PEPFAR, which provided US$75 million for prevention and treatment increase in 2004 alone. In addition to these relatively new contributions, Kenya negotiated a World Bank credit for US$50 million for the period 2000–2005 under the Multi-country HIV/AIDS Programme (MAP) for Africa. The UN System has pledged approximately US$15 million in 2004 for HIV/AIDS initiatives.[40]

Health care system

In 2001, the total per capita expenditure on health care was Intl $114; 7.8 per cent of GDP.[41] Among the countries of Africa, this figure falls within a spending range of Intl $652 in South Africa [8.6 per cent of gross domestic product (GDP)] and Intl $12 in the Democratic Republic of Congo (3.5 per cent of GDP). At 2.0 per cent, the lowest spending as a percentage of GDP is in Equatorial Guinea (Appendix 3).

The WHO overall health system performance score places Kenya 140th out of 191 countries.[42]

Political economy

Kenya is structurally a model African state in that it has multiple ethnic groups and large ethnic and regional variations in development characteristics. Kenya's relative political stability has made it one of the most widely researched and data-rich countries in sub-Saharan Africa.

Kenya gained independence from Britain in 1963, when a unitary constitution was adopted. Since its independence, Kenya has had a parliamentary system with a unicameral legislature. Throughout the 1970s and 1980s, Kenya was often cited as operating a relatively free market in comparison with most other sub-Saharan states. Kenya is one of only a few countries in sub-Saharan Africa in which two ethnic coalitions have taken turns dominating the state apparatus and in which the transition from one to the other has been relatively peaceful.[43]

In 1997, the International Monetary Fund (IMF) suspended Kenya's Enhanced Structural Adjustment Programme due to the government's failure to maintain reforms. A severe drought from 1999 to 2000 compounded Kenya's problems, causing water and energy rationing and reducing agricultural output. As a result, GDP contracted by 0.2 per cent in 2000. The IMF, which had resumed loans in 2000 to help Kenya through the drought, again halted lending in 2001. The return of strong rains in 2001, weak commodity prices and low investment limited Kenya's economic growth to 1.2 per cent. Growth lagged at 1.1 per cent in 2002 because of erratic rains, low investor confidence, meagre donor support and political infighting up to the elections.

In the key 27 December 2002 elections, Daniel Arap Moi's 24 year reign ended, and a new opposition government took on the formidable economic problems facing the nation; progress was made in encouraging donor support, with GDP growth edging up to 1.7 per cent. President Moi stepped down in December 2002 following fair and peaceful elections. Mwai Kibaki, running as the candidate of the multiethnic, united opposition group, the National Rainbow Coalition, defeated Kanu candidate Uhuru Kenyatta and assumed the presidency.[44] Political and ethnic tensions heightened in the run-up to the general elections at the end of 2002. Adding to these problems, the ongoing drought disrupted food distribution and led to major power shortages which slowed economic activity and depressed consumer demand, adversely affecting the country's development.[45]

GDP per capita is Intl $1452. This falls within the range of $8272 (Libya) and $346 (Democratic Republic of the Congo) in the countries of Africa (Appendix 4).

References

1 Report of the United Nations Development Programme 2004 (HDI 2002). Launched by the United Nations in 1990, the Human Development Index measures a country's achievements in three aspects of human development: longevity, knowledge and a decent standard of living. It was created to re-emphasize that people and their lives should be the ultimate criteria for assessing the development of a country, not economic growth. Current values range from 0.956 (Norway, first out of 177 countries) to 0.273 (Sierra Leone, 177th out of 177 countries). Countries fall into one of three groups: countries 1–55 = high development; 56–141 = medium development; 142–177 = low development. See: http://hdr.undp.org/statistics/data/indic/indic_8_1_1.html

2 Nairobi Hospice Annual Report 2003.

3 IOELC interview: Zipporah Ali—1 November 2004.

4 IOELC interview: John Njoka—1 November 2004.

5 Personal communication: Zipporah Ali—1 November 2004.

6 IOELC interview: Bactrin Killingo—2 November 2004.

7 Personal communication: Paul Asige—13 January 2005.

8 Personal communication: Paul Asige—20 January 2005.

9 Coast Hospice Report provided by Nyandia Nderitu—18 January 2005.

10 Personal communication: Florence Kiama—24 January 2005.

11 Information leaflet: *Nyeri Hospice*.

12 Gatherings/meetings.

13 IOELC interview: Stephen Gitonga—22 September 2004.

14 **Allbrook D.** Palliative care in Kenya: report of the International Association of Hospice and Palliative Care Travelling fellowship. *Journal of Pain and Pharmacotherapy* 2003; **17(3/4)**: 185–189.

15 **Grant E, Murray A, Grant A, Brown J.** A good death in rural Kenya? Listening to Meru patients and their families talk about care needs at the end of life. *Journal of Palliative Care* 2003; **19(3)**: 159–167.

16 See also: Murray SA, Grant E, Grant A, Kendall M. Dying from cancer in developed and developing countries: lessons from two qualitative interview studies of patients and their carers. *British Medical Journal* 2003; **326**: 368.

17 'The Diana, Princess of Wales Memorial Fund was created through public donation in the immediate aftermath of the death of the Princess in 1997. A global charity, it continues the Princess's humanitarian work in the UK and overseas. By giving grants to organisations, championing charitable causes and creating new money for the charity sector, the Fund helps the most disadvantaged people change their lives. By the end of 2002, the Fund will have pledged £50 million on good causes'. Diana Palliative Care Initiative (2002) *The Diana, Princess of Wales Memorial Fund*: 21. See: www.theworkcontinues.org

18 Nyeri Hospice Team. *The Development of Nyeri Hospice*. 2002.

19 *Engendering Bold Leadership*. The President's Emergency Plan for AIDS Relief. First Annual Report to Congress, 2005: 115. http://www.state.gov/documents/organisation/43885.pdf

20 Personal communication: Paul Asige—26 January 2005.

21 Personal communication: Florence Kiama—25 January 2005.

22 International Narcotics Control Board. *Narcotic Drugs: Estimated World Requirements for 2004. Statistics for 2002*. New York: United Nations, 2004.

23 'The term *defined daily doses for statistical purposes* (S-DDD) replaces the term *defined daily doses* previously used by the Board. The S-DDDs are technical units of measurement for the purposes of statistical analysis and are not recommended prescription doses. Certain narcotic drugs may be used in certain countries for different treatments or in accordance with different medical practices, and therefore a different daily dose could be more appropriate'. The S-DDD used by the INCB for morphine is 100 milligrams. International Narcotics Control Board. *Narcotic Drugs: Estimated World Requirements for 2004. Statistics for 2002*. New York: United Nations, 2004: 176–177.

24 Kate Jones, Hospice Care Kenya. hospice.care.kenya@virgin.net

25 Foundation for Hospices in Sub-Saharan Africa, see: http://www.fssa.org

26 FHSSA newsletter 17 December 2003.

27 IOELC interview: Jane Appleton—1 February 2005.

28 Personal communication: Nyandia Nderitu—19 January 2005.

29 Personal communication: Stephen Gitonga—19 April 2005.

30 Publicity leaflet. *Nairobi Hospice*. Undated.

31 IOELC interview: Ruth Wooldridge—27 January 2005.

32 IOELC interview: Brigid Sirengo—1 November 2004.

33 Hospice Information Service. *The Bulletin* January 1991; **11**: 1.

34 IOELC interview: David Allbrook—11 February 2005.

35 IOELC interview: Zipporah Ali—2 June 2004.

36 IOELC interview: Bactrin Killingo—2 June 2004.

37 A large majority of Kenyans are Christian, but estimates for the percentage of the population that adheres to Islam or indigenous beliefs vary widely. See: http://www.cia.gov/cia/publications/factbook/geos/ke.htlm

38 This refers to adult mortality risk, which is defined as the probability of dying between 15 and 59 years.

39 See: WHO statistics for Kenya at: http://www.who.int/countries/ken/en/

40 http://www.unaids.org/en/geographical+area/by+country/kenya.asp

41 Total health expenditure per capita is the per capita amount of the sum of Public Health Expenditure (PHE) and Private Expenditure on Health (PvtHE). The international dollar is a common currency unit that takes into account differences in the relative purchasing power of various currencies. Figures expressed in international dollars are calculated using purchasing power parities (PPP), which are rates of currency conversion constructed to account for differences in price level between countries.
http://www3.who.int/whosis/country/compare.cfm?country=s&indicator=strPcTotEOHinIntD2000&language=english

42 This composite measure of overall health system attainment is based on a country's goals relating to health, responsiveness and fairness in financing. The measure varies widely across countries and is highly correlated with general levels of human development as captured in the human development index. See: Tandon A, Murray CLJ, Lauer JA, Evans DB. *Measuring Overall Health System Performance for 191 Countries*. GPE Discussion Paper Series: No 30; WHO.

43 Weinreb AA. First politics, then culture: accounting for ethic differences in demographic behavior in Kenya. *Population and Development Review* 2001; **27(3)**: 437–467.

44 http://www.cia.gov/cia/publications/factbook/geos/ke.htlm

45 World of Information Business Intelligence Report. Kenya: economy, politics and government. *Business Intelligence Report: Kenya* 2001; **1(1)**: 1–46.

Chapter 7

South Africa

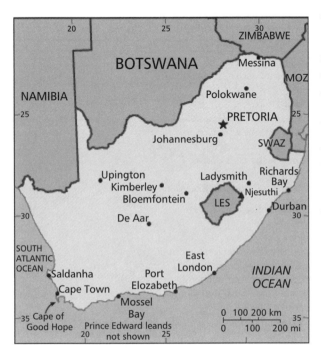

The Republic of South Africa (population 44.76 million) is located at the southern tip of the African continent and covers an area of around 1 220 000 km². Its boundaries border Namibia, Botswana, Zimbabwe, Mozambique, Swaziland and Lesotho.

Pretoria is the capital of South Africa, although Cape Town is the legislative centre and the judicial centre is Bloemfontein. For administration purposes, the country is divided into nine provinces; Eastern Cape, Free State, Gauteng, KwaZulu-Natal, Limpopo, Mpumalanga, North-West, Northern Cape and Western Cape.

According to the United Nations human development index (HDI), South Africa is ranked 119th out of 177 countries worldwide (value 0.666)[1] and fourth out of 45 in African countries for which an index is available. This places South Africa in the group of countries with medium human development.

Palliative care service provision

Current services

In South Africa, around 60 organizations linked to the national association—the Hospice and Palliative Care Association of South Africa (HPCA)—provide a range of services for patients and their families (Table 7.1)[2].

Service types include the following:

◆ Inpatient care

◆ Home care

Table 7.1 Palliative care provision in South Africa: HPCA members/affiliated members, 2004

Date opened	Organization
Pre-1984	Grahamstown Hospice Highway Hospice, Durban Hospice Association of Witwatersrand, Johannesburg St Francis Hospice, Port Elizabeth St Luke's Hospice, Cape Town South Coast Hospice, Port Shepstone Msunduzi Hospice, Pietermaritzburg
1985–1989	Franschoek Hospice, Franschoek Goldfields Hospice Association, Welkom Helderberg Hospice, Somerset West Hospice East Rand Howick Hospice Khanya (Lighthouse Hospice/Amamzimtoti), Umkomaas Knysna/Sedgefield Hospice Naledi Hospice, Blomfontein Pretoria Sungardens Hospice Vryheid Hospice Wide Horizon Hospice, Vereeniging
1990–1994	Chatsworth Hospice Estcourt Hospice Golden Gateway Hospice, Bethlehem Good Shepherd Hospice, Middelburg Hospice Association of Transkei Hospice in the West, Krugersdorp Hospice North West, Klerksdorp Kimberley Hospice Newcastle Hospice Parys Hospice Drakenstein Hospice, Paarl St Bernard's Hospice, East London Stellenbosch Hospice Viljoenskroon Hospice Worcester Hospice Zululand Hospice Association, Empangeni
1995–1999	Breede River Hospice, Robertson Cotlands Hospice, Johannesburg Impilo (Zazile Hope for Life Care Centre) Johannesburg Ladysmith Hospice Association Moretela Sunrise Hospice, North West Nightingale Hospice, De Aar Rustenburg Hospice St Nicholas Children's Hospice, Bloemfontein Sparrow Ministries, Roodepoort Tygerberg Hospice, Bellville Verulam Hospice

Table 7.1 (*Contd.*)

Date opened	Organization
2000–2004	AIDS Care Training and Support, White River
	Arebaokeng Hospice, Tembisa
	Beautiful Gates Ministries, Muizenberg
	Brits Hospice, Brits
	Centurion Hospice, Lyttleton
	Comfi Care, Hartswater
	FWC HIV/AIDS Hospice Shelter, Melville
	Good Samaritan Hospice, Bethulie
	Holy Cross Hospice, Gingindlovu/Emoyeni
	Hospice of White River, Witbank
	Ladybrand Hospice
	Morningstar Hospice, Welkom
	Potchefstroom Hospice
	Philanjalo Hospice, Tugela Ferry
	St Joseph's Care and Support Trust, Sizanani
	Tapologo Hospice, Rustenburg
	Themba Care, Century City
	White Rose Hospice, Witbank

- Day care
- Clinics/drop-in centres
- Hospital support teams
- Education and training
- Patient support groups
- Bereavement care
- Foster parent support groups
- Orphan support groups
- Hospice care for the homeless.[3]

Many of these organizations have branches which provide palliative care services in local settings; examples are shown in Table 7.2.

Not all organizations that provide palliative care in South Africa are members of HPCA. This may partly be due to a desire among international organizations to retain a strong element of independence. *The Dream Centre* (Durban) appears a case in point. Yet without the networks and support of HPCA, establishing a patient base and collaborative relationships can be problematic[4].

In South Africa—unlike most other African countries—palliative care services may be found in hospital settings countrywide (Table 7.3). This feature is reflected in the movement towards a free-standing society for palliative care, a proposal discussed at the HPCA AGM in 2004.

Table 7.2 Examples of hospice/palliative care organizations with local branches

Hospice	Branches
Cotlands, Johannesburg	Cotlands Western Cape Cotlands Turfontein
Grahamstown Hospice	Sunshine Coast Hospice, Port Alfred
Good Shepherd Hospice, Middelburg	Good Samaritan Hospice, Cradock Camdeboo Hospice, Graaf Reinet Living Waters Hospice, Aliwal North
Goldfields Hospice, Welkom	Meloding Hospice, Virginia Kutlwanong Community Hospice centre, Odendaalsrus Thabong Community Hospice Centre, Welkom Bronville Day Care Facility
Hospice Association of Witwatersrand	Soweto Hospice
Pretoria Sungardens	Mamelodi Sungardens Hospice, Mamelodi West
St Francis Hospice, Port Elizabeth	Kouga
St Luke's Hospice, Cape Town	Athlone Constantiaberg/Hout Bay City Bowl False Bay Grassy Park Guguletu Khayelitsha (Michael Mapongwana Hospital) Liesbeeck Lentegeur (Hospital) two wards Mutual Mitchell's Plain West Coast Wynberg

Source: Member Hospices of HPCA, 2004.

Table 7.3 Examples of hospitals with palliative care services/interest

Location	Hospital
Cape Town	2 Military Hospital, Wynberg
Durban	Addington Hospital McCord Hospital Parklands Hospital St Mary's Hospital
Johannesburg	Chris Hani Baragwanath Hospital, Soweto Johannesburg General Hospital
Port Shepstone	Murchison Hospital Port Shepstone Hospital
Pretoria	Pretoria Academic Hospital

In Cape Town, palliative care provision at the 2 Military Hospital is described as follows:

> Situated within a general hospital, the patient has access to palliative care and all its facets from the time of diagnosis of curable and incurable cancer. A major advantage is the availability and affordability of a full multi-disciplinary team, which can provide services and support to other departments, e.g. dietician. Additionally, this particular hospice is combined with a rehabilitation unit, which allows cost effective use of staff as well as space. The issues of loss/grieving/disability and impact on psycho/social functioning are similar. Because of this system, by the time a new symptom develops or some serious event occurs, the patient and family are familiar with palliative care, the ward and the system.[5]

In addition to 2 Military Hospital, St Luke's Hospice (Cape Town) has established close relationships with Groote Schuur Hospital (especially the oncology and pharmacy departments) and Michael Mapongwana Hospital (where a hospice sister runs a day clinic on the premises).[6]

Barbara Campbell-Ker, executive director of the Hospice Association of the Witwatersrand, describes the links with Johannesburg Hospitals:

> As far as the hospitals are concerned, we actually employed one of the palliative care doctors in the Johannesburg General Hospital. The Palliative Care Institute was run by professor Selma Browde—who's well-known as far as palliative care is concerned, and has now partially retired. She asked me if I could possibly help with some funding for the doctor, which I did for five or six months. So, yes, there is a team of a doctor and two nurses in the Johannesburg General Hospital doing palliative care—not just palliative care of the dying, palliative care of everybody; in other words—if a burn victim needs palliative care, if somebody who's really ill with early stages motor neuron; so not just the terminally ill. Then there's a very fine palliative care team in the Chris Hani [Baragwanath] Hospital in Soweto. They've done sterling, sterling work and Dr Rusty Russell [Alison Russell]—she's exemplary in her passion for palliative care. So, yes, palliative care is beginning to be visible in the hospitals as well.[7]

Patient statistics (national), 2003–2004

Between 2003 and 2004, data returned to HPCA indicate that 24 613 patients were cared for, of whom 12 413 had an AIDS diagnosis and 9233 had cancer. Most referrals originated from family, friends or state hospitals (Tables 7.4–7.6).

During 2003–2204, an aggregate of around 48 000 patients utilized hospice and palliative care services in South Africa (Table 7.7).

Table 7.4 Number of patients: HPCA membership, 2003–2004

| Category | No. of patients | | | | | | |
| | Gender | | Race group | | | | |
	Female	Male	Asian	Black	Coloured	White	Total
Existing patients	6474	4144	399	5813	1014	3034	10 618
New referrals	8397	5598	530	7691	1574	3403	13 995
Total patients	14 871	9742	929	13504	2588	6437	24 613

Source: HPCA SA Annual National Statistics 2003–2004.

Table 7.5 Patient diagnoses: HPCA membership, 2003–2004

Diagnosis	No. of patients						
	Gender		Race group				
	Female	Male	Asian	Black	Coloured	White	Total
AIDS	7752	4661	69	10 457	768	194	12 413
Cancer	4878	4355	564	1808	1863	4908	9233
Emphysema	35	32	0	12	8	50	67
Motor neuron disease	13	11	1	1	5	19	24
Cerebrovascular accident	57	50	0	32	42	27	107
Multiple sclerosis	8	11	1	13	3	4	19
Congestive cardiac failure	40	33	2	14	17	30	73
Renal failure	21	24	5	6	9	25	45
Neurological disorders	32	32	5	5	9	45	64
Other	235	209	6	186	105	131	444

Source: HPCA SA Annual National Statistics 2003–2004.

Table 7.6 Source of referrals: HPCA membership, 2003–2004

Source	No. of patients						
	Gender		Race group				
	Female	Male	Asian	Black	Coloured	White	Total
Self	497	237	71	454	39	136	734
Family/friends	2699	1506	331	1481	141	1077	4205
State hospital	3627	1271	240	2169	564	415	4898
Community health centre	696	149	6	311	20	14	845
Primary health centre	1022	639	3	1115	124	28	1661
Private: GP	907	511	59	204	111	832	1418
Private: specialist	635	240	27	26	43	315	875
Social worker	67	21	5	54	5	5	88
Cancer association	26	20	2	12	20	12	46
Faith representative	15	17	2	13	6	11	32
Other hospice	81	41	10	45	11	40	122
Other	819	427	2	463	52	59	1237

Source: HPCA SA Annual National Statistics 2003–2004.

The following extracts from interviews with palliative care workers give an insight into the nature of these services; Barbara Campbell-Ker comments:

> In the Integrated Community Home Based Care programme, we have a community care worker—what you would call an ancillary care worker; it's a base level of three, four, five months of nurse

Table 7.7 Utilization of services: HPCA membership, 2003–2004

| Type of service | No. of patients | | | | | | |
| | Gender | | Race group | | | | |
	Female	Male	Asian	Black	Coloured	White	Total
Home care	12 924	9709	638	12 450	2769	4181	22 633
Day care	1518	871	347	946	323	688	2389
Inpatient	2195	1708	275	999	519	1151	3903
Clinic	1235	1012	675	1304	207	263	2247
Bereavement	3483	2454	287	2169	586	1485	5937
Counselling	5731	4915	153	4063	1247	2050	10 646
Other	382	185	61	494	28	14	567

training with a palliative care component. On the first assessment, when the professional nursing sister goes to the patient's home, she will take a community care worker with her so that the community care worker is well aware of the family dynamics, of the exact problem of the patient, and will work with the professional nursing sister, so that, once that patient has stabilized— symptom managed, pain controlled, any other problems ironed out—that community care worker can do those interim visits: bed-bathing the patient, washing the patient, perhaps cooking breakfast in the morning for the patient—because of course we're not talking first-world; we're talking very much third-world with huge problems of stigma, of no resources whatsoever. So if that family member can get a job—even a part-time job—they will leave the patient unattended, and sometimes in the most appalling conditions. So the community care workers would pop in. We try and let the community care workers work in the area where they live so we divide the area into segments. We also try to have ten community care workers per nursing sister. The nursing sister will do the interim visits and the community care worker will do the regular visits in between. In their kit, the community care worker can't take any of the opioids because in our country, unless you're a professional nursing sister at least, you cannot dispense medicine. That might have to change. Certain dispensing laws are being promulgated in parliament at the moment, but they can take in the very basic aspirin, with the dressings, gloves, aprons, soap, Savlon or Dettol to clean the wounds, but very little besides that. But at least it helps.[7]

Mandla Mtatambi manages the day centre in Inanda, Durban:

The day centre opens here twice a week. Activities in the day centre concern support groups; we give talks and we try to partner with other organizations so they can come and give talks. We find those patients that have been in support groups for some time make the others feel more at home. They talk about how he or she disclosed to her family about her [HIV] status: who did she talk to first? and how did she handle that? The average attendance I would say is 40 to 50 on a Thursday. Then we have opened up on Tuesday. The numbers are a bit less because we had to select for certain areas to come on a certain day, and we have seen positive results. There were people that were said to be pre-terminal or terminal when we initially had contact with them. But finding that the main problem was poor symptom management and hunger, then you know, when those things have been attended to we see people rising up and improving. Some are no longer in the programme; they started with a one-day job and then we feel they can go and hunt for the actual full-time job. So those are the positive results that we are seeing.[8]

Joan de Jong is the executive director of Hospice North West:

Most of our patients live in the poorest of the poor conditions, and our sisters said there were so many mothers dying and very ill, there was no-one to take care of the children. Sometimes they lived with grannies. For example, one granny had arthritis; she had the three-year-old she was looking after, mother had died, and an eight- and a ten-year-old, who were not doing well at school. One day I said to Angie [Sehoke] 'Why are they not doing well at school?' She said, 'Well, granny's got arthritis and she can't pick up the children, so they only go to school on alternate days so that one can stay home and help granny'. And that motivated us—with no money—to go and look at the house next door—which we purchased. The bank wanted to know how we were buying a house, and I said, 'On faith!' They weren't so keen to give us a bond on faith. But they did, and we started a crèche there for our children, a palliative day care crèche. We pay for taxis to fetch them and they bring them in every morning and take them home at about two o'clock, or half past two in the afternoon. With us, they have two meals a day, get vitamins and they're really doing so well; they're all HIV infected, or affected.[9]

Joan Marston is the founder of St Nicholas Children's Hospice, Bloemfontein and Advocacy Officer, HPCA:

I think one of the special challenges is actually just dealing with the dying child, and the emotion and the impact it has on those caring for the children; it's very hard and we're lucky in having tremendous spiritual support, especially from our chaplain, Father Keith, who brings in rituals and support programmes for the staff to help them to cope; so that's one of the big things. The other, of course, is communicating with children. You know, we're very good at communicating with words but children need play and we work in poor communities where people have forgotten to play, or they just feel that there's no fun left in life—and to bring that back into their communication with the children; and then of course there's the abject poverty that most of our children live in, when the basic need is food just to keep them alive 'til the next day; and we also often see children who are sent in—dying of AIDS according to the doctors—and when they come to hospice we find they're dying of starvation; and we actually act very, very aggressively to feed them because we found three quarters of the children that are sent to us dying, if we feed them properly, we actually bring them through. Then of course are the issues of orphanhood. So many children are orphaned—not necessarily that their parents are dead but their parents are very ill and can't care for them, or they're abandoned. We have one little boy whose in our programmes and his mother died of AIDS. His father's infected; and his father one day locked him in the shack and went to Johannesburg and for three months this child who was three years old was fed by neighbours through the window; and it sounds strange that they didn't call anyone in or take him out—but there's often this fear that if they interfere, they will be assaulted or abused or have their shacks burned down. So the neighbours kept on putting food and water through the window for this little child. It was only when somebody doing a project in the community found him that he was brought to us. And he was totally, totally traumatized as you can imagine; covered in sores, skin and bone, and for about two months all he did was sit and rock and cry. But then he started eating and now he's the fattest, chubbiest, happiest little son and he's been fostered by a family. So nutrition is so very important, you know, before you even go in with palliative care interventions, you actually need to take food in to the situations that we're working in.[10]

Challenges facing palliative care development in South Africa have been stated to be:

◆ Raising palliative care awareness for the public, health professionals and ministry of health officials

- Recruiting qualified staff
- Emigration of trained staff
- Funding and resources
- Partnering with government
- Lack of palliative care policy making and integration into practice
- Resistance to change on the part of health professionals
- Smooth referral from clinic and hospital to hospice
- Availability of opioid drugs
- Number of child-headed families
- Denial of the seriousness of the illness
- Transport
- Time taken to admit a patient to a programme
- Poverty
- Lack of volunteers in some regions
- Distances covered by individual services
- Roll out of ARV therapy.[11]

Flora Kobotlo Modiba (founder of Arebaokeng Hospice) and Elna van der Merwe (nursing services manager, Centurion Hospice) speak of some of these challenges. Flora Modiba:

> I had many challenges and problems setting up the service. First, from funding: I didn't have money to set up the proper structure; I had to use what was my salary. I found a lot of resistance from the medical fraternity. The doctors didn't know anything about palliative care and they wouldn't accept instructions from me as a nurse asking them to prescribe morphine for the patient—because at that stage the perception was that morphine was only prescribed for people when you want them to die. They did not understand that it was actually a rescue medicine that makes people more comfortable. So I had a problem with the doctors accepting my expertise in palliative care. And also the referrers: I had problems getting referrals from the clinics and from the doctors because they just did not understand the work that I was doing—and as the bulk of my patients came from lay referrals and I did not have medical reports that substantiated the patients' conditions and diagnoses, at times I had to take blood myself and send it to laboratories so that I could have something in writing that would say a patient is an HIV/AIDS patient. That cost me a lot of money that I didn't have.[12]

Elna van der Merwe:

> I think the biggest challenge for us is not to get into the mentality that we are a hospice and we need your support and your money—because that's true, we all do. But take patients who are at home that are diagnosed quite early in their disease: if their symptoms are under control, then they can live an active life. But, if you do not have a job and you do not have a way of getting an income or a job creation situation, then you are putting that patient back into a situation where he's under stress, because he can't provide for his family. And I think one of our challenges is: how are we going to incorporate the services of hospice into community upliftment projects, where the

community are able to generate an income for themselves? If hospice can play a role in exporting that—whether it be arts and crafts, whether it be cultural aspects of society, whether it's any of those things—if we can help them to export that and earn an income from that, we are actually creating a circle where everyone is doing something for each other. I would really like to see this hospice 10 years from now, where we have say 10 projects that we are marketing overseas—yah, that we can market overseas—that are bringing in an income for this hospice. And I think that we are not just doing something for them, but they are also serving us, and we are helping each other to create a new way of looking at palliative care, because it then makes the whole circle—and until they die—and we give them hope that they feel they are still able to contribute to society in such a special way; it's not just that they are on the receiving side of everything every time, but they are actually giving something back.[13]

Opportunities for palliative care development in South Africa are considered to be:

- Gradual raising of palliative care awareness
- Education and training
- Greater focus upon research
- Structured programmes
- Education for life: behaviour change
- Community involvement and interest
- Growing recognition from the Ministry of Health
- Well developed district health systems as an infrastructure for palliative care development
- Programme of capacity building
- PEPFAR funding
- Involvement of faith-based organizations
- Growth and acceptance of support groups
- Increased cross-cultural awareness
- Expansion of palliative care programmes to include the development of skills: sewing, art
- Growing international recognition of HIV/AIDS in Africa
- International networks.[14]

Edith Khumalo, social worker at Soweto Hospice refers to many of these opportunities:

We do get challenges although there are those days when we feel very [uplifted]. For instance, I'll speak of my part as a social worker: to trace a patient's family; to give support to that patient; when we have money, to get the family and the patient being co-operative; and you feel that you have achieved some success. Dr Thobi [Segabi] has just mentioned: most of our people, when they start getting sick the majority don't just go immediately to seek help from the doctors; they will try this and that. And it's only when they come here, when they are really sick that, you know, they realize how serious their sickness is. They were told—especially most of our female patients, when they go for check-up, especially when they are pregnant—they are immediately told, but because the wife feels she's still OK they don't realize the implications of being HIV positive. Despite the counselling, despite what they were taught, the changing of lifestyle, they'll just go on and on. So when they come here, they haven't even started, you know. They've not applied for this grant, this state grant, which actually helps them to buy good food, so that when they take medication, they are able to become better because they eat healthily.

So what I achieve at times is help from the outside agencies; for instance, our home affairs person has been very co-operative. Most of our sick patients, when they are unable to go to apply for this grant, [the officials] come here to our hospice; they bring their machinery and all that. They have agreed that as long as we have sent somebody home, and that someone has been appointed by the patient herself—who would be given power of attorney—then we can manage to apply for those people. It becomes so great when we know that the grant has been approved and the family is no longer suffering. And at times, you know, people come crying because they cannot accept that; but just talking to them, just talking and counselling, we find a changed person.[15]

A patient who attends a hospice day centre in Cape Town speaks about what hospice means to her:

It is very interesting; it helps you get away from the house. They make you welcome and make you feel part of a family. Sometimes, when I'm feeling sick, I'm happy to just be there and listen to what's going on. I don't feel so lonely. When I stay here, at home, I sometimes feel very, very lonely.[16]

A Cape Town home care patient says:

The hospice staff are wonderful. They encourage me to go on. I think the doctor and nursing staff are marvellous. They treat us like babies; most of all we get love. They have carried me like a baby. It's like the Garden of Eden: beautiful![17]

Patients at the hospice day centre in Soweto speak about why they attend:

I feel quite at home here; we can socialize with each other and we give advice to each other.[18]
The more we come here, the more we get relief from stress because we live in families where we get no social support.[19]
They give us medication because some of it we can't buy on our own.[20]
I very much look forward to coming because it makes me feel good while I am here.[21]

Also in Soweto, a young patient's carer speaks about how the hospice responded to her request for help:

Since I've contacted hospice and told them about my sister's daughter—she has no mother, no father, no ID card, no birth certificate, no money for food, and she's very sick—they gave us food and [incontinence] napkins. They come to see us, and they care about us. It's helped a lot.[22]

To commentators in developed countries, some of the services provided by palliative care organizations—in South Africa and in Africa generally—may seem unfamiliar. In their report (2004) to the Diana Fund, Richard Harding and Irene Higginson address this point:

Although the definition of palliative care is globally relevant, what constitutes palliative care needs and services in sub-Saharan Africa is continent-specific, particularly in the light of poverty and HIV disease. Necessary components include practical care, pain and symptom control, counselling/emotional/psychological support, income generation, financial support for food, shelter, funeral costs and school fees, respite, spiritual care and orphan care.[23]

Integrated Community-based Home Care

At South Coast Hospice, Port Shepstone, an innovative form of care has been developed, in collaboration with networking partners, known as *Integrated Community-based Home Care* (ICHC). This care is available to people living with HIV/AIDS (PLHA), and to their families—and includes the following elements:

- *Clinical management*—providing early diagnosis, including HIV testing, appropriate prophylaxis and treatment of opportunistic infections as well as effective management of pain and symptom control.

- *Nursing care*—promoting and maintaining hygiene and nutrition, teaching the family and microcommunity basic nursing skills and comfort as well as emergency measures, supervising the taking of medication and DOTS (directly observed treatment short course) for TB, teaching and observance of universal precautions.

- *Psycho-spiritual support*—providing counselling and spiritual support, including stress and risk reduction planning, promoting and supporting the acceptance and disclosure of serostatus. Enabling coping in terms of positive living and planning for the future of the family in particular placement of children.

- *Social support*—providing welfare services and legal advice; providing information and referrals between the partners who make up the care network, including poverty alleviation and pastoral and bereavement care; facilitating peer support.

The ICHC model was piloted at seven hospice sites across South Africa in 1999–2000 on behalf of the South African national Department of Health HIV/AIDS Directorate. Research conducted by HASA (now HPCA) and the University of Natal demonstrated the replicability and cost-effectiveness of ICHC and recommended the model be rolled out countrywide. South Coast Hospice was subsequently awarded a research tender by the South African Department of Health to develop Port Shepstone as an HIV/AIDS, TB/STI demonstration site.[24]

In 2002, a review of the South African model of ICHC was undertaken by the Centre for AIDS Development, Research and Evaluation (CADRE) on behalf of the POLICY Futures Group.[25] This research focused on seven hospices located in five of the nine provinces of South Africa. These were: Helderberg, Somerset West (Western Cape); Naledi, Bloemfontein (Free State); Pretoria Sungardens (Gauteng); South Coast, Port Shepstone (KwaZulu-Natal); St Bernard's, East London (Eastern Cape); St Francis, Port Elizabeth (Eastern Cape); and Zululand, Empangeni (KwaZulu-Natal).[25]

The objectives of the research were to:

- Identify and discuss key similarities and differences between the hospice ICHC model and other home-based care models used in South Africa

- Identify and critically review the core elements related to the ICHC model as implemented by the Hospice Association of South Africa (now HPCA)

- Highlight key aspects of best practice related to the hospice ICHC model internal development and transformation, and in relation to its reach into the community.

The report concludes:

- In some hospices, existing systems and structures have been retained and underpin emerging response, whilst in others, systems, structures and infrastructure have been considerably realigned.

- As a whole, hospices are being transformed and expanded as a direct result of the emerging needs of the HIV/AIDS epidemic. Transformation is never easy, especially where new ground is being charted and where human resources need to be managed, but the value of developing and working with models is that this allows transformation to be well considered and systematic. At the same time, the ICHC model is flexible, and any part of it can be adapted to an individual home-based care need or situation

- Within hospice, new models of operation are evolving which incorporate diverse human resources and capacities, and in social and community contexts that are themselves changing, and in circumstances that are constrained by poverty and hardship. However, the underlying ethos of care provision, combined with an understanding of the community contexts, is maintained within the ICHC model

- Hospices are integral to the developing response to HIV/AIDS, and the organization has risen to the emerging challenges. However, continued support is required from other role players in relation to both its internal development and transformation, and in relation to its reach into the community.[27]

Reimbursement and funding for services

Hospices in South Africa are usually registered as not-for-profit organizations. A small amount of money is available from government but, in the main, the hospice has to source its own funds. Barbara Campbell-Ker:

> The spirit can be extremely willing but we are as good as the resources that we have, and we have to find all our money. The Department of Health gives us about two per cent or three per cent of what we require—if we're lucky—and that isn't done just by handing it out, but after completing funding proposals.[7]

This places a considerable burden on hospice organizations which occasionally causes difficulties. Lesley van Zyl, general manager of Highway Hospice (Durban), tells how dwindling funds can impact an organization:

> The challenge for me is always to balance the books. We've gone through some fairly tough periods where we had to retrench staff [make staff redundant] and we moved from being predominantly in-care units—correctly I believe—to care for patients in the community by opening various day centres. We've opened day centres in Chesterville, in Umlazi, in Phoenix and in Inanda, and difficult as it was and as painful as it was, I personally believe it was the right thing to do.
>
> We had two years where we were battling to raise funds and we had to down-size. So, you know, we make a loss year—it's not good; but if you make it in two years, it's worse. By the time we get to the third year you really have to do something. So we reduced our beds from 16 to eight. It was a particularly difficult thing to do; and also I think whenever you are facing the staff and you have to tell them that some of them are going to be without work, that's really tough.[28]

President's Emergency Plan for AIDS Relief (PEPFAR)

During the 2004 financial year (FY), funding of around US$65.42 million was enacted for country-managed programmes in South Africa and $24 million for central programmes. During FY2005, it is anticipated that a total of US$132.1 million will be enacted: US$106.68 million for country-managed programmes and US$25.42 million for central programmes.[29]

In May 2004, HPCA and USAID announced jointly that the PEPFAR had granted initial funding of US$5 million (~35 million South African rand) to HPCA over the next 2 years.

Dr Dirk Dijkerman, USAID South Africa Director, said HPCA's request for funding was successful for many reasons: 'Hospice has been working in South Africa for years, reaching millions of people who are suffering from terminal diseases such as AIDS . . . HPCA's track record and network of organizations throughout South Africa demonstrate its competence and compassion,' said Dijkerman. He indicated that the project's capacity to sustain its activities was well in place through HPCA's ability to leverage complementary funding from local communities, trusts and foundations, combined with strong government partnerships locally, provincially and nationally.

In the press release, Joan Marston explained the ways in which the funding would be used:

- HPCA coordinates the activities of 52 hospices across South Africa which engaged the services of 6,355 people in 2002 and this funding will go a long way in strengthening existing and developing new hospice and palliative care services

- Hospices will benefit from the new structures, but won't receive direct funding. Day-to-day expenses still need to be covered by the ongoing generosity of the public and corporate donors

- One of HPCA's major obstacles lies in the unlocking of available hours of its staff and volunteer base. We have the expertise available, but we need to free up some time. The appointment of provincial palliative care coordinators, trainers and mentors, which will be funded by PEPFAR, will do exactly that. They will oversee the development of hospice and palliative care in their areas and will work with mentorship teams to help hospices and other NGOs, community-based organizations and faith-based organizations to establish new palliative care services

- Mentor hospices which will tutor and guide developing hospices will be identified and exemplar hospices will serve as centres of excellence with outstanding programs, such as bereavement care and home-based care. All hospices will be audited to ensure the care they provide is of the highest quality.[30]

One of the new provincial co-ordinators, Brenda Dass, a nurse and former development manager (outreach programme) at Hospice East Rand, describes her role:

> I'm now employed as the provincial co-ordinator, basically concerned with the mentoring programme. It really works in three ways: there is the mentoring of established hospices; the mentoring of emerging hospices; and the setting up of totally new programmes. Then there's liaison with the different departments involved in HIV/AIDS, the Department of Health, social services and education, as far as the children are concerned. Basically, what we've been doing up to now [August 2004] is identifying the development sites and doing strategic planning around those sites to identify the areas of need. We then set up a team—and the team comprises people with various skills—so we can now send people in to do the development wherever the skill is needed.[31]

André Wagner, HPCA board member responsible for organization development, speaks of another objective which, if achieved, will impact significantly upon hospice development in South Africa:

> One of the objectives of the PEPFAR project is to have, towards the end of the five year period, one hospice in every health district in South Africa—health districts that are identified by the Department of Health. If we look at the Department of Health's breakdown, there are more than 170 health districts in the country and the idea is for us to have a hospice in each of those health districts; and that's why the focus of this project is to develop, to strengthen, existing hospices so that they can be mentors and develop new hospices. The idea is to make sure that all hospices deliver the same level of care—that hospices be accredited—and that's where our standards of care for clinical and management and governance come in.[32]

Alongside this PEPFAR initiative, *A Clinical Guide to Supportive and Palliative Care for HIV/AIDS*[33]—a book that had been published and freely distributed in the USA—became the focus of a working party to adapt it for use in Africa. The working party, led by Liz Gwyther, took the project forward at a 4-day meeting in Cape Town (2003) sponsored by the US State Department and the National Hospice and Palliative Care Organization (the umbrella organization for hospice and palliative care services in the USA). The African edition of the book was due to be sent to the printers in June 2005.[34]

Open Society Institute (OSI)

The Open Society Institute has launched a palliative care initiative in South Africa that is intended to:

- Advance programmes in palliative care education, training and service delivery
- Advocate for their integration into national HIV/AIDS 'treatment and care' programmes

Information about the project states:

> It is well accepted that nothing will have a greater impact on the quality of life of HIV/AIDS patients and families than institutionalising the knowledge we have now to provide pain management, symptom control and psycho-social support in an integrated community based programme for patients and families dying with HIV/AIDS. Integrated community based programmes for the care of patients and families with HIV/AIDS provide a range of services from HIV testing, counselling and prevention, palliative care, social support (food, clothing, housing) orphan care, day care centres, and income generating initiatives.[35]

Reflecting OSI's role as a catalyst, funding has been awarded to three NGOs that have been identified by OSI as leaders in addressing the care of patients and families with HIV/AIDS at the community level. These are:

- Medical Education for South Africa Blacks (MESAB)
- Hospice Palliative Care Association of South Africa (HPCA)
- Foundation for Hospices in Sub-Saharan Africa (FHSSA).

The initiative began in 2002 with OSI funding of US$300 000 to support the work of these organizations. Matched funding from Pfizer USA meant that around US$540 000 was distributed during this year. Liz Gwyther recalls the impact of this funding:

> OSI helped us in that, when our home care programme for AIDS patients was started at South Coast Hospice and we received funding from our Department of Health to replicate that in seven different hospices throughout the country, we asked OSI for funding—to assist those seven hospices that we appointed as mentor hospices to assist another 22 hospices to come to that same standard. Not all of them are there yet but that will be part of this next stage. Stage two is where we have set up provincial development teams because what we found with the initial mentorship is that one or two people within the province were doing all of the mentorship and they found themselves very stretched, and their hospices lost them for a period of time while they were mentoring other organizations. So now we have five strong provincial teams that have a minimum of eight people on the team, with the total interdisciplinary representation including training, advocacy, person living with AIDS, the clinical aspects, the counselling aspects and any other expertise that they feel they need.[36]

The Diana, Princess of Wales Memorial Fund (The Diana Fund)

Among the grants awarded by the Diana Fund to help develop palliative care in South Africa are the following:

2001

+ HPCA—18-month project to establish and run a distance learning diploma in palliative medicine at the University of Cape Town (UCT), including bursaries for selected candidates: £35 000

+ South Coast Hospice—for running an expanded home-based palliative care programme including memory boxes for children: £80 000

+ St Francis Hospice—contribution to strengthen a home-based palliative care programme including training care workers and employing a supervisor: £15 000

+ St Bernard's Hospice—contribution to strengthen and extend pilot home-based palliative care programmes: £15 000

+ Helderberg Hospice—to expand a home-based palliative care programme into two further (rural) communities, including training and capacity building: £15 000

+ Grahamstown Hospice—contribution to home-based palliative care programmes: £15 000

+ Howick Hospice (via Help the Hospices)—contribution to the costs of a home care programme in rural areas: £15 000

+ Naledi Hospice—contribution to costs of expanding home-based care programmes with a special focus on paediatric care, including related training for volunteers, families and professionals: £15 000

+ St Luke's Hospice—cost of employing a second doctor at Khayelitsha day hospice: £9000.

2002

- HPCA—3-year advocacy programme for palliative care, including salary costs of a senior advocacy officer and costs of producing advocacy materials: £129 000
- HPCA—workshop costs for South African conference/trainers meeting: £1224.80 (US$ 2000)
- St Francis Hospice Association—training provided by Dr Lydia Mpanga Sebuyira of Hospice Uganda: £5600
- Bursary to allow two black Africans to attend a conference in 2003 in The Hague to share experiences on setting up national associations for palliative care (via Help the Hospices): £5000.

2003

- HPCA—commission to develop a curriculum for paediatric palliative care in South Africa: £24 135.

UK Forum for Hospice and Palliative Care Worldwide

Since inception, support has been offered to South Africa by the UK Forum for Hospice and Palliative Care Worldwide via the following funds:

- Howick Hospice—short course, HIV/AIDS care and counselling: £337
- Zululand Hospice Association—palliative care course: £644
- Hospice North West—to establish community houses for patients in the last stages of life. The costs include purchase of premises, installation of utilities, equipment for the kitchen, bedrooms and bathroom, and running costs including salaries, administration, food and medicine: £1000
- Onthatile—for the provision of holistic home-based care to the patient with AIDS and the family in the Ga-Rankuwa area. This will be achieved by establishing two teams, each consisting of one registered nurse and 10 caregivers: £2000
- Refilwe community project—to employ a home-based caregiver to work in the small settlements surrounding the hospice. The caregiver will visit people in their homes, bring food or medicine, and if required arrange admittance. The caregiver will also establish relationships with community leaders: £2000.

For FY2005, the following grants were awarded:

- Ladybrand Hospice—short course in palliative nursing for enrolled nurses: £1350
- Overstrand Hospice—for a multiprofessional week: £1500
- St Luke's Hospice—for the 7th International Conference on 'Grief and Bereavement in Contemporary Society': £1500
- Hospice Association of the Witwatersrand—for the certificate course in palliative nursing for professional nurses: £2000.

Opioid availability and consumption

The International Narcotics Control Board[37] has published the following figures for the consumption of narcotic drugs in South Africa: codeine 7587 kg; morphine 156 kg; dihydrocodeine 85 kg; pholcodine 98; dextropropoxyphene 1934 kg; pethidine 283 kg; methadone 1 kg; diphenoxylate 1 kg; and cocaine 4 kg.

For the years 2000–2002, the average defined daily dose consumption of morphine for statistical purposes (S-DDD)[38] in South Africa was 103. This compares with other African countries as follows: Swaziland 1; Egypt 2; Uganda 4; Zimbabwe 13; and Namibia 73. Twenty-nine countries reported no morphine consumption during 2000–2002 (Appendix 1).

Liz Gwyther—education and research coordinator, HPCA, comments:

> I was going to say that our legal system is supportive; but in fact we're just battling a bit with new dispensing laws that really are putting all the dispensing back to the pharmacists; so the doctors are unable to dispense and of course the nurses are not able to dispense. So, having come from that meeting in Arusha where Uganda has just licensed nurses to prescribe and dispense morphine, we seem to be taking a step backwards, in that the dispensing can only happen at the pharmacy level now.
>
> Morphine is available. We don't have a wide range of opioids; we have morphine—and methadone's really only available for weaning addicts, it's not really available as a pain relief medication. There has to be immense motivation to use it anyway as our step three analgesic, and so the prescribing of Schedule 7 medications must be by a doctor. So doctors have to be knowledgeable in prescribing how to use morphine. So that's our biggest barrier right now—the doctor's knowledge. And coming from Port Elizabeth this morning, it's again the nurses who are looking after hospice patients who will say to the doctor, 'You know, doctor, this patient needs to be on morphine,' and 'This morphine does need to be increased' so it makes it quite a tedious way to go.[39]

Marisa Wolheim, executive director of Shanti Nilaya (Hospice in the West) tells how the problems of medication are compounded by distance:

> We have such a struggle in getting medication to our patients because most of our patients are government patients and some of them live 60 kilometres away from main hospital centres; so they don't get enough morphine. Sometimes they sit all day in a hospital—it cost them 60-odd rand to get there—to be told, 'Come back tomorrow, we're too busy'. They just can't do that. Or they're given a little bottle of morphine syrup that's going to last them a week. So we've had to learn to supplement medication, but it's such an expense. Our volunteer co-ordinator took it upon herself to create a fund, a medicine fund, and with this fund we buy extra medication so that when there are patients who are really in need—through our doctor prescribing and so on—we support them and supplement their drugs, because they just cannot have access to proper medication. So that's been a great help, to have a source of income that we know, if there's really a patient that can't afford medication, we can go to that source and lobby for it and say, 'This is the background' and then we buy medication from the fund.[40]

Traditional healers

As in other African countries, Western medicine and traditional healing run side by side. Many patients routinely visit traditional healers before consulting staff trained in Western methods. While such healers focus upon herbal remedies, they also represent indigenous traditions that acknowledge the disease caused when the equilibrium of life has been disturbed. Ancestors feature prominently, forming an unbroken, transcendent link between past, present and future that provides a sense of continuity and belonging. In the context of care at the end of life, there is a growing appreciation that collaboration with traditional healers brings benefits for the patient:

Sr Priscilla Dlamini—founder, Holy Cross Hospice, Gingindlovu:

> I'm also working with traditional healers. My aim in the beginning was to give them knowledge because they were treating these people who are HIV positive, not knowing that they have this [disease]. So it was to make it clear to them that these patients were not going there to be trained as traditional healers but they were sick. And then the traditional healers taught me the traditional uses of the plants. So now we have a project of traditional healing, and we have a garden where we grow those plants I'm using for the immune system.[41]

Flora Kobotlo Modiba:

> My relationship with the traditional healers actually started with a patient. If the patient believes in traditional healing I don't discourage it. Fortunately, in Tembisa, there are a lot of home-based care projects, amongst which we have got one project that is managed by a traditional healer. She actually convinced us that she understands HIV/AIDS is incurable and also, she is a chief of all the traditional healers in Tembisa—and now they all understand that HIV/AIDS is incurable. So she has been able to influence other traditional healers, saying that in their practice they must take care of infection control, they must educate their patients that whatever they do is just to make them comfortable and treat opportunistic diseases—especially sexually transmitted diseases. So she has been of great help to us because, even with the medicines that she is using the patients know that they are more palliative than curative. So we do have a good rapport with the traditional healer because of this common understanding that HIV/AIDS is not curable.[42]

Thembi Nyuswa, a palliative care sister at Highway Hospice, Durban, says:

> People think, you know, something has happened to them because they have failed to appease their ancestors in one way or the other, or they have omitted some rituals, or they've angered their ancestors by doing something they shouldn't have done, and, yeah, this is quite common—and it's very important not to overlook that and to appreciate what they think. Most of the time they would talk about that and they would ask what you think, which is quite interesting, because you would be listening to them, talking about all this. And then they'll suddenly ask you what you think. Then you would say, 'From what I have been taught, it is this way and that way'. At times it helps if we have something in writing—or it could be pictures or a pamphlet—just to prove to them that we conceive illness to be from this and that, but actually this is also the case, and it's scientifically proven so why not try it?—because by the time they come to hospice for help they will have tried all other avenues.[43]

Liz Gwyther:

> It's actually a very exciting cultural environment to explore and I think that St Luke's, Cape Town, has looked at this and has a very strong multifaith spiritual counselling team; and when we're talking about traditional healers—who are also the spiritual leaders in the African culture—I think they are respected by hospice people. The Military Hospice has got quite strong links with traditional healers—and places like South Coast Hospice have a traditional healer that actually looks after the herb garden, because there are a lot of traditional plants that he grows to treat

various ailments. So a lot of our hospices have connections with the traditional healers. We try and make sure that the patient will still be able to get pain medication, for example, but will be able to take whatever else they need on the traditional side—because there are such complex treatments from the traditional healer's point of view. I mean, it's the throwing of the bones; it's the actual calling of the ancestral spiritual medium where the spirit speaks through the traditional healer, in addition to herbal medicines. So it's been getting that understanding that's been important. My impression is that it is still in its infancy, this strong link between hospice and the traditional healer. But the team that includes the multifaith minister—the imam or rabbi or Buddhist or whoever's there—is a stronger team; the link with traditional healers is growing.[39]

National and professional organizations

The Hospice and Palliative Care Association of South Africa (HPCA)

Peter Buckland, in a chapter he wrote on *Hospice in Southern Africa*, notes that the Hospice Association of Southern Africa was formed in 1987 'to represent, facilitate and co-ordinate development and growth of hospice in the region'.[44] He was instrumental in shaping the association during its formative years, having left his post as executive officer of St Luke's Hospice (Cape Town) to help take the Association forward.

By 2002, the association was made up of around 50 member hospices, although large areas of the country were without a palliative care service.[45] Today, the Association has changed its name and geared up for the challenges brought about by the AIDS pandemic and the urgent need for expansion.[46, 47] The director's report of 2004 outlines the structure of HPCA:

A voluntary board of 10 directors, elected by hospices directs the Association. In addition, three directors may be co-opted by the board of directors. A consultant supported by a small office staff manages the day to day affairs of the Association. In response to needs expressed by the membership, the board formed five committees to facilitate development of the hospice movement in South Africa. These five committees are: Advocacy; Fundraising and Public Relations; Organization Development; Education and Research; and Patient Care Services [48] (p. 11).

Josef Lazarus, strategic adviser to the board of HPCA, identifies the significance of these committees in the development of the Association:

I think circumstances often provide a new direction for an organization. In 1997, the then executive director of the national association resigned and I was then asked to do a strategic planning exercise for the national organization, in terms of its future direction. And through that we put a plan in place that actually made the national organization much more development orientated. It decentralized the national organization. As opposed to having a central organi\ation, the national office became a facilitator of hospice development as opposed to a national office that simply represents hospices. Instead of having a CEO who couldn't possibly fulfil all the functions as required in development, because they're so varied, we identified five key portfolios that are required for hospice development; they being patient care, education and training, organizational development, advocacy, and public relations and fundraising.

That has pretty much revolutionized the Hospice Association in South Africa. The people that you've seen here like Liz Gwyther and André Wagner and Joan Marston, they are conveners of those development subcommittees and they've taken full ownership and responsibility for their portfolio with the expertise of their subcommittee. It's become an entirely decentralized organization with only one full time staff member, and that's an administrator. The organization is driven by a team of people with expertise in a particular portfolio. There is a fund to support their activities and hospices are encouraged to engage in further development, extending their services, because there is a fund that supports that development activity specifically.

The Hospice Association was asked to do three major tenders for the national Department of Health—done by these development subcommittees. These development subcommittees now sit on a newly formed steering committee of the Department of Health for palliative care in South Africa and that steering committee is now forming similar subcommittees for operationalizing palliative care throughout South Africa—so that model is now beginning to be replicated by the national Department of Health. It's been a very exciting journey the last five years.[49]

Reports presented by committee leaders at the HPCA AGM in Rustenburg (2004) included the following points.

Advocacy

A desk review of palliative care training and services was carried out in October 2003 and a database was developed for the national Department of Health. Other initiatives include;

- Department of Health plan to integrate palliative care into curriculum of care
- Publication of *Adult Palliative Care Guidelines*. Concept papers written: *Palliative care in South Africa* and *Care of children made vulnerable and orphaned by HIV/AIDS within hospice palliative care programmes*
- Extensive international advocacy activities in Europe, UK, USA [48] (p. 9).

Advocacy officer Joan Marston comments:

It's not enough just to persuade the politicians and the government departments; we're looking at really educating the public, thanks to the Diana Princess of Wales Memorial Fund which, to me, has been the most pro-active funder in Africa. They're a very wise, very insightful funder. They don't put in huge sums of money, but they put it in very strategically, and they're funding the advocacy programme. We're also developing a media campaign and we're busy getting extra funding resources for that, because that's a horribly expensive campaign to do. We've got a number of leading figures who are going to take part in the radio ads, eventually, and TV ads. We've got some print ads developed as well; and yeah, we're going forward with that as well, because you really need to get the public onboard for many reasons—so that they ask for palliative care, they understand they have the right to palliative care, and they volunteer to help with palliative care as well.[10]

Fundraising and Public Relations (one report, 2004)

The major function of the fundraising committee will be

a) to build the capacity of member hospices to do effective fund-raising and

b) to develop standards for the accreditation of fundraising and public relations at member hospices. In addition:

- Each provincial hospice association will identify a person to help build the fundraising capacity of member hospices within the region
- A draft *Fundraising and Guidelines Policy* has been produced. The development of fundraising and PR standards is in process [48] (p. 6).

Patient care services and education (one report, 2004)

Activities include:

◆ Consolidation of the post-graduate palliative medicine course

◆ Inclusion of 28 hospices in HPCA mentor programme; securing funding for second year

◆ Partnership of HPCA with COHSASA (Council for Health and Services and Accreditation for South Africa)

◆ Successful grant applications, including: Elton John AIDS Foundation; Canadian International Development Agency; PEPFAR

◆ Contribution to development of African Palliative Care Association and Arusha conference [48] (p. 7).

Kath Defilippi gives details of the mentorship programme and the model of integrated community home based care endorsed by HPCA.

> I would like to elaborate on the whole concept of mentorship in terms of hospice and palliative care in South Africa, and indeed the entire African context. We've embarked on a mentorship programme here in South Africa. We managed to get funding from the Open Society Institute in 2002, and we're now in the second phase of funding and the second phase of mentorship. We used really well-established, developed hospices to provide guidance and support to emerging or less-developed hospices, within their geographic area; and the reason that we did it was because we felt, in view of the HIV/AIDS epidemic and the enormity of the need for palliative care, that it was really necessary for all the hospices belonging to the Hospice Palliative Care Association of South Africa to really be able to function as a resource that reached out and empowered other organizations, like faith-based and community organizations, to give good home-based care; and I agreed totally with Anne [Merriman] that unless home-based care includes both holistic care and proper pain and symptom control, you can't call it palliative care. We believe that our mission is to promote palliative care—so to graft on pain and symptom control where that's missing, and to graft on holistic care in hospitals with palliative care teams where that is missing; and in each of those instances to do it in a very supportive, facilitatory fashion. So that's really the focus of our mentorship programme.
>
> The initial programme was so successful that we applied and received funding for a second phase. Now in the second phase we're moving from just using individual hospices to provincial or regional hospice associations, and it's also been really providential that it's coincided with the funding from PEPFAR, which means that we've now been able to have provincial palliative care development teams which include a variety of skills, as well as a full-time, employed person paid by the PEPFAR funding. And then having the clinical disciplines represented so that there is physical, emotional, social and spiritual care abilities and experience represented, as well as management, human resources, and even fundraising, and—very importantly—training and education. So we've got a team of about nine to ten people in each of the areas in South Africa where we have a provincial or regional hospice association. There are nine provinces in South Africa. We don't yet have enough hospice services in all of the provinces to warrant a provincial association, but that's our aim, and we certainly hope that within the very near future we will have nine provincial associations and nine provincial palliative care development teams.[50]

Hospice 'twins'

FHSSA has promoted the development of reciprocal 'twinning' arrangements, examples of which can be seen in Table 7.8.

Table 7.8 'Twinned' hospices in South Africa

South African Hospice	Twinned hospice
Brits Hospice	Hospice of the Chesapeake, Millersville, Maryland, USA
Cotlands Johannesburg	Children's hospitals and Clinics Hospice and Palliative Care Services, Minneapolis, Minnesota, USA
Estcourt Hospice	Hospice of the Southern Tier, Elmira, New York, USA
Golden Gateway Hospice, Bethlehem	Hospice of Spokane, Washington, USA
Goldfields Hospice, Welkom	Colorado Hospice Alliance, Loveland, Colorado, USA
Good Shepherd Hospice, Middleburg	Centre for Hospice and Palliative Care, Cheektowaga, New York, USA
Grahamstown Hospice	Hospice of North Central Florida, Gainsville, Florida, USA
Helderberg Hospice	Hospice of the Western Reserve, Cleveland, Ohio, USA
Highway Hospice, Durban	VITAS Chigagoland and VITAS Chicago South, Chicago Illinois, USA
Hospice East Rand, Benoni West	Hospice of the Calumet area, Munster, Indiana, USA
Hospice in the West, Krugersdorp	Alive Hospice, Nashville, Tennessee, USA
Hospice Ladybrand	Nathan Adelson Hospice, Las Vegas, Nevada, USA
Hospice North West, Klerksdorp	Hospices of Henry Ford, St Clare Shores, Michigan, USA
Howick Hospice	Hospice of Siouxland, Sioux City, Iowa, USA
Msunduzi Hospice, Pietermaritzburg	VITAS San Diego, San Diego, California, USA
Naledi Hospice, Bloemfontein	VITAS Corporate, Miami, Florida, USA
St Bernard's Hospice, East London	VITAS Broward, Fort Lauderdale, Florida, USA
St Francis Hospice, Port Elizabeth	Heartland Home Care and Hospice, Dallas, Texas USA
St Joseph's Care and Support Trust (Sizanani Village) Bronkhorstspruit	VITAS Fort Worth, Fort Worth, Texas, USA
St Luke's Hospice, Cape Town	Hospice of Volusia/Fagler, Port orange, Florida, USA
Palliative care dept: Chris Harni Baragwanath Hospital, Soweto	Palliative care team, St Thomas' Hospital, London, UK
Pretoria Sungardens Hospice	Pathways Home Health and Hospice, Mountain View, California, USA
South Coast Hospice, Port Shepstone	Rowcroft Hospice, Torquay, UK Community Hospice, Rensselaer, New York, USA
Tapologo Hospice, Rustenburg	Community Hospice, Rensselaer, New York, USA
Viljoenskroon Hospice	Kansas City Hospice, Missouri, USA
Wide Horizon Hospice, Duncanville	Hospice of the Blue Grass, Lexington, Kentucky, USA
Witwatersrand, Johannesburg	Hospice of the Florida Suncoast, Largo, Florida, USA St Ann's Hospice, Cheadle, UK
Zululand Hospice, Empangeni	Geneesee Region Home Care/Hospice, Rochester, New York, USA

Sources: Abigail Fowlkes Gutierrez (FHSS)—USA twins; Avril Jackson (Hospice information)—UK twins.

Philip Disorbo is chief executive of the Community Hospice, New York. This hospice is engaged in twinning relationships with South Coast Hospice, Port Shepstone, Tapologo Hospice Rustenburg, and Island Hospice in Zimbabwe. Speaking at the 12th International Conference on the Care of the Terminally Ill (Montreal, 2004), he acknowledges the value of twinning but suggests that the goal of the exercise should be to forge closer relationships between hospices—involving joint action—following on from the initial twinning period.

> The partnership is very much a group effort. Once you get into a meaningful partnership you quickly learn that everybody gains. So you quite quickly evolve . . . Twinning itself is becoming outmoded, especially in hospice-to-hospice relationships because the twinning period refers to the initial friendship period, and good though that is, it is not where we need to go. Quite quickly our relationship developed into the working partnership; and the collaborative partnership among these programmes is where such partnerships can become a global HIV/AIDS intervention—and I don't think they need $75,000 of funding.[51]

Palliative care coverage

As yet, palliative care coverage in South Africa is sporadic: comprehensive in some areas but non-existent in others. Services are particularly sparse in the Northern Cape, Mpumalanga and Limpopo. HPCA intends to have a hospice service in each of South Africa's 170 health authorities by 2009.

Education and training

Palliative care education and training is provided at different levels by numerous organizations that include the University of Cape Town (UCT), HPCA and individual hospices.

Importantly, the palliative medicine courses at UCT have become an accessible alternative to courses offered by universities outside of South Africa. Pioneered by Liz Gwyther, who became the first physician in South Africa to be trained in palliative medicine, she explains how the course became established:

> Out of the palliative medicine course that Ilora Finlay and Fiona Rawlinson were running [at the University of Wales], I started looking at the possibility of teaching it here in South Africa, because it was really very expensive to do it in the UK. Apart from the travel, the tuition fees were way above what we pay at our medical schools. So we looked at whether I could initiate the course at the University of Cape Town with the support of the University of Wales. I was really fortunate in that Professor J.P. van Niekerk who was the dean at the faculty of health sciences at UCT, is currently the chairperson of the Hospice Palliative Care Association, and he was my champion at UCT. I was in discussion with Ilora in Wales, and with Ralph Kirsch, who heads the department of medicine at UCT, and he employed me on a retainer of 500 rand a month to develop the course.
>
> I came back from a second meeting in Wales with all the plans and the curriculum and ready to roll, and was told 'you must put it into the dean's circular, it has to be passed by the UCT senate' and there was one further dean's circular for the year. So I put together my motivation for the postgraduate programme in palliative medicine; we put it in the dean's circular, and it was accepted. So we enrolled our first cohort of students: 23 doctors who were currently working in hospices either part-time or full-time, and we started in the January [2001]. So, having been employed on a retainer in April [2000], put it in the dean's letter in November, we were up and running in January. And I was just so naïve, I just thought that this kind of happened, but now that I'm in the University I get colleagues saying, 'How on earth did you get your course approved so quickly?' In fact the accreditation from the course with the South African Qualifications Authority only came

through about three months before our first exams were written. But at least now we have about 60 doctors who are qualified and another 50 or so who are actually in the programme at the moment, and it's developed from being a diploma in palliative medicine to the degree in palliative medicine with a research component, which is where I started with my research interest.[39]

National statistics relating to education and training collected by HPCA and disseminated at the AGM in Rustenburg are to be found in Tables 7.9–7.11; they concern courses, workshops and talks given under the HPCA umbrella.[52]

André Wagner speaks about his role in the development of hospice organizations—and the people within them—and how training has been supported by the introduction of a development fund (Table 7.12):

We have specific funders in South Africa who contribute money; and they want that money to go towards development, so that's why we have the hospice development fund. And we identified

Table 7.9 Training courses, 2003–2004

Province	Participants (n)	Total hours	Location Hospice (n)	Other (n)	Language English (n)	Other (n)
KwaZulu Natal	923	2101	33	19	36	30
Eastern Cape	165	351	4	9	12	2
Western Cape	5420	319	29	50	67	27
Free State	184	1528	9	16	23	11
Northern Cape	0	0	0	0	0	0
Gauteng	1536	5337	65	14	79	2
Northwest Province	197	735	9	12	19	6
Mpumalanga	3	0	1	1	1	0
Limpopo	0	0	0	0	0	0
Total	8428	10371	160	121	237	78

Table 7.10 Training workshops, 2003–2004

Province	Participants (n)	Total hours	Location Hospice (n)	Other (n)	Language English (n)	Other (n)
KwaZulu Natal	480	453	19	15	36	2
Eastern Cape	321	786	12	10	21	9
Western Cape	737	149	33	7	53	9
Free State	667	252	9	24	24	9
Northern Cape	0	0	0	0	0	0
Gauteng	1239	481	65	4	66	5
Northwest Province	48	53	3	10	12	1
Mpumalanga	0	0	0	0	0	0
Limpopo	0	0	0	0	0	0
Total	3492	2174	141	70	212	35

Table 7.11 Talks and presentations, 2003–2004

Province	Participants (n)	Total hours	Location Hospice (n)	Other (n)	Language English (n)	Other (n)
KwaZulu Natal	1528	210	21	32	52	4
Eastern Cape	3009	56	0	23	12	13
Western Cape	5420	319	39	50	67	27
Free State	1750	90	8	55	46	16
Northern Cape	70	2	0	3	3	0
Gauteng	2385	227	30	34	71	7
Northwest Province	3447	45	3	4	8	11
Mpumalanga	0	0	0	0	0	0
Limpopo	0	0	0	0	0	0
Total	17 609	949	101	201	259	78

development areas—like developing boards in the area of being competent governing body members, or developing the fundraising capacity within the hospice, developing the manager in areas of organizational development, or general hospice management—so that's what the fund is for, to develop.

The fund of course is very small so we need to, in some cases, try and benefit a whole region. If one hospice identifies a need we go back and say 'but can't the whole region benefit from it because then we save money?' The fund covers all areas: it covers patient care; education; fund-raising; and public relations; as well as organisational development. So it is about developing skills in all those areas. For me it's quite important to get people developed with quality development opportunities, so I would encourage hospices to make use of recognized tertiary institutions instead of getting someone that would not be able to give them a certificate for what they're doing. So because we're not able to pay market-related salaries, at least we're able to develop people so that should they make a job change, which we don't encourage and which we don't want of course, then at least then they'll have added skills and capacity to go into a new job. So that's what the hospice development fund is about. It doesn't make provision for capital items like buying computers and buying a car and buying a property but it is about developing our staff; and people don't have to pay back, they have to work back.

One of the new things that I've implemented, because of the development needs of our managers, is the Hospice Palliative Care Association bursary fund which at this stage is just in the field of organizational development—where a staff member can get a bursary to study at a university or a college but on a part-time basis. They don't have to pay anything; we pay for the tuition, all they have to do is pass. If they fail, they need to pay back or they need to pay for the repetition of that specific subject—or subjects—themselves; and then they just need to work back the exact number of years that they've had support for.

And that's one that I'm really promoting at the moment because we're getting young people into hospice which is a new thing, and which is exciting—getting younger people that are not retired and who just need to work to supplement their pension—it's people who want to have a career in hospice. So it's to develop them and really make sure that they get a recognized qualification at the end of that activity.[32]

Table 7.12 Requests to HPCA for expertise in development areas

Development area	Requests
Guidance to governing body (board/committee/trust)	13
Establishing a governing/managing body	4
Starting a community-based hospice	2
Starting a hospice within a disadvantaged community	3
Administrative systems and controls	10
Financial systems and controls	10
Job descriptions for hospice posts	15
Strategic planning	13
Staff appraisal/evaluation	24
Fundraising methods and skills	16
Community mobilization	10
Effective use of volunteers	15
Training of volunteer caregivers	8
Training of nurses in palliative care	13
Training of doctors in palliative care	12
Training of educators and trainers	12
Training in bereavement counselling	13
Training in spiritual counselling	11
Setting up and developing a day care system	8
Setting up and developing a home care programme	3
Setting up and developing a bereavement programme	9
Setting up and developing an inpatient unit	3
Keeping statistics on hospice activities	18
Implementation of HOSPAC standards of care	13
Monitoring and evaluation of hospice activities	18
Other	4
Total	280

Source: HPCA SA Annual National Statistics 2003–2004.

Kath Defilippi outlines the significance of a new association with the Council of Health Services Accreditation for Southern Africa (COHASA)

The modus operandi is to first get our own hospice house truly in order, and what's very exciting, I think, is that we are linking accreditation to mentorship, so that we're going to have the back-up of this interdisciplinary, team that includes people with human resource and management experience and interest and skills to support hospices, and to get them into the programme of accreditation. Our aim is to move hospices along as fast as possible to full accreditation, but to do it in a non-threatening, supportive way. Then, to be a mentor hospice and a mentor, not only to hospices but to other organizations—and very importantly to Department of Health organizations—we believe that to fulfil that function effectively a hospice should have full accreditation. And so that's what we're really very excited about at the moment. There's a lot of hard work ahead and probably some resistance, but hopefully not too much.

HPCA have partnered with COHSASA who are a very professional outfit—COHSASA stands for the Council of Health Services Accreditation for Southern Africa—and they are internationally recognized. And so HPCA have signed a formal Memorandum of Understanding with COHSASA and together we've developed hospice standards of care, which is wonderful for us, but it's also very good for them because in fact they have acknowledged that in some ways we have improved their standards. So it's been a real win–win situation. We're very excited at the fact that COHSASA have just trained quite a large group—there were 24 of us—as what they call 'surveyors' and we've done one mock survey in a big group and now we're about to embark on piloting our draft standards in conjunction with the senior surveyor from COHSASA, who will be with a group of us. Then all the people who did the survey training are invited to go along—with COHSASA as an observer—to accredit hospices, and in fact will be evaluated by the very experienced COHSASA team. So, we just believe that it's a quantum leap that we've taken in terms of really working towards quality care, and the fact that we're having it linked to mentorship is what's going to make it achievable and we're confident that it's really going to happen.[50]

At the hospice level, Marisa Wolheim speaks of how the spiritual dimension of care is a central feature of staff training at Hospice in the West:

> When we train people we try and encourage spiritual—not religious—caring; because I think when you go into a patient's home who is dying, and they're so afraid, and you see it in their eyes, you can look past the wound and you can look past the smell and you can talk to that spirit and that god that is within them. There's something that links, and they just know, and everything else becomes less important. And it's such a great opportunity to help people to recognize that our soul and our spirit is part of us all the time, but so often we leave it 'til the last minute. So it's a matter of creating awareness as we go along, to the living and the dying. I think everything that hospice is now, our dying patients have taught us and they are the most valuable lessons and teachers we have.[40]

Elizabeth Scrimgeour[53] illuminates this spiritual domain from the perspective of the patient. In a detailed piece of research, she focuses on the development of what is termed 'sacred spaces'—that which evokes awe and reverence due to its association with spiritual or religious experience. Terminal illness, she suggests, is a sacred experience and she presents qualitative evidence based on patient narratives:

> The patients also talked about experiencing the warmth and nurturing of the God of Grace through visits from friends, the church community, being pain-free and going to day-care. They also find God in flowers, the visits from hospice, sunshine or a back rub. All these aspects are part of and indicative of the spirit or spirituality that makes life worthwhile and engenders a sense of well-being. The patients' spirituality or spiritual experiences with the community and the environment encourages the patients to feel included and worthwhile as part of the body of God. Angie and Margaret experienced their lives as being worthwhile and contributing to the body of God—as contributing to the well-being of their communities when they could share about their illness experiences with their church members. They experienced contributing to the understanding of others about serious illness and identified various coping mechanisms helping to make others more sensitive to the plight of those who are ill. Both Angie and Margaret said that they were pleased that they could contribute in some way to making the illness experience easier for both carers and those who are ill.[54]

Table 7.13 Palliative care workforce capacity (employees): 2003–2004

Category	Employees		Total	Hours/month
	Female	Male		
Medical doctor	15	16	31	1294
Professional nurse	285	5	290	49 361
Staff nurse	59	3	62	9720
Social worker	47	3	50	8205
Social auxiliary worker	11	2	13	1570
Ancillary health carers	103	3	106	16 679
Enrolled nurse assistant	50	0	50	7541
Occupational therapist	2	1	3	257
Therapist (other)	0	0	0	0
Caregivers	188	10	198	27 729
Bereavement carers	8	0	8	983
Spiritual supporters	2	2	4	403
Other	20	7	27	2038
Total	790	52	842	125 780

Source: HPCA SA Annual National Statistics 2003–2004.

Palliative care workforce capacity

National statistics relating to the palliative care workforce capacity in South Africa are shown in Tables 7.13 and 7.14. During 2003–2004, 842 personnel were employed by the membership of HPCA for a total of 125 780 h per month; 1978 volunteers gave 25 806 h per month. During the same period, 695 allied personnel were employed for a total of 85 196 h; 3194 volunteers gave an unspecified amount of time (Tables 7.15 and 7.16).

History and development of hospice–palliative care in South Africa

As the 1970s drew to a close, issues around care of the dying attracted a groundswell of interest in South Africa. Centres of activity developed across the country in places such as Cape Town and Durban, Johannesburg and Port Elizabeth. These initiatives centred on two key features: an affirmation of the value of all human beings—irrespective of race or religion—and an open engagement in the debate surrounding death and the dying process. During her visit to South Africa in 1979, Cicely Saunders added impetus to these developments and, within a year or two, hospice organizations were operating in a variety of settings throughout the country. This section highlights some key events of the early hospice movement in South Africa through the lived experience of people involved in them.

Table 7.14 Palliative care workforce capacity (volunteers): 2003–2004

Category	Volunteers		Total	Hours/month
	Female	Male		
Medical doctor	4	54	58	45
Professional nurse	60	0	60	1108
Staff nurse	6	2	8	71
Social worker	18	0	18	516
Social auxiliary worker	11	0	11	424
Ancillary health carers	32	3	35	2689
Enrolled nurse assistant	9	0	9	356
Occupational therapist	10	0	10	88
Therapist (other)	4	5	9	45
Caregivers	1116	138	1254	16 093
Bereavement carers	196	26	222	2792
Spiritual supporters	82	98	180	773
Other	90	14	104	806
Total	1638	340	1978	25 806

Source: HPCA SA Annual National Statistics 2003–2004.

Table 7.15 Palliative care workforce capacity—allied personnel (employees): 2003–2004

Category	Employees		Total	Hours/month
	Female	Male		
Educator/trainer	61	5	66	7696
Fundraiser/PR	64	6	70	9316
Governance	11	4	15	485
Management	66	8	74	7843
Trust	8	4	12	233
Bookkeeper	39	1	40	4336
Driver	7	23	30	4586
Flower arranger	0	0	0	0
Maintenance	0	6	6	892
Gardener	4	39	43	4503
Cook/housekeeper	27	1	28	4214
Cleaner	69	5	74	8821
Entertainment/activities	0	0	0	0
Receptionist/secretarial/admin	90	7	97	12 944
Shop personnel	90	25	115	15 789
Other	17	8	25	3538
Total	553	142	695	85 196

Source: HPCA SA Annual National Statistics 2003–2004.

Table 7.16 Palliative care workforce capacity—allied personnel (volunteers): 2003–2004

Category	Employees		
	Female	Male	Total
Educator/trainer	53	18	71
Fundraiser/PR	706	139	845
Governance	108	151	259
Management	79	49	27
Trust	13	26	39
Bookkeeper	9	4	13
Driver	38	53	91
Flower arranger	98	2	100
Maintenance	7	33	40
Gardener	41	22	63
Cook/housekeeper	101	2	103
Cleaner	5	0	5
Entertainment/activities	81	23	104
Receptionist/secretarial/admin	230	9	239
Shop personnel	845	69	914
Other	159	21	180
Total	2573	621	3194

Source: HPCA SA Annual National Statistics 2003–2004.

Highway Hospice, Durban[55]

Greta Schoeman was the inspiration behind Highway Hospice Durban, joined at an early stage by Karen Hinton and Stella Thackray.

Greta Schoeman was born in the UK and nursed her father when he developed cancer of the rectum. Having relocated to Durban with her South African husband, she came across *A Way to Die*[56] by Victor and Rosemary Zorza. The book tells of the death of Jane, the Zorzas' 25-year-old daughter, in an English hospice (1977); how her suffering was relieved; and how she described the hospice experience as the happiest time of her life. Inspired by the story of Jane, Greta Schoeman went to Sir Michael Sobell House (Oxford), met the Zorzas, and trained as a hospice nurse before returning to establish a hospice in Durban (1982). She recalls how she came to care for patients in her family home.

> I did have quite an idea. So I donned a uniform, you see, and thought I knew it all, which of course you never do, even today, and went out looking for patients. Well the first patient I got to, she was too sick, she lived way up in Hill Crest and, as I say, I'd got small children so I couldn't spend all my time up there. We'd got a guest cottage at home so I decided that maybe I should open the guest

cottage as a miniature hospice. So I rang up my husband and I said, 'Do you mind if we have patients in?' So he said, 'Well, whatever I say you're going to do it anyway, aren't you?' I said, 'Yes!' So I did. But I must say I had quite a shock when I suddenly realized when the ambulance arrived that this lady was going to die on me and I hadn't sort of thought about all this, but it worked, it worked. And then I quickly put some adverts in the papers and wrote some articles and then the Karens [Hinton] of this world and Stella [Thackray] rallied round and they'd come and help me. That's how we started. And we ran [the hospice] there for 18 months; yes, had about 22 patients I think who died in my house.

Karen Hinton was born in Ellesmere Port in Cheshire, UK and trained at the Birkenhead School of Nursing. She relocated to Durban after marrying her South African husband. She nursed her 23-year-old sister-in-law—who was diagnosed with a brain tumour—for about 2 months before she died. When she heard that Greta Schoeman was beginning a hospice (they belonged to the same church at that time), she contacted her and offered to help. She continues:

> We had a lot of difficulty at Greta's [Schoeman] house. We had our office there and we had this little two-bedded unit and the neighbours were not happy about it. They had visions of the hearse arriving day and night and, again, did not understand the hospice. There were a lot of newspaper articles and one of the headlines was about Greta and the headline involved was 'Come to my house to die'; it was quite an upper suburb where she lived, so neighbours weren't happy. Greta used to go overseas quite regularly to her family and we never actually took too many patients, those of us who were left to hold the fort; but I remember one day we had our meeting at Greta's house and when we came out the neighbours had done a blockade of their cars in protest. So, yeah, we were very naughty, I suppose; but we just ignored people, you know. They couldn't do anything because nobody was charging.[57]

Stella Thackray arrived in South Africa from Perthshire, Scotland (1980):

> I came into hospice by accident. I worked in a doctor's surgery and a lady came in one day with a nurse's uniform on and she said, 'I work for a charity that doesn't have any money, could I possibly give her some sutures: a needle and a suture. An old man had fallen out of bed'. I said to her, 'Where do you work? What is your uniform?' And she told me that there had been a hospice which had just started in Westville and she told me all about it and she said, 'If you'd like to come and help, you're welcome.' So she gave me the address of Greta Schoeman's house in Westville and she said they had a meeting every Monday; and I went there and they had already just started. I think they had been going for about a month, and I just went to the meeting and sat round a table and we discussed a few patients and Greta said to me, 'Would you go and visit this man on Berea?' and I had only been in South Africa for a year, and I said, 'Yes, I'll go', but I didn't even know where Berea was, but that's how I started.[58]

Thembi Nyuswa, the first black sister at Highway Hospice, trained as a psychiatric nurse and found the broad approach associated with hospice care resonated with her view of holistic care:

> When I first came to work for the hospice it was on a part-time basis and I became the first black sister. It was quite different, you know, from the usual kind of nursing that I'd always been involved in. And I discovered that the hospice concept was a very new thing to the average black patient. At that time, all the patients were referred to us from the provincial hospitals. They would get admitted in the hospice inpatient unit and when they went home there was no follow-up system to see how they were doing until they were re-admitted. So, I worked here on and off because I had to

finish my studies; and when I left to do my psychiatric medicine the matron said, 'Thembi, go and finish your studies and come back and start an African home care service', which I was excited about. So I went and finished my studies, got my drivers' licence and there I was: I came back and I started this service.[43]

Hospice Association of the Witwatersrand, Johannesburg[59]

In 1977, the arrival of Margaret Lebish[60] an English nurse with a social work background, added impetus to the developing interest in end-of-life care in the Johannesburg area. The visit was unexpected:

> My brother had emigrated to South Africa with his wife. They had just had their first baby and my sister-in-law had a brain haemorrhage and died, and the baby was just a few weeks old; and so my brother was left alone with a new born baby. I had just finished my nurse training and was actually on my way to Australia, waiting for my documents to come through and I just decided to go to South Africa instead, as I didn't think he'd find it very easy in the circumstances.

It was while seeking work that Margaret Lebish met Sylvia Poss,[61] a social worker at Johannesburg General Hospital, and discovered that they shared a common interest: care for the dying. Before she left England for South Africa, Margaret Lebish worked at St Mary's Hospital, London—an organizsation that included St Luke's, a long-established home for the dying in Bayswater. It was here that the young Cicely Saunders had worked as a volunteer social worker (1948) during what became a formative time for the development of her ground-breaking ideas.[62] More than 25 years later, Margaret Lebish was familiar with the hospice philosophy and a supporter of the hospice movement.

In Johannesburg, Sylvia Poss became involved with the TLC (Tender Loving Care) group that focused on the needs of the terminally ill—and Margaret Lebish was invited to join as a community representative. When she subsequently found employment with the humanitarian organization TOC H,[63] Margaret Lebish found that an inclusive approach to the dying was in keeping with the organization's mission. Consequently, her involvement in the nascent hospice movement increased significantly. She recalls:

> The South African Cancer Association had sent its administrator, Mr Delport, to America to research the hospice movement there. A hospice conference was called by local nurses and doctors at which there were many attendees. Then Sylvia Poss approached me in 1978 and asked if I would be willing to start [hospice development] work in the community, and I had no hesitation in agreeing. I went to TOC H and explained the position. Much to my delight, they agreed to pay my salary for six months to work full time on the project. A new worker was being funded and sent out from the UK who would take over my existing workload and free me up to help establish a hospice in Johannesburg. Arend Hoogervorst eventually became the project chairman where his administrative skills and enthusiasm helped to steer the project in those vital early days.
> In the beginning there was just me, a vision and a simple knowledge of the possibilities. I felt that the UK hospice models of care with which I was familiar were inappropriate to the beginnings of a project in a developing country. I needed a clear model of 'How do we do it here.' So I selected a model of care called the 'consultative group' which consists of a team providing a home care service which follows a patient into hospital if admission becomes necessary. The model was based on the 'Hospice of Marin'[64] in California; its founders were influenced by the work of Elizabeth Kübler-Ross and it was the second home care hospice service to be developed in America. But it

started with a vision, no money and a group of volunteers, and I knew that if they had succeeded, so could we.

The next step was to share the vision and form a steering group for the project. I was invited to speak to a group of social workers and, to my disappointment, the group focused on the fact that I hadn't established the need! Being young and enthusiastic, I was bitterly disappointed that this group didn't catch my vision! As I was leaving, a gentleman approached me and said: 'I think it's a fantastic idea, what can I do to help?' Stan Henen and I had already met at a meeting for community workers in Soweto and Stan was my answer to prayer. He became a member of the steering group and was later to become the hospice administrator.

Over the next six months, the team grew as more people joined us. Dr Brown was chairman of the Hospital TLC group at Johannesburg General Hospital and, with his colleague Dr Browde, was responsible for inviting Cicely Saunders to visit us during her visit to Cape Town. The press publicity from that visit put us on the national map. Others joined: Thelma Avent came to us as a potential user and offered us the use of a room in her garage as an office, free of charge. I approached a gentleman who had recently lost his wife to become our accountant—and so Alistair Bruce joined us. Stan Henen took over public relations. Fr Ronald Cairns, Catholic priest from Alexandra township, joined us as chaplain and Mrs van Heuren Chief Nursing Officer from the Provincial Nursing Service also joined the group. Annette Schmidt [TOC H] joined as our secretary and later, Dion Rhoder [TOC H] joined as a lawyer. Dr Barry from the department of community medicine at the medical school at Witwatersrand University joined as vice chairman. Our core Steering Committee was in place.[65]

Activities became formalized at the TLC meeting held on 9 March 1979. In her historic report to the group, Margaret Lebish writes:

I initially attended the Pathways terminal care symposium where a lot of private discussion and contacts were made. I have also personally approached representatives from the various groups at present concerned with the field of terminal care. My opinions are subjective but my conclusions are as follows:

- There is a general lack of knowledge of existing resources.
- There is a lack of co-ordination and communication among different bodies concerned.
- Existing resources and organisations are specialised in their scope of activity.
- There is no one body sufficiently organised to promote effective action for the establishment and development of comprehensive care facilities for the terminally ill, the bereaved and their families.

I therefore recommend:

- Thanks to the work of organisations like Pathways and TLC the ground seems well prepared for action and for sympathetic response from the public. It is recommended therefore that an independent voluntary organisation be established as soon as possible. It has been suggested that a suitable name for this group would be HOSPICE.
- A preliminary meeting of interested bodies has been called for 15 March at 5 pm to be held at Toc H headquarters, Johannesburg. Anyone interested in attending, please make themselves known to me or to the TLC chairman, Dr Brown.[66]

Records of these meetings in March 1979 throw new light on the early development of palliative care, not just in South Africa but across the African continent, and add weight to the claim that the first formal steps in hospice care were taken not in Harare (Zimbabwe), but in Johannesburg.

In 1979, Arend Hoogervorst arrived in South Africa from Britain to take up the position of TOC H field officer. Among his responsibilities was a commitment to take forward the pioneering work of Margaret Lebish. From 1979 until 1986, he was chair or deputy chairperson of what became known as the Hospice Association's Executive Committee. He takes up the story thus:

> My early role was to act basically as 'gofer', a minute taker, a record keeper a writer, a telephone person; and TOC H's headquarters became the sort of nominal office, so if people were interested they could 'phone or contact people, and I began to be that kind of networker.
>
> We moved into the hospice on the 15th September 1984; prior to that it was a home care programme. Wherever possible we tried to find beds in hospitals or facilities where we could channel home care patients for their last few days and they could get continuity of hospice support. For example, the Kenridge Hospital kept a bed open for us for a short period of time and there were a number of other institutions that tried to help us, but it was an uphill battle. I seem to remember at some stage there being something like 130 or 140 patients being treated.
>
> The big battle was trying to get enough money to buy the first hospice; that was an amazing breakthrough. One of the mining houses gave us 300 000 rand—which was a phenomenal amount of money at that time—and it gave us a base.
>
> I lived in the hospice building at 97 Houghton Drive for about 18 months while we got change of consent to convert the building from a residential building to a nursing structure: the legislation at the time required that there be somebody living in the property while the change went on, so I actually lived in the hospice—in one of the outhouses—and I provided after hours link for various things; that was after I left TOC H.[67]

Among the early pioneers of the Hospice Association of the Witwatersrand were Stan and Shirley Henen. A history of the hospice acknowledges their involvement:

> Stan and Shirley Henen became actively involved with the hospice concept in 1979 and began training caregivers and started operations from their home in Hurlingham, Sandton. Stan was a qualified pharmacist and also worked as an insurance consultant. The Henens and a few loyal and enthusiastic volunteers began 'marketing' the hospice, so much so that by 1984 the first property in Houghton was purchased for R380,000, of which JCI[68] donated R300,000. A 5- to 6-bed unit and hospice pharmacy were opened.[68]

Barbara Campbell-Ker, currently the executive director of Witwatersrand, joined the hospice in 1986 when the organization was looking for a volunteer bookkeeper:

> At that time, we had 16 paid members of staff and innumerable volunteers. I remember distinctly in about 1988 when we admitted our first AIDS patient into the inpatient unit—and of course since then we've come an awfully long way, yes. Things have changed greatly. We were in a wonderful house. About three or four of us shared one of the servant's accommodation at the back, which was our office. Everybody multitasked: if you were a board member you worked in the flea market, you counted money, you mopped, you folded, you licked stamps, you did anything that helped and saved costs and, yes, it was very exciting. Actually it probably was more fun than what we have now, because we've grown so; with such a large staff, eventually you've got to decide you're not a little welfare organization, you're actually a business and you need the business policies, procedures and

principles with the standards. In some way you've got to change focus—because if you have to run a large organization like an organization with 16 staff, it's not going to work. So we've had to make that transition, trying to keep that family approach, but becoming more effective from a business perspective.[7]

A feature of the developing hospice movement was the desire to provide palliative care services in the heart of the large, disadvantaged communities around Johannesburg. Despite all difficulties, a fledgling service began in 1988. Peter Buckland described how this happened in the UK Hospice Bulletin's lead article, published in July 1999:

> The year 1988 was a milestone year for the [hospice] organization: Soweto is a huge community of disadvantaged people on the south western border of Johannesburg. Soweto community representatives met with the board of Hospice Association of Witwatersrand and together they 'workshopped' and made a unanimous decision to extend hospice home care nursing services to the community. Although efforts were initially hampered by social and political upheavals in the area, the first nursing sister was employed. As co-ordinator of the Soweto Hospice programme, Bibi Nkosi worked tirelessly to care for her patients, to establish a base from which to develop the services of hospice, to network with other agencies and to inform ordinary people living in Soweto about hospice.

Today, located in the grounds of Mofolo Clinic, the hospice provides a day care service, home care service and inpatient unit. Archbishop Desmond Tutu, patron of the South African hospice movement, opened the centre in June 1988. Remarkably, the facility was made up of 11 shipping containers that had been combined and adapted for hospice use. There was still much to be done. Hospice co-ordinator Sibongile Mafata:

> When I started in '98 people were not aware of a hospice in Soweto—but it was just two sisters who were working here. We had to work very hard to go out, make people aware that there is a hospice in Soweto; and then with the efforts, the growth started. At that time we were getting cancer patients only, we didn't have HIV/AIDS patients. And slowly, slowly the AIDS patients started coming to our programme. Presently it's unbelievable, the number of AIDS patients—it's about 70 to 80 per cent in comparison to the cancer patients. When I started in '98 we had between 40 and 50 patients. This place was adequate for what we were doing, but now we have really, really grown: everyday there is a growth of something.
>
> As I said, we started being just two nursing sisters, then we grew. We had an extra nursing sister, and then we had a social worker in the problem areas. The social problems are overwhelming. In the beginning, we didn't have an inpatient unit and we had to apply to other places to get a placement for our patients. We started with a four-bedded inpatient unit just to see whether we were going to be sustained, and then we opened the nine beds. So the challenges have been seeing to the growth of hospice in Soweto and also making the community aware. But now, people have really become aware of the hospice. You'll find that the referrals are no longer from hospital only, but by word of mouth, from individuals. People refer each other knowing that there is a hospice, but at the moment our place is inadequate, it's now another challenge.[70]

St Francis Hospice, Port Elizabeth

The inspiration behind St Francis Hospice was Lesley Lawson, an English nurse who trained at Leeds General Infirmary and then experienced community nursing in the USA before arriving in South Africa during the early 1970s. Crucially, she was a member of the audience that heard Cicely Saunders give a lecture on hospice care at the University of Cape Town in 1979; she returned home determined to establish a service in Port Elizabeth. Despite her inexperience, the national Cancer Association was willing to provide support and take the project forward. She recalls:

> This was very much the fledgling time of the hospice movement in South Africa—and in Port Elizabeth we didn't even know the word 'palliative' or have any sort of formal support for patients and families, and in fact not really any expertise for the pain and symptom control and emotional support that is such an important part of our patients' lives, and their families lives; so it was a real learning curve. And the national Cancer Association in Port Elizabeth wanted to establish a home care service, and I was around and they knew that I had an interest, and so they employed me to establish the first hospice home care system in Port Elizabeth. But as we moved along it became clear that if we could also have a back-up inpatient unit it would then provide a fuller service.[71]

The Cancer Association was not so interested in establishing a free standing unit, however, and it fell to local activists to take up the challenge of raising funds and finding premises. At this time, sisters and doctors from the hospital's oncology department featured prominently alongside local ministers and other supporters.

> We were just like sponges. We were just really wanting, hungry for information and picking the brains of people who'd either been to England or who had listened to Dr Cicely Saunders, and we were avidly reading everything that we could. And I was fortunate enough to go a couple of times to England to experience first hand what hospice was all about.
> By 1986 we decided we were ready to find a building and I moved from the Cancer Association to St Francis Hospice. We began in a very small way with just two of us doing home care, and then in 1988 we had gathered enough money, because it was always about money, to be able to open and establish, initially a nine-bedded unit, but as funding got more and more difficult, we had to cut that to six and then latterly to five.[71]

Notwithstanding the difficulties of funding, the hospice was committed to providing care for all those in need. This was an important decision since Port Elizabeth and the Eastern Cape is one of South Africa's least economic areas, with large townships and widespread poverty. Lesley Lawson continues:

> We were always very clear about the fact that part of the philosophy was for the hospice to be available to all, regardless of ability to pay, and that was one of the things that was very, personally, important for me. Coming from England where we have the national health system to a country where there's different levels of care depending on your wealth—or not—it was always very important; and of course, we were in the middle of apartheid during this time. I think that, certainly when we opened our unit one of the things—it was almost like a beacon—was that our inpatient unit was never a segregated unit. At the time hospitals were, and it kind of felt like one way of showing that we cared for all people, with actions, without having to shout things from the rooftops.[71]

By 2002, >60 staff at St Francis Hospice provided home based and inpatient care 24 h a day, 7 days per week. Each month, around 400 patients were seen at home and about 35 were admitted to the inpatient unit.[72]

St Luke's Hospice, Cape Town[73]

Christine Dare was the driving force behind St Luke's Hospice, Cape Town. She had come to know Cicely Saunders when she worked at St Thomas' Hospital (London)[74] and was keen to bring her to South Africa to contribute to the debate on end-of-life care. Finally, Dr Saunders arranged to visit (1979) on condition she could have a public debate with Christian Barnard on euthanasia. Richard Scheffer, a fellow student of Christine Dare in the UCT medical school, recalls how Cicely Saunders came to be in South Africa:

> I was at the University of Cape Town from '74 to '79. While I was there, I sat on a committee called the *Student Visiting Lecturers Organization* which had some money available to bring visiting lecturers to the university for specific projects of interest to the students: and in our class was a girl called Christine Dare who was a physiotherapist by training and had actually trained as a physiotherapist at St Thomas's [London] at the time when Cicely Saunders was a medical student at St Thomas's and they had had known each other. And we had to write an essay on the care of the dying as part of our 3rd year programme and Christine was saying how wonderful it would be if we could get Dame Cicely to come out to South Africa and we said 'well let's go to the Student Visiting Lecturers Organization and see if we can get them to fund the visit'.
>
> And Dame Cicely very kindly agreed to come—because it was a difficult time for South Africa; it was at a time of academic boycott and there weren't many people prepared to visit. And she generated enormous interest amongst medical students. All her lectures were given outside of tutoring time, so they were in our lunch hours or after work and she played to full houses. And also, I think the other interesting thing was: we were a society that was hurting enormously and she spoke *in to* that, in the sense that she tried to address—and I think she gave us ideas to think about—what the meaning of suffering could be. And so for some of us who were finding the situation in South Africa very, very, very stressful, she had some very powerful things to say, not just about dying. So, all in all it was a very successful visit and personally, it made me quite sure that I wanted to do palliative medicine.[75]

The deputy dean of UCT medical school at that time was J. P. van Niekerk—and he acknowledges the special contribution made by Christine Dare:

> In 1979 I was approached by a senior medical student—whom I would later come to know well—to assist in bringing out Dr Cicely Saunders to spread the gospel of hospice. The medical student was, of course, Chris Dare, who went on to start St Luke's Hospice in Cape Town and had a major influence on the development of hospice in South Africa.
>
> She was inspired by what Cicely had done in developing a new concept and determined to follow suit in South Africa. At that stage, Chris was a physiotherapist and applied to do medicine at UCT in order to prepare herself for this task. Since she was missing some of the required background courses for entry, she first commenced with BSc studies. The whole saga of her eventual acceptance was typical of her career, in which the word *No* was something which simply had to be overcome.[76]

Meg Meyers, a trained nurse who was seeking to return to work, was the first person to be employed by the hospice—originally as voluntary services co-ordinator:

> St Luke's Hospice was formed as a company, not for gain, in August 1980. A lot of the medical personnel had realized there was a great hiatus between patients being cared for in a hospital and going home, particularly if they were terminally ill. A lot of people were working and couldn't

afford to care for them so it was felt that there was a need for something like a hospice. And we stayed in a committee stage for about two or three years.

Now I had known Chris [Dare] for a long time through my church connections and eventually, once she had qualified, she would go and give talks and speak to people, and everybody knew she was very enthusiastic about opening a hospice. And then we were given the opportunity in 1983 to rent rooms at the Vincent Pallotti Hospital, which was a private hospital run by nuns, and they felt they'd like to get us started. So we leased their old staff dining room, which was a very large room with a double-sided desk, a rusty filing cabinet and that was about it. But a lady was employed to be the very first voluntary services organizer, because Chris felt that what she needed to do was to train up volunteers and then she could at least have somebody to go and help the patients that she was seeing. And unfortunately the lady came for a morning and then resigned, and it was decided that the board, most of whom came from the same church, should put on their thinking caps and see if they could think of anybody who could help us for the interim. And rumour had it that all four of them thought of me. So—that was the year that I had been planning on going back into work—so Chris approached me and said, could I help out until they could find somebody. So I started in February 1983 as the voluntary services organizer; and we had two volunteer training courses that year, and some of those volunteers are still with us.[77]

In the early days, the hospice had strong links with a local church, and concerns arose relating to both religion and race: religion, due to fears about a Christian-based health organization that would have little relevance to those of other faiths; and race, because the hospice began during the days of the apartheid government which endured until 1994. Meg Meyers:

I think initially there was the fear we were all highly religious and were going to come in and preach hellfire and brimstone, but once they got to realize that that was not the case, things eased. And then I think it was a case of testing the waters. Some of our patients found it a bit difficult when we opened a ward: we had black, white, coloured, everybody in together, sort of thing; and you could feel a little bit of tension, you know. But the interesting thing was we had a wonderful occasion in our female ward: we had one white lady, and this was an extremely foreign thing for her; and she was very sick and in a lot of pain and thought she would rather go home. But there was a delay in the family being able to get her home and so she was there for a couple of days. One evening she was trying to reach the bell—I think she'd vomited or something—and it was the black lady in the bed next to her who came to help her: and she was so caring of her and rang her bell to call the sister, that it changed her whole attitude. And we've had a lot of those sorts of incidents. But everybody is treated the same: it doesn't matter if you've money; it doesn't matter if you haven't got money; it doesn't matter if you're a gangster—we've had lots of those; it doesn't matter where you come from. Everybody is treated with love and compassion; and the bottom line is we want to walk alongside you, we want to control your symptoms, make you comfortable, and allow you to die with dignity. And to me there's no room for racism or antagonism about somebody of a different faith.[77]

Hospice success stories

In South Africa, the successes of the hospice movement have been described in the following terms:[78]

◆ Raised palliative care awareness in the community and among health workers

◆ Patient care: how a concept, previously unknown, has become operationalized

◆ Provision of paediatric care as part of a continuum of care

- Development of a model for community palliative care day centres
- Staff commitment
- Increase in palliative care physicians
- Development of teamwork
- Engagement with the Department of Health
- Education of families and caregivers
- Empowerment of communities
- Mobilization of community caregivers for individual patients
- Networking with the international community
- Income generation
- Creation of a (medicinal) herb garden
- Development of voluntary counselling and testing
- Introduction of the memory boxes
- Distribution of food/social support
- Opportunities for social inclusion
- Gifts from donors premises, materials, funds, skills/time.

Some examples of these successes are given below.

G. K. Moodley—chairperson of Verulam Hospice says:

> I think one of our first successes is the fact that we were able to get the community together to give us the support that we needed to establish the hospice in Verulam in order for us to cater for the needs of terminally ill patients. Secondly, the financial support that we receive on an ongoing basis from people: a very clear indication of their commitment to our goal of establishing our hospice. And, thirdly, the fact that our hospice has been selected by the Global Fund as a site for training nurses and caregivers to serve areas where there are HIV/AIDS patients, is an indication of the recognition of our capacity to run the services on proper lines.[79]

Jackie Schoeman, director of Cotlands:

> Our successes? Treatment! Treatment; it has to be. We discovered antiretroviral treatment and our lives have changed. We still have the chronically ill children that come in from hospital or through our home-based care programmes where it's really too late to do anything; but all those children that were sitting there not getting better—not actually getting worse—going into hospital every few months for some kind of treatment, coming back out again, we've put them all on [ARV] treatment and they're all now sitting in Sanctuary, really well. Children that were four years old, hadn't walked, hadn't talked, are now at school. It's been the most amazing experience. So, yeah, we're big advocates of treatment. I think if I have a regret it's that we didn't do it sooner, but because it's not free and we had to pay, the committee wanted me to secure enough funding to guarantee ongoing treatment prior to starting it, which we did on an annual basis. So we were covered for last year, we're covered again for this year: but yeah, what I've done now is just write it into our running costs: as you budget for water, food, electricity, so we budget for treatment as well.[80]

Zodwe Sithole, home care sister at Highway Hospice:

> Sometimes, if you go to the black communities, when you tell them about hospice they mention that they thought that hospice is for a certain class of people: people who can afford, people

who've got money, people on Medical Aid, especially the white people; they didn't know that even the black people can go to hospice, even if they are not on Medical Aid. So one would start explaining that hospice, regardless of whether you can pay or not, regardless of your colour, as long as you've got a terminal, incurable condition you can be a hospice patient. So I think those are also successes because after you have explained to them, now they say, 'Oh, we can also go to hospice'. And some of the families they also say, 'Thank you very much, sister, we now know what hospice is'.[81]

Marie Backeberg, nursing sister, Centurion Hospice:

I think the success story of Centurion Hospice is that we work as a team, each in our specialized field, not feeling second best to one another, but we can hold hands, and we can get the workers who run the shop, and the sisters and the business people, and we all just give; and one doesn't feel threatened by the other—or feel that you're more important than the other. It's quite a team at the moment.[82]

J. P. van Niekerk, chairperson, HPCA:

I think that the first success [of the hospice movement] is the very work that it does: we have an advocacy programme, but the most important advocacy for everyone to see is the work we do. So there are few families that you could speak to that have not had word of, or experience of, the wonderful support and service they've had through hospices. Now I think that that's a success story. One of the deficiencies is that there are many areas which still do not have such supplies, such facilities and services, and part of our plan is to develop those services in areas that are either underserved or not served at all. So I think that's probably the first and most important success. I think the second aspect that I would consider important is the fact that, in our AIDS epidemic in particular, denial has been a major political barrier; and through the work of our organization, truth and acceptance of reality is happening—we are a very important vehicle in carrying that message across. I think the third one is that all our very extensive training processes, at all levels—volunteers, community caregivers, professional nurses and now doctors at a post-graduate level—that educational influence, spread across the country increases, the value of medical services way beyond the limited services that we can supply.[83]

André Wagner, organization development officer, HPCA:

Definitely, the fact that we have standards for management and governance in place, that is one of our really huge successes; it took us two years to develop those standards but what I also said is that it's not just about doing the standards. Standards go hand-in-hand with policies and procedures, hand-in-hand with other accompanying documents; so what we said is that we're not just going to develop the standards, we're going to develop model policies and procedures to go with those standards: and if the policies and procedures make provision for a specific document—that must be in place. We're also making provision for developing those documents, so it is a major success the fact that we are able to give people the full package.[32]

Ethical issues

From the survey of palliative care personal at the HPCA AGM at Rustenburg, a number of ethical issues were identified (Table 7.17):

Some of these issues are amplified below:

South Africa has a very liberal constitution, probably one of the most liberal constitutions in the world, and a very advanced human rights constitution. We have abortion on demand,

Table 7.17 Identified ethical issues

Category	Issue
Patient issues	Confidentiality
	Stigmatization
	Social exclusion
	Disclosure of diagnosis
Service issues	Health service disempowerment
	Inadequate resourcing
	Distribution of resources
	Relationship between quality and coverage
	Myths associated with morphine
	Dispensing of opioids (new legislation)
	Access to care
	Euthanasia
Cultural/social issues	Poverty
	Cultural/tribal beliefs

Rustenburg survey 2004.[84]

and the euthanasia debate is going to come up within the next ten years—and the northern European, the Dutch model, I could foresee being proposed. That's speculation on my part. But they've made the transition from at the beginning of life to permit abortion on demand, and so I see no reason that the human rights lobby might not push for euthanasia on demand or some version of that in due course. That will be a major ethical issue. The issues of confidentiality and disclosure with regard to HIV are really topical—not new because they have applied to tuberculosis in the past and have been negotiated. We've got models for these things and I think we should explore our history before we develop new ways to deal with this.[85]

I really think that the major ethical issue has been access to care and access to antiretrovirals; and then, the place of women in society that have made them the kind of victims, as it were, in Africa, of the epidemic. Then we need to look at the children's rights because our social services are not as strong as our health care services, and children are being abandoned to really horrific circumstances when their parents die from the AIDS epidemic . . . And one of the issues that I've discovered in my career as a GP—and also in hospice—is that medical care, and also traditional life, has been very autocratic. So it's the doctor telling you what's good for you, you know, 'Take this medicine', and it's the chief and the traditional leaders saying, 'This is what we'll do'.[39]

I think the ethical issues are beginning to be appreciated now with the impact of HIV/AIDS on hospice care in this country. Historically, hospices in this country were primarily established to provide care for the terminally ill cancer patient, and there was genuine support from the public for this. I think the onset of the HIV/AIDS pandemic has eroded the donor base, you know, that is why it's become dependent now on overseas funding to take care of the HIV/AIDS aspect of hospice work in this country.[86]

Life/oral histories

Marie Backeberg—*nursing sister, Centurion Hospice*: interviewed by Michael Wright, 13 August 2004. Length of interview (Centurion group): 32 min.

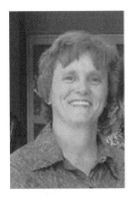

Marie Backeberg tells of her nursing background and of her work as a wound care practitioner. Her mother had died of cancer and when she sought to relocate her practice, she approached Centurion Hospice as she considered that her nursing skills could be of value to the patients. Since her move to the hospice, she has been elected to the committee and now makes a broader contribution to the life of the organization. Among many successes of hospice she considers that teamwork features prominently, pointing to the willingness of staff to work together in a collaborative, non-hierarchical way for the good of the patients.

Dr Alan Barnard—*GP and hospice physician, St Luke's Hospice, Cape Town*: interviewed by Michael Wright, 12 August 2004. Length of interview: 26 minutes.

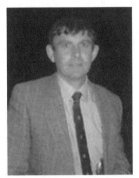

Alan Barnard is a GP who trained at UCT and for the past 15 years has practised in the southern suburbs of Cape Town. He has a long-standing interest in palliative care and provides part-time cover for St Luke's Hospice. He is currently taking the UCT masters degree in palliative medicine and pursuing an interest in research. He speaks of the family physician's role in palliative care, of the impetus brought about by the new (PEPFAR) funding, and of the need to keep sight of other disease categories alongside HIV/AIDS. On the question of ethics, he refers to issues around confidentiality and disclosure—especially for HIV patients—and perceives a growing interest in the euthanasia debate.

Peter Buckland—*chief executive, North Shore Hospice, New Zealand; formerly executive officer of St Luke's Hospice, Cape Town and the Hospice Association of the Witwatersrand*: interviewed by Michael Wright, 2 September 2004. Length of interview: 14 min.

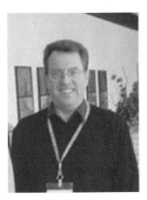

At the beginning of the 1980s, Peter Buckland ran a personnel recruitment company in Cape Town. He became aware of the hospice movement about the time that his father died, and when the hospice subsequently advertised for an administrator he decided to apply. After his appointment in 1985, he spent 7 years at St Luke's at a time when the organization grew from small beginnings into a much larger organization with home care, day care and an inpatient unit. He then took up a post with the newly formed national association—the Hospice Association of South Africa—and supported the developing hospice movement at a time of countrywide growth. In 1996, he moved as chief executive to the Hospice Association of the Witwatersrand at the time when Soweto Hospice was in the process of being established. Three years later, he left South Africa for New Zealand. He remembers reading *A Way to Die*—written by Victor and Rosemary Zorza about the death of their daughter in an English hospice—and speaks of the impact it made on him. Despite the passage of time and the changes along the way, he tells how he retains an idealistic vision of the essence of hospice care: of a patient-oriented service where staff also have time to be alongside the family offering care and support.

Sue Cameron—*HPCA board member and manager, Centre for Palliative Learning, Pretoria Sungardens Hospice*: interviewed by Michael Wright, 26 April 2005. Length of interview: 31 min.

After studying for a degree in Psychology and English, Sue Cameron became involved with the hospice movement after a friend informed her of a local meeting that was called in 1987 to found a hospice in Pretoria. Though reticent, she went along and quickly found that she related to both the aims and philosophy of palliative care. As local activity gathered momentum, she recalls the initial resistance from the medical profession; expansion into the informal settlements; the issues raised by caring for patients with AIDS; and problems of stigmatization. As the hospice became grounded in the local community, thoughts turned next to the question of training. From small beginnings, the Centre for Palliative Learning at Sungardens Hospice has grown into one of the largest training facilities in the country, with the home care programme becoming adopted as the national training programme for home-based care. Sue Cameron is currently a member of the HPCA board with a joint responsibility (with Kath Defilippi) for patient services. She reflects on the support that has been forthcoming from local communities, often from people with very little themselves; on the relationships that have developed between palliative caregivers and spiritual healers; and on the challenges facing the future development of palliative care—in particular, the major issues of funding and coverage.

Barbara Campbell-Ker—*executive director, Hospice Association of the Witwatersrand*: interviewed by Michael Wright, 11 August 2004. Length of interview: 48 min.

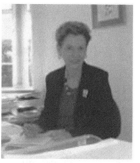

Barbara Campbell-Ker became a volunteer accountant at the Witwatersrand Hospice Association in 1986. By 1992, she had become a full-time member of staff in charge of finance and administration. In the intervening years, she had under-taken a role with the national hospice association and become chairperson of the provincial association covering Gauteng, Limpopo, Mpumalanga and North West Province—previously known as

Transvaal. She recalls the late 1980s when Witwatersrand had 16 paid members of staff and outlines the transition to the organization that operates today: a large NGO covering an area which encompasses 7 million people. She outlines the services provided by the association, including two distinct types of home care, and acknowledges the challenge of running an organization that receives only 3 per cent of its funding from government. Turning to the national picture, she then speaks of the vision for South Africa and the development of a strategy that takes account of training needs, standards development, the place of mentoring and the availability of PEPFAR funding.

Jeanette Daniel—*community palliative care nurse, St Luke's Hospice, Cape Town*: interviewed by Michael Wright, 6 August 2004. Length of interview: 24 min.

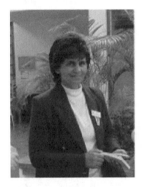

Jeanette Daniel speaks of how she came to work at the hospice after experiencing the sudden death of her mother. At that time, she worked in the psychiatry department of a local hospital. Moving to a part-time post on the ward of St Luke's, she saw the difference the hospice made in the lives of patients and their families. Eventually, she moved into the community, where she has worked for the past 12 years. As coverage grew, she moved to a new service in the Grassy Park area—her own locality—and helped establish a new clinic/drop-in centre, which has become a focal point locally. She speaks of issues around pain relief, euthanasia and spirituality, and of the valuable, harmonious relationships which have been established with both Muslim and Christian sections of the local community.

Brenda Dass—*provincial (PEPFAR) co-ordinator Limpopo, Gauteng and Mpumalanga*: interviewed by Michael Wright, 12 August 2004. Length of interview: 29 min.

Brenda Dass began her work in palliative care as a community nurse in 1990 and, after a period teaching auxiliary nurses, became nursing services manager for Hospice East Rand. She is currently employed as a PEPFAR Provincial Co-ordinator, a position which is directly related to the HPCA mentoring programme. Her provincial responsibility covers a vast expanse of land that includes large rural areas, most of them without palliative care provision. Activities include: the mentoring of established hospices; the mentoring of emerging hospices; and the setting up of new hospice programmes. Phase 1 began in 2003, supported by OSI, phase 2 in 2004. Current work involves the identification of development sites and the areas of need; these needs are then met by a team of people that possess the required skills. She is currently working with six development sites, 12 emerging hospices and six new programmes. Liaison with the Department of Health, the development of a buddy system and the availability of ARVs are seen as key factors in the drive to combat HIV/AIDS.

Rosemary de Jager—*home care co-ordinator, Highway Hospice, Durban*: interviewed by Michael Wright, 8 August 2004. Length of interview (Highway group): 1 h 33 min.

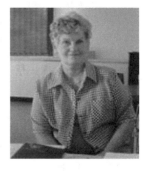

Rosemary de Jager joined Highway Hospice in 1986, first as a volunteer and shortly afterwards as a member of staff when her husband was retrenched. She contrasts the role of the home care sister in the early years of hospice compared with the present day—when pressures are greater, the care more sophisticated and the training more detailed. These changes mirror the increasing demands being placed upon hospice and the need to care for AIDS patients alongside cancer patients. Given the demands of the work, care for staff is a high priority. Support, therefore, has been carefully structured within a closely bonded home care team, with added support, if required, from a psychologist who visits on a regular basis.

Joan de Jong—*executive director, Hospice North West*: interviewed by Michael Wright, 12 August 2004. Length of interview (with Angie Sehoke): 24 min.

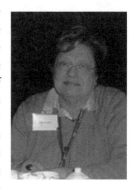

Joan de Jong recalls how she joined Hospice North West after previous experience as director of Lifeline—a telephone counselling service. Over the course of the next 8 years, the hospice grew from the small beginnings with a director, one nurse and a clerical assistant to an organization with 17 staff that has become widely known in the locality. Sixty volunteers assist the nurses and each of them receives a (very small) stipend. Home-based care is flourishing, and day care centres have become established in the local townships. Transport is essential, however, since many patients live in the poorest areas some distance from the hospice. Among the successes of the hospice is a crèche that operates daily to ensure that children do not need to stay off school to help grannies care for younger children.

Kathleen Defilippi (1)—*chairperson of APCA; HPCA board member and chief executive officer, South Coast Hospice, Port Shepstone*: interviewed by David Clark, 5 June 2004. Length of interview: 58 min.

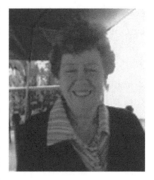

Kath Defilippi first became interested in hospice care in 1979 as a result of hearing a talk given by Dr Cicely Saunders at a symposium on death and dying. At the time, she was taking an advanced nursing course in Johannesburg, South Africa. It was not until a few years later, however, following a move to the South Coast area in KwaZulu Natal, that she was able to develop this interest further. Together with others in the area, she began to get involved in the care of terminally ill patients. At this time, the apartheid regime was at its height. She began to realize, however, that a particular model of care was needed, one well suited to local circumstances:

> . . . like all the hospices in South Africa . . . we had inherited the British model and that was the hallmark, [but] very soon I realized that the people in our part of the world who had the greatest need for pain and symptom control and holistic care actually lived in the outlying areas and they were black people, and we were a group of white, middle-class white women at that stage, you know, all volunteers, and that, you know, it just didn't make sense to have this sort of wonderful little, comfortable service for people who certainly needed it but not nearly as badly as others who had virtually no access to health care at all.

There could also be problems when patients cared for in the hospital facility were established on good pain relief, but then had to return home where no morphine was available. In response to this, they began to build a rural outreach programme. For a long time, they had very little funds to support their operation, relying on donations of money, time, materials and goodwill. In this way, the South Coast Hospice was able to expand the 5 million rand organization that it had become by 2004.

Initially, almost all of the patients had cancer, but in the 1990s they began to see an increasing number with HIV/AIDS. They began to address the question of how they could care for people in such growing numbers. They strengthened and widened their links with the primary health care teams and the hospitals. They described the model as 'Integrated Community-based Home Care'. Kath Defilippi describes the complex social problems faced by their patients: poverty, starvation, unemployment, substance abuse and sexual abuse.

She also describes the wider development of hospice and palliative care in South Africa, drawing on her experience as a board member of the national association—first in the Hospice Association of South Africa, later renamed the Hospice Palliative Care Association of South Africa. She describes the isolation of South Africa from the wider palliative care community during the years of apartheid. She reflects on the importance of bringing together both 'quality' and 'coverage' in the development of palliative care services in South Africa. She concludes with a discussion of her role in the work of the African Palliative Care Association, of which she is the first President, and also some observations on the impact of PEPFAR funding on the developing palliative care scene in South Africa and other countries in the region.

Kathleen Defilippi (2)—*chairperson of APCA; HPCA board member and chief executive officer, South Coast Hospice, Port Shepstone*: interviewed by Michael Wright, 12 August 2004. Length of interview: 10 min.

In this interview, Kath Defilippi focuses on the concept of mentorship and its relevance to the hospice movement in South Africa and in the broader African context. Funding was provided by the Open Society Institute in 2002 to develop a programme that utilized well-established, developed hospices to provide guidance and support to emerging or less-developed organizations within their geographic area. Underpinning this initiative was a forward-looking response to the HIV/AIDS epidemic that enabled hospices belonging to HPCA to function as a resource that could reach out and empower other faith-based and community organizations to provide quality home-based care that includes pain and symptom control. After a successful first phase, funding became available for a second phase, beginning in 2003—an initiative that has coincided with the PEPFAR funding. This has enabled HPCA to recruit provincial palliative care development teams and a full-time PEPFAR provincial co-ordinator. The aim is to have a provincial association in each of South Africa's nine provinces, linked to nine provincial development teams. Crucially, this is linked to a three-stage accreditation system developed in partnership with the Council of Health Services Accreditation for Southern Africa.

Sr Priscilla Dlamini—*founder, Holy Cross Hospice, Gingindlovu*: interviewed by Michael Wright, 12 August 2004. Length of interview: 40 min.

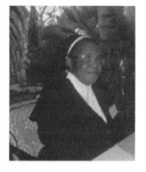

Sr Priscilla Dlamini has a background in nursing and founded Holy Cross Hospice in 1999, converting a block of stables to a 40-bed inpatient unit with 20 adult and 20 paediatric places. She speaks of the difficulties posed by around 470 child-headed families in the locality and of the project's support for young family members by the provision of a crèche and day centre. Around 25 carers provide home-based care to around 200 patients, although the inpatient unit is available for sole-surviving family members or carers who are exhausted. The hospice is self-supporting and, where appropriate, modern medicines are used alongside herbal and homeopathic treatments; some morphine is available prescribed by sympathetic doctors. A social care project supports children by ensuring death certificates are provided for their parents, thereby giving access to government grants. Orphans are further supported by the construction of two-roomed pre-fabricated houses imported from The Netherlands. A target figure of 215 houses has been set, and these houses arrive in containers carrying 15 at a time. Links have been established with the University of Zululand for the provision of counselling and psychological support. Sister Priscilla speaks of the challenges she has faced initiating and sustaining these projects and of the generosity of the local communities and international donors.

Stella Dubazana—*child care manager, Cotlands Hospice, Johannesburg*: Interviewed by Michael Wright, 11 August 2004. Length of interview: 30 min.

Stella Dubazana has a background in nursing and began work at Cotlands paediatric hospice in 2001 in a search for more job satisfaction. She is now the hospice's child care manager, having undergone palliative care training at Pretoria Sungardens Hospice—and speaks of her new role as her 'passion'. She tells of the children's backgrounds and of the

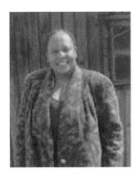

combined difficulties caused by sickness and poverty. She draws attention to the hospice facilities and the relationships established with local hospitals and other child-focused organizations. Outlining the nature of the relationship between the hospice and the child's family, she says, 'We say to them, "we'll take care of the child for you", but the family remains the first people that can tell us what we can do; we never take decisions for them'. This relationship is supported by the provision of funding so that family members can visit; financial support is also available when funeral arrangements become necessary. In the community, families are also supported by outreach workers who, once they become involved with a child, maintain support wherever the child is located. Finally, Stella Dubazana speaks of the needs of staff and the ways in which support is given to those involved with children who die.

Dr Sarah Fakroodeen—*palliative care physician, Highway Hospice, Durban*: interviewed by Michael Wright, 8 August 2004. Length of interview (group): 1 h 33 min.

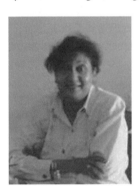

Sarah Fakroodeen studied at the Royal College of Physicians and Surgeons in Dublin (Ireland) and followed her initial studies with a post-graduate course in obstetrics. She subsequently travelled to South Africa to see her father and never returned to Ireland. She eventually saw a post advertised at the hospice and was appointed day centre doctor, part-time. She found herself suited to the work and took the palliative medicine diploma at Cardiff, followed by the Master's course at the University of Cape Town. She highlights a number of issues: getting palliative medicine recognized as a medical specialty; communicating with GPs regarding a patient's quality of life; ensuring symptom relief and maintaining an accepting, non-judgemental approach towards religious diversity. She sees patient care and the difference it makes to people's lives as being the major success of the hospice.

Dr Elizabeth Gwyther (1)—*HPCA board member; education and research co-ordinator*: interviewed by David Clark, 4 June 2004. Length of interview: 30 min.

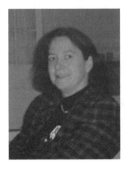

This interview focuses chiefly on the impact of PEPFAR funding on the palliative care scene in South Africa. The country is one of 12 in Africa to be eligible for support and the first to receive palliative care funding from PEPFAR. The foundation of the proposal to PEPFAR is the Hospice Palliative Care Association's Mentorship Programme, where hospices with established programmes and people with the technical expertise, the knowledge and skills assist smaller programmes or new and emerging home-based care and hospice programmes to develop their own palliative care components. That mentorship programme has been supported for the past two and a half years (up to June 2004) by Open Society Institute and is being used as the vehicle for the PEPFAR funding, of which the first year's grant is US$2 million.

The aim of the Mentorship Programme is to deliver quality palliative care to patients and families, looking at organizations that have a component of clinical palliative care but that also have good management, good governance and financial accountability. The idea is to develop those organizations. This involves looking at the holistic care of patients and families, together with pain and symptom control and with psycho-social and spiritual support. The mentorship programme started with standards of clinical care, to which were added standards of management and good governance. There are different levels of accreditation: pre-entry level, entry level, intermediate level and those that get full accreditation. This covers the range of services that hospices offer: home-based care services, inpatient services, day hospice, spiritual counselling, bereavement counselling, education and training.

Liz Gwyther discusses the key elements of palliative care and their definition. She outlines the process of applying for PEPFAR funds and the short time scale involved.

There are six objectives for the programme of PEPFAR-funded work: (1) to build capacity in the national office; (2) to strengthen services; (3) to develop new hospices; (4) advocacy; (5) palliative care research and training; and (6) monitoring and evaluation. The interview concludes with reference to the work of the newly created African Association of Palliative Care and the role of South Africa within it.

Dr Elizabeth Gwyther (2)—interviewed by Michael Wright, 7 August 2004. Length of interview: 51 min.

Liz Gwyther tells how she was a contemporary of Christine Dare at the UCT Medical School. After qualifying, she first practised in Zimbabwe before returning to the Cape in the early 1980s as the hospice service at St Luke's was gathering momentum. She referred her first patient to St Luke's in 1983 and collaborated intermittently with the hospice during the next 10 years. As her interest developed, she became directly involved in hospice care during the 1980s and obtained a diploma in palliative medicine from the University of Wales. She subsequently explored the possibilities of establishing a palliative medicine course at UTC, an initiative which eventually commenced with a first intake of 23 doctors; around 60 have since qualified. After serving as chairperson of the Helderberg board, she became CEO at St Luke's Hospice, Cape Town in 2001 at a time when the service was being expanded to include HIV/AIDS patients. She refers to the developments that focused on the needs of patients, orphans and families; comments on how morphine is prescribed and dispensed; and raises the ethical issues surrounding access to care and the positions of women and children. Finally, she acknowledges the strengthening relationships between hospice personnel, traditional healers and the leaders of different faiths,

Bonnie Haack—*director, Human Resources and Training, Cotlands, Johannesburg*: interviewed by Michael Wright, 11 August 2004. Length of interview: 21 min.

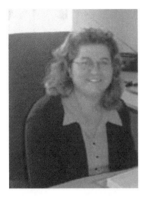

Bonnie Haack joined the staff of Cotlands in 1994 as pre-school teacher and principal. At that time, there were around 45 staff involved with sanctuary (the residential unit) and the hospice was in the process of development. As the number of personnel increased, she developed an interest in staff issues and devised a programme of meetings that was accessible to a staff body that worked shifts. Today, the Cotlands organization employs around 150 staff spread across several sites as far afield as Cape Town and East London in addition to Johannesburg. In caring for children, staff are seen as a major resource, and related issues are given high priority. She tells how the movement towards hospice care was a 'paradigm shift' that prompted a detailed review of practice. Central to this review was a debate about non-hospice staff and their relationship with children in the hospice. Subsequently, those who wished to be involved were included, and experience has shown the lasting effects of human contact. Among the many successes of Cotlands, Bonnie Haack considers that the team approach and the willingness of staff to undertake extra roles for the well-being of the children is a strength of the organization.

Arend Hoogervorst—*former chairperson, Executive Committee, Hospice Association of the Witwatersrand*: interviewed by Michael Wright, 19 May 2005. Length of interview: 50 min.

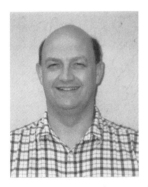

During his school days in England, Arend Hoogervorst became associated with TOC H and related well to the Christian yet non-denominational ideals of the organization. After representing the youth components of TOC H during a visit to South Africa, he was invited to return for a 2-year period as field officer after finishing his degree in Environmental Science. Consequently, he arrived in Johannesburg in January 1979 to take over from Margaret Lebish (McGettrick) and take forward her pioneering work. During 1979, he became chairperson of the Association's Executive Committee and continued as chair or deputy chairperson until 1986. He speaks about the early growth of the Hospice Association; of community and hospital collaboration; of the role of NGOs such as the National Cancer Association and Care for the Aged; and the valuable support of Lifeline staff, social workers and the Sisters from Holy Cross Convent—seconded from Kenridge Hospital. He recalls the move to secure hospice buildings on Houghton Drive and how, for around 18 months, he lived in the property since legislation at that time required the premises to be inhabited during any request for change of use. Among many challenges, Arend Hoogervorst remembers how a disparate group of people came together with an irresistible determination to provide better care for the terminally ill, and to make this care accessible to those who needed it.

Karen Hinton (1)—interviewed by Michelle Winslow, 28 June 2002. Length of interview: 56 min.

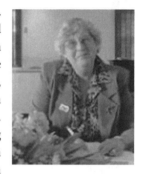

Karen Hinton grew up in Ellesmere Port in Cheshire, UK. She trained as a nurse in Birkenhead and in 1969 met and married her South African husband. She moved to South Africa in 1970, continued her nursing career, and after the birth of her children became involved with Greta Schoeman, who was seeking help to establish a hospice in Durban. In 1982, Greta started Highway Hospice from her own home. Karen Hinton discusses the early days of the service, working with local doctors, and Greta's UK visit to gain experience in palliative care. In 1984, following a fundraising campaign, an inpatient unit opened. This was during the apartheid era but the political system was disregarded and patients from all backgrounds were admitted, predominantly with cancer but increasingly with AIDS. She talks about issues involved in caring for AIDS patients, particularly economic hardship, and then reflects on the hospice's growth and development, treatment and pain relief, staff and volunteers, education, and involvement with the Hospice Association of South Africa. At the time of interview, Karen was Education Manager at Highway Hospice and Chairman of the KwaZulu Natal Hospice Association.

Karen Hinton (2)—*chairperson: Hospice Association of KwaZulu Natal; quality assurance adviser, Highway Hospice, Durban*: interviewed by Michael Wright, 8 August 2004. Length of interview (Highway group): 1 h 33 min.

Karen Hinton has been at Highway Hospice since it opened in 1982 and in those days was instrumental in forming the shape of the hospice in association with Greta Schoeman. Until 2004, she mainly focused on education, serving also on the national subcommittee for patient care and education and being a member of the team which developed the certificate course for professional nurses. Recalling the development of the hospice movement in South Africa, she points to the role played by nurses as a counter to the contemporary focus upon palliative medicine. Turning next to the changing hospice provision, she describes how the 'British model' of hospice care—an inpatient unit and accompanying home care service—did not meet the needs of the whole community. The reduction of inpatient beds, therefore, did not just reflect the financial problems of the day, but also a growing realization that the service had to be amongst and accessible to the whole community. Bringing this about has been one of the biggest challenges of recent times.

Theresa Hlongwa—*nursing sister, manager of Umlazi day centre, Highway Hospice, Durban*: interviewed by Michael Wright 9 August 2004. Length of interview: 25 min.

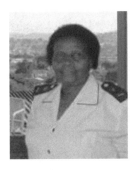

Theresa Hlongwa trained as a nurse at Edendale Hospital and then qualified a midwife at King Edward VIII Hospital. She undertook further training in community health nursing science and took a bachelor's degree in nursing administration at the University of South Africa. Since her retirement as a professional nurse, she has become involved in hospice work as a home care sister and manager of the hospice day centre in Umlazi, near Durban. She regards poverty as a major challenge and has worked hard to ensure that the centre remains open despite the interest of local gangsters who have stripped the centre of its equipment. Yet Theresa Hlongwa has won the confidence of the local community and she regards it as a major success that residents recognize her car and stop her in the street to ask for help spontaneously.

Goonam Jacob—*social worker, Highway Hospice, Durban*: interviewed by Michael Wright, 8 August 2004. Length of interview (Highway group): 1 h 33 min.

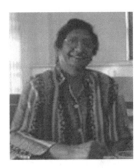

After retiring from her previous employment at the beginning of 2003, Goonam Jacob joined Highway Hospice as a volunteer social worker having previously studied death and dying as part of a Master's degree course. From her work in the Indian community, she refers to the denial that is commonplace about AIDS—notably that Indian families are not affected. The reality, however, has become painfully obvious and this is causing huge distress, not only physically and emotionally but also conceptually. When these factors combine with cultural practices such as women remaining in their homes when a family member is dying, getting support and counselling to those who need it can be problematic.

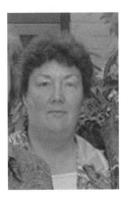

Jackie Jackson—*nursing sister, Pretoria Sungardens, previously employed at Centurion Hospice*: interviewed by Michael Wright, 13 August 2004. Length of interview (Centurion group): 32 min.

Jackie Jackson recalls the groundswell of energy during the mid-1990s that led to the establishment of Centurion Hospice. Local support was considerable: the municipality donated grounds and local activists raised funds to build the premises. Initially, the hospice opened a day centre, but provision now includes counselling, home-based care and an inpatient facility. Early challenges centred on the recruitment of staff with the medical and nursing skills to take the hospice forward. Jackie Jackson has since moved to Pretoria Sungardens Hospice which is the mentor hospice for Centurion.

Edith Khumalo—*social worker, Soweto Hospice*: interviewed by Michael Wright, 10 August 2004. Length of interview (Soweto group): 34 min.

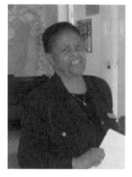

Edith Khumalo was a retired social worker when Sibongile Mafata approached her to work at Soweto Hospice; she was pleased to respond. She tells of the extreme pressures brought about by unemployment and poverty; of the hardships of life in the squatters' camps; of the paralysing effects of sickness and AIDS; and the complex search for relatives when itinerant workers—often from rural areas—die in the city. She speaks too, of the problems of bereavement, especially for children, and of the ways in which the hospice supports those who are affected. This frequently involves the provision of food parcels, assistance with funeral expenses, help with documentation and grant applications. Despite the challenges, she is optimistic about the support which can be given and considers her present role to be the most fulfilling of her professional career.

Lesley Lawson—*co-founder and director of nursing services, St Francis Hospice, Port Elizabeth*: interviewed by Michael Wright, 26 April 2005. Length of interview: 48 min.

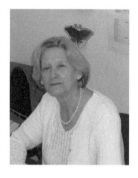

Lesley Lawson trained as a nurse in England and experienced community nursing in the USA before arriving in South Africa in the 1970s. After hearing a lecture by Cicely Saunders at the University of Cape Town (1979), she returned home to Port Elizabeth determined to found a hospice programme. With support from the Cancer Association of South Africa, she first established a home care service at the beginning of the 1980s and then co-founded St Francis Hospice—which came to include an inpatient unit—in 1986. She speaks about the early challenges faced by these services: of fundraising and the development of expertise, of incorporating psycho-social care alongside physical care and of operating a non-segregated unit during the days of apartheid. She highlights what she sees as key ingredients of hospice care—respect for the individual and patient autonomy—and reflects upon the demands brought about by factors such as poverty, the AIDS pandemic and child-headed families. Turning to the needs of staff, she outlines a strategy of support designed to ensure that the stresses of the service do not become overwhelming. As she looks to the future, Lesley Lawson is encouraged by the gradual spread of palliative care into the rural areas, and sees strengths in the adaptability of the service, the commitment of staff and the leadership of the national association.

Josef Lazarus—*strategic adviser to the HPCA board*: interviewed by Michael Wright, 13 August 2004. Length of interview: 33 min.

Josef Lazarus initially trained as a priest and then sought a practical application to his life, and so became involved in the national training of health professionals in South Africa's eight medical schools. When he led a development unit at the University of Natal, he became interested in the community dimension of medicine which eventually led to his involvement in the hospice movement (1994). In 1997, he was asked to undertake a strategic planning exercise for HPCA that focused on developmental aspects of the service. Key portfolios were established in patient care, education and training, organizational development, advocacy and fundraising; and people were appointed to those subcommitters who had the appropriate expertise. Joe Lazarus speaks of the Hospice Development Fund and its overall impact on the hospice movement; he also refers to the PEPFAR funding and how these funds will be used for capacity development and the establishment of regional (hospice) centres of excellence in each of South Africa's health districts.

Margaret Lebish (McGettrick)—*former TOC H-funded hospice project worker, Johannesburg:* interviewed by Michael Wright, 25 March 2005. Length of interview: 58 min.

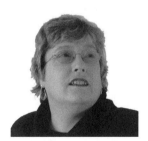

Margaret Lebish arrived in South Africa to support her brother whose wife had died after a brain haemorrhage in the autumn of 1976. She was aware of the hospice movement in Britain and, when she worked in London, had experience of end-of-life care at St Mary's Hospital (Paddington) which also linked with St Luke's Hospital, Bayswater.[87] After arriving in South Africa, she met the hospital social worker Sylvia Poss who was involved with the Tender Loving Care group: a special interest group based at Johannesburg General Hospital that focused on care of the dying. As interest in the hospice ideal developed, TOC H continued to pay the salary of Margaret Lebish while she encouraged local interest. This led her to present a paper at a meeting of the TLC group on 9 March 1979 which formally proposed the establishment of a hospice in Johannesburg. This proposal was accepted and led to the formation of a steering group that included Stan Henen—a local activist who became a key figure in the Witwatersrand hospice until the early 1990s. Margaret Lebish reflects upon the early development of what became the Hospice Association of the Witwatersrand, the contributions of key individuals, and the role of TOC H at this formative time.

Sibongile Mafata—*co-ordinator, Soweto Hospice*: interviewed by Michael Wright, 10 August 2004. Length of interview (Soweto group): 34 min.

Sibongile Mafata trained as a nurse and was appointed co-ordinator of the new hospice facility in Soweto in 1998. She had previously worked at Chris Hani Baragwanath

Hospital, and also as a First Aid Instructor, but she missed the hands-on nursing and interaction with patients. At first, Soweto Hospice developed slowly since little was known about the nature of hospice care. As awareness increased, the number of patients rose dramatically. The first patients mostly had a cancer diagnosis but, today, the majority of patients are living with AIDS. She considers that a major success of the organization is the way in which the local community has supported the hospice, which is struggling to meet the demands now being placed upon it; in the future, she hopes for an expansion of the inpatient unit.

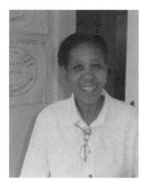

Joan Marston—*HPCA board member; advocacy officer; founder of St Nicholas Children's Hospice Bloemfontein*: interviewed by Michael Wright, 21 September 2004. Length of interview: 28 min.

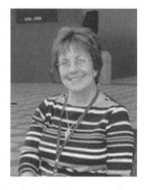

Joan Marston is a nurse by profession and began working in a hospice as a volunteer in Bloemfontein. As she worked as a nurse, she saw the over-riding need for a children's service. She was instrumental in securing premises and establishing an 18-bed inpatient unit, supported by six day care centres and a home care programme that reaches 750 children. She recalls how children need play as well as words and how this dimension has been built into the service. Three-quarters of the children are dying at presentation, so an aggressive policy of food provision has become an essential part of the service. Remarkably, children have a matter of fact way of thinking about spirituality and the afterlife that challenges more sophisticated articulations. Joan Marston then speaks of her advocacy role, promoting hospice and palliative care throughout South Africa and the support received from the Diana, Princess of Wales Memorial Fund: a very pro-active funder. Among many successes has been the government commitment to hospice and palliative care.

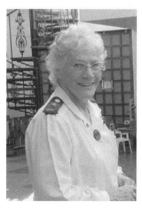

Meg Meyers—*director of nursing, St Luke's Hospice, Cape Town*: interviewed by Michael Wright, 7 August 2004. Length of interview: 54 min.

Meg Myers was born in the country now known as Zambia and, with her family, relocated to Cape Town when she was about 11 years old. She trained as a nurse and, throughout her professional life, enjoyed nursing patients and being integrally involved in their care. She became involved with the hospice movement through her connection with the local church, which Christine Dare, the founder of St Luke's, also attended. Eventually, she became St Luke's first employee, and has remained with the hospice ever since. Meg Myers speaks of the issues and challenges which faced the hospice as it began to become established: raising funds; securing pain relief; promoting a racially integrated service; confronting the AIDS epidemic; and maintaining a broad patient base that includes all life-limiting conditions. She considers that the success of St Luke's is due to the commitment of staff and their generous gifs of time and expertise. She thinks that staff who are drawn to the hospice have a distinct empathy with dying people and, as a result, the hospice develops a dedicated team that generates a spirit of service and belonging.

Flora Kobotlo Modiba—*founder, Arebaokeng Hospice*: interviewed by Michael Wright, 13 August 2004. Length of interview: 20 min.

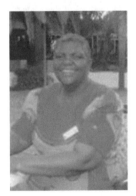

Under the guidance of Flora Kobotlo Modiba, Arebaokeng Hospice was registered as a non-profit organization in 2000 and the first patients were cared for in 2001. When the hospice opened, she was working full time and caring for hospice patients on her day off, helped by one other caregiver. She became aware of the hospice movement when she worked with cancer patients and, after undergoing a palliative care training course, decided to begin a service in her local community. She speaks of several challenges: obtaining funds; networking with health organizations and personnel; gaining access to patient records; and challenging the myths around morphine. Some local doctors support the hospice, and good relationships have been established with traditional healers in the area. An orphan programme has begun and a day centre is operational. A regular supply of food is the orphans' most urgent need, so children are fed before they leave the centre. Plans are in hand to provide food parcels for the orphans' extended families as a means of keeping the children in their communities rather than seeing them admitted to orphanages. In the future, Flora Modiba looks forward to the mentorship scheme and discussions have already taken place about the hospice's involvement.

G. K. Moodly—*chairperson, Verulam Regional Hospice Association*: interviewed by Michael Wright, 12 August 2004. Length of interview (with C. N. Pillay): 34 min.

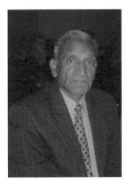

G. K. Moodly, a retired school principal, tells how Verulam Hospice has developed day care and home care services that reach out to the poorest areas of Verulam. The hospice relocated to a new building in 2004 and he is pleased that this will be the venue for HIV/AIDS training provided by South Coast Hospice. Networks have been established with other organizations, including: Victoria Hospital; the Senior Citizens Day Care Centre; the Child and Family Care Centre; and the Lighthouse Crisis Centre—with beneficial effects. G. K. Moodly recalls the challenge of recruiting volunteers, since initially the philosophy of hospice was largely unknown and no salary was payable. Gradually, however, the number of personnel increased and the hospice has expanded. Although fundraising is a constant issue, there have been pleasant surprises. One such surprise was the anonymous donation of a new 4 × 4 vehicle from members of the business community.

Mandla Mtatambi—*palliative care nurse, manager of Inanda day centre, Highway Hospice, Durban:* interviewed by Michael Wright 9 August 2004. Length of interview: 52 min.

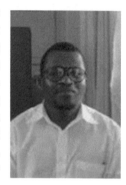

Mandla Mtatambi received his nurse training in the South African gold mines and, thereafter, worked in government hospitals and clinics. He attended a lecture on death and dying as part of a course in psychiatric nursing; an experience that eventually led him to Highway Hospice. In 2000, he began working as a hospice home care nurse in Umlazi before becoming involved with the Inanda project in 2003. He describes Inanda as a community of >18 000 people that includes informal settlements of self-erected accommodation. In such settings, widespread poverty combined with the absence of clean water and effective sanitation systems are a constant source of health problems. The hospice provides home-based care and day care. The day centre opens 2 days each week and 101 patients attended weekly in 2004. Food is provided and, if necessary, a family will bring a patient in a wheelbarrow to secure a meal. Support groups help patients living with AIDS to combat the stigma, and the social inclusion is greatly appreciated. Although ARVs are beginning to be dispensed from Mahatma Ghandi Hospital, the roll out programme is slower than what had been anticipated. Mandla Mtatambi speaks of the rights of passage around death and dying and of the importance of respecting the diverse spiritual perspectives of the patients.

Thembi Nyuswa—*palliative care nurse, Highway Hospice:* interviewed by Michael Wright, 8 August 2004. Length of interview: 22 min.

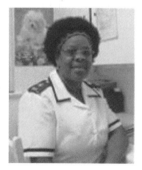

Thembi Nyuswa tells how she was the first black nurse to work for Highway Hospice at a time when the hospice concept was still very new. Charged with introducing an African home care service, she obtained a drivers' licence and began her visits in a donated Toyota Stallion. It was a fulfilling experience and Thembi Nyuswa tells how she valued the time spent with patients and the ways in which the service was received. She recalls the sense of shock that her presence occasionally caused during the transition to post-apartheid

South Africa; a striking contrast to the supportive, family atmosphere of the hospice environment. A central feature of the hospice's support for staff has been the regular group meetings/de-briefings based on a strong concept of teamwork. The successes of hospice include: better pain relief for patients; comprehensive family support; a growth in volunteers; dialogue with traditional healers; and a widespread acceptance of the hospice concept.

Jennifer Padayachee—*nursing sister, manager of Phoenix day centre, Highway Hospice, Durban*: interviewed by Michael Wright, 9 August 2004. Length of interview: 37 min.

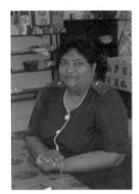

Jennifer Padayachee joined Highway Hospice after her father died of cancer in 1999. She previously worked as a midwife but has since followed the palliative care course at Highway Hospice. She speaks of the challenges faced by the community of Phoenix—of the poverty, the crime and the drug abuse—and how the hospice supports terminally ill people. This involves confronting the myths around morphine and raising hospice awareness within the community. Her responsibilities include the home care service and Phoenix day care centre. In 2004, the day centre operated in a shopping mall in premises donated free of charge. Although a temporary arrangement, this has had many benefits: accessibility; space for meetings/therapies; low costs; and a customer base for sale items. Eventually, a permanent location is expected at the nearby Mahatma Ghandi Hospital. Jennifer Padayachee speaks highly of the local interest, the fundraising activities and the increasing involvement of the community—all contribute to her feeling of fulfilment. She is aware, however, of the risks associated with her role and appreciates the support of the home care team at Highway Hospice.

Dr C. N. Pillay—*president, Chatsworth Hospice*: interviewed by Michael Wight, 12 August 2004. Length of interview (with G. K. Moody): 34 min.

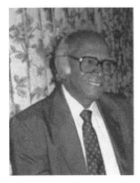

C. N. Pillay is a retired surgeon who served the Chatsworth community as head of the department of surgery at the local hospital from 1969. Prompted by the lack of provision for people with cancer who were deemed incurable, C. N. Pillay conducted an audit and established the need for a hospice. Chatsworth Hospice opened in 1991 amid huge support. Today, Chatsworth Hospice provides a wide range of services to patients of all races whose condition is considered to be incurable. The majority of patients are of Indian origin and most have a cancer diagnosis. As only 5 per cent of patients present with AIDS, the work of the hospice in this area is mostly preventive and concerned with behaviour change. Spiritual care features prominently and begins at an early stage. Among the successes of the hospice, C. N. Pillay speaks of the broad community involvement and mentions in particular the schools week: an initiative that raises children's awareness of the hospice and brings them onto the premises.

Dr Richard Scheffer—*medical director, Rowcroft Hospice, UK*: interviewed by Michael Wight, 24 March 2005. Length of interview: 42 min.

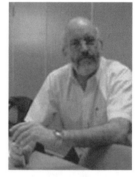

Richard Scheffer was born in Empangeni, Zululand. After a course in social work, he took up a teaching post at the University of Natal but subsequently changed direction to pursue a career in medicine. It was at medical school (University of Cape Town) that he met Christine Dare and responded to her desire to bring Cicely Saunders to South Africa by taking her request to the Student Visiting Lecturers' Organization, on which he served. During her visit, Cicely Saunders famously engaged in a public debate on euthanasia with Dr Christian Barnard, an event which attracted widespread interest. Richard Scheffer recalls how he was determined to specialize in palliative medicine after he heard Cicely Saunders give an inspiring lecture. After qualifying as a doctor, he took up a post in the Durban area and became involved in Highway Hospice before leaving South Africa in 1983.

Greta Schoeman—*founder, Highway Hospice, Durban*: interviewed by Michael Wright, 9 August 2004. Length of interview: 50 min.

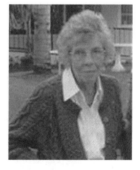

Greta Schoeman was 12 years old when she became aware of her father and grandmother's cancer diagnosis. She nursed her father intermittently during the next 20 years and recalls how poorly pain was controlled in those days. She trained as a paediatric nurse and, after her marriage to an orthopaedic surgeon, she returned with him to his home in South Africa. It was in Durban that she came across Victor Zorza's book about the death of his daughter in an English hospice, whereupon she returned to England, met the Zorzas and subsequently undertook a hospice care training course at Sir Michael Sobell House (Oxford). Back home in South Africa, she determined to begin a hospice service, and opened the guest wing of her home as an inpatient unit, eventually caring for 22 patients there during the next 18 months. Eventually, a suitable property became available and the hospice moved to its current site and expanded as neighbouring properties became available. Greta Schoeman goes on to speak of the challenges which confronted the developing service, of ways in which the multidisciplinary team was built and strengthened, and of how the hospice ideal proved a unifying and motivating force for those involved. Finally, she tells of her own cancer diagnosis and her experience of being cared for in the hospice she had founded.

Jackie Schoeman—*director, Cotlands, Johannesburg*: interviewed by Michael Wright, 11 August 2004. Length of interview: 32 min.

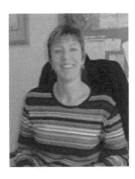

Jackie Schoeman has a background in social work and, after working in residential settings, became director of the Cotlands organization. She speaks of the different needs of children, of the paramount importance of home and family, but also of the roles played by Cotlands sanctuary (residential care) and hospice. Until ARVs became available, the emotional demands upon hospice staff were particularly high, and care for staff remains a top priority. Everyone is heartened, however, by the improvements brought about by ARVs and the way children receiving ARV therapy return to school and lead active lives. Such medication is expensive, but the costs have been incorporated into the organization's business plan to ensure continuity and maintain the children's quality of life. Jackie Schoeman speaks of the need to raise funds and how the organization is in constant touch with donors to generate a sense of belonging. A current challenge is to find foster placements for children who are HIV positive. Potential carers are apprehensive at the thought of imminent loss. Yet, in fact, ARVs have improved the life of expectancy of such children. Among an expanding range of programmes, end-of-life care is seen as an important aspect of Cotland's provision and, in 2003, the organization opened another hospice in the Western Cape.

Rosemary Schütler—*social worker, Highway Hospice, Durban*: interviewed by Michael Wright, 8 August 2004. Length of interview (Highway group): 1 h 33 min.

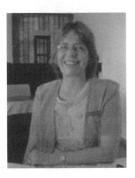

Rosemary Schütler joined Highway Hospice as a social worker in 1999. She was aware of the hospice ideal and had seen the service develop during the previous decade when Greta Schoeman and her volunteers used to speak to her elderly clients—some of whom were eventually admitted to the inpatient unit. She tells of the value of the interdisciplinary team meetings and of the introductory course that assists new staff to come to terms with their work with the dying and bereaved. The number of deaths is often high: a recent audit showed that in 1 month, 80 patients had been referred to hospice and 25 of these had died during the same month. She highlights the impact of bereavement, and recalls a 10-year-old boy who had already experienced the death of eight family members. Amongst the suffering, however, are many high points, and Rosemary Schütler outlines the ways in which hospice has made a difference to the lives of individuals.

Dr Thobi Segabi—*palliative care physician, Soweto Hospice*: interviewed by Michael Wright, 10 August 2004. Length of interview (Soweto group): 34 min.

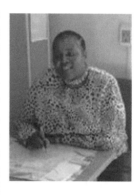

When Thobi Segabi was working as a GP, she found an increasing number of people with AIDS were consulting her for treatment. As a result, she decided to become involved with Soweto Hospice so she could influence a larger group of infected people. She subscribes to the concept of the multidisciplinary team and appreciates how issues can be approached from a variety of perspectives. She speaks of the difficulties communicating with those who believe they are bewitched, but is encouraged by the ways in which many patients are ultimately able to accept their diagnosis and deal with unfinished business. Thobi Segabi finds this activity to be a fulfilling part of her work, and is encouraged by the improvements brought about by antiretroviral drugs.

Angie Sehoke—*palliative care nurse, Hospice North West*: interviewed by Michael Wright, 12 August 2004. Length of interview (with Joan de Jong): 24 min.

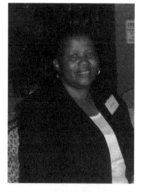

Angie Sehoke previously worked as a theatre nurse and knew little about Hospice North West when she applied for a post there. Yet in the 5 years since her appointment, she has found the work to be particularly rewarding. Many patients live in poverty, a situation exacerbated by their lack of documentation which precludes them from government assistance. Although all disease categories are catered for, around 90 per cent of patients are HIV positive. In the context of personal relationships—where women are usually powerless—an outreach programme of education attempts to change behaviours and 'keep the negatives, negative'. Angie Sehoke thinks the hospice can be a resource to other organizations and looks forward to further opportunities for training and education.

Zodwe Sithole—*palliative care nurse, Highway Hospice, Durban*: interviewed by Michael Wright, 12 August 2004. Length of interview: 18 min.

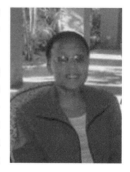

Zodwe Sithole recalls how Highway Hospice supported her sister after she was diagnosed with breast cancer and how the care encompassed the whole family. Despite her nursing background, it was the first time she had come into contact with palliative care and, from that moment, she decided to seek work in a hospice in order to 'make a difference'. She lived in

Johannesburg at the time and, when a project co-ordinator was required for Soweto Hospice, she was subsequently offered the post. Little was known about palliative care then, so she visited local institutions advocating for hospice and explaining the benefits of the service to physicians and nurses. When her husband's work caused a relocation to Durban, she joined the staff of Highway Hospice and continues her advocacy work in the community and among Department of Health officials. Her hope for the future is that the work of volunteers will be recognized by the payment of a stipend.

Stella Thackray—*palliative care nurse, Highway Hospice, Durban*: interviewed by Michael Wright, 9 August 2004. Length of interview: 13 min.

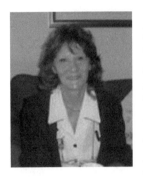

Stella Thackray recalls how she came to Durban from Perthshire, Scotland, in 1980. Two years later, she came into contact with the newly formed Highway Hospice after a request for sutures to care for a patient who had fallen out of bed. She was subsequently invited to a hospice meeting where she was asked by Greta Schoeman to see a patient—and has been involved with hospice ever since. Stella Thackray tells how, in the early days, the hospice was located in Greta Schoeman's home and nurses worked voluntarily, caring for patients who lived close to their own homes. She speaks of the changes that have occurred in the intervening years: the development of the inpatient unit; the growth in personnel; and the development from nursing care to include other disciplines. Among the successes of the hospice, she prioritizes the way in which the organization has reached out to all sections of the community and responded to the needs of the patients and their families.

Elna van der Merwe—*nursing services manager, Centurion Hospice, Pretoria*: interviewed by Michael Wright, 13 August 2004. Length of interview (Centurion group): 32 min.

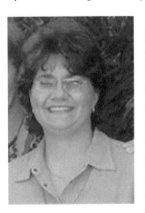

After living in Mozambique and Lesotho, Elna van der Merwe returned to South Africa and, seeing a board that promoted the work of Centurion Hospice, telephoned to see if she could be of assistance. Her fortuitous call answered a need at the time and, after working for the hospice as a nurse, she eventually took up the post of nursing services manager. She speaks of the challenges faced by the hospice: developing an inclusive service; staff training; and bereavement care after the death of a patient. These challenges are exacerbated by the drain on resources caused by the number of trained staff who leave South Africa and of the pressures this places on human resources. She is anxious to develop a hospice culture where patients do not merely receive from the hospice, but are able to contribute as participating members of a wider community. She reflects upon the process of mentoring and how it impacts upon the life of the hospice, and concludes by suggesting that in essence, the success of Centurion hospice is due to the 'servant attitude' that has been developed there.

Alta van der Wetering—*nursing sister, Centurion Hospice, Pretoria*: interviewed by Michael Wright, 13 August 2004. Length of interview (Centurion group): 32 min.

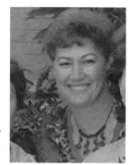

Alta van der Wetering tells how she came to work at the hospice at a time when there was a shortage of nursing skills. Among the many challenges confronting the hospice, she considers funding to be a particular issue due to the constraints that a shortage of funds places on the range and quality of hospice services. She points to the importance of prayer in the day to day life of the organization and how, repeatedly, those prayers are answered at a time of need.

Professor J. P. van Niekerk—*chair of HPCA, manager of PEPFAR project*: interviewed by Michael Wright, 13 August 2004. Length of interview: 34 min.

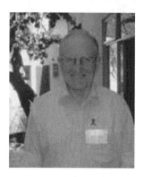

J. P. van Niekerk was deputy dean of the medical faculty at the University of Cape Town when Chris Dare, a medical student and friend of Cicely Saunders, sought help to bring her to South Africa (1979). As the hospice movement gathered momentum, he joined the board of St Luke's, but later relinquished the position when he became chair of the national organization—named then the Hospice Association of South Africa (HASA). He speaks of the conceptual and practical challenges that have faced the movement over the years, and how the service has broadened to include patients with HIV/AIDS. As he looks to the future, he itemizes the successes so far: the inclusive nature of the service; raised public awareness; widespread education and training programmes; the production of standards; and a comprehensive strategy for development. The next step is to use the PEPFAR funding to build capacity and roll out the programme of expansion in collaboration with South Africa's provincial governments in order to ensure that all areas of the country receive the benefits of palliative care.

Lesley van Zyl—*general manager; Highway Hospice, Durban*: interviewed by Michael Wright, 8 August 2004. Length of interview (Highway group): 1 h 33 min.

From her background in nursing, Lesley van Zyl undertook further studies that led to diplomas in financial management and personnel. She is currently the general manager of Highway Hospice and tells of the major changes in service provision: the movement away

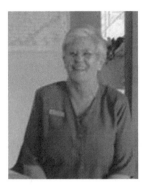

from inpatient provision to community care and the establishment of day centres in Phoenix, Umlazi and Inanda. This movement was accompanied by a painful process of retrenchment which saw the inpatient facility reduced from 16 beds to eight, together with a corresponding reduction in staff. Successful fundraising over the previous 2 years, however, means the hospice is buoyant and optimistic about the future. Among a group of around 400 volunteers, recent initiatives have included the training of 24 community home-based caregivers who support the social workers and cover an area within walking distance of their homes. Plans for the future include the introduction of special family care workers who will support those families without documentation—such as birth certificates and identity forms—and as a result are denied access to government support.

André Wagner—*HPCA board member; organization development officer*: interviewed by Michael Wright, 22 September 2004. Length of interview: 30 min.

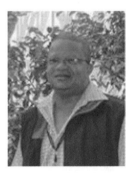

André Wagner became associated with the hospice movement in South Africa after he founded the Helderberg AIDS centre and looked for support for patients coming towards the end of their lives. At that time, he was working in local government and had a background in organizational development related especially to human resources. Before long, Liz Gwyther suggested he became more involved in the palliative care movement and he subsequently became a board member of HPCA, with a full-time commitment from June 2004. André Wagner's priority has been to develop standards in management and governance to stand alongside clinical standards developed in 1998.

Marisa Wolheim—*executive director, Shanti Nilaya, Hospice in the West*: interviewed by Michael Wright, 13 August 2004. Length of interview: 20 min.

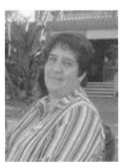

Marisa Wolheim was part of a group that was inspired by the work of Dr Elizabeth Kübler-Ross. It was a high point, therefore, when Kübler-Ross visited the hospice during 1994. The building was donated by the spiritualist church and, initially, this led to some misconceptions about the relationship between the organization and the church. Funding has also been a problem. Yet despite expansion and increased demands, the service remains free of charge. A strength of the hospice has been the in-house training, and Marisa Wolheim speaks of the benefits of the self-awareness course undertaken by new employees and volunteers. Other courses include counselling and caring for the carers, and these have been provided for the Department of Health and a wide range of other groups. The hospice has a strong spiritual tradition, and this is evident in the training of staff and the engagement with patients.

Public health context

Population

South Africa's population of around 44.76 million is served by 11 official languages, including Afrikaans, English, Ndebele, Pedi, Sotho, Swazi, Tsonga, Tswana, Venda, Xhosa and Zulu.

Religious groups include Christian 68 per cent, Muslim 2 per cent, Hindu 1.5 per cent, indigenous beliefs and animist 28.5 per cent.[88]

Epidemiology

In South Africa, the WHO World Health Report (2004) indicates an adult mortality[89] rate per 1000 population of 598 for males and 482 for females. Life expectancy for males is 48.8; for females 52.6. Healthy life expectancy is 43.3 for males; and 45.3 for females.[90]

South Africa has the largest number of individuals affected by AIDS in the world. Estimates suggest that between 4.5 million and 6.2 million people were living with HIV/AIDS at the end of 2003. In the same year, up to 520 000 adults and children are thought to have died from the disease (Table 7.18).

UNAIDS reports:

> South Africa has a population of 44.8 million people and the largest economy in the Southern African Development Community. The national HIV infection rate among pregnant women attending antenatal services in 2003 was 27.9%, with variation among the country's nine provinces from as high as 37.5% in KwaZulu-Natal to as low as 13.1% in the Province of Western Cape. Over the past four consecutive years, the rate of HIV infection among young people below the age of 20 has remained stable.
>
> South Africa has a national strategic framework for 2000–2005. In 2003, the government approved a Comprehensive National Plan on HIV and AIDS Care, Management and Treatment,

Table 7.18 South Africa HIV and AIDS estimates, end 2003

Adult (15–49) HIV prevalence rate	21.5 per cent (range: 18.5–24.9 per cent)
Adults (15–49) living with HIV	5 100 000 (range: 4 300 000–5 900 000)
Adults and children (0–49) living with HIV	5 300 000 (range: 4 500 000–6 200 000)
Women (15–49) living with HIV	2 900 000 (range: 2 500 000–3 300 000)
AIDS deaths (adults and children) in 2003	370 000 (range: 270 000–520 000)

Source: 2004 Report of the global AIDS epidemic.

which aims among other things to provide access to antiretroviral treatment to more than 1.4 million South Africans by 2008.

The degree of commitment to tackle the epidemic in South Africa is high. The South African government fulfils the 2001 Abuja commitment to allocate 15% of government expenditure to health. In 2003, South Africa allocated US$1.7 billion from its national treasury to fight HIV/AIDS over a three-year period.

On the policy front, South Africa has a national strategic framework for 2000–2005. In 2003, the government approved a Comprehensive National Plan on HIV and AIDS Care, Management and Treatment, which aims among other things to provide access to antiretroviral treatment to more than 1.4 million South Africans by 2008.

South Africa has a multisectoral National AIDS Council (NAC) chaired by the deputy president. Civil society and private sector engagement in shaping, influencing and implementing policies and programme interventions is dynamic and robust, facilitated largely by South Africa's open and progressive constitutional democracy.

There is a plethora of international bilateral organizations, foundations and NGOs working in HIV/AIDS. Most of these organizations bring additional resources to the national response against HIV/AIDS. Among the lead HIV/AIDS funding contributors in South Africa are the Global Fund to fight AIDS, Tuberculosis and Malaria and the American Government Emergency Plan for AIDS Relief. Bilateral donors bring additional resources to complement government and civil society efforts.[91]

Health care system

In 2001, the total per capita expenditure on health care[92] in South Africa was Intl $652; 8.6% of GDP (Appendix 3).

The WHO overall health system performance score places South Africa 175th out of 191 countries.[93] This composite measure of overall health system attainment is based on a country's goals relating to health, responsiveness and fairness in financing. The measure varies widely across countries and is highly correlated with general levels of human development as captured in the human development index. In this case, however, there is a disparity between South Africa's low score on the health system achievement scale and higher ranking with regard to the human development index (119th out of 177 countries).

Political economy

South Africa is a middle-income, emerging market with an abundant supply of natural resources; well-developed financial, legal, communications, energy and transport sectors; a stock exchange that ranks among the 10 largest in the world; and a modern infrastructure supporting an efficient distribution of goods to major urban centres throughout the region. However, growth has not been strong enough to lower South Africa's high unemployment rate; and daunting economic problems remain from the apartheid era, especially poverty and lack of economic empowerment among the disadvantaged groups. High crime and HIV/AIDS infection rates also deter investment. South African economic policy is fiscally conservative, but pragmatic, focusing on targeting inflation and liberalizing trade as means to increase job growth and household income.[88]

GDP per capita is Intl $7538 (Appendix 4).

References

1 Report of the United Nations Development Programme 2004 (HDI 2002). Launched by the UN in 1990, the HDI measures a country's achievements in three aspects of human development: longevity, knowledge and a decent standard of living. It was created to re-emphasize that people and their lives should be the ultimate criteria for assessing the development of a country, not economic growth. Current values range from 0.956 (Norway, first out of 177 countries) to 0.273 (Sierra Leone, 177th out of 177 countries). Countries fall into one of three groups: countries 1–55 = high development; 56–141 = medium development; 142–177 = low development. See: http://hdr.undp.org/statistics/data/indic/indic_8_1_1.html

2 During the association's annual general meeting held in Rustenburg in 2004, delegates who attended a parallel session presented by Michael Wright were invited to complete a questionnaire that focused on palliative care service types, education and training, challenges, opportunities and service successes. A self-select sample returned 34 questionnaires and the data therein have helped to inform this report.

3 Palliative Care in South Africa: a survey of delegates at the HPCA annual general meeting, Rustenburg, South Africa, 2004.

4 The Dream Centre opened in 2002. Publicity material describes it as a palliative care centre with a 240-bed inpatient facility that provides institutional home-based care. Collaboration has been established with McCord Hospital, Durban, and the centre operates as a mission in association with Ambassadors of Christ, Canada. Staff and services are stated to include medical doctors, nursing staff, social workers, psychologists, physiotherapists, occupational therapists, HIV counsellors, spiritual counsellors, support group services, income generation projects, and antiretroviral treatment programmes.[86]

By October 2004, however, the facility was little used, with two-thirds of the beds remaining empty. IRIN, part of the United Nations Office for the Coordination of Humanitarian Affairs, reports:

According to the centre's management, the low usage is because the concept of step-down-care, which functions as an intermediary between hospital and home-based care, is relatively new and has not been integrated into provincial hospitals' response to the HIV/AIDS pandemic. Although the centre is funded by the South African Department of Health, there has been 'a lack of proper cooperation' between provincial hospitals and the Dream Centre, said Dr. Henry Sunpath, the medical director.

There are less than a handful of step-down-care institutions in the entire country, added Vincent Chitray, one of the Dream Centre's social workers. Most provinces operate drop-in-centres that provide immediate aid, rather than practical long-term assistance. The Centre integrates palliative care and rehabilitation, which it provides to HIV/AIDS patients until they are ready to return to their homes, and offers terminal care to patients in the last stages of the disease. 'We provide care for those who need care the most and for whom no [customised] care system exists', Sunpath explained. After the Dream Centre opened in July 2002, Sunpath visited all provincial hospitals to introduce the concept of step-down-care to doctors, nurses and other healthcare workers. With beds remaining empty and public hospitals showing little initiative to collaborate, Sunpath and Dream Centre general manager Les Harris have asked the KZN Department of Health to intervene and organise a meeting with the province's hospital managers.[86]

5 IAHPC newsletter, October 2003. See:
   http://www.hospicecare.com/newsletter2003/october2003/page7.html

6 Personal communication: Meg Meyers—23 March 2005.

7 IOELC interview: Barbara Campbell-Ker—11 August 2004.

8 IOELC interview: Mandla Mtatambi—9 August 2004.

9 IOELC interview: Joan de Jong—12 August 2004.

10 IOELC interview: Joan Marston—21 September 2004.

11 Palliative Care in South Africa: a survey of delegates at the HPCA annual general meeting, Rustenburg, South Africa, 2004.

12 IOELC interview: Flora Kobotlo Modiba—13 August 2004.

13 IOELC interview: Elna van der Merwe—13 August 2004.

14 Palliative Care in South Africa: a survey of delegates at the HPCA annual general meeting, Rustenburg, South Africa, 2004.

15 IOELC interview: Edith Khumalo—10 August 2004.

16 IOELC interview: Patient A—7 August 2004.

17 IOELC interview: Patient B—7 August 2004.

18 IOELC interview: Patient C—11 August 2004.

19 IOELC interview: Patient D—11 August 2004.

20 IOELC interview: Patient E—11 August 2004.

21 IOELC interview: Patient F—11 August 2004.

22 IOELC interview: Carer G—11 August 2004.

23 **Harding R, Higginson I.** *Executive Summary. Palliative Care in Sub-Saharan Africa: An Appraisal.* London: The Diana, Princess of Wales Memorial Fund and King's College London, 2004: 4.

24 **Defilippi K.** South Coast Hospice: Integrated Community-based Home Care. *South Coast Hospice information leaflet*, April 2002.

25 Part of the Washington-based Futures Group International, the POLICY Project aims to facilitate the development of policies and plans that promote and sustain access to high-quality family planning and reproductive health (FP/RH) services. The project also addresses HIV/AIDS and maternal health policy issues. See: http://www.policyproject.com/index.cfm

26 Centre for AIDS Development, Research and Evaluation (Cadre) on behalf of the POLICY Project. Integrated Community Home-based Care in South Africa: A review of the model implemented by the Hospice Association of South Africa. National Department of Health Government of South Africa, 2002. Report available in full at: http://www.policyproject.com/pubs/countryreports/SA_Hospice.pdf

27 See: http://www.eldis.org/cf/search/disp/docdisplay.cfm?doc=DOC12596&resource=f1

28 IOELC interview: Lesley van Zyl—8 August 2004.

29 *Engendering Bold Leadership*. The President's Emergency Plan for AIDS Relief. First Annual Report to Congress, 2005: 115. http://www.state.gov/documents/organization/43885.pdf

30 Press Release: R35 Million USAID for Hospice Palliative Care. See: http://216.239.59.104/search?q=cache:dYK7ioo5vPIJ:www.sn.apc.org/usaidsa/press81.html+&hl=en

31 IOELC interview: Brenda Dass—12 August 2004.

32 IOELC interview: André Wagner—30 September 2004.

33 **O'Neill JF, Selwyn PA, Scheitinger H** (eds). *A Clinical Guide to Supportive and Palliative Care for HIV/AIDS.* US Department for Health and Human Services, 2003 edition.

34 Personal communication: Elizabeth Gwyther—24 March 2005.

35 Palliative Care in South Africa: improving the care of patients with HIV/AIDS. Open Society Institute (undated).

36 IOELC interview: Elizabeth Gwyther—4 June 2004.

37 International Narcotics Control Board. *Narcotic Drugs: Estimated World Requirements for 2004. Statistics for 2002.* New York: United Nations, 2004.

38 'The term *defined daily doses for statistical purposes* (S-DDD) replaces the term *defined daily doses* previously used by the Board. The S-DDDs are technical units of measurement for the purposes of statistical analysis and are not recommended prescription doses. Certain narcotic drugs may be used in certain countries for different treatments or in accordance with different medical practices, and therefore a different daily dose could be more appropriate'. The S-DDD used by the INCB for

morphine is 100 mg. International Narcotics Control Board. *Narcotic Drugs: Estimated World Requirements for 2004. Statistics for 2002.* New York: United Nations, 2004: 176–177.

39 IOELC interview: Liz Gwyther—7 August 2004.

40 IOELV interview: Marisa Wolheim—12 August 2004.

41 IOELC interview: Sr Priscilla Dlamini—12 August 2004.

42 IOELC interview: Flora Kobotlo Modiba—13 August 2004.

43 IOELC interview: Thembi Nyuswa—8 August 2004.

44 **Buckland P. Hospice in Southern Africa. In: Saunders C, Kastenbaum R** (eds), *Hospice Care on the International Scene.* New York: Springer Publishing Company, 1997: 48.

45 **Gwyther E.** South Africa: the status of palliative care. *Journal of Pain and Symptom Management* 2002; **24(2)**: 236–238.

46 **Defilippi K.** Palliative care issues in sub-Saharan Africa. *International Journal of Palliative Nursing* 2000; **6(3)**: 108.

47 Foundation for Hospices in Sub-Saharan Africa. *Challenging Times.* Liverpool: NY, USA, 2000.

48 Hospice Palliative Care Association of South Africa. Annual Report. Presented to members at the 17th annual general meeting, Rustenburg, 14 August 2004.

49 IOELC interview: Josef Lazarus—13 August 2004.

50 IOELC interview: Kathleen Defilippi—12 August 2004.

51 **Disorbo P.** Twinning—what have we learned. Presentation at the 15th International Congress on Care of the Terminally Ill, Montreal; 20 September 2004.

52 Hospice Palliative Care Association South Africa. *Annual National Statistics 2003–2004.* HPCA, 2004: 34–36.

53 Elizabeth Scrimgeour is chief executive officer of Drakenstein Hospice (Paarl).

54 Elizabeth Scrimgeour. *Honouring Sacred Spaces: Voicing Stories of Terminal Illness.* Unpublished thesis submitted in part fulfilment of the requirements for the degree of Master of Theology, University of South Africa, 2002: 126.

55 Highway Hospice Association, Durban. See: http://www.hospice.co.za/site/

56 **Zorza R, Zorza V.** *A Way to Die.* London: André Deutsch, 1980.

57 IOELC interview: Karen Hinton—28 June 2002.

58 IOELC interview: Stella Thackray—9 Aug 2004.

59 Hospice Association of the Witwatersrand. See: http://196.35.64.114/

60 Since her marriage, Margaret Lebish has been known as Margaret McGettrick.

61 Sylvia Poss is the author of *Towards Death with Dignity: Caring for Dying People*, published by Allen and Unwin, 1981.

62 See the forward written by David Clark in: Saunders C. *Watch with Me: Inspiration for a Life in Hospice Care.* Sheffield: Mortal Press, 2003: vii.

63 TOC H is a Christian organization formed by 'Tubby' Clayton who was an army chaplain during the First World War. The stated aim of the organization is to 'build a fairer society by working with communities to promote friendship and service, confront prejudice and practise reconciliation'. See: http://www.toch.org.uk/

64 A history of the Hospice of Marin states: 'Hospice of Marin has a rich legacy of being the second hospice established in the United States [after Connecticut] and the first hospice on the West Coast. It was established by Dr. William Lamers Jr, Reverend John Thornton, and Barbara Hill Gonce in the early 1970s and with a growing staff of professionals and expanding community support, officially incorporated in March of 1975'. Hospice of Marin has grown from an all-volunteer organization to its present staff of more than 150 employees committed to providing the full range of hospice services in Marin, Sonoma, and San Francisco counties. See: http://www.volunteersolutions.org/marin/org/1333734.html

65 Personal communication: Margaret McGettrick—25 March 2005.

66 Report by Margaret Lebish to the TLC Group on Recent Activities: 9 March 1979.

67 IOELC interview: Arend Hoogervorst—19 May 2005.

68 The Junior Chamber International is a worldwide federation of young professionals and entrepre-
neurs between the ages of 19 and 40. The mission statement of JCI is 'To contribute to the
advancement of the global community by providing the opportunity for young people to develop
the leadership skills, social responsibility, fellowship, and entrepreneurship necessary to create positive change'. See: http://www.jci.cc/members/info.php?lang_id=1&info_id=1000&sidebar_id=1000

69 The Hospice Association of the Witwatersrand. In: *The Hospice Movement in South Africa: A Brief
History*. 2002: 61.

70 IOELC interview: Sibongile Mafata—10 August 2004.

71 IOELC interview: Lesley Lawson—26 April 2005.

72 Lewis P. *Background Details of St Francis Hospice Palliative Care Services in East Cape Townships for
Terminally Ill Cancer and AIDS Patients*. 2002.

73 St Luke's Hospice, Cape Town. See: http://www.stlukes.co.za/

74 St Luke's Hospice. A brief history of St Luke's Hospice. In: St Luke's Hospice Information Booklet
(undated).

75 IOELC interview: Richard Scheffer—24 March 2005.

76 van Niekerk JP. Recollections. In: *The Hospice Movement in South Africa: A Brief History*. 2002: 1.

77 IOELC interview: Meg Meyers—7 August 2004.

78 Palliative Care in South Africa: a survey of delegates at the HPCA annual general meeting,
Rustenburg, South Africa, 2004.

79 IOELC interview: G. K. Moodly—12 August 2004.

80 IOELC interview: Jackie Schoeman—11 August 2004.

81 IOELC interview: Zodwe Sithole—12 August 2004.

82 IOELC interview: Marie Backeberg—13 August 2004.

83 IOELC interview: J. P. van Niekerk—12 August 2004.

84 Palliative Care in South Africa: a survey of delegates at the HPCA annual general meeting,
Rustenburg, South Africa, 2004.

85 IOELC interview: Alan Barnard—12 August 2004.

86 IOELC interview: C. N. Pillay—12 August 2004.

87 British History Online states: 'St. Luke's hospital for advanced cases was opened in Osnaburgh
Street, St. Pancras, in 1893 as a branch of the West London Mission. It moved to Hampstead in 1901,
to Pembridge Square, North Kensington, in 1903, and to a new building with 48 beds in Hereford
Road in 1923. Affiliated to St. Mary's in 1948, it had 42 beds for pre-convalescence and terminal care
in 1981'.

British History Online. Source: Paddington: Public Services. A History of the County of Middlesex:
Volume IX, T.F.T. Baker (Editor) (1989). URL: http://64.233.183.104/search?q=cache:
gea5aSyV-esJ:www.british-history.ac.uk/report.asp%3Fcompid%3D22673+St+Luke%27s+hospi-
tal+for+advanced+cases,+Bayswater&hl=en

88 See: http://www.cia.gov/cia/publications/factbook/geos/sf.html

89 This refers to adult mortality risk, which is defined as the probability of dying between 15 and 59
years.

90 See: WHO statistics at: http://www.who.int/countries/zaf/en/

91 http://www.unaids.org/en/geographical+area/by+country/south+africa.asp

92 Total health expenditure per capita is the per capita amount of the sum of Public Health
Expenditure (PHE) and Private Expenditure on Health (PvtHE). The international dollar is a

common currency unit that takes into account differences in the relative purchasing power of various currencies. Figures expressed in international dollars are calculated using purchasing power parities (PPP), which are rates of currency conversion constructed to account for differences in price level between countries.http://www3.who.int/whosis/country/compare.cfm?country=s&indicator=strPcTotEOHinIntD2000&language=english

93 Tandon A, Murray CLJ, Lauer JA, Evans DB. *Measuring Overall Health System Performance for 191 Countries*. GPE Discussion Paper Series: No 30; WHO.

Chapter 8

Uganda

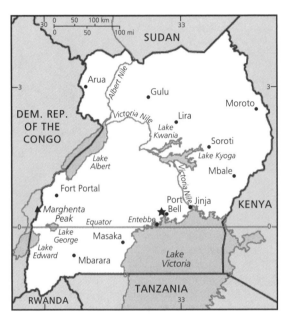

Uganda (population 25 million) is a landlocked country in Eastern Africa that covers an area of 236 040 km². Its boundaries border Democratic Republic of the Congo, Kenya, Rwanda, Sudan and Tanzania. The capital Kampala (population 1.28 million) is situated near Lake Victoria.

The country became independent of Britain in 1962 and has been governed by President Yoweri Museveni since 1986. Conflicts over the past 15 years have disrupted the lives of many Ugandans, particularly in the north.

According to the United Nations human development index (HDI),[1] Uganda is ranked 146th out of 177 countries worldwide (value 0.493) and 18th out of 45 African countries for which a value is available. This places Uganda in the low human development group.

Palliative care service provision

Current services

In Uganda, eight palliative care organizations deliver some 155 services (Table 8.1).

Hospice Africa Uganda (HAU)

HAU was founded in 1993 to care for cancer and HIV/AIDS patients and give support to family members.[2] In the past, most referrals came from hospitals; now, an increasing number originate from community vigilantes (trained carers who identify patients in the community in need of the hospice's services). Hospice Africa Uganda also incorporates *Mobile Hospice Mbarara* and *Little Hospice Hoima*, both established in 1998[3] (Table 8.2).

Kitovu Mobile Home Care

This NGO was founded by the Medical Missionaries of Mary in 1987 as a response to the AIDS pandemic. Patients frequently self-refer by presenting themselves at one of the

Table 8.1 Palliative care provision in Uganda, 2004

	Inpatient unit	Paediatric inpatient unit	Hospital unit	Hospital support service	Home care	Day care	Paediatric day care	Paediatric clinic	Clinic/drop-in center	Mobile clinic	Total
Association François-Xavier Bagnoud					1						1
Hospice Africa Uganda				2	1	1			1		5
Mobile Hospice Mbarara				2	1	1				2	6
Little Hospice Hoima				2	1	1				2	6
Mildmay International		1		1			1	1	1		5
Joy Hospice, Mbale	1			1	1				1		4
Kitovu Mobile Home Care					1					124	125
PC Unit: Lira Regional Referral Hospital			1	1	1						3
Total	1	1	1	9	7	3	1	1	3	128	155

Table 8.2 Patients cared for by Hospice Africa Uganda 1993–2004

	Date of inception	Total patients since inception	Patients in programme March 2004
Hospice Africa Uganda	September 1993	4218	285
Mobile Hospice Mbarara	January 1998	1176	179
Little Hospice Hoima	June 1998	450	151
Grand total		5484	615

Table 8.3 Activity report: Kitovu Home Care and Mildmay International (Uganda)

	Date of inception	Total patients registered	Total active patients
Kitovu Home Care*	August 1987	12 000	3600
Mildmay International[†]	September 1998	7545	5000

* Figures published September 2003.

† Figures at March 2004[5].

centres. Other referrals come from family members, parish priests, community volunteers, local hospitals, TASO (in Masaka) or Hospice Africa Uganda after patients return home (Table 8.3). Palliative care has been grafted onto their support service since 2000.

The Mildmay Centre

The centre opened in Kampala in September 1998, having previously received an invitation from the Uganda AIDS Commission to establish an AIDS care and training centre on land donated by the government (Table 8.3).[4]

Joy Hospice

Joy Hospice opened in Mbale in 2001 to care for AIDS and cancer patients; provision includes a five-bed inpatient unit, home care service and clinic.[6]

The Palliative Care Unit; Lira Regional Referral Hospital

This service consists of a one-bed facility supplemented by a hospital support service and home care service.[7]

Association François-Xavier Bagnoud (AFXB)[8]

AFXB began a home care service in Luwero in January 2003.[9]

The palliative care gains made in Uganda have been recognized by WHO:

In the last ten years, thanks to NGO initiatives, progressive government involvement and the support of the WHO country office, Uganda has been able to include palliative care in the government health agenda which has resulted in the allocation of resources, improved morphine availability, and the provision of training at all levels of care and to undergraduate and post graduate health professionals. It has integrated palliative care into the existing health system at a district level and is planning to extend the programme to other districts and eventually to the rest of the country.[10]

WHO also recognized the valuable contribution of research undertaken in Uganda by Ekiria Kikule:

> A needs assessment study recently undertaken in Uganda (Kikule, 2000), showed that the distribution of terminally ill patients was 73% HIV/AIDS, 22% cancer, 3% both and 2% other diseases. The majority of patients preferred to be cared for at home and, in fact, 87% of the caregivers were family members who were very supportive. Among the various needs shared by patients and their caregivers, the major ones were food and welfare. Poverty and sickness combined to put families in a critical situation. Patients experienced pain and other symptoms quite often and 65% declared them a problem. The main fears expressed by the patients were fear of death and abandonment. The study concluded that the home is the best place to care for the terminally ill.[11]

Reimbursement and funding for services

Hospice Africa Uganda received a pledge of 50 million shillings from the Ministry of Health for the financial year (FY) 2003–2004;[12] this was supplemented by income raised from donors and fundraising activities such as sponsored walks, luncheons and a flea market. Donors have included: Hospice Africa (UK), the British High Commission, the Government of Ireland, the States of Jersey, Singapore and Canada, CORDAID (The Netherlands), CAFOD (England), SCIAF (Scotland) and the Nuffield Foundation, the Diana Princess of Wales Memorial Fund (Diana Fund) and the RAF (UK). Rotarians worldwide have contributed; DANIDA and USAID are committed during 2004. APSO, VMM (Ireland) and VSO have supported expert volunteers, and the diploma course was supported by the UK Forum for Hospice and Palliative Care Worldwide. In the UK, funds are raised from two charity shops and private individual donors. In future, the hospice aims to raise 10 per cent of its running costs in Uganda.[13]

Mobile Hospice Mbarara[14] has been supported by CAFOD, the 3H International Rotary Grant from the USA (with assistance from Hospice Africa, Rotary Clubs of Coventry and Manchester) the Andrew Mitchell Christian Charitable Trust and the Diana, Princess of Wales Memorial Fund. Little Hospice Hoima has received support from GOAL, Ireland and friends, Elizabeth Taylor Foundation (USA), Global Cancer Concern (UK) and the Andrew Mitchell Christian Charitable Trust (UK). The Rotary Club of Hamilton, Victoria (Australia) has provided a car for home care.

Patients are asked to pay 5000 Ugandan shillings per week (towards the total weekly cost of 25 000/=) for care. Sixty per cent of patients have this contribution waived because of their poverty.

President's Emergency Plan for AIDS Relief (PEPFAR)

During the 2004 FY, funding of around US$80.58 million was enacted for country-managed programmes in Uganda and US$10.18 million for central programmes. During FY2005, it is anticipated that a total of US$124.34 million will be enacted: US$112.82 million for country-managed programmes and US$11.52 million for central programmes.[15]

The Diana, Princess of Wales Memorial Fund

The Diana Fund has both supported in-country developments and, at the same time, commissioned Hospice Africa Uganda to advocate for palliative care in Central and East Africa.

In Uganda, grants have been awarded:

- To continue the work of Mbarara Mobile Hospice: salaries, vehicle running costs, office overheads and evaluation: 2-year grant, £60 000 (Hospice Africa Mbarara)
- To consolidate the HBC programme in three districts: staff salaries, transport costs, drugs and training: 3-year grant, £81 995 (Medical Missionaries of Mary, CAFOD[16])
- For capacity building in end-of-life/palliative care for the HBC programme in Kampala; training, welfare fund, transport, drugs: 3-year grant, £14 200 [Nsambya Home Care Services (St Francis)]
- For palliative care nurse specialist training: £14 168 (Hospice Uganda).

In Central and East Africa, Hospice Africa Uganda became the Diana Fund's partner agency in a 3-year project which attracted funding of £300 000. During this period, Hospice Africa Uganda would:

- Provide technical support and advice on the identification of countries with the capacity and political will to initiate palliative care services
- Provide guidance and training to such countries
- Set up and run a distance learning Diploma in Palliative Care for African countries
- Set up a resource centre of palliative care materials for Africa, at Makindye, Kampala
- Improve services within Uganda so that a model can be developed that works for the poorest and that can be duplicated in other African countries.

Anne Merriman comments:

> In 2001, the Diana, Princess of Wales, Memorial Fund in London, invited Hospice Africa Uganda to be their technical experts in assisting other African countries to start or strengthen palliative care services using the public health approach and integrating with existing health systems. Working with World Health Organisation, this initiative has brought the Hospice training programmes to several other African countries.[17]

Opioid availability and consumption

Data from the International Narcotics Control Board[18] show the following figures for narcotic consumption in Uganda, 2002: codeine 27 kg (down from 83 kg, 1998); morphine 9 kg (up from 2 kg, 1993); pethidine 8 kg (as in 1998, but down from 22 kg in 2001).

For the years 2000–2002, the average defined daily dose consumption of morphine for statistical purposes (S-DDD)[19] in Uganda was 4. This compares with other African countries as follows: Swaziland 1; Egypt 2; Zimbabwe 13; Botswana 53; Namibia 73; and

South Africa 103. Twenty-nine countries reported no morphine consumption during 2000–2002 (Appendix 1).

Morphine for cancer and HIV/AIDS patients is provided free of charge by the government. In March 2004, a Statutory Instrument[20] was signed by the Minister of Health authorizing palliative care nurses and clinical officers to prescribe morphine as part of their clinical practice: a ground-breaking innovation.

Morphine is supplied by HAU in tablet and liquid forms. The slow-release morphine tablets (MST)—donated by NAPP (UK)—are in 10 and 30 mg strengths. Liquid (oral) morphine is the most frequent form of pain control and is prepared in 1, 10 and 20 mg/ml strengths. Pharmacist Peter Mikajjo comments:

> We prepare [liquid morphine] in a very simple way whereby it cannot take a lot of time and cannot be costly. Morphine is prepared out of morphine powder: there are actually two types—either morphine sulphate or morphine hydrochloride—but basically we are using morphine sulphate and we prepare enough that can be used in a week.[21]

HAU founder Anne Merriman is clear about the role played by morphine in palliative care:

> I think support care can be put in if you don't have morphine but I don't think palliative care is there . . . When I met Dame Cicely a few years back, I said to her 'You know something: there was support care in Uganda before I went, and there were really caring people doing it'. And she said 'that's why I started the modern hospice movement. The support care was there—people were dying with people caring for them—but they weren't controlling pain; that's why I started it, and that's the difference I made'. So my definition now is: support care without pain control is support care; pain control without support care is anaesthesiology . . . to have palliative care you have to have pain control *plus* support care.[22]

A key contributor to the debate surrounding morphine has been Jack Jagwe, who describes his role as follows:

> My role in Hospice Africa Uganda is that of the senior advisor on policy, drugs and advocacy. Policy concerns how palliative care relates to Government health policies so that we don't have any conflict. The second one is about drugs, how to access palliative care drugs and most specifically the availability of morphine to patients in palliative care. And the third one is advocacy—to try and convince Government and top health policy makers about the value of having palliative care for so many patients in our country who are dying from HIV/AIDS and cancer.
>
> First of all: I'm a physician by training, and I've been in the Government services for 30 years 'til my retirement—and I got interested when Dr Anne Merriman came to Uganda in 1993. By then I was the Deputy Director of Medical Services in charge of clinical services and also in charge of essential grants in the country. That's when she came and mentioned that we should have drugs like morphine available for these people. And after that, when I retired officially from the Government, I became Chairman of the National Drug Regulatory Body in Uganda. Since then I've been interested in palliative care and in 1998 when she organized a national workshop I was appointed Chairman of a task force which worked out a national policy on palliative care. That draft was thoroughly discussed and eventually submitted to the Ministry of Health, and it was incorporated into the Health Strategic Plan of 2001–2005.[23]

If morphine is required by patients in the Kitovu Mobile Home Care programme, a referral is made to the programme doctor. Once the doctor prescribes the morphine, the patient or a family member can collect the medicine from nurses at a nearby centre.

National and professional organizations

Palliative Care Association of Uganda (PCAU)

This national association was founded in 1998. It is chaired by Dr Lydia Mpanga; Julia Downing is co-editor of the PCAU journal with Anne Merriman, and the organization has >180 members. Aims include:

- Introducing and maintaining standards
- Bringing together key players and stake-holders
- Establishing a journal
- Quarterly CME update
- Publications
- Advocacy
- Co-ordination of education and CME throughout the 56 districts of Uganda.

Palliative care coverage

Hospice Africa Uganda provides a palliative care service to patients and their families within a 20 km radius of the hospice, and promotes this care throughout Uganda and in other African countries.

Mbarara Mobile Hospice covers a radius of 20 km encompassing the area of Mbarara and beyond. It also has outreach services and roadside clinics.

Joy Hospice provides a travel-to service that covers 15 districts of Uganda (population 100 000).

Mildmay is an internationally recognized referral centre that has accepted patients countrywide from Uganda and also from Kenya, Rwanda, Democratic Republic of Congo and Eritrea.

The Palliative Care Unit; Lira Regional Referral Hospital provides a hospital referral service; a home care service operates within a bicycle ride of the hospital.

Kitovu Mobile Home Care covers the 26 subcounties of Masaka, Rakai and Ssembabule districts.

Association François-Xavier Bagnoud covers three subcounties of Luweero: Semuto, Makulubita and Kasangombe.

Education and training

Hospice Africa Uganda

A total of 1121 health professionals and 553 non-health professionals have attended HAU palliative care courses since 1994 (Table 8.4).

Table 8.4 Training courses: Hospice Africa Uganda, Mbara, Hoima 1994–2004

Venue	Organization	Target group	Courses (n)	Hours per course (n)	Participants (n)
Kampala	HAU	Health professionals	22	45–56	672
Kampala	HAU	Volunteers	12	24–40	311
Kampala	HAU	Professionals: non-health	1		42
Kampala	HAU	Health professionals: train the trainers	8		97
Districts	HAU	Health professionals		42	519
Districts	HAU	Professionals: non-health			203
Districts	Mbara	Health professionals	12	48	344
Districts	Mbara	Professionals: non-health	5	24	122
Districts	Mbara	Volunteers	1	24	16
Districts	Hoima	Health professionals	3		88
Districts	Hoima	Professionals: non-health	11*		294

* Of the 11 courses organized by Little Hospice Hoima, five were for district community volunteers, one for Hospice community volunteers and five for different NGOs in Hoima district.

Sources: Hospice Africa Uganda, and Clare Fitzgibbon (for Mbara and Hoima).

In addition, in-service training is given to the HAU team and to health professionals who support the work of the hospice. Certificates of Practice are given to clinicians who follow up the courses, present case studies and pass an oral examination.

Hospice Africa Uganda provides teaching sessions for undergraduate and post-graduate doctors at Makerere University (from 1993) and Mbarara University of Science and Technology (MUST) Medical School (since 1998)—along with courses for pharmacy and nursing students.

The hospice has also been sharing expertise with HIV/AIDS organizations to ensure that palliative care is grafted onto community-based home care services.[24,25] Anne Merriman:

> Every village and every family in Uganda has experienced the death of a loved one from AIDS. Many of these patients have died at home. Many have also had cancer. The AIDS home care teams are under a lot of strain trying to spread themselves to cater for the increase in those dying at home. These teams are excellent at counselling and basic medications; however, for those patients with extreme pain and symptoms, the lack of knowledge of the methods of control, and the use of medications, have prevented pain and symptom control. Hospice has introduced palliative care and the modern methods of pain and symptom control which are working in the home. The training of personnel in this specialty is a major part of the work of Hospice Uganda.[26]

All three hospice organizations are working with the Ministry of Health to provide training programmes for 56 districts about to receive oral morphine through an initiative that has already introduced oral morphine to 15 districts during the first phase.

In 2002, HAU established a distance learning Diploma in Palliative Care in conjunction with Makerere University. Twenty participants enrolled on the first course (including

Table 8.5 Students enrolled on the distance learning Diploma course from outside Uganda, 2002–2003

Country	Doctors (n)	Nurses (n)	Clinical officers (n)	Total
Cameroon		1		1
Malawi	1			1
Tanzania	1	1	2	4
Zambia			1	1
Zimbabwe		2		2
Total	2	4	3	9

nine from outside of Uganda, Table 8.5). Facilities include the resource centre and 14-room residential centre (Kateregga House) at Makindye. A second course with 18 participants began in 2003.

Course director Michelle McGannon comments:

The diploma is training people to provide holistic care within the palliative care setting, and it's so important to look at *all* the elements that are involved in that. Also, it's an African diploma for an African audience; I think that's the most important thing that I could say about it—it's trying to give people, not just the clinical skills, but the skills to be able to pass on that knowledge. We have modules on management, organization and palliative care, so they can have information on what is most appropriate for their particular setting or country; and management styles—to give all-round tuition and help them to develop a service.[27]

A course participant, Ndikintum George Mbeng (from Cameroon) comments:

The distance learning course is a very good way of teaching palliative care to health professionals in Africa, and it equips the students with the knowledge to train other health professionals. The compulsory residential weeks are very helpful because you have to come on site, see the practices and whatever.[28]

Training courses have also been delivered by HAU in other African countries, including: Ethiopia, Tanzania, Malawi, Nigeria, Kenya and Zambia.

To support the development of education and training, a resource centre has been established with support from the Diana Fund. Centre manager Ronnah Abinaitwe spent a month at St Christopher's Hospice, London, in preparation for her innovative role;[29] she here describes the library resources:

We have many books on pain and symptom control; I've classified them separately according to the different subjects. We have a few publications from the Ministry of Health, Uganda, because some of them apply to us; some publications from the WHO; and other publications from the UNDP—this will help especially the researchers to know what they want. Then I have shut cupboards with journals. Most of the journals are palliative care journals—only some of them don't come very regularly because we don't always have the money to subscribe to them; but then we have the *British Medical Journal* and the *Lancet*, which come free for us. So we always get at least a copy every week of the two journals; we have quite a collection. Near the main entrance we have the information material that hospice publishes. We have the famous blue book by Dr Merriman and we have a few other manuals—trainers' manuals that we usually give to the people that come for training.[30]

Training has recently come into sharper focus as a result of a research project undertaken by Ekiria Kikule which sought to identify the palliative care needs of terminally ill patients in Uganda. Among a sample of 173 participants registered in palliative home care programmes, three needs were identified: the control or relief of pain and other symptoms; counselling; and financial assistance for basic needs such as food, shelter and children's school fees. Significantly, the home was the preferred setting for care, although all participants had access to health care services within 5 km of their homes.[31]

The Mildmay Centre

The Mildmay International Study Centre (MISC) aims to develop initiatives that will introduce the knowledge and skills needed to provide comprehensive, holistic rehabilitation and palliative care for people living with HIV/AIDS. Training programmes are provided for government bodies, NGOs, faith-based organizations and companies in Uganda and the surrounding region. Programmes include:

- ◆ One-day HIV/AIDS awareness seminars
- ◆ One-and two-week residential courses
- ◆ Modular courses of up to 18 months duration, such as

    a Diploma in HIV/AIDS Care and Management in association with Manchester University, UK

    a 1-year course delivered upcountry by two mobile training teams

- ◆ Placement schemes.

Julia Downing (MISC director), speaking in June 2004, comments:

> We have had over 3000 people on our short courses over the last three years, from about 45 of the districts in Uganda and from 22 countries—mainly Uganda, but we have regional programmes as well for people from within Africa. And then at our centre in Kampala we have a specialist outpatient referral centre/clinic, and so we have clinical placements as well, and we have people from all over coming on the clinical placements and the training programmes. On the year-long programme in the districts, we've had—and I counted that just a few days ago—about 220 people on that course. And the Diploma courses, obviously the numbers get smaller as the course gets more demanding, but from the Diploma course, we've just graduated 23 people on Friday, and we have a further 24 undertaking it.[32]

Edith Akankwasa, manager of the innovative mobile training team (MTT) writes:

> The aim of the MTTs is to build capacity amongst health workers to deal effectively with the care needs of patients living with HIV and AIDS (PLWHAs) in the rural communities. Each multidisciplinary training team consists of a doctor or clinical officer, a nurse, a counsellor and a driver. The teams take trainees through a year's modular training programme addressing issues such as clinical care, communication skills, teaching skills, Proposal writing and management skills.[33]

Association François-Xavier Bagnoud (AFXB)

AFXB provides training for its staff and in Uganda this has been in association with the Mildmay Centre.[34]

PROMETRA Uganda

PROMETRA Uganda is an NGO which promotes traditional medicine and the role it plays alongside Western models. President/director Yahaya Hills Sekagya writes:

> PROMETRA Uganda initiated a program for training and empowering traditional healers in the care and management of patients with cancer, HIV/AIDS and other diseases using traditional methods. The training covers areas of basic anatomy, herbal identification, preparation, administration, diagnosis, danger signs and referrals. Traditional medicine and healers are an alternative resource in rural and poor communities as they are available, accessible, affordable, and in every village
>
> Traditional healers have actively participated in hospice trainings, willingly share information with each other regarding medicinal plants for opportunistic infections, [and have] developed unique yet appropriate methods of communally looking after the sick. They have committed themselves to working as a team and are a strong resource for local communities.[35]

Palliative care workforce capacity

Hospice Africa Uganda: the staff list for 2003–2004 details 107 staff. This includes 18 staff in the *Mobile Hospice Mbarara* team and seven staff at *Little Hospice Hoima*. In March 2003, 88 of these were permanently employed members of staff.[36]

Joy Hospice: one medical director; one clerical officer; four enrolled nurses; one trainee nurse.

Palliative Care Unit, Lira Regional Referral Hospital: staffed by two nurses.

The Mildmay Centre: in November 2003, 127 people were employed (123 Ugandans).[37]

History and development of hospice–palliative care in Uganda

Hospice Uganda

HUA is the model hospice for *Hospice Africa*—an NGO founded in 1993 to promote hospice developments in the countries of Africa which lack palliative medicine. Objectives are:

- To provide a palliative care service to patients and families within a 20 km radius of the Makindye premises and to promote this care throughout Uganda
- To carry out education programmes in palliative medicine to health professionals at undergraduate and post-graduate levels
- To encourage the initiation/consolidation of palliative care in other African countries by providing a training facility at Hospice Uganda.

HAU opened on 23 September 1993 based in a two-bedroom house loaned by Nsambya Hospital. At this time, funds were only available for the following 3 months, although a 10-year-old Land Rover had been donated by the British High Commission. Hospice headquarters subsequently moved to alternative accommodation, donated free of charge by Henry Mary Kateregga, before securing the current premises at Makindye with the help of the organization Ireland AID[38] in 1994.

The key person behind HAU was Anne Merriman, a doctor from Liverpool who had previously worked in Singapore and Kenya. She recalls how she came to work in Uganda:

> Dame Cicely had written to me [in 1991] and in October she had edited a book; have you ever seen that journal *Contact*—published by the Christian Council of Churches, Geneva? Well they had a volume dedicated to palliative care and she asked me to write an article about what we were doing in Nairobi, which I did; and it went out free to most of the developing countries, and I started to get letters from different parts of Africa begging me to do what we were doing in Nairobi in their countries, and I realized there was this big need.
>
> So what I wanted to do was to set up a hospice that would be a model from which other countries could say, 'Look it works in our situation'—because Africans went to Europe, they went to America, and they came back saying, 'Oh it's not affordable: it's wonderful but we'll never be able to afford that'. So what I wanted to do was set up a model that was affordable and to show them that it could work in the African situation. So I went home and I worked at home for a year. During that time, we approached people about writing a constitution and my friends came together to form the Board of Hospice Africa, and that was registered in August 1993 as a charity. Meanwhile, in January '93, we started doing a feasibility study. We visited Zimbabwe then we went to Nigeria and we did Uganda; and we really felt Uganda was the best place. And the reason was: one, that the Government was trusted and we would be able to get funding from outside. Secondly, they had a huge AIDS epidemic. You could see the people suffering even driving along the road, it was so big at that stage; it's gone right down now but it was very big then. And also the Ministry of Health were fully behind us and promised to get in the morphine: I said I wouldn't come in without morphine and they promised to get it in, and they did. It was a big struggle, but we got it.
>
> I made a lot of enemies trying to get morphine in because, although the Minister was behind me, people like the pharmacists were very against what I was doing. Also, we had a lot of trouble getting the Ministry of Health on board. In fact we didn't get it on board 'til five years later, in '98, when we held the big conference for the stakeholders in palliative care and we got the finance from SCIAF—the Scottish Catholic International Aid Fund.
>
> I think we had two days discussing things and Jan Stjernswärd came as the motivator. We ended up employing Dr Jagwe as an advocate: he's five sessions a week. And the people from the Ministry formed a group that would look at the needs of palliative care and see what they were going to do. As a result, palliative medicine was put into the five-year strategic plan in the year 2000. We were the first country in Africa to do that—and it wasn't only written into it, it's been taken up seriously and they have moved forward on it. So the five years since '98 has been much better working with the Ministry of Health.[39]

In January 1998, the service was extended with the founding of *Mobile Hospice Mbarara*. An outreach clinic was established and supplemented by the inception of roadside clinics for those outside of the 20 km catchment area.

Clare Fitzgibbon, a Macmillan nurse consultant, was heavily involved in the establishment of Mobile Hospice Mbarara. Having taken early retirement, VSO placed her in Mbarara (together with her husband) where she had previously worked in a country hospital during the 1970s.

> We went out in October 98. Locked up our house, left our keys with the neighbour, squared it with our three children, and went out to Mbarara.

I made it very clear that I wouldn't lead; it was important that Ugandans led. So I'd work along side them as a nurse consultant, working with the clinical team (which was then two nurses) charged with establishing palliative care in the curriculum at Mbarara University of Science and Technology.

Within the first three months we'd prioritized that we needed a doctor and we needed another nurse before we could possibly extend beyond Mbarara. We sat down together and prioritized what we could do with what we had and what we might plan to do. Bereavement training: although there was a huge awareness, one of the problems in even doing a primary visit was, where have the people gone? Out into the distant villages—back home. So that in itself was a difficulty. But we agreed to set at least one visit as a standard.

One of my roles was to assess the need in the district. By looking at referrals and new patients that weren't able to return, we realized it was because of the distance and lack of money; and we know what a difference one has made, being able to establish those mobile clinics back in 1999.

In June 1998, a third service was founded—*Little Hospice Hoima*—to demonstrate how a simple service could be introduced using existing health facilities and personnel. As a result, an affordable service reached out to the villages, supported by community volunteers who helped to identify those in need.[40]

The Mildmay Centre

Mildmay International is a UK-based Christian organization which was established during the nineteenth century for the relief of suffering. In 1988, Mildmay opened the first palliative care service in Europe for people living with HIV/AIDS at the Mildmay Mission Hospital, London. After a study tour to Africa in 1991, Mildmay developed training programmes in East Africa, funded by the British Council. This in turn led to an invitation from the Uganda AIDS Commission to set up a care and training programme in Uganda. The Centre opened in 1998 and Mildmay has an agreement with the Ministry of Health to manage the Centre and its activities until 2008. Julia Downing:

> The Mildmay Centre was developed in order to provide and demonstrate good-quality holistic, comprehensive, outpatient care for patients with HIV/AIDS-related health problems, and to teach and train health workers throughout Uganda and the region in such care.[41]

Joy Hospice

Following work as a GP in Oxfordshire, Janet White arrived in Uganda in 1988 in response to what she considered to be a call from God. She worked in Kenya between 1994 and 1998, whereupon she was invited by the Deliverance Church to return to Uganda and establish a medical service in Mbale. The following year, a second clinic was established in Buwasunguyi. By this time, the majority of patients were presenting with advanced cancers and end-stage AIDS. As a result, Janet White began to nurse patients in her home in Mbale. Recognizing the gap in provision, she subsequently obtained and renovated a house to create a 5-bed inpatient unit and home care service that opened on 31 August 2001. Janet White:

> Patients are mainly seen as outpatients, sometimes with a brief admission for symptom control. Occasionally, a patient and family choose to remain at hospice until death occurs. As the service

expands, more home visits will take place. Two factors have delayed the home visiting programme: patients are scattered over seven districts and many live over 50 km from hospice, and the hospice vehicle was involved in an accident in November 2002 and has been written off.[42]

Kitovu Mobile Home Care

Sister Ursula of the Medical Missionaries of Mary founded Kitovu Mobile Home Care in response to a growing awareness of the AIDS epidemic. As the disease became increasingly apparent, myths and fears developed around the infection. Many of those initially affected were considered to be suffering punishments for past thefts, and suffered stigmatization and marginalization. Some sold their homes and possessions to make restitution, falling into extreme poverty, children dropped out of school, and patients were abandoned at the hospital doors. Nurse Rose Nabatanzi comments:

> The patients realized there was a need for them to be cared for and they created centres where they could come together and wait for the nurses to come.[43]

In this scenario, Sr Ursula initially cared for infected people with a small team of nurses, gradually increasing the provision to include community volunteers, local co-ordinators and psycho-social support. Food, soap and sugar were provided alongside medicines and, with the introduction of morphine in 2000, the home care developed into a palliative care service. Today, each centre is visited every 2 weeks. Each team carries a supply of medicines and patients are treated for diseases such as malaria and opportunistic infections associated with HIV/AIDS.

Kitovu palliative care physician and medical consultant Mary Simmons explains the impact morphine has made on both patients and health workers:

> Pain and symptom relief not only benefits the patients, but the family and even our staff. The suffering of caregivers is intensified when they see their patient suffering. Their relief is obvious when the patient no longer suffers. As for our staff, they repeatedly tell me how grateful they are for palliative care. Before we had morphine, they felt helpless in the face of the suffering of their patients. Now they know something can be done.[44]

Significantly, greater attention is being paid to the complexities in offering palliative care for people with HIV infections. Kathleen Defilippi and colleagues:

> A major aim is to assist those suffering at home, in situations where, as in Uganda and elsewhere in mid-Africa, up to 57 per cent of the population will never have access to a health worker. In this context, anti-retroviral (ARV) treatments *and* palliative care must be delivered hand in hand, thereby extending quality of life to the poorest people. This requires thinking about palliative care within a preventative and public health model in which care can be delivered across the complete trajectory of the disease and in which well-constructed home-based palliative care services can serve as an important platform for education, primary disease prevention and also the support of patients receiving active treatment.[45]

Association François-Xavier Bagnoud (AFXB)

AFXB is an international organization that sponsors research, programmes and field work in areas such as palliative care, care for AIDS orphans in Africa, humanitarian rights and paediatric HIV/AIDS care. The association is named after François-Xavier Bagnoud, a young helicopter pilot committed to rescuing people, who died at the age of 24 during a mission in Mali, West Africa. In 1989, his mother, the Countess Albina du Boisrouvray, joined by her son's family and friends, established and financed the activities of the Association François-Xavier Bagnoud to perpetuate the compassion and generosity that guided François' life.[46]

AFXB began its operations in Uganda (1990) with the goal of assisting the people of Luwero to develop community-based capability to meet the needs of orphans in their care. With support from Mildmay International and the Ministry of Health, the palliative care service began in January 2003. Medical director Robert Kalyesubula and his colleagues state:

> [Palliative] care is given alongside other supportive programs of income generation activities and provision of education to orphans and vulnerable children. Since the palliative care program started 30 PLWAs have benefited from oral morphine and adjuvant drugs for alleviation of pain . . . The medical team visits these patients every two weeks and they can also attend to emergencies following calls from the community volunteers. Providing palliative care has alleviated pain and has enabled PLWAs to die in dignity.[47]

Traditional and Western medicine

In Uganda, palliative care is trying to bridge the gap between traditional and Western medicine in a way that affirms the values of each tradition. Lydia Mpanga Sebuyira, director of clinical services at HAU explains:

> People prefer to be seen by a traditional healer, someone who understands their language, understands their background and who actually looks at the whole of them. And we've found that in what they call the Western medical tradition, people are just so busy that they don't have time to think about the whole person. So when palliative care comes along and says 'we're trying to be holistic as well', we try to inject back into our practice the kind of things people have been looking for and haven't found. So I think health professionals are saying, 'We'd like to learn that, but how do we put it into practice?'[48]

This point is echoed by Yahaya Hills Sekagya, a traditional healer and Western-trained physician:

> We all walk to the future in the footsteps of our ancestors; and our ancestors have influence on us. In African spirituality, our ancestors can cause disharmony in our life. They are also responsible for a lot of happiness in our life—but when they cause disharmony, we become more conscious of them and we turn back to them. For example: one of the disharmonies I normally experience with my patients is when an ancestor has died and we don't care about the grave of that ancestor. He can come and cause a disharmony in a person; and it doesn't need much.
>
> When we do the Western investigations and we don't see the cause of disease, as a traditional healer we go into the spiritual cause, and we find that the ancestor is disgruntled about an issue. And to get treatment, you just need to do what is needed. Go dig the grave and the madness will go. You do not need any medicines—the Western approach—but you will have solved the issue. So when we are looking at somebody who is sick, we are viewing him as somebody who is in disequilibrium, and accessing how to treat and restore him to equilibrium requires accessing the subconscious levels, which in spirituality we do.[49]

Ethical issues

Within the International Observatory on End of Life Care, we have chosen a particular framework/template for global ethical analysis. This is the so-called Four Principles approach to health care ethics. The principles are:

Beneficence: the obligation to provide benefits and balance benefits against risks

Non-maleficence: the obligation to avoid the causation of harm

Respect for autonomy: the obligation to respect the decision-making capacities of autonomous persons

Justice: obligations of fairness in the distribution of benefits and risks.

This is not to say that other, or even competing, frameworks for ethical analysis are not relevant. Elsewhere, we have discussed in great detail that particular issue, as well as the various strengths and weaknesses of the approach—and, indeed, whether or not the approach is at all worthwhile.[50]

We may note, however, that the approach is used worldwide and that it has gained remarkable acceptance since 1979, when it was first introduced.[51] This may at least be taken as a sign of the global potential of the approach. Furthermore, and highly relevant in our context here, scholars have used it in analysing the African ethical 'map'.[52,53] In so doing, they have managed to highlight both similarities to, and differences between, 'African' ethical thinking and the ethical thinking represented by the Four Principles approach.

The African world-view, religion, the vital force principle, and the principles of beneficence and non-maleficence

Peter Kasenene[52] claims that there is such a thing as a common African-ness that characterizes the culture and world-view of Africans—notwithstanding the fact that there are remarkable differences in values among Africans; urban and rural, educated and illiterate, Christian or traditionalist.

As far as religion is concerned, Anne Merriman reports that in Uganda, 'it's about 90 per cent Christian, 10 per cent Muslim, and the Muslim religion is very integrated with the Christian religion—they even marry Christians and don't insist that they change their religion'. We may note that what has been named *the vital force principle* within African thinking has a profound religious meaning in that 'this vital force is hierarchical, descending from God through ancestors and elders to the individual', and, that 'whatever increases life or vital force is good; whatever decreases it is bad'.[52]

That also means there is a direct link between the vital force principle and the principles of beneficence and non-maleficence: 'Following the vital force principle, everyone has a duty to do good to his or her neighbour, especially to friends, relatives and clansmen', and the very same principle 'establishes the duty not to cause harm, injure or do anything that reduces the vital force of the individual members of the community or threatens its collective existence'.[52] In summary, then, this very important aspect of African thinking does indeed appear to be congruent with the two first principles of the Four Principles approach to health care ethics.

The role of justice

Due to the communal nature of African societies, observes Kasenene,[52] 'justice is highly valued', and 'justice is first and foremost a social affair', meaning that 'an offence against an individual is an offence against the community, and for the good of the community everyone's needs must be attended to without discrimination. Health care is, consequently, made available to everyone according to his or her needs'.[52]

The Ugandan Government's policy of making morphine available to all patients who need it, free of charge, across districts, is a very clear example of this. The interview with dispenser Peter Mikajjo is revealing as far as the details of this policy are concerned. Also, Jack Jagwe—who has earlier been in government services for some 30 years—has much to say on this policy. In the words of the interviewer, 'almost uniquely among certain of the countries in Africa, [Uganda has] managed to have morphine availability and its regulations integrated into Government policy'.

Perhaps intuitively, we tend to think of justice in terms of treating people equally. Yet that idea seems to go only half way since people often have different needs, and thus treating them equally could mean that some people will not get enough of what they need. Hence, according to what has been called Aristotle's formal theory of justice, philosopher and physician Raanan Gillon notes, 'equals should be treated equally and unequals should be treated unequally in proportion to the morally relevant inequalities'.[54] Surely a morally relevant inequality is the one between those who are not sick and those who suffer from a life-limiting illness like cancer or AIDS, and who therefore will be in need of good pain control, for example in the form of morphine.

The issue of patient autonomy

The principle of autonomy may be said to be of less importance in the African setting than in, say, most European societies (although this is arguably not so if one compares it with some southern European societies such as Spain, for instance.[55] Claims Kasenene: 'In African culture . . . beneficence has a higher value [than autonomy], which justifies paternalistic interventions either by the doctor . . . or by the family'.[52] Now paternalism has been defined thus by the philosopher Gerald Dworkin: 'By paternalism, I . . . understand roughly the interference with a person's liberty of action justified by reasons referring exclusively to the welfare, good, happiness, needs, interests or values of the person being coerced'.[56] Also, more succinctly, another philosopher, Derek Parfit, says of it: 'We are paternalists when we make someone act in his own interests'.[57]

That people are sometimes treated paternalistically should also be seen in the light of the so-called *communalism principle* of African traditional ethics, according to which 'to be is to belong, and an individual exists corporately in terms of the family, clan and whole ethnic group'.[52] There is thus a strong current of collectivism in African societies— something than runs counter to the occasionally quite extreme individualism of Western societies, an individualism that is a pre-supposition of what we may call 'the ideology of autonomy' (seen most starkly, perhaps, in the euthanasia and so-called 'right to die' movements). In concrete terms, this collectivism or communalism comes to the surface when relatives 'want the doctor or nurse to let them know what the patient is suffering from'.[52] Additionally, observes Kasenene, 'individual autonomy is not respected when the community believes that the person is acting against himself or herself'.[52]

That the *principle of beneficence* thus has the upper hand is something that comes across very clearly in the interviews with Anne Merriman, Ekiria Kikule and Michelle McGannon. They all point to the Ugandan practice of not telling patients about diagnosis and prognosis when they face terminal illness. Anne Merriman mentions the case of a doctor, even, who was not told: 'recently [a doctor] died . . . he had an operation, was diagnosed as cancer of the stomach, nobody told him the diagnosis, they told it to the family, they didn't tell him—but he knew, of course he knew'. Michelle McGannon frames the issue of truth-telling in terms of patient confidentiality: 'I think sometimes that really ties in with the confidentiality, they'll go and tell a relative possibly instead of telling the actual patient first of all'.

Apparently, the lack of respect for autonomy as far as disclosure of diagnosis and prognosis is concerned must also be seen in relation to a culture that denies death. To quote Anne Merriman in her reference to Jack Jagwe—a colleague who happens to be one of the other interviewees: 'we teach end-of-life ethical issues. One of them is that people can't accept that people are going to die. Dr Jagwe, you heard me teasing him today about death, he's a year older than me and I keep saying to everybody, "Now look, when you reach my age, you should be able to know that death's gonna come any time, you know", "Oh, God forbid", says Dr Jagwe . . . the doctors have the feeling about death, they won't acknowledge that it happens, the senior doctors in particular won't acknowledge that it happens. So if a patient goes into the hospital and they're seen to be terminally ill, they will do everything to resuscitate them'.

Finally, another way to look at these issues is through the *principle of non-maleficence*. Patients are not told the truth because doing so is perceived as harming them psychologically—including taking away hope—as well as culturally (compare this with the culture of death denial).

Hospice success stories

Hospice Africa Uganda

Anne Merriman describes the major achievements of HAU in the following terms:

> I could never have envisaged that the thing would have grown so rapidly. We started, but I never thought of the future—you just saw what was on your doorstep and what needed to be done. But I think one of the achievements is: although we had a struggle getting into the curriculum for undergraduates, we were teaching in the university here since '93 and every doctor that's come out since then knows what we're talking about and is converted. So we've got a group of these doctors who want to prescribe morphine and their senior doctors are telling them not to, but that will all change. We've Dr Jagwe who is trying to change them and he's doing a good job with advocacy, but, you know, it's taking a long time. So I think that's one of the major achievements.
>
> The other achievement is the fact that we've demonstrated that palliative care works and people who've come on our training programmes are really committed to it. When patients come

here, not only do they have the medicines—they're in their case with them—the doctors start them the minute they see them. They see the patient's pain relieved within an hour—before they leave. If they find a patient or a patient comes in here with severe pain which they've had for months, within an hour they're relieved of their pain and when you can see that, and see it as a reality, you get a deep joy, you know? And so people are really uplifted in their vocation as health workers because they're seeing things happen which they never saw before.[58]

A hospice patient confirms the discovery of a better quality of life:

Hospice helped me a lot; they helped me in so many ways. My father really praises God for hospice. I was going to hospital every day and feeling bad. But when I start with these people [hospice] they brought everything here; and I'm feeling well, and I've put on weight.[59]

Little Hospice Hoima

During 2003–2004, the hospice's achievements include:[60]

◆ Acquisition of land for a new headquarters of LHH in Hoima town

◆ Establishment of a community volunteers programme

◆ Sensitization of the community regarding the work of LHH

◆ Increase in pain control for patients

◆ Improved report writing due to staff development activities

◆ Founding of a journal club.

Mobile Hospice Mbarara

Program manager Martha Rabwoni writes:

Mobile Hospice has continued to expand in both the infrastructure and the personnel. We are very grateful to God who has given us the grace to care for our patients. We have seen many patients in their homes, in hospitals and at roadside clinics. Patients are also examined in the back of our vehicle if the roadside clinic does not provide adequate privacy. The patients in turn have cared for us with a lot of prayers, appreciation and support which have helped us to keep working and sharing our knowledge and skills.[61]

Regarding HAU training, Fatia Kiyange comments:

We've got the distance learning Diploma course affiliated to Makerere University off the ground; it's running very well. We are having students from different countries in Africa, that's really an achievement for training. We've got the Clinical Palliative Care Course off the ground, it's running—and we do that with the Ministry of Health, so that is also an achievement. We've trained and introduced oral morphine and pain control in 14 districts of Uganda and the morphine is there, they are dispensing it, the Ministry has purchased it and it's free of charge. So that is as a result of our training here, so that's also a major success. And even our major referral hospital: for years they have continued to refer patients, but we have active people now who have been trained to give the service, and they are giving the service there.[62]

The Mildmay Centre

Successes at the Mildmay Centre are seen in terms of:

◆ Communicating the goals and services of the Centre to the people of Uganda (and beyond) such that >7000 patients have come forward to be registered; around 5000 are actively involved with the service at any particular moment

- Changing attitudes—with the assistance of ARVs—regarding the value of a family's investment in a child's recovery, previously seen to be futile[63]
- The range of education/training courses being taken up from people both within and outside of Uganda[64]
- The delivery of education/training courses in country districts by innovative mobile teams[65]
- Public awareness raising of the inclusive nature of the service which, due to the quality of the premises, could be misinterpreted as being exclusively for the privileged
- Management of a service that has grown rapidly in a short space of time.[66]

Among these many successes, a particular cause for celebration occurred on 23 July 2003 when 85 trainees from eight districts of Uganda graduated from the HIV/AIDS palliative care and rehabilitation course. Joy Edith Angulo, mobile training team co-ordinator, writes:

> The trainees at the end of the course designed and presented project proposals to potential donors. It is hoped that these projects will be implemented within the next six months and thus help to develop HIV/AIDS care services in the districts. Some of the districts have also formed palliative care teams within their districts and initiated HIV/AIDS clinics in various health centres and hospitals. The palliative care teams within the districts are also working together to strengthen the services provided.[67]

Life/oral histories

Derek Atkins—*centre director*: *The Mildmay Centre, Kampala*: Interviewed by Michael Wright, 11 March 2003. Length of interview (Mildmay group): 45 min.

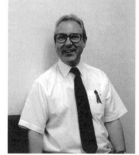

Derek Atkins speaks of patient provision at the Centre and of the administrative demands inherent in a growing organization. He draws attention to: the taboo of HIV testing for children; the ethical issues surrounding truth-telling; the potential impact of a positive test on parents; and the support need of families. Successes include the organization's capacity to meet seamlessly the demands of a growing patient base.

Ronnah Abinaitwe—*manager, Resource Centre, HAU*: interviewed by Michael Wright, 10 March 2004. Length of interview: 32 min.

Ronnah Abinaitwe tells how she graduated in Library and Information Science at Makarere University and now manages the resources centre at Hospice Africa Uganda. This centre has been developed to include computer work stations, bookshelves, storage

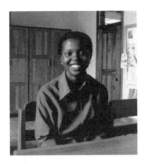

space and a meeting area—all with hand-made furniture from a group of German Fathers in Hoima. As the first person appointed to the centre, Ronnah has learnt how to combine library and resource management skills, and has been helped in this respect by a placement with Avril Jackson at Hospice Information in London. The centre is heavily used by hospice staff and by a wide range of students and visitors—frequently from other African countries. She sees herself as part of the hospice team and looks forward to the day when the centre expands to include multiple copies of key books to take pressure off the popular titles.

Julia Downing—*director, Mildmay International Study Centre, Kampala*: interviewed by David Clark, 2 June 2004. Length of interview: 36 min.

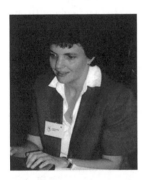

Julia Downing has wide experience of HIV/cancer care and palliative care in the UK both clinically and in the field of education. She worked in a mission hospital in Zambia and, when a post was advertised for a vacancy in Uganda, returned to Kampala as the Director of Mildmay Study Centre (2001). The Centre now offers a wide variety of courses and reaches into the rural areas via mobile education teams. These initiatives are underpinned by Julia's doctoral studies: an evaluation of the mobile training team programme in the rural setting. She underlines the Centre's focus on paediatrics, the importance of counselling, and the role played by religious leaders in rural areas—and of the need for cultural sensitivity in the face of different tribal traditions. Finally, she describes the background to the Cape Town Declaration and her role in the newly formed African Palliative Care Association.

Winnie Elem—*palliative care nurse: Lira Regional Referral Hospital, Northern Uganda*: interviewed by Michael Wright, 11 March 2003. Length of interview: 10 min.

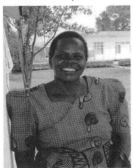

Winnie Elem speaks of her work at the Lira Regional Referral Hospital (288 beds) where she and her colleague receive referrals to their palliative care unit. Referred patients have either HIV/AIDS or cancer. The unit has one bed for acute cases and they each see around five patients per day. Morphine is available. A community home care service is provided within a radius of 5 km from the hospital—a distance generally considered to be within walking distance (or preferably a bicycle ride).

Clare Fitzgibbon—*Macmillan nurse consultant, Mobile Hospice Mbarara*: interviewed by Michael Wright, 8 July 2005. Length of interview: 38 min.

During the 1960s, Clare Fitzgibbon was working as a theatre sister when she saw a programme about Africa that caused her to change direction and, in 1964, to relocate to a country hospital in Mbarara, Uganda. She stayed until 1972, by which time she had married her husband, Brian (a teacher), and given birth to three sons. Their joint interest in Africa continued and they determined to seek the opportunity to retire early and thereafter offer their skills in the developing world. During the course of her career, Clare Fitzgibbon became a Macmillan nurse and by the early 1990s had heard of the initiatives taking place in Uganda, supported by Anne Merriman. When the Fitzgibbons retired in 1998 and subsequently approached VSO for a placement, they were amazed to find themselves bound for Uganda and Mbarara, an occurrence they regarded as divine intervention. Clare Fitzgibbon tells of her work with the clinical team charged with establishing palliative care education in the curriculum of Mbarara University of Science and Technology; of her struggle with the local language; the issues around truth-telling; and the constraints imposed by limited resources. Her perceived successes include a growing expertise in the use of drugs; the increased empowerment of staff; and the inception of the Mbarara mobile hospice service.

Dr Jack Jagwe—*senior adviser, national policy, drugs and advocacy, HAU*: interviewed by Michael Wright, 10 March 2004. Length of interview: 29 min.

Jack Jagwe speaks of his 30 year involvement with the Government of Uganda and of his role as Deputy Medical Director responsible for clinical services. He has a strong commitment to palliative care, and in 1998 was appointed chairman of the task force which formulated the national palliative care policy which became incorporated into the government's strategic plan, 2001–2005. He recalls how morphine was available during the 1960s and 1970s but then became unavailable during Uganda's period of political turmoil. Oral morphine was introduced with the inception of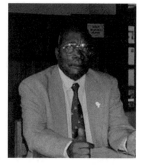
palliative care under the auspices of the Joint Medical Store. He speaks of Uganda's 20 year experience of HIV/AIDS and of the open way in which the disease has been confronted, right down to the village level. Based on his personal experience, Jack Jagwe is enthusiastic about convincing professionals and ministers of the benefits of palliative care both in Uganda and in other African countries. Finally, he tells of the major successes in Uganda: of the government's acceptance of the need for palliative care; of morphine availability; of the new generation of doctors leaving medical school with an understanding of palliative care; and of the distance learning course validated by the prestigious African University of Makerere.

Dr Ekiria Kikule—*deputy director and research co-ordinator, HAU*: interviewed by Michael Wright, 10 March 2004. Length of interview: 1 h 9 min.

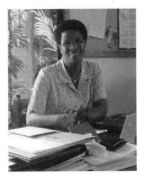

Ekiria Kikule met Anne Merriman and Jan Stjernswärd when she took a Master's degree in public health. She was invited to join the hospice as a researcher and became executive director in 2002. She tells of her commitment to hospice after being influenced by a succession of home visits, her sister's painful death from cancer and another sister's relief from suffering after taking morphine. She highlights ethical issues surrounding palliative care: of truth-telling and breaking bad news; of relationships with traditional healers (herbalists); and of the benefits of collaborative working. As a result, herbalists are encouraged to assist with the provision of natural ingredients, such as laxatives, whereas hospice retains an input into pain relief. Turning to the future for Hospice Africa Uganda, she speaks of the component roles of service, training and modelling—and of the strain arising from the demands on the organization due to its unforeseen success and growing requests to 'scale up'. Although the hospice is not based on one particular faith, she considers that many staff are drawn to the service because of their personal faith, a feature which is manifest in many ways, not least in the generous gifts of time. In future, closer co-operation with faith-based organizations is expected to help the hospice reach the poorest people in very remote areas, although a current priority is also to secure essential funding.

Fatia Kiyange—*education administrator, HAU*: interviewed by Michael Wright, 10 March 2004. Length of interview: 22 min.

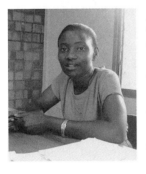

Fatia Kiyange trained at Makerere University and tells of her background in social work and social administration, and how she eventually arrived at Hospice Africa Uganda (department of education and training) in April 2000. At that time, the education block had not been constructed and the small team worked in one room of the hospice. Nevertheless, there was a comprehensive range of courses which targeted medical students, spiritual leaders, health professionals and volunteers—and which now form the core of the expanded provision. She speaks of the value of the sensitization programmes, of the challenges posed by reactionary (senior) health professionals and the strategies used to develop palliative care throughout the country. As the courses developed, the department scaled up to a staff of 10, and Hospice Africa Uganda became regarded as a significant training institution. The aim is now to integrate palliative care into all 56 districts in Uganda, with an accompanying training programme to support these clinical innovations.

Dr Emmanuel Luyirika—*director of medical services: The Mildmay Centre, Kampala*: interviewed by Michael Wright, 11 March 2003. Length of interview (Mildmay group): 45 min.

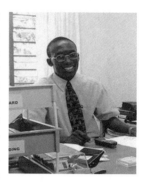

Emmanuel Luyirika speaks about the work of the centre since it opened in 1998. Focusing exclusively on AIDS patients, this encompasses a broader remit than hospice/ home-based care organizations, since team members are involved in a continuing process of sustaining life, dealing with opportunistic infections and helping people return to work—as well as providing care at the end of life. Currently, 7545 patients are registered with the organization, 5000 of which are regular patients—half of them children. Networks have been established countrywide and patients are also drawn from neighbouring countries. Challenges faced by the new organization relate to the affordability of ARVs and the reluctance of some families to invest in a child with a life-limiting disease. Successes relate to the public welcome now given to AIDS patients and the obvious signs of improvement in human lives—weight gain, hope and the capacity to return to work.

Michelle McGannon—*co-ordinator, distance learning Diploma in Palliative Care, HAU*: interviewed by Michael Wright, 10 March 2004. Length of interview: 33 min.

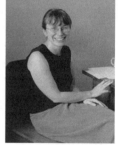

Michelle McGannon speaks of her role as co-ordinator of the distance learning Diploma in Palliative Care: a course she helped to establish which has attracted widespread interest. She intends to remain in Uganda until October 2004, by which time she will have completed >3 years in Kampala, having previously been with the hospice during 1998/1999. She comments on the high standards of professionalism among the staff. A key feature of the distance learning course is that it is African in nature, located within an African University, with modules written by African-based educators. As a result, every element is culturally and clinically appropriate to Africa. Importantly, modules include an education element so that students can pass on their skills in their own country. Interest for the October 2004 intake is high. In future, the department is looking to build on the current successes, capitalize on the enthusiasm of the students, fine-tune the curriculum and provide more clinical support. In 5 years time, it is hoped to offer a Bachelor's course—and a Master's course in 10 years.

Margaret Mawanda—*public relations officer: the Mildmay Centre, Kampala*: interviewed by Michael Wright, 11 March 2003. Length of interview (Mildmay group): 45 min.

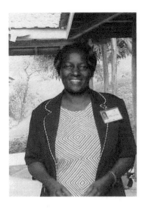

Margaret Mawanda recalls the opening of the Mildmay Centre by Princess Anne, and how many thought that Princess Diana had been involved too, due to her well known interest in patients with HIV/AIDS. The buildings are impressive, and this aspect of the centre gave rise to a widely held misunderstanding: that the centre was designed and intended for whites. She tells of the determined—and successful—public relations effort to change this misapprehension and how the centre has now been warmly accepted by patients and the local community.

Dr Anne Merriman (1)—*founder and director, medical services and education, Hospice Africa Uganda*: interviewed by Michael Wright, 9 March 2004. Length of interview: 1 h 18 min.

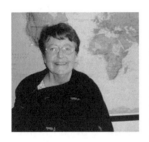

Anne Merriman recalls her childhood as a member of a religious family in Liverpool. When 4 years old, she declared an interest to work in Africa and as she grew up, became profoundly affected by the death of her 11-year-old brother from cancer. After leaving school, she joined the Medical Missionaries of Mary, a religious order founded in 1937 to care for the sick in Africa. After an unfulfilling time working in a laboratory, she was accepted by the sisters for medical training and thereafter undertook a 9 year placement in Nigeria. Changes within the Catholic Church after Vatican II—combined with the illness of her mother—caused her to leave the Order after 20 years service and return to Liverpool. There she practised geriatric medicine. As she became committed to palliative medicine, she organized a conference with Cicely Saunders that began a series of developments in the Knowsley and Liverpool area. After her mother died, she moved to Singapore where she focused on the needs of an ageing population. Starting in 1985 with a group of volunteers, she commenced a palliative care home care service to meet the needs of patients who were not benefiting from conventional chemo- or radiotherapy. This followed on research carried out from the national University of Singapore (NUS) where she was working in Community Medicine. This eventually became a palliative home care service under the Community Chest (Social Services) and commenced from her 22nd floor flat. As her contract with the NUS came to an end, Gillian Petrie Hunter suggested she develop the newly established service in Nairobi, a commission she accepted in 1990 on condition the government procured oral morphine. Despite the potential in Kenya, she became frustrated by excessive bureaucracy and eventually moved to Uganda (1993) to set up a model service capable of implementation in other resource-poor countries. She goes on to speak of the challenges she faced, how they were overcome and how palliative care was eventually incorporated into the government's 5-year strategic plan. She then reflects on the spiritual dimension of health care, of her hopes for the future and of the relationship between supportive care and palliative care—drawing particular attention to the benefits of grafting pain control onto existing supportive care networks, and the essential task of procuring affordable morphine.

Dr Anne Merriman (2)—*founder, director, medical services and education, Hospice Africa Uganda*: interviewed by David Clark, 20 July 2004.

In a short interview, published in full on the website of the International Observatory on End of Life Care, Anne Merriman speaks about the impact of HIV/AIDS in Africa. In the past, support has been available for treatment and behaviour change relating to HIV/AIDS but, until recently, there has been little forthcoming for the dying. Many want to die at home, but that is not always possible. Poverty, lack of food to take with medicines, a dearth of trained personnel and the inaction of governments provide barriers to palliative care development. Yet countries like Zimbabwe and Kenya have shown what can be done. Since 1993, Hospice Uganda has developed a model of care that can be utilized in other resource-poor countries of Africa. With the impetus provided by the PEPFAR initiative, developments will begin to happen more quickly and on a broader front. A significant development has been the establishment of the region-wide African Palliative Care Association (APCA) which held its first meeting in June 2004 in Arusha, Tanzania; representatives attended from 20 African countries. These developments, together with a wider accessibility to morphine, will provide significant opportunities for palliative care development in the future.

Peter Mikajjo—*dispenser, HAU*: interviewed by Michael Wright, 10 March 2004. Length of interview: 28 min.

Peter Mikkajjo tells of his background working in a mission hospital, of his interest in pain, and how he moved to Hospice Africa Uganda in 2001. He describes how morphine powder is supplied by the Joint Medical Store, how he mixes the powder into a solution and then dispenses liquid morphine in three different strengths, coloured appropriately. He goes on to speak of the internal procedures required to monitor the use of morphine and how prescriptions are balanced with the records of morphine dispensed at the end of each day. In addition, patients sign a 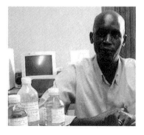 record sheet to confirm their morphine use, and each week these records are returned to the pharmacy and reconciled with the stocks issued.

Rose Nabatanzi—*palliative care nurse: Kitovu Mobile Home Care*: interviewed by Michael Wright, 11 March 2003. Length of interview: 11 min.

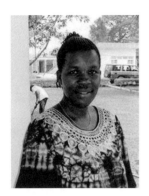

Rose Nabatanzi tells how Sister Ursula of the Medical Missionaries of Mary founded Kitovu Mobile Home Care in response to a growing awareness of the AIDS epidemic. As the disease became apparent, myths and fears developed around the infection. The early sufferers were thought to be punished for past thefts and consequently became stigmatized and marginalized. Sufferers sold their homes and possessions in an attempt to make restitution, falling into extreme poverty; their children dropped out of school and relatives were abandoned at the hospital doors. In this scenario, Sr Ursula cared for infected people with a small team of nurses, gradually increasing the provision to include community volunteers and local co-ordinators. Food, soap and sugar were provided alongside medicines and, with the introduction of morphine in 2000, home care developed into a palliative care service. Today, the service covers 124 centres throughout three districts of Uganda.

Dr Lydia Mpanga Sebuyira—*director, Clinical Services, HAU*: interviewed by Michael Wright, 21 September 2004. Length of interview: 37 min.

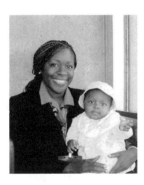

Lydia Mpanga Sebuyira was born in Uganda but spent extended periods in England, where she studied medicine at Oxford University. After working in a hospice in Sunderland, she returned to Kampala and bumped into Anne Merriman—wearing a Hospice Uganda T-shirt—on one of the wards. As a result of that meeting, she became a visiting consultant at the hospice while lecturing at the medical school for the next 5 years. As she prepared to take some of Anne Merriman's responsibilities, her husband was offered a position in South Africa—and Lydia subsequently took up a position at St Francis Hospice, Port Elizabeth. She recalls the impression that the South Africa experience made upon her: the struggle against poverty; the stigmatization of HIV/AIDS patients; and the role of the local church—factors which impacted upon her advocacy role. Returning to Uganda in 2003, she has rejoined the hospice team as Director of Education; a position that looks increasingly beyond the borders of Uganda to other African countries which request assistance.

Dr Yahaya Hills Sekagya—*general secretary, National Integrated Forum for Traditional Health Practitioners, Uganda; President PROMETRA Uganda*: interviewed by Michael Wright, 9 September 2004. Length of interview: 20 min.

Yahaya Hills Sekagya outlines an African concept of illness that integrates the spiritual and physical domains of person-hood with strong ancestral connections. As a traditional health practitioner who is also a Western-trained physician, he articulates the benefits and drawbacks of each approach and speaks of the possibilities for collaboration—an activity that is already proving beneficial in Uganda. He reflects on the practical problems of reaching the poor in remote rural areas, and of the difficulties of dispensing modern medicines in such circumstances. Against this background, he advocates for a better understanding of how herbal remedies and Western treatments can complement one another.

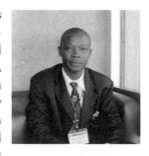

Dr Janet White—*founder, medical director: Joy Hospice*: interviewed by Michael Wright, 11 March 2003. Length of interview: 12 min.

In this interview, Janet White recalls how she founded Joy Hospice (*Jesus first, Others second, You last*) in 2001. She first came to Uganda with the Deliverance Church in 1988 and thereafter combined medical and educational work. After a spell in Kenya (1994–1998), she was invited by the church to return to Uganda and establish a medical service in Mbale. The following year, a second clinic was established in Buwasunguyi. By this time, the majority of patients were presenting with advanced cancers and end-stage AIDS. As a result, Janet White began to nurse patients in her home in Mbale. Recognizing a gap in provision, she then obtained and renovated a house, creating a 5-bed inpatient unit, and launched a palliative care service on 31 August 2001.

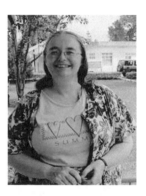

Public health context

Population

Uganda has an estimated population of 25 million of which 66% is Christian (Roman Catholic 33%, Protestant 33%), 16% Muslim, and 18% subscribe to indigenous beliefs.[68]

Epidemiology

In Uganda, the WHO World Health Report (2004) indicates an adult mortality[69] rate per 1000 population of 505 for males and 431 for females. Life expectancy for males is 47.9; for females 50.8. Healthy life expectancy is 41.7 for males; and 43.7 for females.[70]

At the end of 2003, UNAIDS suggested that in Uganda, up to 880 000 adults and children were living with HIV, and that up 120,000 AIDS-related deaths had occurred during this year (Table 8.6).

Government action has helped reduce the prevalence of AIDS from 30 per cent of the population in the early 1990s to an estimated 6 per cent in 2002. This package of support

Table 8.6 Uganda HIV and AIDS estimates, end 2003

Adult (15–49) HIV prevalence rate	4.1 per cent (range: 2.8–6.6 per cent)
Adults (15–49) living with HIV	450 000 (range: 300 000–730 000)
Adults and children (0–49) living with HIV	530 000 (range: 350 000–880 000)
Women (15–49) living with HIV	270 000 (range: 170 000–410 000)
AIDS deaths (adults and children) in 2003	78 000 (range: 54 000–120 000)

Source: UNAIDS 2004 report on the global AIDS epidemic.

has focused on prevention and care, and includes awareness raising, education, condom distribution, and voluntary testing and counselling. UNAIDS reports:

> AIDS is the leading cause of death for those aged 15–49 years. The overall antenatal HIV prevalence rate in 2002 was reported to be 6.5%. The country has an orphan population of more than two million, nearly half as a result of HIV/AIDS. Single, widowed surviving mothers and elderly widowed grandmothers have now become the predominant heads of households.
>
> Even within this grim picture, Uganda has become a beacon of hope and an example of accomplishments in the area of HIV/AIDS for many countries all over the world. The government and the people of Uganda have consistently pursued a policy of openness about HIV/AIDS, backed by the strong political commitment and leadership of President Yoweri Museveni. By mainstreaming HIV/AIDS prevention and control into different sectors, in national plans, including the National Poverty Eradication Action Plan, all segments of society in all parts of the country have been encouraged to play a role. In addition, the government has been successful in mobilizing additional resources for HIV/AIDS.[71]

Health care system

In its *World Health Report, 2003*, WHO noted that the total per capita expenditure on health care in Uganda was Intl $57; 5.9 per cent of GDP[72] (Appendix 3).

The WHO overall health system performance score places Uganda 149th out of 191 countries.[73]

The Government of Uganda has adopted a national health policy[74] and endorsed a 5-year plan which began in 2001[75] that includes palliative care in its remit. As a result, the possibilities for growth—in both service provision and professional education—have been significantly improved.[76] The Ministry of Health works closely with palliative care stake-holders and during 2004 has co-ordinated a network of services that includes: Ministry of Health clinical services and AIDS control programmes, WHO field Office (Kampala), Hospice Africa Uganda, Mildmay International, TASO and Makerere University.[77]

Stjernswärd and Clark comment on Uganda's Health Strategic plan as follows:

> Uganda is the only country in Africa that has made palliative care for people with AIDS and cancer a priority in its National Health Plan where it is classed as 'essential care' . . . Uganda has

established all the foundation measures as recommended by WHO. A clear national policy has been established, education in palliative care is incorporated into the undergraduate curricula of doctors and nurses, health professionals at all levels are exposed to courses and workshops in pain relief and palliative care and affordable morphine has been made easily available and is produced generically in the country.[78]

Ekiria Kikule, executive director of HAU comments on the role of the government in Uganda:

> When this present government came in, in 1986—remember the civil war—they had already seen the scourge of AIDS during their bush struggle, so they came in knowing there's a problem. And they came in openly and said, 'Look, we have a problem, we need help. What do we do?' They also started from a need, I mean people saying, 'My husband is sick with HIV/AIDS' or 'I have lost one—nursing one—maybe you have the disease' And they would sit and ask themselves: 'What do we do? How do we do it?'
>
> I remember I was in London in 1988 and Princess Anne came to visit and of course the BBC was there, and I felt very proud to see my President on the BBC being interviewed. There were all these cameras and whatever, but I remember a reporter asking President Museveni 'You are talking about AIDS openly, don't you think that somebody's going to turn it into a political issue and discredit your government?' And he said 'I don't care, somebody might; but what I know is that we have a problem, our people are dying, and we want help. Anybody who has any kind of help to help us fight this,' he says, 'we need it'. And for me I really felt proud. This is a man who was so secure and was not about to turn an epidemic into a political thing. The Government was behind anybody who had anything to offer.[79]

Political economy

Uganda has substantial natural resources, including fertile soils, regular rainfall and sizable mineral deposits of copper and cobalt. Agriculture is the most important sector of the economy, employing >80 per cent of the work force. Coffee accounts for the bulk of export revenues. Since 1986, the government—with the support of foreign countries and international agencies—has acted to rehabilitate and stabilize the economy by undertaking currency reform, raising producer prices on export crops, increasing prices of petroleum products and improving civil service wages. The policy changes are especially aimed at dampening inflation and boosting production and export earnings.[68]

GDP per capita is in Uganda Intl $964 (Appendix 4).

References

1 **Report of the United Nations Development Programme 2004 (HDI 2002).** Launched by the United Nations in 1990, the Human Development Index measures a country's achievements in three aspects of human development: longevity, knowledge and a decent standard of living. It was created to re-emphasize that people and their lives should be the ultimate criteria for assessing the development of a country, not economic growth. Current values range from 0.956 (Norway, first out of 177 countries) to 0.273 (Sierra Leone, 177th out of 177 countries). Countries fall into one of three groups: countries 1–55 = high development; 56–141 = medium development; 142–177 = low development. See: http://hdr.undp.org/statistics/data/indic/indic_8_1_1.html

2 **Merriman A.** Hospice Uganda: 1993–1998. *Journal of Palliative Care* 1999; **15**(1): 50–52.

3 **Merriman A.** History of Palliative care in Uganda. Hospice Africa Uganda Aspects: 1993–2003. In: *Conference proceedings—Palliative Care: Completing the Circle of Care*, 16–17 September 2003.

4 The Mildmay Centre, Uganda: background information. Mildmay International: 3.

5 IOELC interview: Emmanuel Luyirika—11 March 2003.

6 IOELC interview: Janet White—11 March 2003.

7 IOELC interview: Winnie Elem—11 March 2004.

8 See: http://www.afxb.org/en/index.php?link=program&sub1=uganda

9 **Robert K, Bekunda R, Dorothy N.** Integrating palliative care in the care of PWLAs—AFBX experience. In: *Conference proceedings—Palliative Care: Completing the Circle of Care*, 16–17 September 2003.

10 Community Health approach to palliative care for HIV/AIDS and cancer patients in Africa: WHO joint project cancer and HIV/AIDS programmes. Progress Report. August 2002.

11 WHO report: Community Health Approach to Palliative Care for HIV/AIDS Patients, 2004: 8. Available to download at: http://whqlibdoc.who.int/publications/2004/9241591498.pdf

    The extract cites: **Kikule E.** A good death in Uganda: survey of needs for palliative care for terminally ill people in urban areas. *British Medical Journal* 2003; **327**(7408): 192–194.

12 **Kikule E.** A word from the executive director. In: *Eleventh Annual Report: 1 April 2003 to 31 March 2004*. 33. 17.

13 **Hospice Uganda.** *Some Facts about Hospice Uganda.* January 2004.

14 **Mobile Hospice Mbarara.** January 2004.

15 *Engendering Bold Leadership.* The President's Emergency Plan for AIDS Relief. First Annual Report to Congress, 2005: 115. http://www.state.gov/documents/organization/43885.pdf

16 See: http://www.cafod.org.uk

17 **Merriman A.** Hospice Africa Uganda: 10th Anniversary (1993–2003). In: *Conference proceedings—Palliative Care: Completing the Circle of Care*, 16–17 September 2003.

18 **International Narcotics Control Board.** *Narcotic Drugs: Estimated World Requirements for 2004. Statistics for 2002.* New York: United Nations, 2004.

19 'The term defined daily doses for statistical purposes (S-DDD) replaces the term defined daily doses previously used by the Board. The S-DDDs are technical units of measurement for the purposes of statistical analysis and are not recommended prescription doses. Certain narcotic drugs may be used in certain countries for different treatments or in accordance with different medical practices, and therefore a different daily dose could be more appropriate'. The S-DDD used by the INCB for morphine is 100 mg. International Narcotics Control Board. *Narcotic Drugs: Estimated WorldRequirements for 2004. Statistics for 2002.* New York: United Nations, 2004: 176–177.

20 **Ministry of Health, Republic of Uganda.** *Statutory Instruments 2004: 24 The National Drug Authority (Prescription and Supply of Certain Narcotic Analgesic Drugs) Regulations, 2004.* Ministry of Health, 2004.

21 IOELC interview: Peter Mikajjo—10 March 2004.

22 IOELC interview: Anne Merriman—9 March 2004.

23 IOELC interview: Jack Jagwe—10 March 2004.

24 **Otterstedt C.** The hospice concept as an addition to care and counselling of people dying of HIV/AIDS in Africa. *Hospice Information Service* 1999; **7**(3): 3–4.

25 **Kennedy A.** Journey to Kampala—the AIDS crisis in Uganda. *Hospice Information Service* 1999; **7**(2): 12–13.

26 **Merriman A.** Preface to third edition. In: *Palliative Medicine—Pain and Symptom Control in the Cancer and/or AIDS Patient in Uganda and Other African Countries.* Kampala: Hospice Africa Uganda, 2002: v.

27 IOELC interview: Michelle McGannon—10 March 2004.

28 Personal communication: Ndikintum George Mbeng—11 March 2004.

29 **Jackson A.** Hospice information welcomes visitor from Africa. *Hospice Information Service* 2003; **2**(3): 16.

30 IOELC interview: Ronnah Abinaitwe—10 March 2004.

31 **Kikule E.** A good death in Uganda: survey of needs for palliative care for terminally ill people in urban areas. *British Medical Journal* 2003; **327**(7408): 192–194.

32 IOELC interview: Julia Downing—2 June 2004.

33 **Akankwasa A.** Palliative care in the districts through the mobile training teams. In: *Conference proceedings—Palliative Care: Completing the Circle of Care*, 16–17 September 2003.

34 Personal communication: Remigious Bekunda—18 November 2004.

35 **Sekagya YH.** Traditional medicine/healers contributing to the circle of care. In: *Conference proceedings—Palliative Care: Completing the Circle of Care*, 16–17 September 2003.

36 **Nyakoojo SB.** Human Resources Department report. Hospice Africa Uganda. *Eleventh Annual Report: 1 April 2003 to 31 March 2004*: 33.

37 The Mildmay Centre, Uganda: background information. Mildmay International: 2.

38 See: http://www.fias.net/Donor%20Page/Ireland-Donor.htm

39 IOELC interview: Anne Merriman—9 March 2004.

40 **Wheatley S.** Little Hospice Hoima celebrates five years. *Hospice Information Service* 2003; **2(3)**: 9.

41 **Downing J.** Welcome from the Mildmay Centre, Uganda. In: *Conference proceedings—Palliative Care: Completing the Circle of Care*, 16–17 September 2003.

42 **White J.** Experiences of an in-patient unit with community outreach. In: *Conference proceedings—Palliative Care: Completing the Circle of Care*, 16–17 September 2003.

43 IOELC Interview: Rose Nabatanzi—11 March 2004.

44 **Simmons M.** The integration of palliative care using oral morphine into an existing home care programme. *PCAU Journal of Palliative Care* 2003; **6**(3): 28.

45 **Defilippi K, Downing J, Merriman A, Clark D.** A palliative care association for the whole of Africa. *Palliative Medicine* 2004; **18**: 583–584.

46 See: http://www.afxb.org/en/index.php?link=about&sub1=history

47 **Robert K, Bekunda R, Dorothy N.** Integrating palliative care in the care of PWLAs—AFBX experience. In: *Conference proceedings—Palliative Care: Completing the Circle of Care*, 16–17 September 2003.

48 IOELC interview: Lydia Mpanga Sebuyira—21 September 2004.

49 IOELC interview: Yahaya Hills Sekagya— 19 September 2004.

50 For an exposition on The Four Principles approach to health care ethics at the end of life: Hegedüs K, Materstvedt LJ. Ethical perspectives on end of life care. In: Wright M, Clark D (ed.), *Voices from Central and Eastern Europe: Perspectives on Palliative Care*. Observatory Publications (forthcoming).

51 **Beauchamp TL, Childress JF.** *Principles of Biomedical Ethics*. New York: Oxford University Press, 1979.

52 **Kasenene P.** African ethical theory and the four principles. In: R. Gillon (ed.), *Principles of Health Care Ethics*. London: John Wiley & Sons, 1994: 183–192.

53 **Bailhache N.** The four pillars of medical ethics. *Hospice Uganda Journal of Palliative Care* 2000; **2**(2): 26–27.

54 **Gillon R..** Value judgements about equity in health. In: Oliver A, Cookson R, McDavid D (ed.), *The Issues Panel for Equity in Health—Discussion Papers*. London: The Nuffield Trust, 2001.

55 **Núñez Olarte JM, Guillen DG.** Cultural issues and ethical dilemmas in palliative and end-of-life care in Spain. *Cancer Control* 2001; **8**: 46–54. (Full text/free download: http://www.moffitt.usf.edu/pubs/ccj/v8n1/pdf/46.pdf)

56 **Dworkin G..**Paternalism. *The Monist* 1972; **1**: 64–84.

57 **Parfit D.** *Reasons and Persons*. Oxford: Clarendon Press, 1984.

58 IOELC interview: Anne Merriman—9 March 2004.

59 Patient: Hospice Uganda—11 March 2003.

60 **Kasigwa B.** Little Hospice Hoima. In: Hospice Africa Uganda. *Eleventh Annual Report: 1 April 2003 to 31 March 2004.* 63.

61 **Rabwoni M.** Mobile Hospice Mbarara. In: Hospice Africa Uganda. *Eleventh Annual Report: 1 April 2003 to 31 March 2004.* 52.

62 IOELC interview: Fatia Kiyange—10 March 2004.

63 IOELC interview: Emmanuel Luyirika—11 March 2003.

64 IOELC interview: Margaret Mawanda—11 March 2003.

65 IOELC interview: Julia Downing—2 June 2004.

66 IOELC interview: Derek Atkins—11 March 2003.

67 **Angulo JE.** Graduation and conclusion of the HIV/AIDS palliative care and rehabilitation course for 85 trainees from 8 districts of Uganda at the Mildmay Centre. *PCAU Journal of Palliative Care* 2003; **6**(3): 10.

68 See: http://www.cia.gov/cia/publications/factbook/geos/ug.html

69 This refers to adult mortality risk, which is defined as the probability of dying between 15 and 59 years.

70 See: WHO statistics for Uganda at: http:/www.who.int/countries/uga/en

71 See http://www.unaids.org/en/geographical+area/by+country/uganda.asp

72 Total health expenditure per capita is the per capita amount of the sum of Public Health Expenditure (PHE) and Private Expenditure on Health (PvtHE). The international dollar is a common currency unit that takes into account differences in the relative purchasing power of various currencies. Figures expressed in international dollars are calculated using purchasing power parities (PPP), which are rates of currency conversion constructed to account for differences in price level between countries.http://www3.who.int/whosis/country/compare.cfm?country=s&indicator=strPcTotEOHinIntD2000&language=english

73 This composite measure of overall health system attainment is based on a country's goals relating to health, responsiveness and fairness in financing. The measure varies widely across countries and is highly correlated with general levels of human development as captured in the human development index. Tandon A, Murray CLJ, Lauer JA, Evans DB. *Measuring Overall Health System Performance for 191 Countries.* GPE Discussion Paper Series: No. 30; WHO.

74 Ministry of Health, Republic of Uganda. *National Health Policy.* Kampala: Ministry of Health, 1999.

75 Ministry of Health Republic of Uganda. *National Sector Strategic Plan 2000/1–2004/5.* Kampala: Ministry of Health, 2000.

76 **Jagwe JGM.** The introduction of palliative care in Uganda. *Journal of Palliative Medicine* 2002; **5**(1): 160–163.

77 Hospice Africa Uganda. *Eleventh Annual Report: 1 April 2003 to 31 March 2004.* 5.

78 **Stjernswärd J, Clark D.** Palliative medicine—a global perspective. In: Doyle, D Hanks G, Cherny N, Calman K (ed.), *Oxford Textbook of Palliative Medicine.* Oxford: Oxford University Press, 2003: 1209.

79 IOELC interview: Ekiria Kikule—10 March 2004.

Chapter 9

Zimbabwe

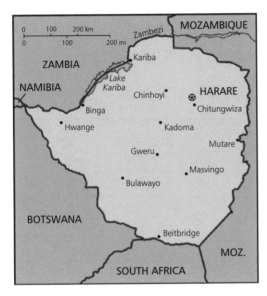

Zimbabwe (population 12.84 million)[1] is a landlocked country in Southern Africa that covers an area of 390 580 km². Its boundaries border Zambia, Botswana, South Africa and Mozambique. The river Zambezi forms a natural boundary with Zambia. In full flood between February and April, the Victoria Falls forms the world's largest curtain of falling water.

According to the United Nations human development index (HDI), Zimbabwe is ranked 147th out of 177 countries worldwide (value 0.491)[2] and 19th out of 45 African countries for which an index is available. This places Zimbabwe in the group of countries with low human development.

Palliative care service provision

Current services

In Zimbabwe, 13 organizations provide a total of 34 palliative care services (Table 9.1).

Bekezela Community Home Based Care

This NGO was founded in 1994. Around 140 patients were cared for during 2003 and about 200 patients have registered in 2004 (to March 21).[3]

Dananai Home Based Care (Murambinda)

Dananai was founded in 1992 as a home-based care organization. Focusing on HIV/AIDS patients, it has since extended its service to include education, palliative care and care for orphans. Around 740 patients are registered with the organization.[4]

Family AIDS Caring Trust (FACT)

FACT was Zimbabwe's first AIDS service (1987). Today, FACT undertakes peer education and training; facilitates community responses to AIDS patients and orphans; and mobilizes local resources and volunteers.[5]

Table 9.1 Palliative care provision in Zimbabwe, 2004

	Free-standing unit	Hospital unit	Hospital support team	Home care	Day care	Clinic/drop-in centre	Total
Bekezela Home Based Care				1			1
Dananai Home Based Care (Murambinda)			1	1			2
FACT Mutare				1			1
Island Hospice, Bulawayo			1	1			2
Island Hospice, Harare			1	1		2	4
Island Hospice, Mutare			1	1			2
Island Hospice branches				6			6
Lubancho House, Hwange				1			1
Mashambanzou	1			1	1	1	4
Methodist Church of Zimbabwe (Epworth Project)				1		1	2
The Mildmay Centre			1	1	1	1	4
Morgenster Mission Hospital			1	1			2
Seke Rural Home Based Care				1			1
Thembelihle Halfway Home	1			1			2
Total services	2		6	19	2	5	34

Island Hospice

This NGO has centres in Harare (established 1979), Bulawayo (1981) and Mutare (1985), and incorporates six autonomous branches throughout the country.[6] Services range from a full palliative home care service—including palliative nursing support, counselling and volunteer services—to simple nursing care. In 2002, 287 patients were registered with *Island Hospice, Harare* (excluding patients seen at Chitungwiza and in the community-based projects). During 2003, *Island Hospice, Bulawayo* cared for 160 patients,[7] and *Island Hospice, Mutare* cared for 368.[8]

During 2004, 1400 patients were cared for countrywide by the Island Hospice organization, of which 919 (66 per cent) were female and 481 (34 per cent) were male. In the same year, 587 new patients were seen and a total of 529 patients died.

Lubancho House

Established in 1989, Lubancho House focuses on home-based care (primarily AIDS patients), children and youth (primarily orphans) and community mobilization. Around 2500 patients are currently registered (March 2004). Patients are seen weekly by a member of staff and three times per week by a community volunteer.[9]

Mashambanzou Care Trust

Mashambanzou hospice offers a wide range of services, including: a drop-in centre; pre- and post-test counselling; a terminal care centre (for 22 patients); home-based care; and bereavement support and counselling. Referrals come via Harare clinics, other care organizations or word of mouth. In 2000, four home-based care teams visited 8350 patients; 40 per cent were male, 60 per cent female. Thirty-two per cent were new patients. In the same year, 1506 orphans received assistance.[10]

The Mildmay Centre Harare Children's Hospital

This organization is designed to care for children affected by HIV/AIDS. Based at Harare Hospital, children are referred from other health centres, from doctors or from Mildmay's outreach centre in Kuwadzana (a high density area). At present, 250 children aged from birth to 16 years are registered with the project. The day care centre can accommodate 15 children.[11]

Morgenster Mission Hospital

This developing service began in March 2003 and cares for up to 150 patients.[12]

Seke Rural Home Based Care

This NGO arose from the need to provide home-based and palliative care services to terminally and chronically ill people in the district of Manyame. When the programme began in February 2002, 112 patients registered. In January 2003, the number had grown to 1778; by March 2004, it was 4575. The service can accommodate 5000.[13]

Thembelihle Halfway Home

This home was founded in February 2003 to provide inpatient and home-based care for terminally ill HIV/AIDS patients. The inpatient unit provides transitional care for 1 or 2 weeks as patients move from hospital to home. During this time, patients receive pain relief, counselling and support, and family members are taught how to give basic care in the home. *Halfway Home* opened with two wards and 24 beds in July 2003, and by May 2004 had increased to six wards and 72 beds. Patients are referred from private hospitals, government hospitals and clinics.[14]

In her 2002 report to the Diana Fund, Anne Lloyd Williams writes of Zimbabwe:

> I visited two of island Hospice's four satellite programmes in Harare's high-density areas—Chitungwiza and Chiedza. I found both models very impressive. Hundreds of patients are in active care throughout a combination of different systems, all benefiting from support of the hospice outreach team. In Chitungwiza there is a small hospice unit based in the district hospital, which also provides backup for clinics in the area and carries out home visits where required. In Chiedza, the hospice works through 30 different community-based organisations (CBOs) encompassing a network of volunteer carers each looking after 20–25 patients. I visited one of the CBO day clinics in Chiedza; the hospice team was providing consultations and drugs in a large open shack roofed with plastic sheeting. Later we visited some patients in their homes, some of whom were in a pathetic condition due to poverty.[15]

Two years later, WHO comments on the overall development of palliative care in Zimbabwe:

> Zimbabwe has a long tradition in palliative care provided by the hospice movement, however this is still not widely integrated into the health system. There is no exclusive national policy concerning palliative care although palliative care policies are included in the following documents: the Home Based Care Policy, the Discharge Policy and the Ten Year Plan produced by the Committee for Prevention and Control of Cancer in Zimbabwe (PCCZ). Like Hospice Uganda, Island Hospice in Zimbabwe provides training at various levels in palliative care within the community, within the country and to neighbouring countries.[16]

Reimbursement and funding for services

Island Hospice is a charity that depends increasingly on foreign donors for financial support. Services to patients and their families are free, although a small amount of income is recovered from medical aid societies if patients subscribe to private medical schemes. In 2004, the UK Forum for Hospice and Palliative Care Worldwide granted Bulawayo Island Hospice Service £2000 to increase the salaries of the nursing staff. The following year, the Diana Fund awarded £51 712 to Island Hospice, Harare, to build on the present training in palliative and bereavement care both in Harare and more generally throughout the country.

Lubancho House is funded by Catholic Relief Services.

Mashambanzou Care Trust is supported by NORAD, Danida, the US Embassy, Plan International, Beit Trust, Terre des Hommes, Canadian Public Health Authority, Dutch Reformed Church and the European Union.

In the financial year 2002, USAID/OFDA provided >US$1 million to Catholic Relief Services (CRS) to support food assistance in 20 rural hospitals targeting approximately 150 000 people. In co-operation with the Zimbabwe Association of Church-related Hospitals (ZACH), CRS provides daily food distributions in 14 rural districts. ZACH also provides 45 per cent of all hospital beds in Zimbabwe and 68 per cent of all rural hospital beds.[17]

In 2005, the UK Forum for Hospice and Palliative Care Worldwide granted £1500 to support the studies of Eunice Garanganga (MSc in Palliative Care).

Opioid availability and consumption

The International Narcotics Control Board[18] has published the following figures for the consumption of narcotic drugs in Zimbabwe (2002): codeine 235 kg; morphine 10 kg; dextropropoxyphene 49 kg; tilidine 1 kg; pethidine 35 kg.

For the years 2000–2002, the average defined daily dose consumption of morphine for statistical purposes (S-DDD)[19] in Zimbabwe was 1 (Appendix 1).

Island Hospice, Harare uses the WHO pain ladder and keeps a supply of morphine for patients who are unable to collect the drug from the government hospitals of Pariryanetwa and Harare. A local firm produces morphine whenever powder can be imported, although availability is erratic. The hospice doctor writes a prescription after discussion with a nurse. The Ministry of Health and the Drug Control Council have given permission for a hospice nurse to prescribe drugs falling within the Dangerous Drugs Act providing the prescription is validated by a hospice doctor. *Island Hospice, Bulawayo* does not prescribe morphine. The service liaises with the patient's doctor who prescribes the necessary morphine. *Island Hospice, Mutare* does not prescribe morphine.

Bekezela Community Home Based Care has access to doctors at Inyati District Hospital. These doctors prescribe morphine in injectable and MST forms; volunteers administer paracetamol and aspirin.

Dananai Home Based Care (Murambinda) has access to three doctors at Murambinda Mission Hospital, who may prescribe liquid morphine.

Family AIDS Caring Trust (FACT) has three qualified nurses who have responsibility for morphine prescription, supervised by a volunteer doctor.[20]

Lubancho House is limited to the administration of paracetamol; morphine is difficult to access and the hospital supply is frequently exhausted.

Morgenster Mission Hospital does not prescribe morphine to home care patients. If a patient is taking morphine on discharge from hospital, relatives are able to collect repeat prescriptions (tablets and syrup) as required.

National and professional organizations

Hospice Association of Zimbabwe (HOSPAZ)[21]

HOSPAZ is a registered public voluntary organization (PVO) whose mission is to provide national co-ordination, training and advocacy to support organizations in their provision of hospice and palliative care. All organizations describing themselves either as palliative care providers or home-based care groups have been invited to register with HOSPAZ, and a database of members is currently being constructed. Palliative care standards have been devised by HOSPAZ and approved by the Ministry of Health, although there is no implementation policy as yet.

Table 9.2 Hospices twinned with Island Hospice, Harare

Twinned hospice	Activity
Hospice of Central New York; Liverpool, NY	Awareness-raising events, community fundraisers, sponsorship of visitors from Island to come to Hospice CNY; sponsorship of Island staff members to attend international conferences; on-going communication and interaction*
Community Hospice; Rensselaezr, NY	Staff and Community fundraisers, sponsorship of visitors from Island to come to Community Hospice*
Hospice of the Valleys; Tredegar, Wales	'Exchange visits, where we raise a little money by selling their books and pictures. We also exchange literature'. (Ref: *Hospice Twinning, HtH*)

* *Source*: Abigail Fowlkes Gutierrez.

Hospice 'twins'

The Foundation for Hospices in Sub-Saharan Africa (FHSSA) has actively promoted the development of reciprocal 'twinning' arrangements. Island Hospice, Harare is twinned with three hospices: two in America and one in Wales (Table 9.2).

In 2003, the FHSSA announced its 31st twinning match. In the same publication, Val Maasdorp, acting director of Island Hospice writes:

> Island Hospice and Bereavement Service in Zimbabwe and Hospice of Central New York have been 'involved' since 1985, almost 20 years!! Like any relationship, at times it goes through periods of 'non-attention', generally when things get too busy, stressed or fraught, and other priorities are serviced. But it is precisely at times like that when we most need to reach out and relate to others, and to me that is the beauty of our twinning with you guys so very far away. These twinnings should not just be about money: rich twin giving to poorer twin, there is also so much to be gained on the non material side. Whilst visiting in October, I was struck by the very different challenges we all face. The African Hospice ones may appear more apparently difficult, acute, and emotionally stressful, but your path is a different one with challenges I don't envy!! . . . Attempting to maintain an appropriate service with a 'developed world' standard in a 'developing world' country is a daily battle on all fronts. So, although set against a very different environment, because they are committed to the same basic goals, the interest and support I gained from my few days with your hospice staff was so very meaningful. I found myself re-energized to come back and tackle each day's problems with an air of 'OK. Let us see what is going to be thrown our way today!!'[22]

In addition, HOSPAZ is twinned with the Ohio Hospice and Palliative Care Organization, Arlington, Ohio, USA.

Palliative care coverage

Bekezela Community Home Based Care covers five out of 14 wards within the district of Bubi (population: 56 000).

Dananai Home Based Care (Murambinda) covers north Buhera, population 150 000.

Family AIDS Caring Trust (FACT) has developed a regional role supporting local organizations in their response to the AIDS epidemic.

Island Hospice and Bereavement Service Harare covers a population of 1.5 million and Chitungwiza—1 million. Comprehensive services are generally available in the larger centres of Harare and Bulawayo. *Island Hospice, Bulawayo* covers Bulawayo municipality—a radius of about 15 km from the hospice; and *Island Hospicem Mutare* covers a population of 176 630.

Lubancho House covers four chiefdoms which spread from Victoria Falls to Lupane. A doctor is on the board of trustees and patients have access to medical support at Hwange Colliery Hospital.

Mashambanzou Care Trust utilizes four home-based care teams, each with a sister and counsellor, which cover the greater Harare area, Porta Farm and Epworth.

Morgenster Mission Hospital covers a population of around 200 000; the home-based care programme covers 60 000.

Seke Home Based Care serves all 21 wards of Manyame Rural District (population 150 000).

Thembelihle Halfway Home cares for patients in Bulawayo.

Education and training

Ministry of Health

A 10-year cancer control plan initiated by the Ministry of Health (1994) was taken forward by Island Hospice who trained health professionals in all provinces. This was an extension of the work begun by the Committee for Prevention and Control of Cancer in Zimbabwe (PCCZ). The training of these workers is to be funded by Catholic Relief Services in the future.

Catholic Relief Services

The new CRS project covers the five dioceses of Hwange, Gokwe, Chinoyi, Mutare and Bulawayo, and aims to develop palliative care expertise amongst health professionals and community groups. With a budget of US$1 million, it is a significant project for Island Hospice. A project manager, a monitoring and evaluation officer, a finance manager and two trainers have been recruited to supplement current staff. Trainees have been drawn from government employees and church-employed health workers, and skills have been developed using the 'train the trainer' approach.

The outcomes of this training reveal a mixed story. Ambitious initiatives have been undertaken: a doctor and his wife established a home-based care service; and properties have been purchased so the dying have a place to stay after being evicted from their lodgings (there is a taboo around death in a rented property). Yet many newly qualified nurses have left the country and only around 30 out of 250 are left. Once trained, community and health workers can also find work in the health/NGO sectors.

Bekezela Community Home Based Care began a major initiative in September 2003, and has since trained five groups of volunteers.

Family AIDS Caring Trust (FACT) began to provide professional training to hundreds of AIDS organizations across Africa during the 1990s. Rather than seek organizational expansion, FACT took a strategic decision to strengthen existing organizations to promote a more effective approach to the epidemic. Where necessary, FACT has worked with community groups to help establish new, locally owned NGOs.

Lubancho House volunteers were trained by the project facilitators, who themselves were trained by CONNECT—the Family Therapy Institute, Harare. Palliative care training was given by Island Hospice Harare.

Mashambanzou Care Trust has trained 250 volunteers in most of the high-density areas around Harare.

The Mildmay Centre has completed an in-house training programme for its staff. A training programme for health workers and volunteers—which includes a clinical placement scheme—is currently being developed.

Island Hospice, Harare has a well developed training programme for various groups of health workers (Table 9.3).

In addition, Island Hospice has provided education and training to:

◆ The HIV/AIDS Quality of Care Initiative (HAQOCI) based at the Medical School, University of Zimbabwe. This is mainly for doctors and nurses being trained in opportunistic infections; a manual has been written to support the programme

◆ Regional community-based groups, funded by the Canadian International Development Agency's Southern Africa AIDS Training Programme (SAT2).[23] In 2003, these groups included health workers from Zambia, Mozambique and Tanzania

◆ Rural-based State Registered Nurses (SRNs) and other health professionals

◆ Health professionals in Chitungwiza

◆ Trainee teachers.

Sambulo Mkwananzi, training manager at Island Hospice, speaks of the complexities of working with patients, and of the need for knowledge and understanding to combat stigmatization:

> [Another] thing we are doing is to work closely with faith-based centres, whether they be the hospital or the health care commissions of a different faith, because they are also responding to HIV and AIDS by developing their own home-based care groups. Again, we try and bring in the palliative care element, you know—the relief of suffering; and it's usually the same issues of basic symptom control and spiritual matters, issues that cause emotional pain, how to deal with children of parents who are dying, or children who are sick. If I could tell a story that touched me two weeks ago? We saw two 17 year olds, but I was particularly touched by one boy who had been HIV positive since birth but he wasn't aware because his mother died and his father died. So the siblings who were very healthy—both of them married—had marginalized him and seen him as being the odd one, 'Why are you sick?' you know, 'Our parents had us and we're both healthy'. And, this 17-year-old boy was really puzzled; and he asked me and said, 'Why did it happen? I don't understand it'. And I, you know, was explaining in a simple way about how, even if both parents are positives, not all children are who are born. I told him the rate and how it happens. And you could see in his face that he was now beginning to work it out, where he had previously thought it's his fault somehow. It was so touching. And these are just simple things—about talking to caregivers, asking, 'Had you ever spoken about it?' 'No, we just prayed'. So issues like that, when you train and you follow-up. Yes, there are successes.[24]

Table 9.3 Training programmes for health and community workers provided by Island Hospice Harare

Group	No. per year	Training	Funding	Follow-up
Caregivers (volunteer)	50	Palliative care and HIV related. Five modules. Trainees are asked to donate their time to the organization providing counselling and patient care	Trainees self-funding	Bi-monthly supervision and training
Community volunteers drawn from Red Cross, Kellogg Foundation and churches	20–30	Four modules: module 1 = 2 days; module 2 = 2 days; module 3 = 1 week; module 4 = 1 week; practical work—HIV related. Includes paediatric focus and use of 9-cell bereavement table[25]	Free to trainees	2 days
Pastors		2 days		1 day
Student nurses (who study oncology) Years 1–3	50			
SRN training		As requested		
Medical students Year 5	138	2 mornings (6 h), once per year.		
Post-basic nurses (senior, experienced staff)		2 mornings (6 h), once per year. Basic pain and symptom control		
Nurse aides		1 week, mornings only (25 h) once per year		
NGOs working with orphans	77	Palliative care and bereavement awareness to nine NGO partners.	Firelight Foundation USA	Ongoing programme
Home-based care organizations	45	2 × 5 day modules for selected volunteers	Firelight Foundation USA	Ongoing programme
AIDS support organizations	114	6 × Caring for the Carer workshops with three partners	Firelight Foundation USA	Ongoing programme

Source: Island Hospice, Harare.

HOSPAZ regard education and training as a core activity. In 2003, an initial programme—part of the WHO palliative care initiative in consultation with the Ministry of Health—included the training of nurses from a clinic in Goromonzi. In clinics such as these, opioids are unavailable and the training takes note of this. The next step is to train doctors, who could then prescribe morphine. This is a 'train the trainer' programme where doctors and nurses are expected to impart these skills to community workers.

A variety of home-based care manuals have been published in Zimbabwe. HOSPAZ has developed 'care cards' to simplify information for rural community workers, and these are currently being piloted.

Palliative care workforce capacity

Bekezela Community Home Based Care has one executive director; two programme directors; one driver; and 128 volunteers.

Dananai Home Based Care Service (Murambinda) is made up of Sr Onya Cunliffe (trained nurse), three assistants (Red Cross-trained nurse aides), three volunteer doctors and 350 volunteers.

Family AIDS Caring Trust (FACT) has a team of 52 staff and 600 volunteers.

Island Hospice Harare had around 125 staff and volunteers in 2003 based at headquarters or in the high-density communities (Table 9.4).

Island Hospice Bulawayo has a staff of 10; *Island Hospice Mutare* has two SRNs; six caregivers (qualified); six caregivers (part qualified); two administrative staff; and one messenger.

Lubancho House has 20 staff accountable to a board of trustees, including: one co-ordinator; one project officer; four heads of department (one a nurse); one accountant; one administrative secretary; one receptionist; facilitators/trainers (one a nurse); and 200 volunteers.

The Mildmay Centre employs around 23 staff (March 2004).

Morgenster Mission Hospital has one doctor responsible for the home care programme, one accounts clerk and around 400 volunteers (working in close co-operation with 10 district nurses).

Seke Rural Home Based Care has one director; one home-based care co-ordinator; one home-based care field officer; one social worker; one palliative care nurse; one

Table 9.4 Personnel working for Island Hospice and Bereavement Service, 2003

Full time	Doctors	Nurses workers	Social staff	Admin staff	Ancillary	Volunteers	Massage therapists
Full time		12	8	8	4		
Part time	1	2	2	2		85	3
Total	1	14	10	10	4	85	3

finance officer; one bookkeeper; one advocacy officer; one secretary; one office orderly; one security guard; 44 supervisors; and 400 secondary caregivers. Manyame District has 10 clinics and two district hospitals. Patients are usually referred to Chitungwiza General Hospital for medical support.

Thembelihle Halfway Home employs 26 staff, including a manager, nurses, nurse aids, cleaners and cooks. Volunteers support the home-based care service.

History and development of hospice–palliative care in Zimbabwe

Prior to the advent of the hospice movement which began in Zimbabwe in 1979, care for the dying was given by herbalists and traditional healers. An ill person would be moved to a *musasa*[26] on the outskirts of the village. The traditional healer would direct care which was mainly provided by elderly women in the form of hygiene, nutrition, psychosocial and spiritual support. Modern nursing was introduced to Zimbabwe in 1890. Only acute care was offered, however, until the advent of Island Hospice in 1979.[27] Traditional healers are still an important part of the culture, and many patients will alternate between these and allopathic health services.[28]

Island Hospice

In 1977, Maureen Butterfield and her husband watched helplessly as their daughter, Frances, died of cancer. The inadequate levels of care that Frances and her parents received caused a grieving Maureen Butterfield to source something better for others in a similar position. She travelled to St Christopher's Hospice (London) where she learned more of the services and facilities, and considered the concept 'well suited, with slight adaptations, to the needs of the section(s) of the population which were most familiar to me'.[29,30] She returned to Zimbabwe eager to pursue ways of establishing a hospice service. A crowded public meeting in May 1979 resulted in the establishment of Island Hospice Service—among the first of its kind in Africa—that developed 17 regional branches by 1997.[31] The name was taken from the words of John Donne:

> No man is an island, entire of itself. Every man is a part of the continent, a piece of the main, and each man's death diminishes me because I am involved in mankind.[32]

In a country which became independent from Britain in 1980, the developing service operated in a receding colonial framework where whites still held social and financial power. Yet over the next 24 years, the organization changed from 'a charitable institution, relying on volunteers, initially with patients who were elderly, middle class and mostly white',[33] to something more attuned to the wider population of Zimbabwe. David McElvaine, a former Senior Administrator of Island Hospice writes:

> Zimbabwe's pre-independence history also had a marked effect on public opinion regarding death and bereavement. The bloody and protracted struggle for independence had personally affected hundreds of thousands of people. The need for skilled bereavement care was at its zenith when Island Hospice was formed. These large-scale events, coupled with our early focus on public

relations and education were strong contributory factors to our successful establishment and have remained crucial to our continued functioning.[31]

At the outset, Island Hospice was a specialized unit with qualified and experienced staff who delivered care to a relatively small number of people. As the reputation of the service spread, 'the patient profile changed. There were more black patients and they tended to be younger (conforming to the pattern of cancer in Africa), lived in small, overcrowded houses and spoke Shona'.[34]

As the effects of HIV/AIDS became apparent, Island Hospice broadened its base to include patients with AIDS. Speaking at Island's 25th anniversary celebrations in January 2004, social worker Rona Martin recalls the impact of the AIDS epidemic on the service:

> Twenty five years ago who could have known how the spread of HIV/AIDS would change the face of hospice care in Africa? Our first AIDS patient was in 1986 and we continued to take patients with HIV referred in the usual way. However, as with the rest of the country, we were slow to realize and respond to the full impact of the pandemic. It became clear, however, that in order to reach our increasing numbers of families in need, we would have to change the way we work. Carla Lamadora, former Director and now Director of HOSPAZ, the new umbrella organization, was instrumental in getting us into community based work. Island had always worked in the community with its home based care, but now with the increased need it became necessary to partner with other groups committed to home care. Our first base in the community was Mabvuku. Training, always a part of our work with medical students, nurses and caregivers, became increasingly important. Our separate training department was formed in 1996 to respond to demand. Spreading skills in palliative and home based care through training and mentoring continues to be seen as the way forward.[35]

While celebrating 25 years of hospice care in Zimbabwe, the anonymous writer of an article in *Progress in Palliative Care* (2004) highlights the modern day challenges:

> Operating a hospice is not easy anywhere, but in the past three years Island has had to deal with challenges above and beyond the call of normal hospice duty. In 2000 the country began experiencing increasing political instability and polarisation. When certain areas of the city become impassable due to strikes, stayaways and turmoil, staff safety becomes a concern. Zimbabwe has one of the fastest shrinking economies in the world, with official inflation running in excess of 400%. The population is experiencing shortages of essentials such as transport, fuel, basic foods, etc. Economic hardships have increased the brain drain, and many professionals are leaving the country. Medication is expensive, if available, and medical bills are above the reach of many of the population. This strains already weakened health and welfare systems and adds to the pressure on an established and well-respected organisation like Island.
>
> All of this inevitably affects service delivery. There are clinical supervision meetings in fuel queues; nutritional supplements have to be sourced in order to safely implement certain medication regimes; administration and accounting functions have become extremely challenging as almost daily rebudgetting is necessary and accounting systems struggle with the increasing number of zeros appearing (need a four digit number to equate to one US$); foreign donors have to be patient with the massive changes in budget items.
>
> But there are many positives. Island staff have learned to become flexible and creative in dealing with these never ending difficulties and see the challenges as 'today's special'. Many non-traditional hospice services are undertaken as and when necessary. Like a positive form of an opportunistic infection. Island takes any opportunity it can to diversify its service and improve access to it by all sectors of the population. Relationships with our committed donors and partners are strong. And, of course, work is never boring or hum drum. I ask you, who would want to work anywhere else?[36]

Family AIDS Caring Trust (FACT)

This NGO was founded in 1987 by Geoff Foster, a paediatrician at the government hospital in Mutare. As he saw some of the earliest cases of HIV/AIDS, he realized that Zimbabwe's limited health services were becoming overwhelmed. At the same time, AIDS prevention programmes and office-based counselling for HIV-positive people were largely ineffective. Consequently, Geoff Foster developed an alternative vision—of an organization which would work with local communities, develop culturally appropriate models of prevention and home care, address religious beliefs on disease causation, and decrease the stigma associated with AIDS.

FACT began by engaging local church, political, health and business leaders and built up a broad volunteer and funding base within the local community. Issues of sexuality, female subordination and other taboo topics were confronted and openly discussed. Programmes were directed towards target groups, including: sex workers; single women; truckers; youth; rural inhabitants; and people living with AIDS.[5]

Mashambanzou Care Trust

Sister Noreen Nolan of the Little Company of Mary founded the Mashambanzou Care Trust in 1989. She had spent time in the rural areas and saw the impact AIDS was beginning to have on Zimbabwean society. Consequently, she founded a ward for terminal care at St Anne's Hospital—a private centre in a well-to-do neighbourhood of Harare. Yet it became clear that pressing need for care existed in the high-density areas where the majority of people live. With the assistance of the Norwegian aid association, NORAD, Mashambanzou purchased a property on the outskirts of Harare to respond to the epidemic from a broader base.[37]

The Mildmay Centre

The Mildmay Centre opened an outpatient clinic at Harare Hospital in April 2003; the day care centre opened the following month. The project is designed to be a model of care for children affected by HIV/AIDS, and focuses on intensive rehabilitation after diagnosis/illness. Children who have been referred for intensive support in the day care centre are transported from their homes to the centre and then taken home at the end of the day. Where necessary, children are admitted to a ward in the hospital. ARVs are not currently available, but it is planned to begin an ARVs programme during 2004. Nevertheless, many children have been able to return to school.[38]

Morgenster Mission Hospital

Dr Breugem founded the palliative/home care service in 2003 after receiving training from Island Hospice. She subsequently trained a body of volunteers (now ~400) who work in home care and orphan care programmes and also distribute care kits, bandages, gloves and bleach. There is close liaison with district nurses (10) based at five clinics, where patients can also access medical support. Although the programme is weighted towards physical care, and as yet there are no social workers or nurses, Dr Breugem is mindful of incorporating psycho-social care as the service becomes established.

Hospice success stories

Bezekela Community Home Based Care regard the development of home-based care centres, the training of caregivers and the provision of kits for the sick as major successes of the service.

Dananai Home Based Care (Murambinda). Sister Onya Cunliffe considers that the success of the organization centres on the delivery of a person-oriented service, where limited resources are directed to the patients in their homes.

Family AIDS Caring Trust (FACT). Featuring prominently among the successes of FACT is a well-motivated body of volunteers; links have also been developed with local churches, thereby allowing the organization to reach the poor in remote areas.

Island Hospice. In the 25years that Island Hospice has been in operation, the organization's greatest success has been to maintain a high level of quality care in the face of growing hardships. Val Maasdorp:

> We are very aware of not letting our standards drop and this is increasingly difficult given the high demand on the service and the decreasing numbers of experienced staff. The organization is at the cutting edge of palliative care in the country and has created several innovative programmes, including bereaved children's groups, memory books and many training programmes. It has also managed the transition from low numbers to large numbers in community care, and has effectively decentralized its work. This is partly due to AIDS, economics and staffing problems.[39]

Lubancho House. Sr Nehwati considers that the success of the service has been to raise the awareness of AIDS and to mobilize communities to take responsibility for their patients. The service is now keen to de-centralize and delegate management to village level substations.

Seke Rural Home Based Care measures success by the number of patients who have registered for home care—up from 112 in 2002 to 4575 in 2004; by the appreciation shown to the organization by the local council, the department of social welfare, the New Start Centre, Churches and traditional leaders; by the work of Seke's Advocacy and Care committees which operate in the 21 wards; and by the successful lobbying of the World Food Programme, which provided 5 kg of rice per patient per month for a period of 3 months.

In addition, Seke Rural Home Based Care had an audience with the Parliamentary Portfolio Committee on Health during an awareness-raising field visit by committee members. Discussions centred on the unavailability of drugs, and treatment in home-based care. Veronica Kanyongo writes:

> We presented a position paper and policy analysis which highlighted the gaps in the National HIV and AIDS Policy, Community Home Based Care Policy and the Discharge Plan Guidelines. The Parliamentarians promised to use the recommendations made by Seke Rural Home Based Care and other stakeholders to review these documents.[40]

Eunice Garanganga sums up the success of hospice care in Zimbabwe:

> We have lots of successes. To start with, I just want to mention that Zimbabwe was the first country to bring hospice into Africa, and that has grown; it has given us strength to go on, just knowing

that we are Mother Hospice. I can quote South Africa: I remember one time at a conference, they said, 'You are really Mother Hospice', because of the fact that we were the first in Africa. And we have grown in the sense that training started in 1983 when doctors at the medical school came to say, 'We don't know how to break bad news, can you come and do some lectures with final medical students on breaking bad news?' So that was our opportunity to sell everything in hospice, sell everything in palliative care. So we started training even in pain control, breaking bad news, communications skills, symptom management, in 1983.

Going back to what we have achieved so far. We've realized the numbers are huge in home-based care, and we are grafting palliative care onto home-based care groups so that the quality remains very good. So again, in Africa, we were the first to come up with standards for home-based care, and we are proud of that. And from there we have had an association, the Hospice Association of Zimbabwe; it's a mother body that oversees all the other hospice branches, and we have accommodated home-based care groups because we want to graft palliative care into their activities so that palliative care remains very high, palliative care remains acceptable.

We have also embarked on a rural model: this was initiated by WHO. The WHO chose five countries in Africa and Zimbabwe's one of them, to initiate palliative care and see how to go about it through the Ministry of Health. At some stage the funds were not there and HOSPAZ sought the funds so that this project can go on, and we can see how to graft palliative care onto a district hospital. The training—the hospital, the health professionals—is going on at the moment. We are going to evaluate and see if it can be taken to another area. We are going to learn a lot, so even through difficult circumstances we are taking strides to try and maintain our palliative care standards in Zimbabwe.[41]

Ethical issues

In Zimbabwe, a belief that deceased relatives control family affairs impacts upon attitudes towards illness. While accepting the nature of contemporary, Western medicine, illness is thought to originate in avenging ancestral spirits and its remedy, therefore, lies in rituals of appeasement.[28,34] As a result, many Zimbabweans initially consult traditional healers, and movement between these parallel systems often results in late presentation of disease.

Life/oral histories

Maureen Butterfield—*founder, Island Hospice and Bereavement Service, Harare*: interviewed by Jennifer Hunt, 7 June 2003. Length of interview: 30 min.

Maureen Butterfield tells how she heard of the hospice ideal from a young nurse who was caring for her daughter, Frances. At that time, she did not understand what she heard but, after Frances died, she visited St Christopher's while staying with friends in the UK. On her return to Rhodesia (as Zimbabwe was then called), Maureen Butterfield attended a conference run by the Compassionate Friends and determined to found a hospice in her own country. She received strong support from her friend, John McMaster, who helped her to plan and establish Zimbabwe's first hospice service. After 7 years involvement, Maureen Butterfield moved to South Africa and no longer has any 'hands on' experience. Nevertheless, she holds firmly to the belief that the value of the hospice approach is in the integration of the physical and psychological aspects of care, combined with good communication and a focus on both the patient and the family. In the context of a wounded and divided Africa, she considers this approach has a special appropriateness and lasting significance.

Sambulo Mkwananzi (1)—*training manager, Island Hospice and Bereavement Service, Harare; board member APCA*: interviewed by David Clark, 4 July 2004. Length of interview: 13 min.

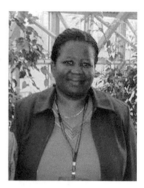

Sambulo Mkwananzi trained as a nurse at Lancaster Royal Infirmary (UK) and, after subsequent training as a health visitor, worked in London for the next 11 years. She moved to Zimbabwe in 1994 and took up a post at the Ministry of Health that focused on palliative care training and awareness raising in partnership with Island Hospice; eventually, she moved to Island Hospice as training manager. She was invited to attend the conference that led to the Cape Town Declaration, and became a member of the APCA steering committee, later to be elected to the board. Speaking after the inaugural meeting of APCA in Arusha (2004), she tells of her enthusiasm for the new organization and the challenges for the future,

Sambulo Mkwananzi (2)—*training manager, Island Hospice and Bereavement Service, Harare; board member APCA*: interviewed by Michael Wright, 20 September 2004. Length of interview (with Eunice Garanganga): 45 min.

Sambulo Mkwananzi speaks of her role at Island Hospice and of the challenges facing the hospice movement in Zimbabwe. Due to the AIDS pandemic, more people are seeking help to care for sick relatives and great demands are made on the education and training service. She speaks of the drain on resources caused by professionals who are themselves ill, and of the loss of trained staff to better paying organizations. In partnership with HOSPAZ, the hospice focuses on the training needs of rural communities where relatives care for family members with few resources. Turning to spiritual issues, she speaks of the African perspective, of the place of the ancestors in indigenous beliefs, and of the importance of being welcomed into the next world by those who have

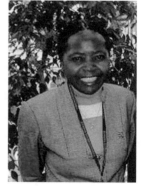

gone before, a belief which brings a sense of peacefulness to many. Ritual is frequently required and it is important to be aware of its meaning to individuals and families. In essence, the hospice acknowledges the belief systems of those who are being cared for. Finally, she tells how the hospice is working with other agencies such as the Red Cross to provide much needed services to the poor in rural areas.

Eunice Garanganga—*clinical and technical adviser, Hospice Association of Zimbabwe (HOSPAZ)*: interviewed by Michael Wright, 20 September 2004. Length of interview (with Sambulo Mkwananzi): 45 min.

Eunice Garanganga worked in an Accident and Emergency Department before joining Island Hospice in 1986. Once she began to care for patients, the work became more than a job and she has been involved with hospice ever since. Due to the late presentation of patients and the ravages of AIDS, she tells how palliative care is needed from the point of diagnosis. As the needs of the patients increase, however, international funding has decreased due to the place of Zimbabwe on the world stage. Of the 17 rural branches of Island Hospice that operated in the late 1980s, she considers that nine offer a service today but only four are fully functional. She speaks of the disparity of home-based care, from services that offer only prayer to those which provide 'hands on' care; in this context, the need for training and standards is seen to be paramount. Finally, she speaks of collaboration with traditional healers, of the place of herbal medicines and the cultural need to maintain hope rather than prepare people for death.

Public health context

Population

Zimbabwe's population of 12.84 million (2002) is 98 per cent African (Shona 82 per cent, Ndebele 14 per cent) and < 1 per cent aqre white. Around 50 per cent of the population subscribes to syncretic religion (part Christian, part indigenous beliefs); 25 per cent are Christian; 24 per cent hold indigenous beliefs; and 1 per cent are Muslim.

Epidemiology

In Zimbabwe, the WHO World Health Report (2004) indicates an adult mortality[42] rate per 1000 population of 821 for males and 789 for females. Life expectancy for males is 37.7; for females 38.0. Healthy life expectancy is 33.8 for males; and 33.3 for females.[43]

Predictions suggest that life expectancy will fall further in the coming years—from a life expectancy of 56 in early 1970s.[44] This fall is mainly attributable to the soaring AIDS death rates.

Most patients present with advanced disease having tried alternative herbal treatments or traditional healers.[27]

A 1995 survey[45] classified 45 per cent of Zimbabwean households as 'very poor' with an income below the level of subsistence. Around 70 per cent of Zimbabweans reside in rural areas and it is these areas which have the highest percentage of poverty, estimated at 71 per cent of households. The high cost of rented accommodation exacerbates the over-crowding in high-density areas, contributing to the spread of communicable diseases. Throughout Zimbabwe, the incidence of suicide, mental illness, child abuse and domestic violence is on the increase.[46]

In hospitals, the major causes of death include TB, malaria and respiratory infections. The Ministry of Health prioritizes diseases in its National Health Strategy 1997–2007, where HIV/AIDS, sexually transmitted diseases and TB head the list above malaria and reproductive diseases.

Zimbabwe is one of the worst HIV/AIDS-affected countries in Southern Africa. Estimates suggest that in Zimbabwe, between 1.5 and 2 million people were living with

Table 9.5 Zimbabwe HIV and AIDS estimates, end 2003

Adult (15–49) HIV prevalence rate	24.6 per cent (range: 21.7–27.8 per cent)
Adults (15–49) living with HIV	1 600 000 (range: 1 400 000–1 900 000)
Adults and children (0–49) living with HIV	1 800 000 (range: 1 500 000–2 000 000)
Women (15–49) living with HIV	930 000 (range: 820 000–1 000 000)
AIDS deaths (adults and children) in 2003	170 000 (range: 130 000–230 000)

Source: 2004 Report on the global AIDS epidemic

HIV/AIDS at the end of 2003. In the same year, up to 230 000 adults and children are thought to have died from the disease (Table 9.5).

UNAIDS reports:

> There are considerable discrepancies in HIV prevalence rates according to geographical location, age and sex. Young women and those living in semi-urban growth points, mining areas and commercial farms are most vulnerable.
>
> In 1987, the National AIDS Coordination Programme (NACP) was established to lead the national response. In 1999, the National AIDS Policy and National Strategic Framework 1999–2004 were launched, followed by an Act of Parliament that established a multisectoral National AIDS Council (NAC) in 2000.
>
> In 1999, Zimbabwe became the first country in the world to introduce a 3% levy on all taxable income to finance HIV/AIDS activities. By December 2003, approximately US$2 million had been raised through the AIDS levy and about US$1 million has been disbursed and utilized.
>
> Civil society and the private sector are playing an important role in the national response. Most donor support for prevention mitigation and home-based care is channelled though NGOs. In 2004, it was estimated that external assistance to the Zimbabwean HIV/AIDS response amounted to about US$60 million, significantly less than aid provided to some neighbouring countries.
>
> The government, together with the NAC, has set aside US$600 000 in 2003 and US$2.5 million in 2004 solely for the procurement of antiretroviral drugs, while external donor funding for antiretroviral drugs has remained very limited. Only 5000 persons (less than 1% of those eligible) are currently on antiretroviral drugs in Zimbabwe.
>
> Zimbabwe is currently ineligible for financial assistance from the IMF and World Bank because of debt arrears, nor is Zimbabwe a PEPFAR focus country.[47]

Health care system

Post-independence saw a rapid increase in education and health facilities in rural areas, but developments were threatened by increasing demands on the health sector and dwindling government health expenditure. Nevertheless, it is estimated that 85 per cent of the population live within 8 km of a health facility.[48]

WHO recognizes the following strengths and opportunities in Zimbabwe:[49]

- Training of hospice workers and community volunteers
- Integration of palliative care into the mainstream health care system
- Oncology and HIV/AIDS policies (developed as early as 1992)
- Publication of guidelines, training manuals and booklets on the care of the terminally ill
- The community home-based care policy launched in 2001.

Concernscentre on:

- Lack of support for home-based care patients
- Lack of access to national AIDS levy for AIDS patients
- Procurement and distribution of drugs
- Implementation of an effective policy on morphine
- Lack of resources and inadequate equipment
- Staff recruitment, motivation and retention.

In 2001, the total per capita expenditure on health care was Intl $142; 6.2% of GDP[50] (Appendix 3).

The WHO overall health system performance score places Zimbabwe 155th out of 191 countries.[51]

Political economy

Independence was gained from Britain after around 90 years of colonization and from minority white rule in 1980 after a protracted war of liberation.[52] During the 1990s, a combination of high inflation, an expanding population and illnesses related to HIV/AIDS threatened the achievements of immediate post-independence. The introduction of the Economic Structural Adjustment Programme (ESAP) designed to protect the social sector, resulted in a harsh economic reality for many Zimbabweans. At the end of 2003, inflation was estimated at around 600 per cent.[53,54]

The country's political, economic and social instability over the past decade has exacerbated the devastation caused by recurrent droughts and the AIDS epidemic. Imports are limited, and even basic commodities such as over-the-counter drugs, cotton wool and bandages are either unavailable or beyond the reach of most.

GDP per capita is Intl $2271 (Appendix 4).

References

1 WHO. The World Health Report 2004.
2 Report of the United Nations Development Programme 2004 (HDI 2002). Launched by the United Nations in 1990, the Human Development Index measures a country's achievements in three aspects of human development: longevity, knowledge and a decent standard of living. It was created to re-emphasize that people and their lives should be the ultimate criteria for assessing the development of a country, not economic growth. Current values range from 0.956 (Norway, first out of

177 countries) to 0.273 (Sierra Leone, 177th out of 177 countries). Countries fall into one of three groups: countries 1–55 = high development; 56–141 = medium development; 142–177 = low development. See: http://hdr.undp.org/statistics/data/indic/indic_8_1_1.html

3 Personal communication: Sithokozile Masunye, Edward Chigodoro and Gift Sibanda—25 March 2004.

4 Personal communication: Sr Onya Cunliffe—23 March 2004.

5 FACT, see: http://www.schwabfound.org/schwabentrepreneurs.htm?schwabid=298

6 See: http://site.mweb.co.zw/islandhospice/

7 Personal communication: Sr Daphne Clarke—25 March 2004.

8 Personal communication: John and Diana Russell—31 January 2004.

9 Personal communication: Sr Nehwati—31 March 2004.

10 Mashambanzou Care Trust, see: http://www.ekhaya.org/zimbabwe/mashambanzou.html

11 Personal communication: Veronica Moss and Catherine O'Keefe—31 January 2004.

12 Personal communication: Dr Breugem—5 April 2004.

13 Personal communication: Veronica Kanyongo—19 March 2004.

14 Personal communication: Almah Mangena —24 May 2004.

15 **Anne Lloyd Williams**. *Report on Visit to Zimbabwe, October 2002.*

16 WHO report: Community Health Approach to Palliative Care for HIV/AIDS Patients, 2004: 19–20. Available to download at: http://whqlibdoc.who.int/publications/2004/9241591498.pdf

17 For USAID non-food assistance to Zimbabwe see: http://www.zimrelief.info/index.php?sectid=5

18 International Narcotics Control Board. *Narcotic Drugs: Estimated World Requirements for 2004. Statistics for 2002.* New York: United Nations, 2004.

19 'The term *defined daily doses for statistical purposes* (S-DDD) replaces the term *defined daily doses* previously used by the Board. The S-DDDs are technical units of measurement for the purposes of statistical analysis and are not recommended prescription doses. Certain narcotic drugs may be used in certain countries for different treatments or in accordance with different medical practices, and therefore a different daily dose could be more appropriate'. The S-DDD used by the INCB for morphine is 100 mg. International Narcotics Control Board. *Narcotic Drugs: Estimated World Requirements for 2004. Statistics for 2002.* New York: United Nations, 2004: 176–177.

20 Personal communication: Pardon Muyambo—19 March 2004.

21 Personal communication: Carla Lamadora—13 November 2003.

22 African Hospice Foundation News, December 2003.

23 This is the second phase of the South Africa AIDS Training programme which has assisted in improving the capacities of community organizations in Southern Africa to develop effective and efficient programmes for those most vulnerable to HIV/AIDS. See the Canadian International Development Agency website at http://www.acdi-cida.gc.ca/cida_ind.nsf/0/3579da86ef71bbf9852565c9006915ec?OpenDocument

24 IOELC interview: Sambulo Mkwananzi—20 September 2004.

25 See: **Hunt J.** The nine-cell bereavement table: a tool for training. *Bereavement Care* 2002; **21**(3): 40–41.

26 A temporary home.

27 See: **Munodawafa A.** Zimbabwe. In: Ferrell B, Coyle N (ed.), *Textbook of Palliative Nursing.* New York; Oxford University Press, 2001: 718–726

28 See: **Levy L.** Communication with the cancer patient in Zimbabwe. In: Surbane A, Zwitter M (ed.), *Communication with the Cancer Patient. Information and Truth.* New York: The New York Academy of Sciences, 1997: 133–141

29 IOELC interview: Maureen Butterfield—7 June 2003.

30 See: **Jennifer Hunt** From Micro to Macro. A Comparative Analysis of Views on how India and Zimbabwe use the British Hospice Model. Unpublished MA Dissertation: Reading University (UK), 2003.

31 **McElvaine D.** Zimbabwe: the Island Hospice experience. In: Saunders C, Kastenbaum R (eds), *Hospice Care on the International Scene.* New York: Springer Publishing Company, 1997: 52–53.

32 **Donne J.** *Devotions upon Emergent Occasions.* New York: Vintage Books, 1999.

33 **Stjernswärd J**, Clark D. Palliative medicine—a global perspective. In: Doyle D, Hanks G, Cherney N, Chalman K (ed.), *Oxford Textbook of Palliative Medicine,* 3rd edn. Oxford: Oxford University Press, 2003: 1199–1224.

34 **Williams S.** Global perspective: Zimbabwe. *Palliative Medicine* 2000; **14**: 225.

35 **Rona Martin**: speech delivered at the celebrations marking the 25th anniversary of Island Hospice—22 January 2004.

36 **Anon.** International Perspective. Island hospice and Bereavement Service (Island) hits a quarter century 'not out' in 2004. *Progress in Palliative Care* 2004; **12**(1): 30–31.

37 Mashambanzou Care Trust, see: http://www.ekhaya.org/zimbabwe/mashambanzou.html

38 Personal communication: Veronica Moss and Catherine O'Keefe—31 January 2004.

39 Personal communication: Val Maarsdorp—10 November 2003

40 Personal communication: Veronica Kanyongo—19 March 2004.

41 IOELC interview: Eunice Garanganga—20 September 2004.

42 This refers to adult mortality risk, which is defined as the probability of dying between 15 and 59 years.

43 See: WHO statistics for Zimbabwe: http://www.who.int/countries/zwe/en//

44 **Larry Elliott**. The lost decade. *The Guardian*, 9 July 2003.

45 1995 Poverty Alleviation Survey (PASS) cited in National Health Strategy for Zimbabwe 1997–2007.

46 Ministry of Health and Child Welfare, Zimbabwe. *National Health Strategy for Zimbabwe 1997–2007.* Harare: Government Printer, 1999: 54–56.

47 See: http://www.unaids.org/en/geographical+area/by+country/zimbabwe.asp

48 Foundation for Hospices in Sub-Saharan Africa, see: http://www.fssa.org

49 WHO report: Community Health Approach to Palliative Care for HIV/AIDS Patients, 2004: 21. Available to download at: http://whqlibdoc.who.int/publications/2004/9241591498.pdf

50 Total health expenditure per capita is the per capita amount of the sum of Public Health Expenditure (PHE) and Private Expenditure on Health (PvtHE). The international dollar is a common currency unit that takes into account differences in the relative purchasing power of various currencies. Figures expressed in international dollars are calculated using purchasing power parities (PPP), which are rates of currency conversion constructed to account for differences in price level between countries. http://www3.who.int/whosis/country/compare.cfm?country=s&indicator=strPcTotEOHinIntD2000&language=english

51 This composite measure of overall health system attainment1 is based on a country's goals relating to health, responsiveness and fairness in financing. The measure varies widely across countries and is highly correlated with general levels of human development as captured in the human development index. Tandon A, Murray CLJ, Lauer JA, Evans DB. *Measuring Overall Health system Performance for 191 Countries.* GPE Discussion Paper Series: No. 30; WHO.

52 See: Herbst J. Zimbabwe. In: Lipset S (ed.), *The Encyclopedia of Democracy.* London: Routledge, 1995, Vol. IV.

53 The Jewel Bank. The financial world: inflation. *Zimbabwe Independent*, 5 to 11 December 2003: 1.

54 **Rachel Smith**. As Zimbabwe shops with stolen cash, millions starve. *The Independent*, 23 December 2003.

Part 4

Hospice–palliative care service development in Africa: countries with localized provision

We identified 11 countries with localized hospice–palliative care provision (Fig. 1). Countries in this category are characterized by: the development of a critical mass of activists in one or more locations; the establishment of a hospice–palliative care service—often linked to home-based care; the growth of local support; the sourcing of funding; the availability of morphine; and the provision of training by the hospice organization.

This group of countries comprises: Botswana, Republic of the Congo (Congo-Brazzaville), Egypt, Malawi, Morocco, Nigeria, Sierra Leone, Swaziland, Tanzania, The Gambia and Zambia. We report on each of these countries in turn.

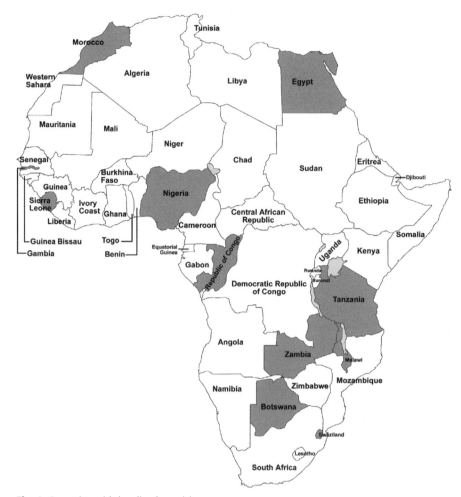

Fig. 1 Countries with localized provision.

Botswana

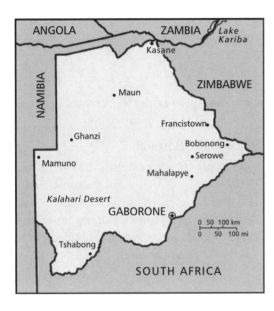

Botswana (population 1.77 million) is a landlocked country in Southern Africa that covers an area of 600 000 km². Its boundaries border Zambia, Zimbabwe, South Africa, Namibia and Angola. Formerly the British protectorate of Bechuanaland, Botswana adopted its new name on independence in 1966. The economy, one of the most robust on the continent, is dominated by diamond mining.

According to the United Nations human development index (HDI), Botswana is ranked 128th out of 177 countries worldwide (value 0.589)[1] and 10th out of 45 in African countries for which an index is available. This places Botswana in the group of countries with medium human development.

Palliative care service provision

Current services

Botswana is in the unusual position of being an African country that is not financially resource poor. It is poor, however, in specialized human resources, and notably in the field of palliative care.

In Botswana, 10 palliative care services are delivered by three organizations: Holy Cross Hospice, Gaborone; Ramotswa Hospice at Home; and the Light and Courage Centre, Francistown (Table 10.1).

Holy Cross Hospice

This faith-based organization was founded in 1994 as a day care centre and to provide home-based care in response to the AIDS epidemic. It now offers home-based services,

Table 10.1 Palliative care provision in Botswana, 2004

	Free-standing unit	Hospital unit	Hospital support team	Home care	Day care	Clinic/drop-in centre	Total
Holy Cross Hospice, Gaborone				1	1	1	3
Ramotswa Hospice at Home, Ramotswa	1			1	1	1	4
Light and Courage Centre, Francistown				1	1	1	3
Total services	1			3	3	3	10

day care for adults and orphans, and includes a drop-in centre for patients. In March 2004, 30 adults and seven orphans were registered with the day care centre.

Ramotswa Hospice at Home (Bamalete Lutheran Hospital)

The hospice was founded in 1992, initially to provide day care for the elderly and chronically ill. It soon became used for HIV-positive patients and for some cancer patients. The hospice operates a home-based care service, offering nursing and counselling to approximately 48 patients at any one time. Daily respite care is available when necessary. A day care centre operates twice weekly where patients are fed; they can also partake in occupational pursuits such as beadwork and sewing.

Light and Courage Centre

The service was established as a day care centre in 1998 by the Francistown Multisectoral AIDS Committee as a response to the growing AIDS crisis. The Centre had, by September 2003, provided day care and support to >210 registered clients who have an AIDS-defining illness. Those who are asymptomatic are able to access information and counselling, but are not considered as day care clients. A maximum of 40 clients at any one time receive holistic care from this faith-based organization. Home visits are limited to those who would normally attend the day centre but are too unwell.

In its project report 2004, WHO noted that Botswana's strengths lay in factors such as: the community home-based care programme; policies already in place (for care and support, for ARVs); and the commitment of government. Weakness included: the lack of trained human resources; lack of understanding of palliative care among health providers; inadequate capacity to train for palliative care; shortage of health professionals and social workers; increased burden of care/burn-out among caregivers; and an inadequate number of hospices, halfway houses and day care centres. Crucially, the report states:

> Botswana has relatively more resources and better health infrastructure than the other countries involved in this project, but has not reached a health status in accordance with its level of resources.[2]

Reimbursement and funding for services

Holy Cross Hospice has received funding from community donations, international organizations and embassies—NORAD, Norwegian Church Aids and the US Embassy, as well as a grant from the Botswana government. A 2-year grant was provided by the Bristol Myers Foundation (2001–2003) to develop core services and systems. All services are free.

Ramotswa Hospice at Home depends for its funding on the hospital to which it is attached; that in turn obtains faith-based funds for its operations and receives contributions from the Botswana government. All donations for the hospice are channelled through the hospital administration. Services are provided free to patients.

Light and Courage Centre is supported by a large number of donations from individuals, local businesses and international donors. The centre has mainly been dependent on government funding and commits to fulfil government economic and social policies. Major donors include the Francistown City Council (children's programme), UNAIDS (income generation), the government of New Zealand (printing costs), the government of Japan (vehicle), Skillshare Africa (staff costs) and the government of Botswana–African Comprehensive HIV/AIDS Partnerships/Botswana Network of AIDS Service Organizations (general running expenses and equipment).

President's Emergency Plan for AIDS Relief (PEPFAR)

During the 2004 financial year (FY), funding of around US$17.88 million was enacted for country-managed programmes in Botswana and US$6.51 million for central programmes. During FY2005, it is anticipated that a total of US$43.10 million will be enacted: US$35.33 million for country-managed programmes and US$7.74 million for central programmes.[3]

Opioid availability and consumption

The International Narcotics Control Board[4] has published the following figures for the consumption of narcotic drugs in Botswana: codeine 3 kg; morphine 1 kg; pethidine 2 kg.

For the years 2000–2002, the average defined daily dose consumption of morphine for statistical purposes (S-DDD)[5] in Botswana was 22 (Appendix 1).

Since 2002, morphine has been used in the adult oncology ward at the Princess Marina Hospital, yet pain control in the general health system is limited to pethidine- and paracetamol-based treatments. Syringe drivers are not common.

Holy Cross Hospice provides some medications for its patients. Only mild analgesics (paracetamol) are used for pain relief.

Light and Courage Centre is supportive of ARV therapy but does not offer opioid treatments.

Ramotswa Hospice has a weekly visit from the hospital doctor who prescribes morphine as necessary.

National and professional organizations

African Comprehensive HIV/AIDS Partnerships (ACHAP)

This is a joint initiative between the Government of Botswana, the Bill & Melinda Gates Foundation and the Merck Company Foundation/Merck & Co., Inc. to prevent and treat HIV/AIDS in Botswana through a public–private partnership. ACHAP's focus is to support the goals of the government to decrease HIV incidence and significantly increase the rate of diagnosis and treatment of HIV/AIDS in Botswana by rapidly advancing prevention programmes, health care access, patient management and treatment of HIV. The partnership was formally announced on 10 July 2000. Both donor foundations are dedicating US$50 million over 5 years towards the project. Merck also donates two antiretroviral medicines for the treatment programmes.[6]

Botswana Network of AIDS Service Organizations (BONASO)

Non-governmental and community-based organizations are invited to submit proposals to BONASO for review. BONASO assists in identifying innovative grass roots level ideas that may be scaled up or adopted in other communities.

There is no national hospice/palliative care body in Botswana and there are no known twinning arrangements.

Palliative care coverage

Holy Cross Hospice covers three areas around Gaborone: Tlokweng, Old Naledi and urban Gaborone (population ~300 000).

Ramotswa Hospice serves the Ramotswa area only (population 25 700).

Light and Courage Centre services Francistown (population 100 000).

Education and training

Ministry of Health/WHO

A palliative care conference was hosted in Gaborone in 2002.

Ministry of Health/ACHAP

The national ARV programme was launched in January 2002; 11 sites are currently operational with a further 21 planned to be active by the end of 2004. A programme offering training for home-based care programmes is run by the Ministry, and implemented by the city councils. These services are not considered palliative care.

Holy Cross Hospice

This hospice does not provide training. Training of volunteers was undertaken by a trainer from South Africa. Bristol Myers funding helped develop a model which may be used to train more volunteers. Palliative care knowledge is obtained from the limited literature resources that are currently available.

Light and Courage Centre

The centre provides training and education not only to its own clients and their care-givers, but also to members of the community to reduce the stigma associated with AIDS. Community members are educated in issues relating to HIV/AIDS through presentations and workshops at schools, public awareness campaigns, and through the drop-in service available to all members of the public wanting information and advice. Training in crafts is provided for patients and family carers. A teacher provided by the Ministry of Education offers literacy lessons for clients. Computer lessons have been offered by a volunteer Methodist Minister who has since joined the staff.

Ramotswa Hospice at Home

Staff have received training in monitoring ARV treatments by the Ministry of Health and ACHAP. One member of staff attended a terminal care nursing and bereavement course in Swaziland in September 1994. No other hospice or hospital member of staff has any palliative care training. There is some sharing of knowledge with occasional vis-its to hospices in South Africa. Training of volunteers and caregivers is done by the staff.

African Comprehensive HIV/AIDS Partnerships

HIV/AIDS sector staff have been trained in project management, proposal writing, monitoring and evaluation by ACHAP which provides the National AIDS Coordinating Agency (NACA) with financial, logistical, technical and administrative support.

Palliative care workforce capacity

Holy Cross Hospice

Full-time staff include: one director/health administrator; three nurses; one day care manager (nurse trained); two social workers; three drivers; one accounts officer; one receptionist; one administrative assistant; and one cleaner. In addition, there are two volunteer doctors who attend the clinic at the day centre and are on call for advice. Fifteen volunteers work 5 days a week from 8.00 am to 1.00 pm in the centre kitchen and in the community. They receive a stipend for this work.

Light and Courage Centre

The centre is headed by one co-ordinator assisted by two nurses/development workers who are responsible for the day-to-day operations of the centre and the medical assess-ment of the clients. There is a financial administrator. A social worker helps to assess clients and links with clinic social workers to provide practical needs for clients. Other staff include: a driver/general assistant; a welfare educator; a craft teacher; a cook; an assistant cook/cleaner; and a gardener.

Ramotswa Hospice at Home

Staff salaries are paid by the Bamalete Lutheran Hospital (BLH) that receives a grant from the government of Botswana. All staff are full time and comprise: one administrator/principal registered nurse; one administrative assistant/family nurse practitioner; two SRNs/counsellors; one SRN at the day centre; one registered nurse/counsellor; and one cleaner. A hospital-based doctor is scheduled to attend the day care clinic each Thursday. There are 12 volunteers working with the home-based team and three volunteers working at the hospice centre; all are part time and receive a stipend. Hospice staff rotate throughout the hospital and are not permanently located at the hospice.

History and development of hospice–palliative care in Botswana

Botswana's public health system coped effectively with most of the basic health needs of the nation until the HIV/AIDS epidemic hit the country. Specialist oncology treatments, including radiotherapy and chemotherapy, were introduced by the private sector as late as 1999. Two years later (2001), the first oncology ward was opened at Princess Marina Hospital. There are no official cancer statistics, but experienced health professionals estimate the most common cancers to be Kaposi's sarcoma and cancers of the cervix, prostate, lung, breast and head and neck.[7,8]

Despite Botswana's dynamic and aggressive approach to treating AIDS, there are gaps in the field of palliative care provision for patients living with other terminal conditions. The Ministry of Health does not provide palliative care support for people dying from cancers, AIDS and other illnesses, although there are signs of increasing interest in this field. Whilst effective pain control with the use of morphine was introduced into the adult oncology ward in 2001, pain control in the health system is limited.

Ideas of witchcraft are common and are generally directed at women—who are often blamed for the death of a husband or relative. Cultural understandings identify an external cause of an illness. For example, cancer of the oesophagus is attributed to eating something that has caused choking. Use of both traditional and allopathic care is common.

Holy Cross Hospice

In 1994, concerned members of the community, the Anglican Church and Dr Moffat (Superintendent of Princess Marina Hospital and an Anglican priest) drafted a constitution to establish an organization which it was hoped would address the growing threat of AIDS in Gaborone. In October 1995, the registered Holy Cross Hospice established itself on donated land. An Australian nurse, sponsored by the Episcopalian Church in the USA and linked to the Anglican Church in Botswana, was the first nurse at the hospice. She networked with the clinics and the Princess Marina Hospital and accompanied doctors on their rounds in the community. Terminally ill patients were referred to the centre. NORAD donated a vehicle to enable home-based care to be delivered. Language was a barrier, however, and soon afterwards a Botswanan nurse was employed. Gradually, more staff were employed and local volunteers began to help in the kitchen and by sewing and craft-making. At that time, about 10 patients were registered, mainly suffering from symptomatic HIV. Volunteers from the Anglican Church in the UK also offered practical help.

Funding has been a constant problem, and several nurses have resigned due to poor salaries. 'Nurses were paid less than government hospitals, and as it's a stressful job anyway there was little incentive to stay'.[9] The service now sustains a drop-in centre, day care centre and home-based care. It continues to look after children orphaned by the deaths of either or both parent(s) who were registered hospice patients.

Light and Courage Centre

In 1998, in response to the ever-increasing number of infected individuals in Francistown, the Light and Courage Centre was established by the Francistown Multisectoral AIDS Committee (DMSAC) as a day centre to provide support and information to community members infected and affected by HIV/AIDS. The roots of the present centre lie with the appointment of Angelina Magaga as Acting Co-ordinator in March 2000 and the arrival in July 2000 of Olwen Donald as nurse/development worker.

In May 2001, the facilities were handed over to the Light and Courage Centre Trust, a community-based organization managed by a Board of Trustees drawn from both the business sector and the wider community of Francistown (Deed of Trust No. 482 /2000 dated 30 November 2000). DMSAC, however, is still responsible for the co-ordination of all HIV/AIDS activities and is therefore still involved with, and supportive of, the centre.[10]

The centre is mindful of the increasing number of persons who could benefit from its services—and that it is the only one of its kind in Francistown. The organization, therefore, is in the process of acquiring more land and extending its facilities to expand its programme.

Ramotswa Hospice at Home

Christa Kiebelstein, a nurse who worked with the Bamalete Lutheran Hospital, and Dr Ian Kennedy shared a vision of establishing a hospice at the hospital. The latter was the medical superintendent at the hospital and, according to Kiebelstein, 'has been shaping the medical landscape in Botwana during his 30 years service as MO.[11]

The Matron of the hospital at that time was Johanna Kalake. 'She played a very important part as Matron of the BLH at Ramotswa in getting the hospice on the way. She has retired as Matron, but lives in Ramotswa just near the Bamalete Lutheran Hospital. She is now 64 years old, but still working at a clinic of the District Council.'[11]

This hospice started by caring for the elderly and chronically ill, but was rapidly adapted to providing care for HIV-positive patients as well. Cancer patients comprise a significant proportion of the registered patients. The hospital provides the referral system for the hospice. Patients who have incurable cancer or who have been diagnosed HIV positive are advised to go to the hospice, situated in the grounds of the hospital. The main focus is on home care, although those who require facilities and care unavailable at home are brought daily for respite care. Baths, medical care, occupational interests and rehydration are available.

Hospice success stories

Holy Cross Hospice

Hospice staff believe it is successful in helping people cope with their chronic illnesses by helping them accept their condition.

Light and Courage Centre

The centre lists several achievements including capacity building and efficient operating systems. The organization's networking relationships ensure good community coverage. Patients have been helped to return to productive and economically viable activities, and the centre believes it has been instrumental in reducing stigma and discrimination for AIDS patients. Craft activities augment income generation, and the drop-in centre is regarded as an effective means of disseminating information to the population. Significantly, the holistic model is replicated by other organizations which recognize its value.

Ramotswa Hospice

At Ramotswa Hospice, success lies in the continuity of care provided. Bereavement support is offered after the death of the patient, particularly when children are involved. Helping patients adhere to their ARV programme brings great rewards. 'Many people are recovering, that's why we have a very small number of patients here at the moment—because a lot of them have recovered and they have gone back to work'.[12]

Public health context

Population

Botswana has an estimated population of 1.77 million of which 85 per cent subscribe to indigenous beliefs and 15 per cent are Christian.

Epidemiology

In Botswana, the WHO World Health Report (2003) indicates an adult mortality[13] rate per 1000 population of 786 for males and 745 for females. Life expectancy for males is 40.2; for females 40.6. Healthy life expectancy is 36.0 for males; and 35.4 for females.[14]

In a report (2004)[15] that focuses on a community health approach to palliative care in five African countries, the WHO noted that the prevalence of HIV/AIDS in adults is higher in Botswana (38.8 per cent in 2002) than other project countries (Ethiopia, Tanzania, Uganda and Zimbabwe). The prevalence of HIV/AIDS, however, is higher in the other four countries than most countries in the world. In the project countries, Kaposi's sarcoma is among the most common cancers because of its association with AIDS. Head and neck cancer and lymphoma are common in males and, like most developing countries, the most common cancers in females are cancers of the cervix and breast.

At the end of 2003, UNAIDS suggested that up to 380 000 adults and children were living with HIV in Botswana, and that up 43,000 AIDS-related deaths had occurred during this year (Table 10.2).

Table 10.2 Country HIV and AIDS estimates, end 2003

Adult (15–49) HIV prevalence rate	37.3 per cent (range: 35.5–39.1 per cent)
Adults (15–49) living with HIV	330 000 (range: 310 000–340 000)
Adults and children (0–49) living with HIV	350 000 (range: 330 000–380 000)
Women (15–49) living with HIV	190 000 (range: 180 000–190 000)
AIDS deaths (adults and children) in 2003	33 000 (range: 25 000–43 000)

Source: UNAIDS 2004 report on the global AIDS epidemic.

UNAIDS reports:

> Since the first HIV/AIDS case diagnosis in 1985, the overall prevalence rate has risen dramatically. Surveillance results show a rise from 18.1% in 1992 to 35.7% in 1998 and 37.3% in 2003.
>
> In 2003, in more than two thirds of the country the prevalence was over 30%, and in over one third of the country it exceeded 40%. The highest prevalence is among 25–29 year old adults. Prevalence in the older age groups appears to be increasing, while prevalence among 15–19 year olds has remained fairly stable.
>
> The government, driven by the president's efforts, has put in place a strong multisectoral response through the National AIDS Council (NAC). The National AIDS Coordinating Agency (NACA) provides technical support to the NAC and coordinates the national response. Strong political commitment has led to the integration of HIV/AIDS into national development planning and budgeting (National Development Plan 9). The National Strategic Plan on HIV/AIDS (2003–2009) was developed to foster a broad-based mechanism to achieve an expanded multisectoral response.
>
> To effectively monitor and evaluate the response, the Botswana HIV Response Information Management System was developed. The system seeks to gather data from all levels of the response. Civil society and the private sector have become increasingly involved in the national response, and in 2003 the private sector coordination unit was set up by the NACA with key support from the UN and other development partners. The Country Coordinating Mechanism, originally established to manage the Global Fund resources, was mandated to manage additional donor funds, PEPFAR in particular.[16]

Health care system

In 2001, the total per capita expenditure on health care was Intl $381; 6.6% of GDP[17] (Appendix 3).

The WHO overall health system performance score places Botswana 169th out of 191 countries.[18]

Concluding the country report on Botswana, WHO note:

> The demand for palliative care services in Botswana is increasing—primarily due to the expanding HIV/AIDS epidemic and secondly due to chronic diseases, such as cancer. While current palliative care services have been found to be somewhat inadequate in this investigation, the gaps to be

bridged have been identified and the government of Botswana is committed to providing quality health care services to its entire population. The government has already established a suitable base for strengthening palliative care services by its primary health care delivery system, CHBC programme, national HIV/AIDS activities, National Drug Act, cancer management protocols, and strong partnership among the government, civil society and private sector.[19]

Political economy

GDP per capita is Intl $5747 (Appendix 4).

Botswana has maintained one of the world's highest growth rates since independence in 1966. Through fiscal discipline and sound management, Botswana has transformed itself from one of the poorest countries in the world to a middle-income country with a per capita GDP of US$8800 in 2003. Two major investment services rank Botswana as the best credit risk in Africa. Diamond mining has fuelled much of the expansion and currently accounts for more than one-third of GDP and for nine-tenths of export earnings. Tourism, subsistence farming and cattle raising are other key sectors. On the downside, the government must deal with high rates of unemployment and poverty. Unemployment officially is 21 per cent, but unofficial estimates place it closer to 40 per cent. HIV/AIDS infection rates are the highest in the world and threaten Botswana's impressive economic gains. Long-term prospects are overshadowed by the expected levelling off in diamond mining production.[20]

References

1   Report of the United Nations Development Programme, 2004 (HDI for 2002). Launched by the United Nations in 1990, the Human Development Index measures a country's achievements in three aspects of human development: longevity, knowledge and a decent standard of living. It was created to re-emphasize that people and their lives should be the ultimate criteria for assessing the development of a country, not economic growth. Current values range from 0.956 (Norway, first out of 177 countries) to 0.273 (Sierra Leone, 177th out of 177 countries). Countries fall into one of three groups: countries 1–55 = high development; 56–141 = medium development; 142–177 = low development. http://hdr.undp.org/statistics/data/indic/indic_8_1_1.html

2   WHO report: Community Health Approach to Palliative Care for HIV/AIDS Patients, 2004: 8. Available to download at: http://whqlibdoc.who.int/publications/2004/9241591498.pdf

3   *Engendering Bold Leadership*. The President's Emergency Plan for AIDS Relief. First Annual Report to Congress, 2005: 115. http://www.state.gov/documents/organization/43885.pdf

4   International Narcotics Control Board. *Narcotic Drugs: Estimated World Requirements for 2004. Statistics for 2002*. New York: United Nations, 2004.

5   'The term *defined daily doses for statistical purposes* (S-DDD) replaces the term *defined daily doses* previously used by the Board. The S-DDDs are technical units of measurement for the purposes of statistical analysis and are not recommended prescription doses. Certain narcotic drugs may be used in certain countries for different treatments or in accordance with different medical practices, and therefore a different daily dose could be more appropriate'. The S-DDD used by the INCB for morphine is 100 mg. International Narcotics Control Board. *Narcotic Drugs: Estimated World Requirements for 2004. Statistics for 2002*. New York: United Nations, 2004: 176–177.

6   Adapted from African Comprehensive HIV/AIDS Partnerships draft report: background information. Updated February 2003.

7 Personal communication: Dr Paleske—27 February 2004.

8 Personal communication: Sr Cecilia Tommy—29 February 2004.

9 Personal communication: Josephine Makate—24 February 2004.

10 Chairperson's report for general Meeting December 2000–September 2003.

11 Personal communication: Christa Kiebelstein—5 February 2004.

12 Personal communication: Katsetse Maruaeng—27 February 2004.

13 This refers to adult mortality risk, which is defined as the probability of dying between 15 and 59 years.

14 See: WHO statistics for Botswana at: http://www.who.int/countries/bwa/en/

15 WHO report: Community Health Approach to Palliative Care for HIV/AIDS Patients, 2004: 21. Available to download at: http://whqlibdoc.who.int/publications/2004/9241591498.pdf

16 See http://www.unaids.org/en/geographical+area/by+country/botswana.asp

17 Total health expenditure per capita is the per capita amount of the sum of Public Health Expenditure (PHE) and Private Expenditure on Health (PvtHE). The international dollar is a common currency unit that takes into account differences in the relative purchasing power of various currencies. Figures expressed in international dollars are calculated using purchasing power parities (PPP), which are rates of currency conversion constructed to account for differences in price level between countries. http://www3.who.int/whosis/country/compare.cfm?country=s&indicator=strPcTotEOHinIntD2000&language=english

18 This composite measure of overall health system attainment is based on a country's goals relating to health, responsiveness and fairness in financing. The measure varies widely across countries and is highly correlated with general levels of human development as captured in the human development index. Tandon A, Murray CLJ, Lauer JA, Evans DB. *Measuring Overall Health System Performance for 191 Countries*. GPE Discussion Paper Series: No. 30; WHO

19 WHO report: Community Health Approach to Palliative Care for HIV/AIDS Patients, 2004: 41. Available to download at: http://whqlibdoc.who.int/publications/2004/9241591498.pdf

20 See: http://www.cia.gov/cia/publications/factbook/geos/bc.htlm

Chapter 11

Republic of the Congo (Congo-Brazzaville)

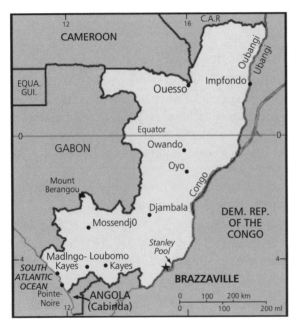

Republic of the Congo (population 2.99 million people) is a country in Western Africa, bordering the South Atlantic Ocean that covers an area of 342 000 km². Its boundaries border the countries of Gabon, Cameroon, Central African Republic, Democratic Republic of the Congo and Angola. The capital of Republic of the Congo is Brazzaville.

According to the United Nations human development index (HDI), Republic of the Congo is ranked 144th out of 177 countries worldwide (value 0.494)[1] and 15th out of 45 in African countries for which an index is available. This places Republic of the Congo in the group of countries with low human development.

Palliative care service provision

Current services

There appears to be just one hospice–palliative care organization operating in Congo-Brazzaville: L'Association Congolese Accompagner (ACA) (Table 11.1).[2]

ACA was founded in 1996 by Soeur Eliane Julienne Boukaka, of the Congregation Occiliatrise. ACA cares for incurably ill persons, particularly those with AIDS and cancer, and offers support in the hospital and in the home. About 50 persons are in the care of ACA on a given day.

Reimbursement and funding for services

ACA funding is mainly derived from the 100 volunteers who, as members of the association, give financial support each month. The service is free to patients at the point of delivery.

Table 11.1 Palliative care provision in the Republic of the Congo, 2004

	Free-standing unit	Hospital unit	Hospital support team	Home care	Day care	Clinic/drop-in centre	Total
L'Association Congolese Accompagner (ACA), Brazzaville			1	1			2

In 2005, the UK Forum for Hospice and Palliative Care Worldwide awarded a grant of US$2265 to Association Azur Developpement for a workshop on palliative care for HIV/AIDS patients.

Opioid availability and consumption

Obtaining supplies of appropriate drugs is the biggest challenge faced by the ACA service; these are either unavailable or too expensive. Some pain-relieving drugs are sent from an association called Les Amis de Brazzaville, based in France. Small amounts of morphine are sometimes available.

No figures were published by the International Narcotics Control Board[3] for the consumption of narcotic drugs in Congo (2002).

For the years 2000–2002, the average defined daily dose consumption of morphine for statistical purposes (S-DDD)[4] in Republic of the Congo was 0 (Appendix 1).

Palliative care coverage

ACA covers seven zones of the city of Brazzaville and is the only palliative care service in Congo.

Palliative care workforce capacity

ACA has a compliment of about 10 doctors and nurses and is supported by 100 volunteers.

History and development of hospice–palliative care in Congo-Brazzaville

See interview summary below for Sister Eliane Boukaka.

Hospice success stories

The principle successes reported are the sense of appreciation shown by the patients who are cared for and the rapport that is established with them.

Life/oral histories

Sister Eliane Boukaka—*L'Association Congolese Accompagner*: interviewed by David Clark, 4 June 2005, assisted by Marilene Filbet. Length of interview: 18 min.

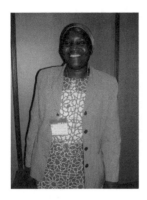

The Association started in Brazzaville in 1996, but the war of 1997 frustrated all efforts, until the work began again in 1999. The situation now is very difficult with few resources. Sister Eliane was struck by the loneliness of the patients and families, who are abandoned by physicians, and who have very poor pain control. The initiative began with 10 volunteers and now there are >100 volunteers, working in 12 teams, who follow the patients at home. The Association has volunteer help from some doctors and nurses who also assist in the management of the centre. The patients have no resources to pay. At the moment, the Association has no medications, and these are expensive to obtain in the pharmacy. The generic drugs can sometimes be obtained, including morphine. Members of the team sometimes buy drugs with their own resources. However, physicians need training in the use of morphine. Many patients are affected by HIV disease and are at home with no treatment, suffering from bed sores and numerous other problems. Visiting physicians are themselves burnt out and unable to provide medication and food, often feeling very useless. The Association has an ambition to open a hospice unit for palliative care with 10 beds, and is seeking support for this from international donors. There is also a great need for medications and other materials.

Public health context

Population

Republic of the Congo's population of around 2.99 million people is made up of the following ethnic groups: Kongo 48 per cent, Sangha 20 per cent, M'Bochi 12 per cent, Teke 17 per cent, Europeans and other 3 per cent.

Religious groups include: Christian 50 per cent, animist 48 per cent and Muslim 2 per cent.[5]

Epidemiology

In Republic of the Congo, the WHO World Health Report (2004) indicates an adult mortality[6] rate per 1000 population of 474 for males and 410 for females. Life expectancy for males is 51.6; for females 54.5. Healthy life expectancy is 45.3 for males; and 47.3 for females.[7]

Republic of the Congo is a country in Western Africa that has been severely affected by the HIV/AIDS epidemic. Estimates suggest that in Republic of the Congo, between 39 000 and 200 000 people were living with HIV/AIDS at the end of 2003. In the same year, up to 20 000 adults and children are thought to have died from the disease (Table 11.2).

UNAIDS reports:

> The Republic of the Congo is a post-conflict country that has been engaged in consistent development since 2003. It is classified by the World Bank among the countries with the lowest income (Global Fund guidelines 2004). The only significant prevalence study was undertaken between November and December 2003. Highly contrasting rates were observed around the country: 1.3%

Table 11.2 Republic of the Congo: HIV and AIDS estimates, end 2003

Adult (15–49) HIV prevalence rate	4.9 per cent (range: 2.1–11.0 per cent)
Adults (15–49) living with HIV	80 000 (range: 34 000–180 000)
Adults and children (0–49)living with HIV	90 000 (range: 39 000–200 000)
Women (15–49) living with HIV	45 000 (range: 19 000–100 000)
AIDS deaths (adults and children) in 2003	9700 (range: 4900–20 000)

Source: 2004 Report on the global AIDS epidemic.

in Impfondo and Djambala, 10.3% in Sibiti and 3.3% in Brazzaville. The Southern region has the highest rates: Sibiti, Dolisie (9.4%), Pointe-Noire (5.0%) and Madingou (4.7%). In general, adults over 30 years had the highest infection rate, almost 10% of 35–49 year old men, and 7% of women 25–39 years old are living with the disease. (National AIDS Committee [Comité National de Lutte contre le SIDA, CNLS] Study Centre for Public Health Development, CREDES, 2003). The National Strategic Framework (NSF) 2003–2007 was adopted in December 2002. The CNLS was officially launched by the head of state in July 2003. Congo held a resource mobilization meeting in July 2003. The MAP is being formulated and the country submitted a request to the fourth round of the Global Fund.

UNAIDS facilitated a joint visit by five heads of UN agencies (WHO, World Bank, UNICEF, UNDP, WFP) and the Country Coordinator to the minister in charge of coordinating governmental action, in order to address national HIV/AIDS issues. UNAIDS facilitated information sharing through feedback sessions following consultants' missions, the sharing of best practices documents, publications by all cosponsors, and oral presentations to large audiences for communicating the latest information on HIV/AIDS. UNAIDS supported the elaboration of a national strategic framework and sectoral and departmental operational plans. UNAIDS facilitated the organization of the resource mobilization round table, the development of the country Global Fund proposal, and participated in facilitating the achievement of the requirements for the country to benefit from MAP funding. PAF resources were utilized in collaboration with UNDP to develop and reinforce partnerships with religious bodies and associations of people living with HIV. UNAIDS and the World Bank are facilitating and supporting the NAC in developing a monitoring and evaluation system with the participation of all partners.[8]

Health care system

In 2001, the total per capita expenditure on health care was Intl $22; 2.1% of GDP[9] (Appendix 3).

The WHO overall health system performance score places Republic of the Congo 166th out of 191 countries.[10]

Political economy

After the September 1958 referendum approving the new French constitution, French Equatorial Africa was dissolved. Its four territories became autonomous members of the

French Community, and Middle Congo was renamed the Congo Republic. Formal independence was granted in August 1960.

In 1997, Congo's democratic progress was derailed due to tensions before the presidential elections scheduled for July that year. In early October, the Lissouba government fell. Soon thereafter, Sassou declared himself President and named a 33 member government. In January 1998, the Sassou regime held a National Forum for Reconciliation to determine the nature and duration of the transition period. The Forum, tightly controlled by the government, decided elections should be held in about 3 years, elected a transition advisory legislature, and announced that a constitutional convention would finalize a draft constitution. In November and December 1999, the government signed agreements with representatives of many, though not all, of the rebel groups. The December accord, mediated by President Omar Bongo of Gabon, called for follow-on, inclusive political negotiations between the government and the opposition. During the years 2000–2001, Sassou-Nguesso's government conducted a national dialogue (Dialogue Sans Exclusif), in which the opposition parties and the government agreed to continue on the path to peace. A new constitution was drafted in 2001, approved by the provisional legislature (National Transition Council), and approved by the people of Congo in a national referendum in January 2002. Presidential elections were held in March 2002, and Sassou-Nguesso was declared the winner. Legislative elections were scheduled for May and June 2002.[11] Southern-based rebel groups agreed to a final peace accord in March 2003.

The Republic of Congo is one of Africa's largest petroleum producers, with significant potential for offshore development. The economy is a mixture of village agriculture and handicrafts, and an industrial sector based largely on oil. Oil has supplanted forestry as the mainstay of the economy, providing a major share of government revenues and exports. In the early 1980s, rapidly rising oil revenues enabled the government to finance large-scale development projects, with GDP growth averaging 5 per cent annually, one of the highest rates in Africa. The 12 January 1994 devaluation of Franc Zone currencies by 50 per cent resulted in inflation of 61 per cent, but this has subsided since. Economic reform efforts continued with the support of international organizations, notably the World Bank and the IMF. In October 1997, Denis Sassou-Nguesso publicly expressed interest in moving forward on economic reforms and privatization and in renewing co-operation with international financial institutions. However, economic progress was badly hurt by slumping oil prices in December 1998, which worsened the republic's budget deficit. The current administration faces difficult economic problems of stimulating recovery and reducing poverty.[12]

GDP per capita is Intl $1936 (Appendix 4).

References

1 Report of the United Nations Development Programme 2004 (HDI 2002). Launched by the United Nations in 1990, the Human Development Index measures a country's achievements in three aspects of human development: longevity, knowledge and a decent standard of living. It was created to re-emphasize that people and their lives should be the ultimate criteria for assessing the development of a country, not economic growth. Current values range from 0.956 (Norway, first out of

177 countries) to 0.273 (Sierra Leone, 177th out of 177 countries). Countries fall into one of three groups: countries 1–55 = high development; 56–141 = medium development; 142–177 = low development. See: http://hdr.undp.org/statistics/data/indic/indic_8_1_1.html

2 Personal communication: Sr Kahaalena and Sr Eliane—21 April 2005.

3 International Narcotics Control Board. *Narcotic Drugs: Estimated World Requirements for 2004. Statistics for 2002.* New York: United Nations, 2004.

4 'The term *defined daily doses for statistical purposes* (S-DDD) replaces the term *defined daily doses* previously used by the Board. The S-DDDs are technical units of measurement for the purposes of statistical analysis and are not recommended prescription doses. Certain narcotic drugs may be used in certain countries for different treatments or in accordance with different medical practices, and therefore a different daily dose could be more appropriate'. The S-DDD used by the INCB for morphine is 100 mg. International Narcotics Control Board. *Narcotic Drugs: Estimated World Requirements for 2004. Statistics for 2002.* New York: United Nations, 2004: 176–177.

5 See: http://www.cia.gov/cia/publications/factbook/geos/cf.html

6 This refers to adult mortality risk, which is defined as the probability of dying between 15 and 59 years.

7 See: WHO statistics at: http://www.who.int/countries/cog/en/

8 http://www.unaids.org/en/geographical+area/by+country/congo.asp

9 Total health expenditure per capita is the per capita amount of the sum of Public Health Expenditure (PHE) and Private Expenditure on Health (PvtHE). The international dollar is a common currency unit that takes into account differences in the relative purchasing power of various currencies. Figures expressed in international dollars are calculated using purchasing power parities (PPP), which are rates of currency conversion constructed to account for differences in price level between countries. http://www3.who.int/whosis/country/compare.cfm?country=s&indicator=strPcTotEOHinIntD2000&language=english

10 This composite measure of overall health system attainment is based on a country's goals relating to health, responsiveness and fairness in financing. The measure varies widely across countries and is highly correlated with general levels of human development as captured in the human development index. Tandon A, Murray CLJ, Lauer JA, Evans DB. *Measuring Overall Health System Performance for 191 Countries.* GPE Discussion Paper Series: No. 30; WHO.

11 United States Government. *Background Notes to Countries of the World.* Washington DC: US Governmet, 2003.

12 http://www.cia.gov/cia/publications/factbook/geos/cf.html

Chapter 12

Egypt

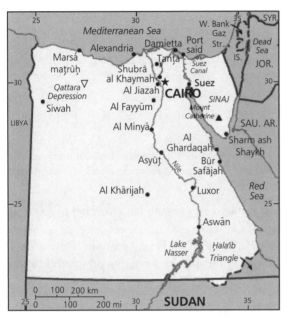

Egypt (population 76 117 421) is a country in Northern Africa which covers an area of 1 001 450 km², bordering the Mediterranean Sea, between Libya and the Gaza Strip, and the Red Sea north of Sudan, and includes the Asian Sinai Peninsula. Its boundaries border Israel, Libya, the Palestinian Authority Gaza Strip and Sudan.

The regularity and richness of the annual Nile River flood, coupled with semi-isolation provided by deserts to the east and west, allowed for the development of one of the world's great civilizations.

According to the United Nations human development index (HDI), Egypt is ranked 120th out of 177 countries worldwide (value 0.653).[1] This places Egypt in the group of countries with medium human development.

Palliative care service provision

Current services

In Egypt, it appears that supportive care with elements of hospice–palliative care may be linked to the development of other services. We have taken the view that where a service is in the process of development from (largely) physical care to a broader form of holistic care that approximates to the WHO definition of palliative care, then it should be included in our study.

In Egypt, three organizations provide hospice–palliative care services (Table 12.1).

The Cairo Evangelical Medical Society provides hospice facilities at the Cairo Evangelical Medical Hospital and at Elhadara Elromany, in Alexandria.

Table 12.1 Palliative care provision in Egypt 2005

	Free-standing unit	Hospital unit	Hospital support team	Home care	Day care	Clinic/drop-in centre	Total
Cairo Evangelical Medical Hospice	1			1		2	4
Elhadara Elromany, Alexandria	1						1
National Cancer Institute (NCI),Cairo University		1					1
Total services	2	1		1		2	6

Dr Naguib Elnikhaily reports on the services at Cairo Evangelical Medical Hospice, developed and opened in 2001/2002:

> At first there were four beds, now eleven; we have a waiting list, we may double the number of patients in each room. We also have a home care programme: 'Care with Love' and two outpatient clinics and are aiming for a day care service.[2]

In February 2005, inpatient numbers averaged 8–9. Naguib Elnikhaily has plans for up to three more projects in the south east of Cairo.[3]

The emphasis in government hospital oncology units is on pain relief. During 2004, however, palliative care became included in the oncology nursing programme at the National Cancer Institute (NCI).[4]

Reimbursement and funding for services

The NCI is a government-funded facility. An estimated 65 per cent of patients are treated free of charge; the remainder have health insurance which covers their treatment costs.

Cairo Evangelical Medical Hospice provides privately funded inpatient hospice and home care. Patients are required to cover their own costs, but fees are reportedly kept to a minimum.

Opioid availability and consumption

The International Narcotics Control Board[5] has published the following figures in 2002 for the consumption of narcotic drugs in Egypt: codeine 296 kg (down from 1983 kg in 1998); morphine 5 kg (down from 12 kg in 2000); pethidine 87 kg (up from 30 kg in 1999).

For the years 2000–2002, the average defined daily dose consumption of morphine for statistical purposes (S-DDD)[6] in Egypt was 2 (Appendix 1).

National and professional organizations

Although there are many NGOs involved in general health care in Egypt, currently none are dedicated to palliative care.

National Cancer Institute (NCI), Cairo University. This government organization is actively engaged in planning and developing services.

The *Cairo Evangelical Medical Society*, a Christian organization, supports and runs one private hospice in Cairo and another recently opened in Alexandria.

Palliative care coverage

There are six university-based hospital oncology units around the country committed to providing pain relief. The main oncology unit at NCI based at Cairo University is taking the lead actively to develop services within the NCI by building on their work in the pain relief units. In addition, there are eight small cancer centres in various parts of the country.

Cairo Evangelical Medical Hospice receives patients from the local area, most of whom self-refer or are referred by family members.[7]

Egypt has national guidelines for the management of acute pain and chronic cancer pain. Guidelines for symptom management, end-of-life care and home-based hospice care are currently being developed.

Education and training

The Eastern Mediterranean Regional Office (EMRO) based in Cairo, as a WHO office, aims to promote health in the 22 states of the region, of which Egypt is one. At present, EMRO is proposing to develop a training programme as part of a plan to promote palliative care services in these states, since palliative care services remain underdeveloped.[8]

A palliative care training programme is being developed at NCI; this aims to provide basic training as part of the general medical education for doctors, nurses and other professionals.[9]

At the Cairo Evangelical Medical Hospice, Naguib Elnikhaily has organized training courses provided by visiting nurses from the UK.[2]

Palliative care workforce capacity

As of February 2005, no data are available for numbers of government-funded medical and related professionals specifically involved in palliative care in Egypt.

Cairo Evangelical Medical Hospice has one medical director, one senior nurse and four assistant nurses.[7]

Nursing and medical staff involved in developing palliative care at the NCI are keen to seek government and WHO support to initiate a needs assessment.[10]

History and development of hospice–palliative care in Egypt

Palliative care in Egypt is in the early stages of development. For many years, the major support for patients with life-threatening illness, most particularly cancer, has been via oncology units specializing in pain relief.[11] Tawfik reports that in the early 1990s he located a single clinic that focused on training a member of the patient's family in pain relief with the help of the supporting doctor.

Dr Nagwa Elkateb (NCI) reports that at present there is much debate about how and in what form palliative care might become established in Egypt: solutions are still unclear. She explains:

> We have good guidelines on opioids, but we have to assess the needs in Egypt—motivated by the workshop [Larnaca Middle East Cancer Consortium (MECC) conference, February 2004], but we don't know the needs. Do we need supportive care, palliative care? Do we start with cancer or other diseases? Maybe we don't need other hospices? Maybe a terminal care unit in each hospital?'[12]

There is felt to be a need for some input from experienced international organizations who can offer support and guidance.[4]

Ethical issues

Egypt has a strong cultural tradition of family support. When a family member is diagnosed with a life-threatening disease, the family will assume the care for their relative. However, as Dr Helmy at NCI notes, in addition to the problem of financial support for providing services there remains a lack of adequate knowledge about the importance of palliative care. Dr Elkateb explains that there is a great need to educate 'families about home palliative care' and not to rush into an inappropriate approach. As she notes, 'we have a shortage of nurses; and we need to teach families [about palliative care]. We have a high respect for families'.[12]

As several authors have noted in their observations around the world, different cultural approaches to death and dying may present considerable challenges in developing palliative care services that are sensitive to, and appropriate for, the different communities they serve.[13] There is a continuing ethical challenge and debate concerning openly discussing diagnosis and prognosis with patients. As in other parts of the world, cultural and religious traditions create a marked resistance to discuss openly with a patient the fact of their imminent death. The family will tend to protect their relative and talk with the medical professionals directly, regardless of whether the patient would wish to know their prognosis and prepare themselves for death.[14]

Life/oral histories

Dr Naguib Elnikhaily describes how he became interested in palliative care after he was treated for cancer at the Cleveland Clinic in the USA and saw a hospice unit there. On his return to Cairo, he discussed it with the hospital and started the Cairo Evangelical Medical Hospice with only four beds.

Public health context

Population

Egypt's population of around 76 117 421 is made up of the following ethnic groups: Eastern Hamitic stock (Egyptians, Bedouins and Berbers) 99 per cent, Greek, Nubian, Armenian other European (primarily Italian and French) 1 per cent.

Religious groups include: Muslim (mostly Sunni) 94 per cent, Coptic Christian and other 6 per cent.[15]

Table 12.2 Egypt HIV and AIDS estimates, end 2003

Adult (15–49) HIV prevalence rate	<0.1 per cent (range: <0.2 percent)
Adults (15–49) living with HIV	12 000 (range: 5000–30 000)
Adults and children (0–49) living with HIV	12 000 (range: 5000–31 000)
Women (15–49) living with HIV	1600 (range: 500–3200)
AIDS deaths (adults and children) in 2003	700 (range: 200–1600)

Source: 2004 Report of the global AIDS epidemic.

Epidemiology

In Egypt, the WHO World Health Report (2003) indicates an adult mortality[16] rate per 1000 population of 240 for males and 157 for females.[17] Life expectancy for males is 65.3; for females 69. Healthy life expectancy is 57.8 for males; and 60.2 for females.[18]

In 2000, there were an estimated 55 003 cancer cases in Egypt and 34 429[19] cancer deaths. These figures suggest a considerable palliative care need among patients with cancer—and do not include end-of-life care for patients with other diseases.

Unlike some African countries, Egypt has a very low prevalence of HIV/AIDS (0.2 per cent). Estimates suggest that between 5000 and 31 000 people were living with HIV/AIDS at the end of 2003. In the same year, up to 1600 adults and children are thought to have died from the disease (Table 12.2).

UNAIDS reports:

> Data on HIV/AIDS in Egypt, while limited, suggest low prevalence (far less than 1% in the general population). However, current surveillance methods and barriers to HIV testing suggest that a substantial number of cases may go undetected. In addition, many of the behavioural risk factors and social determinants of HIV identified in other regions also exist in Egypt and have been documented in studies. Without a concerted effort to prevent transmission, Egypt is likely to suffer an increase in the incidence of HIV/AIDS.[20]

Health care system

In 2001, Egypt's total per capita expenditure on health care was Intl $153; 3.9% of GDP[21] (Appendix 3).

The WHO overall health system performance score places Egypt 63rd out of 191 countries.[22]

Political economy

Since the mid-1990s, there had been a lack of substantial progress on economic reform; this has limited foreign investment in Egypt and kept the annual GDP growth during 2001–2003 in the range of 2–3 per cent.

In late 2003 and early 2004, Egyptian officials proposed new privatization and customs reform measures, but the government is unlikely to pursue these initiatives vigorously to avoid a public backlash over potential inflation or layoffs associated with the reforms. Monetary pressures on an overvalued Egyptian pound caused the government to float the currency in January 2003, leading to a sharp drop in its value and consequent inflationary pressure. The existence of a black market for hard currency is evidence that the government continues to influence the official exchange rate offered in banks. In September 2003, Egyptian officials increased subsidies on basic foodstuffs, helping to calm a frustrated public but widening an already deep budget deficit.

Egypt's balance of payments position was not hurt by the war in Iraq in 2003, as tourism and Suez Canal revenues fared well. The development of an export market for natural gas is a bright spot for future growth prospects, but improvement in the capital intensive hydrocarbons sector will do little to reduce Egypt's persistent unemployment.[16]

GDP per capita of Egypt is Intl $3901 (Appendix 4).

References

1 Report of the United Nations Development Programme 2004 (HDI 2002). Launched by the United Nations in 1990, the Human Development Index measures a country's achievements in three aspects of human development: longevity, knowledge, and a decent standard of living. It was created to re-emphasize that people and their lives should be the ultimate criteria for assessing the development of a country, not economic growth. Current values range from 0.956 (Norway, first out of 177 countries) to 0.273 (Sierra Leone, 177th out of 177 countries). Countries fall into one of three groups: countries 1–55 = high development; 56–141 = medium development; 142–177 = low development. See: http://hdr.undp.org/statistics/data/indic/indic_8_1_1.html

2 Naguib Elnikhaily in discussion: MECC conference, Larnaca, Cyprus—February 2004.

3 Personal communication: Naguib Elnikhaily—February 2005.

4 Personal communication: Nagwa Elkateb—February 2005.

5 International Narcotics Control Board. *Narcotic Drugs: Estimated World Requirements for 2004. Statistics for 2002.* New York: United Nations, 2004.

6 'The term *defined daily doses for statistical purposes* (S-DDD) replaces the term *defined daily doses* previously used by the Board. The S-DDDs are technical units of measurement for the purposes of statistical analysis and are not recommended prescription doses. Certain narcotic drugs may be used in certain countries for different treatments or in accordance with different medical practices, and therefore a different daily dose could be more appropriate'. The S-DDD used by the INCB for morphine is 100 mg. International Narcotics Control Board. *Narcotic Drugs: Estimated World Requirements for 2004. Statistics for 2002.* New York: United Nations, 2004: 176–177.

7 Personal communication: Fouad Bekeheit—20 April 2005.

8 Al-Shahri M. Brown S, Ezzat A. Khatib O. Palliative care initiative for the Eastern Mediterranean Region: a proposal. *Annals of Saudi Medicine* 2004; **24(6)**: 465–468.

9 Personal communication: Ahmed Helmy—February 2005.

10 Personal communication: Ahmed Helmy and Nagwa Elkateb—February 2005.

11 **Tawfik MO.** Egypt: status of cancer pain and palliative care. *Journal of Pain and Symptom Management* 1993; **8(6)**: 409–411.

12 Nagwa Elkateb in discussion: MECC conference, Larnaca, Cyprus—February 2004.

13 **Musgrave C.** Rituals of death and dying in Israeli Jewish culture. *European Journal of Palliative Care* 1995; **2(2)**: 83–86.

14 **Gatrad AR, Sheikh A.** Palliative care for Muslims and issues before death. *International Journal of Palliative Nursing* 2002; **8(11)**: 526–531.

15 http://www.cia.gov/cia/publications/factbook/geos/eg.html

16 This refers to adult mortality risk, which is defined as the probability of dying between 15 and 59 years.

17 See The World Fact book http://www.cia.gov/cia/publications/factbook/geos/eg.html

18 See: WHO statistics for Egypt at: http://www.who.int/countries/en/

19 **Ferlay J, Bray F, Pisani, P, Parkin DM.** GLOBOCAN 2000: Cancer incidence, mortality and prevalence worldwide. V1.0 *IARC Cancerbase No.5* Lyon: IARC Press, 2001.

20 http://www.unaids.org/en/geographical+area/by+country/egypt.asp

21 Total health expenditure per capita is the per capita amount of the sum of Public Health Expenditure (PHE) and Private Expenditure on Health (PvtHE). The international dollar is a common currency unit that takes into account differences in the relative purchasing power of various currencies. Figures expressed in international dollars are calculated using purchasing power parities (PPP), which are rates of currency conversion constructed to account for differences in price level between countries. http://www3.who.int/whosis/country/compare.cfm?country=s&indicator=strPcTotEOHinIntD2000&language=english

22 This composite measure of overall health system attainment is based on a country's goals relating to health, responsiveness and fairness in financing. The measure varies widely across countries and is highly correlated with general levels of human development as captured in the human development index. Tandon A, Murray CLJ, Lauer JA, Evans DB. *Measuring Overall Health System Performance for 191 Countries.* GPE Discussion Paper Series: No. 30; WHO.

Chapter 13

Malawi

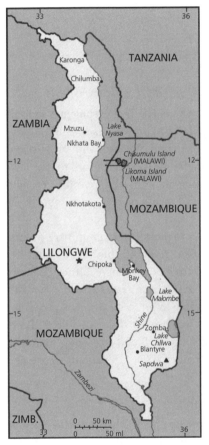

Malawi (population 11.87 million) is a landlocked country in Southern Africa that covers an area of 118 400 km². Its boundaries border Mozambique, Tanzania and Zambia. Lake Nyasa, around 580 km long, is the country's most prominent feature. Formerly the British protectorate of Nyasaland, Malawi became independent in 1964. Lilongwe is the capital and the country is divided into 27 districts for administrative purposes. After three decades of one-party rule under President Hastings Kamuzu Banda, the country held multiparty elections in 1994.

According to the United Nations human development index (HDI), Malawi is ranked 165th out of 177 countries worldwide (value 0.388)[1] and 33rd out of 45 in African countries for which an index is available. This places Malawi in the group of countries with low human development.

Palliative care service provision

Current services

Five palliative care organizations are known to exist in Malawi and deliver some 12 services (Table 13.1).

Palliative care services may also be provided by St Luke's Hospital, Zomba and Ekwendeni hospital, near Mzuzu.

Table 13.1 Palliative care provision in Malawi, 2004

	Free-standing unit	Hospital unit	Hospital support team	Home care	Day care	Clinic/drop-in centre	Total
Lighthouse				1		1	2
Tiyanjane Clinic	1	1				1	3
Umodzi Clinic	1	1				1	3
Mulanje Mission Hospital	1	1					2
St. Anne's Hospital	1			1			2
Total services	4	3		2		3	12

Lighthouse, Lilongwe

The service was founded in 1997 in direct response to the HIV/AIDS epidemic and initially provided a hospital discharge/home visiting service to prevent readmissions. It has since grown into a multiservice organization. A home-based care team with professional staff and about 300 volunteers visit patients and families who cannot afford to take relatives to the clinic. Patients are identified by community home-based care volunteers who work closely with Lighthouse home-based care nurses. On average, 150 patients are registered with the home-based care scheme.

This programme links with 13 local chiefs in order to mobilize community resources. The Voluntary Counselling and Testing (VCT) Centre offers these services to the public. An HIV clinic is open 5 days per week. Testing is done here, although many patients are referred for ARVs and further care having been tested elsewhere. A full medical history is taken by a clinical officer who is able to prescribe drugs as necessary. A day care ward attends to critically ill patients waiting for the clinic. Procedures include resuscitation, rehydration and emotional support. Blood grouping and cross-matching can be done here. From January to September 2003, 115 patients were cared for in the day ward.

Tiyanjane Clinic, Queen Elizabeth Hospital, Blantyre

This clinic was started in July 2003 to facilitate follow-up after discharge of HIV-positive patients from the adult wards at the hospital. From January 2004, there has been a counselling and testing service attached to the clinic. The service links closely with the network of existing home-based care organizations in the area so as not to duplicate services in this resource-limited region. The clinic receives referrals for hospital patients about to be discharged by clinicians who cannot give quality time to those patients identified as requiring palliative care, symptom control or counselling. The clinic is mainly regarded as an HIV service, but provides symptom control and assessment of cancer patients. It is located in the grounds of the hospital.

Umodzi Pediatric Clinic, Queen Elizabeth Hospital, Blantyre

This clinic grew out of the recognition that the force-feeding approach used in the children's malnutrition ward at Queen Elizabeth Hospital was inappropriate, particularly with HIV-infected children. The service provides a designated service for children with AIDS and cancer up to the age of about 14. A weekly morning clinic is run on support group lines, with mothers and children able to share experiences and receive counselling. About 10 children are seen each week. From May 2002 to May 2004, 375 children were seen at the clinic. At present, continuity of care is dependent on local faith-based home-based care groups. The development of an home-based care service organized by the clinic is being considered.

Mulanje Mission Hospital, Mulanje

The beginnings of a palliative care programme started here in early 2003 after a local palliative care training session. Recognition that pain in many AIDS and cancer patients remained uncontrolled without morphine became the catalyst to do something different. The unit is within the gynaecology department and benefits from the gynaecologist's interest in palliative care. The gynaecology department identifies at least four or five new cases of inoperable cervical cancer every month. This is the most common female cancer in Malawi besides AIDS-related Kaposi's sarcoma. A referral system for terminally patients was initiated within the hospital in December 2003, and a weekly palliative care clinic now operates.

Referrals come from the government district hospital, the local clinics and mainly from the outpatients department at Mulanje Mission Hospital. Most patients present late with advanced undiagnosed illness that requires palliation. There are approximately 50 patients registered with the palliative care clinic at any time. Each of the 71 villages in the catchment area has identified an home-based care volunteer who currently works with the primary health care team in identifying patients who may benefit from palliative care. They will form the core of the planned outreach programme. An ARV programme started in April 2004, and by May 2004 had 10 registered patients.

St Anne's Hospital, Nkhotakota

Palliative care here is hospital based, and was started in 2002. The hospital is a 144-bed rural general hospital catering for all comers; historically, it is also the referral centre for district-wide maternity services. General palliative care is complemented by specialist nerve blocks and palliative surgery when necessary. Approximately 10 inpatients per week receive palliative care accumulating to 500 per year. Patients have either end-stage AIDS, cancer, or end-stage cardiac or renal failure. Outpatients requiring palliative care number approximately 15 per week, and 750 per year. Home-based care, which in Malawi means home-based support rather than palliative care, is run by 80 community volunteers. Fifty-six volunteers have received formal training and carry simple medications; they are based within the catchment area of one of the three health centres in the district. The number of patients registered for home-based support is currently 320. The patient is admitted to hospital when any significant problems arise.

Palliative care is beginning to be recognized by the Malawi government, and activity is currently focused on the following policies and guidelines:

- The National HIV/AIDS policy, launched on 10 February 2004
- National Palliative Care Guidelines—being developed by the Care and Support Working Group under the National AIDS Commission
- National Antiretroviral (ARV) Guidelines.

An ARV programme began in Malawi in April 2004. The Malawi government has committed to providing free ARV treatments to 50 per cent of the HIV-positive population. It is costly to do CD4 counts here, so clinical symptomatology determined by WHO is used as the criteria for treatment. *Médecins Sans Frontières* operate ARV programmes, at Thyolo and Chiladzulo.

While the government is accepting of the palliative care concept, the establishment of such services has fallen to individuals and NGOs.

A visit by the consultant Anne Lloyd-Williams and subsequent collating of country information[2,3] enabled The Diana, Princess of Wales Memorial Fund (Diana Fund) to prioritize support for palliative care development in Malawi. Aware of the lack of resources and the absence of trained staff, strategies for intervention have focused upon advocacy, education and training, and the management of change.

Reimbursement and funding for services

Lighthouse

Money from the Diana Fund supported the establishment of this service that is operated as a trust. Funding is complicated, with many donors allocating funds for specific programmes. For example:

- Some salaries are paid by the Ministry of Health, others by the Diana Fund, the Nuffield Foundation and the Centers for Disease Control (CDC)
- At the VCT Centre: CAFOD pays for salaries and activities, CDC pays for test kits
- In the home-based care programme, capacity building is funded by Family Health International (FHI). Clinical officers at the clinic are funded by GTZ (German Aid)
- The University of North Carolina operates an STI and AIDS prevention research programme and offers one clinician 4 days per week to work in the clinic
- The CDC has agreed to sponsor staff training.

Tiyanjane Clinic

The clinic operates as a part of the Queen Elizabeth Hospital, from which it receives funding. The Diana Fund awarded a grant to the hospital to establish a paediatric palliative care resource centre, pain management advice and training, and provision of basic home care kits. An award was made by the UK Forum for Hospice and Palliative Care Worldwide to support Jane Bates' studies for a Master's degree in Palliative Medicine.

Umodzi Clinic

A small charitable fund was established some years ago by Friends of Sick Children (FOSC) to sustain the activities of the paediatric clinic. Extra nurses have been employed to increase the ratio of nurses to patients in this setting. Funds from the Diana Fund are channelled through this trust fund.

Mulanje Mission Hospital

Church donations from the USA have helped to establish this service. General expenses and salaries are met by the Church of Central Africa Presbyterian (CCAP) Hospital which receives money from the Church in different countries including the USA, Canada, Germany and the UK. Financial support at present is minimal but allows for drugs to be given free to patients who are not in a position to pay. Technical support is required for data collection, and it would be helpful for the palliative care clinic to be separate from the gynaecology department. There are no funds at present to provide a vehicle for home visits.

In 2004, the UK Forum for Hospice and Palliative Care Worldwide awarded a grant to Mulanje Mission Hospital to provide: training for 72 volunteers (one for each village in which the service operates); the development of an outreach service in the community; the supervision of volunteers; and a weekly clinic.

St Anne's Hospital

Palliative care provision is not separately funded. All services fall under the hospital administration and are financially supported by the hospital. Services are free to clients, although they do have to pay for inpatient days. Most of the palliative care medication is free, or at minimal cost.

Opioid availability and consumption

Data from the International Narcotics Control Board[4] give no opioid consumption figures for Malawi to 2002 (Appendix 1).

Current in-country information suggests there is no injectable morphine in Malawi, although the Ministry of Health distributes morphine tablets (MST). Morphine solution for oral use has recently been introduced as a result of a close relationship with the Ministry of Health and Lighthouse, which has lobbied for its introduction. Lighthouse orders the parabene powder from the UK which is mixed with the preservative propylene glycol by the government Central Medical Stores pharmacists. Supplies of the oral morphine are distributed by this department to hospitals and clinics around Malawi where palliative care is practised. Supplies have been uninterrupted since the introduction of this system, and indicate the benefit of co-operation between government and the private sector.

Lighthouse

Tables 13.2–13.4 indicate the distribution of morphine by Lighthouse from January to July, 2004. Prescriptions for morphine are signed by clinical officers. WHO analgesic ladder step two drugs are usually unavailable, and often drugs for patients are bought from private pharmacies.

Tiyanjane

The clinic obtains its supplies of morphine from the Central Medical Stores organized by Lighthouse. For the period February 2004 to August 2004, 11 l (11 g) were used. MST tablets—available from the pharmacy at Queen Elizabeth Hospital—are also prescribed.

Umodzi

Since January 2003, the clinic has had access to the morphine solution made up to a solution of 5 mg in 5 ml by the pharmacist at Central Medical Stores. During 2003, 15 l (15 g) were drawn by this clinic and distributed to a couple of mission hospitals, an home-based care project in one area of Blantyre, and Tiyanjane Clinic. Umodzi clinic itself used 3 l (3 g).

Table 13.2 Distribution of morphine tables by Lighthouse, Lilongwe, January to July 2004

Month	Tablets (*n*)	Patients (*n*)
January	1101	41
February	1277	39
March	1117	44
April	1512	65
May	960	40
June	556	32
July	410	20

Table 13.3 Distribution of morphine strong solution (10 mg/ml) by Lighthouse, Lilongwe, January to May 2004

Month	Home-based care patients (ml)	Clinic patients (ml)	To partners (ml)	Patients (*n*)	Balance month end (ml)
January	600	240	0	2	
February	420	210	0	3	
March	420	840	0	3	
April	840	210	0	3	
May	210	840	3000	2	1510
Total	2490	2340	3000	13	1510

Table 13.4 Distribution of morphine in weak solution (1 mg/ml) by Lighthouse, Lilongwe, January to July 2004

Month	Home-based care patients (ml)	Clinic patients (ml)	Patients (n)
January			3
February	1260	840	4
March	210	1890	2
April	3200	4000	4
May	4200	2100	6
June	1680	–	3
July	1900	–	4

Morphine is prescribed by the doctor or the clinical officer. Nurses do not assess pain according to any visual analogue scales or pain charts, and are often unwilling to acknowledge pain in children. Most referred children present with discomfort (thrush, itching) rather than severe pain.

Mulanje

Pain control in this programme proceeds from step one to step three of the WHO analgesic ladder because of the unavailability of codeine. Often patients do not continue with oral morphine as they dislike the taste and they revert to step one analgesics, resulting in poor pain control. Patients are given aspirin, paracetamol, ibuprofen, oral morphine and some antibiotics.

St Anne's

This hospital unit collects 4 l of strong morphine (50 mg/5 ml) every three months from Lighthouse. Morphine is provided in three different strengths; 5, 10 and 20 mg per 2 ml, for ease of administration. The WHO pain ladder approach is followed. Step two analgesics are available from donors and include Solpadol, Codydramol, Tramadol, Cocodamol and occasionally simple codeine on its own.

National and Professional Organizations

No national palliative care organizations are known to exist in Malawi. However, the UK Forum for Hospice and Palliative Care Worldwide has given support to the African Palliative Care Association to help establish a national palliative care association in Malawi.

Palliative care coverage

Lighthouse covers different catchments with different services. The home-based care service works in specific parts of Lilongwe City (400 000 people). The VCT unit sees mainly people from Lilongwe District (1.5 million) whilst the clinic currently manages patients from all of the central region and (for ARVs) beyond (~4 million people).

Tiyanjane receives referrals from hospital ward clinicians that cannot give quality time to those HIV patients identified as requiring palliative care. Upon discharge, the patient is referred to the clinic. Further links with home-based care providers in the community ensure minimal duplication of services. Both Tiyanjane and Umodzi clinics cover Blantyre district, which has a population of 850 000.

Umodzi Clinic works with children referred by the paediatric department at the hospital. Where possible, most are sent home for home care, with return visits to the clinic as necessary. Links with home-based care providers ensure that follow-up and monitoring by community groups continue. Queen Elizabeth Central Hospital is a referral centre for paediatric cancer for the whole of Malawi's southern region, which has a population of 4.6 million (1998 estimate).

Mulanje Mission Hospital. The catchment area for the palliative care service encompasses 71 villages comprising about 70 000 people. This falls within the Mulanje district that has a population of around 250 000. Although there is a government district hospital in the area, many members of this community come to this private health facility for medical help. Dr Sue Makin is the only gynaecologist in the district. She identifies at least four or five new cases of advanced, inoperable cervical cancer on admission every month. Each week, a visit to the government hospital identifies additional similar cases. In a recent survey of the villages, it was established that there were >1000 HIV-positive patients in this area.

St Anne's Hospital is situated in Nkhotakota district which is 4300 km^2, and contains just over 250 000 people. The population density is 54 people/km^2, mostly comprising rural subsistence farmers or those who fish. Most earn less than US$1 per day.

Education and training

Lighthouse

One of the clinical officers, Lameck Thambo, is currently undertaking the Distance Learning Diploma in Palliative Care through Hospice Africa Uganda. He attended a 3-week course in 2002 to develop skills in palliative care and rehabilitation of people living with HIV/AIDS at the Mildmay Centre in Kampala, Uganda. He provides ongoing palliative care in-house training and heads the national palliative care training team. Several training sessions for health professionals have been conducted by this core training team from September 2002 until May 2004. A total of 61 trained health professionals have received training, including 17 clinical officers, three doctors and 41 nurses.

Tiyanjane

Neither the doctor nor the nurse working in this clinic has any formal palliative care training. There is scope for introducing education in palliative care and morphine use as Queen Elizabeth Central Hospital is a teaching hospital. There is a nursing school here, but palliative care has yet to be introduced into the curriculum.

Umodzi Clinic

Dr Lavy and Sr Nyirenda have both completed the Distance Learning Diploma in Palliative Care with Hospice Africa Uganda. Counselling training is provided by ICOCA, a local faith-based counselling organization. The specific area of communicating with dying children has yet to be addressed, and expertise is unavailable in this country. The concept of health professionals using play as a means to communicate with ill children is unusual here and will need external training.

Mulanje Mission Hospital

The palliative care clinical officer, Suave Gombwa, is expected to enrol shortly with the Distance Learning Diploma in Palliative Care through Hospice Africa Uganda. No training is undertaken here although the need for training has been identified for community volunteers in order to provide better home-based care. The lack of human resources makes this impossible at the moment.

St Anne's Hospital

At present, due to financial constraints, palliative care is disseminated only through practical in-house training. Ideally, it would be worth getting the trainers from Lighthouse to come to train St Anne's staff and the health centre workers. Dr Wiggins is a member of the national training team. He obtained a Master's degree in palliative care and policy at King's College, London in 2000. He was a community advisor in palliative care with the Greenwich community palliative care team, 1994–2001.

Palliative care workforce capacity

Lighthouse employs a diverse cross-section of people to assist with the many programmes. Administrative staff number 21, including: receptionists, a management adviser, security workers and an accountant. The VCT Centre is staffed by one co-ordinator and nine counsellors. The home-based care programme is headed by a co-ordinator, one deputy co-ordinator and four community nurses. Twice a week, a clinical officer accompanies the nurses on home visits. There are four clinical officers employed at the HIV clinic as well as one doctor and one director. All are full time. There are also three doctors and two clinical officers on attachment from the University of Carolina research programme, and three nurses in attendance at the clinic and day care ward.

Tiyanjane Clinic is staffed by one doctor and one nurse, both of whom are learning about palliative care as they work. Much of the counselling is done by the nurse. This releases the doctor to attend to pain assessment and symptom control. Ongoing monitoring is undertaken by home-based care providers in the community.

Umodzi Clinic has added to its original staff complement of one part-time medical director and one part-time palliative care nurse, with one clinical officer and two nurses, all of whom are full time.

Mulanje Mission identifies limited human resources as one of its areas of greatest need. This nascent palliative care scheme draws on the interest and skill of Dr Makin and one clinical officer. Another clinical officer heads the ARV programme.

Because of the staff shortages in Malawi, *St Anne's Hospital* has encouraged all its employees to become familiar with palliative care. There is no room to develop specialist teams without affecting already existing services. The palliative care unit has capacity for 56 nurses but is staffed with only 14. Many health professionals leave the country to seek higher salaries abroad. The vacant positions are filled by patient attendants (who have received 3 weeks training) and ward attendants (who get 2 weeks training). There is one medical assistant and eight clinical officers. They have 3 years of training (diploma in clinical training). Currently, four of them are doing their first year post-qualification training. Dr Wiggins is the only doctor. Follow-up care is provided by 80 community volunteers. The volunteer drop-out rate is low at 7 per cent.

History and development of hospice–palliative care in Malawi

Lighthouse

During the mid and late 1990s, there was severe congestion on the wards of Lilongwe Central Hospital (LCH) due to the increasing number of HIV/AIDS patients; beds were being shared and there were many more admissions than discharges. Into this scenario entered Nicky Hargreaves, a UK physician who went to Malawi to study respiratory pathogens in HIV via bronchoscopy and, as part of her work, ran a clinic in Lilongwe. When she began to follow-up non-attending patients at home, she discovered they were suffering terrible symptoms, with little support, and were unable to access hospital services effectively. As a result, she joined a group of Malawian health professionals and, together, they founded the Lilongwe home-based care service.

Among those who paid home visits were two nurses, Olive Kadzakumanja and Agnes Kuluwangu, who volunteered to follow-up patients discharged from the wards; health problems, therefore, were handled at home instead of the patient returning to hospital.

Traditionally in Malawian communities, neighbours and friends would care for the ill and dying, so these nurses used the existing system by working with the neighbours. The nurses gave basic nursing care training to the volunteers, and gradually the numbers grew as people became more interested in caring for the increasing numbers of ill and dying.

Nicky Hargreaves guided the home-based care group through its early stages and secured financial support at a time it was most needed. Importantly, she stayed on after her research project ended to co-ordinate HIV work in Lilongwe; a time that proved crucial to the development of palliative care services. Dr Charlie Bond comments:

> Nicky did not lead from the front but allowed a group of well motivated Malawians to evolve and lead the project. I think it is safe to say, however, that there would be no home-based care, no Lighthouse, and probably no palliative care service at its current state of development without her involvement. I joined her in Malawi in 1998 when she invited me out for 4 months to do some palliative care education and capacity building with Lilongwe home-based care. We both visited Hospice Uganda, met Anne Merriman, and spent time with the services in Kampala, learning what we could to take back to Malawi. Anne was extremely helpful and supportive and later visited Lilongwe.[5]

There was an old building in the hospital grounds that had been used for dermatology, and this was refurbished to encompass the joint facility of home-based care and the clinic. It was named Lighthouse as a symbol of hope for HIV/AIDS people. At that time, the term hospice was unknown in Malawi, and the use of opioids and narcotics was looked upon with suspicion. Dr Anne Merriman subsequently visited Malawi to sensitize the government to the use of opioids and morphine, in particular for severe pain in terminally ill patients. She recommended that Lighthouse become known as a hospice and that it should take the palliative care lead in the country.

Tiyanjane Clinic

Tiyanjane Clinic was developed by Jane Bates who had trained as a General Practitioner in the UK and worked in South Africa in a district hospital. That environment encouraged her interest in HIV/AIDS and she came to Malawi specifically to work in this field of medicine. The clinic was developed in response to the perceived gap between hospital discharge and an unsupported home environment.

Umodzi Clinic

This grew out of the realization that dying children and their families required much more than force-feeding and nutritional monitoring on the malnutrition ward. Liz Molyneux was Professor of Paediatrics and head of department at Queen Elizabeth Hospital (2002) and used her position to enable the development of a more holistic approach to chronically ill children than a brief regimented feeding programme. She wrote a proposal and the Diana Fund agreed to fund the project.

Dr Vicky Lavy was working in other departments of the hospital at the time but had undertaken a 6-month palliative care course in the UK in 1993. Her interest and abilities in this field led her to her current position as medical director for the programme. The addition of nursing and clinical officer staff makes possible the extension of the work into home-based care and follow-up support for families.

Mulanje Mission Hospital

The palliative care programme here started early in 2003 with a 1-week training session in Mulanje taught by Dr Tim Wiggin, Dr Vicky Lavy, Sr Nyirenda and Lameck Thambo. The early days of this service depended upon the enthusiasm of the gynaecologist and a clinical officer at the hospital. They identified the need for a major increase in expertise in this field in order for the service to provide a proper palliative care facility. Of the nurses who attended national training programmes, many are ill themselves and others have left the hospital, creating a skill gap. The need for counselling patients and relatives has yet to be addressed due to lack of personnel. Dr Makin:

> If we are really going to provide palliative care that would be a wonderful asset to have somebody like [a counsellor] who could speak Chichewa . . . then I think our programme would really take off.[6]

St Anne's Hospital

Palliative care at this hospital was made possible with the provision of free morphine via the Diana Fund in Malawi in 2001. The palliative care training started by Lameck Thambo and his team has provided a sustained supply of morphine and of palliative care skills training. As the number of trained practitioners is small, provision of pain relief is erratic.

Hospice success stories

Lighthouse

The national palliative care training programme led by this organization is considered to have been a big achievement, and many health professionals in the country have been encouraged to become involved in this work. The services offered by Lighthouse are well known and accepted within the community, and most significantly by the government of Malawi. The Ministry of Health works closely with this organization in policy development, and acknowledges the importance of palliative care. Most importantly, the introduction of morphine and ensuring easy and sustained access to pain control is regarded as the greatest success of Lighthouse.

Tiyanjane

Although this clinic is new and limited in its services, it is beginning to provide continuity of care for terminal patients discharged from hospital with very few resources. It utilizes existing community support systems.

Umodzi Clinic

The clinic has overcome initial resistance to dealing differently with dying children, and referrals have increased. The hospital clinicians are increasingly grateful to be able to refer children for meaningful care. Dr Lavy believes that the service baseline in Malawi is so low that any help given is considered a major achievement.

Mulanje Mission Hospital

The development of relationships with families is seen as an important step in establishing this service. Dr Sue Makin:

> Last Thursday a relative of a patient who had died came over here specially to tell us he had died. That says we had a connection with them, and that we really cared about him, so I consider that a success.[6]

St Anne's Hospital

Staff at this unit feel progress has been made in establishing palliative care as an accepted form of medicine for all patients.

Ethical issues

The common Malawian approach of being indirect about breaking bad news makes this aspect of palliative care difficult. Dr Lavy:

> Almost always the family would not want the person with the illness to know. The way would not be to tell someone this is what will happen to you, and I've heard it time and time again with nurses giving false reassurances . . . and you know it will NOT be fine actually.[7]

Life/oral histories

Umodzi Clinic

The impact of HIV/AIDS upon children and families in Malawi formed much of Dr Lavy's motivation to develop this service:

> There is a sense of hopelessness in Malawi about HIV/AIDS, so I just want to provide something especially for them that says 'you're worth something'[7]

Mulanje Mission Hospital

The initial palliative care training at this hospital in 2003 inspired Suave Gombwa, a clinical officer, to become interested in palliative care. He had heard of palliative care during his medical training but it was never well explained and never put into practice:

> I had some patients in the male ward who had stage 4 WHO HIV staging. They had very nasty burning pain of the legs. I didn't know what to do with the patient and I was just giving pain killers, and each time . . . the patient was saying it's not changing. I still have the pain. And in that week we had the training of that palliative care where I learnt about neuropathic pain. That's when I learnt about amytryptaline for treating neuropathic pain. We gave the patient a very low dose. That patient by the very next day was well, now becoming mobile, praising the drug. He knew he wouldn't be cured because he was stage 4 HIV. At that time, there were no ARVs so palliative care was the only hope for the patient . . . after that I was very interested in this palliative care . . . now I could do something for the patient.[8]

Public health context

Population

Malawi's population of around 11.87 million is made up of the following ethnic groups: Chewa, Nyanja, Tumbuka, Yao, Lomwe, Sena, Tonga, Ngoni, Ngonde, Asian and European.

Religious groups include: Protestant 55 per cent, Roman Catholic 20 per cent, Muslim 20 per cent, indigenous beliefs 3 per cent, and other 2 per cent.[9]

Epidemiology

In Malawi, the WHO World Health Report (2003) indicates an adult mortality[10] rate per 1000 population of 657 for males and 610 for females. Life expectancy for males is 39.8; for females 40.6. Healthy life expectancy is 35.0 for males; and 34.8 for females.[11]

Malawi is one of the worst HIV/AIDS-affected countries in Southern Africa. Estimates suggest that in Malawi, between 700 000 and 1.1 million people were living with HIV/AIDS at the end of 2003. In the same year, up to 120 000 adults and children are thought to have died from the disease (Table 13.5).

UNAIDS reports:

> Malawi has been successful in mobilizing resources for HIV/AIDS control. In 2003, Malawi signed an agreement with the Global Fund for the allocation of US$196 million over the next five years.

Table 13.5 Malawi HIV and AIDS estimates, end 2003

Adult (15–49) HIV prevalence rate	14.2 per cent (range: 11.3–17.7 per cent)
Adults (15–49) living with HIV	810 000 (range: 650 000–1 000 000)
Adults and children (0–49) living with HIV	900 000 (range: 700 000–1 100 000)
Women (15–49) living with HIV	460 000 (range: 370 000–570 000)
AIDS deaths (adults and children) in 2003	84 000 (range: 58 000–120 000)

Source: 2004 Report of the global AIDS epidemic.

Through its Multi-country AIDS Program (MAP), the World Bank also approved an allocation of US$35 million for Malawi over four years. However, with an increasing epidemic burden, especially the need to deal with the growing numbers of HIV-positive people, there is still need for additional external support. A Poverty Reduction Strategy Paper was launched in April 2002. Key challenges include: i) the need to further mainstream HIV/AIDS into the core policies and activities of all sectors; ii) better rationalization and coordination of interventions by the several partners; iii) capacity building of NAC and of implementing partners at national, district and community levels.[12]

Health care system

In 2001, the total per capita expenditure on health care was Intl $39; 7.8% of GDP[13] (Appendix 3).

The WHO overall health system performance score places Malawi 185th out of 191 countries.[14]

Political economy

Landlocked Malawi ranks among the world's least developed countries. The economy is predominantly agricultural, with about 90 per cent of the population living in rural areas. Agriculture accounted for nearly 40 per cent of GDP and 88 per cent of export revenues in 2001. The economy depends on substantial inflows of economic assistance from the IMF, the World Bank and individual donor nations. In late 2000, Malawi was approved for relief under the Heavily Indebted Poor Countries (HIPC) programme. In November 2002, the World Bank approved a US$50 million drought recovery package, which is to be used for famine relief. The government faces strong challenges, e.g. to develop fully a market economy, to improve educational facilities, to face up to environmental problems, to deal with the rapidly growing problem of HIV/AIDS and to satisfy foreign donors that fiscal discipline is being tightened. The performance of the tobacco sector is key to short-term growth as tobacco accounts for > 50 per cent of exports.[9]

GDP per capita is Intl $501 (Appendix 4).

References

1 Report of the United Nations Development Programme 2004 (HDI 2002). Launched by the United Nations in 1990, the Human Development Index measures a country's achievements in three aspects of human development: longevity, knowledge and a decent standard of living. It was created to re-emphasize that people and their lives should be the ultimate criteria for assessing the development of a country, not economic growth. Current values range from 0.956 (Norway, first of 177 countries) to 0.273 (Sierra Leone, 177th out of 177 countries). Countries fall into one of three groups: countries 1–55 = high development; 56–141 = medium development; 142–177 = low development. See: http://hdr.undp.org/statistics/data/indic/indic_8_1_1.html

2 **Anne Lloyd Williams**. *Visit to Malawi in April 2001*. Report to the Diana, Princess of Wales Memorial Fund, 15 May 2001.

3 Faith Mwangi-Powell. Country Summary—Malawi. (Undated).

4 International Narcotics Control Board. *Narcotic Drugs: Estimated World Requirements for 2004. Statistics for 2002*. New York: United Nations, 2004.

5 Personal communication: Charlie Bond—3 October 2005.

6 Personal communication: Sue Makin—19 May 2004.

7 Personal communication: Vicky Lavy—18 May 2004.

8 Personal communication: Suave Gombwa—19 May 2004.

9 See: http://www.cia.gov/cia/publications/factbook/geos/mi.html

10 This refers to adult mortality risk, which is defined as the probability of dying between 15 and 59 years.

11 See: WHO statistics for Malawi at: http://www.who.int/countries/mwi/en/

12 http://www.unaids.org/en/geographical+area/by+country/malawi.asp

13 Total health expenditure per capita is the per capita amount of the sum of Public Health Expenditure (PHE) and Private Expenditure on Health (PvtHE). The international dollar is a common currency unit that takes into account differences in the relative purchasing power of various currencies. Figures expressed in international dollars are calculated using purchasing power parities (PPP), which are rates of currency conversion constructed to account for differences in price level between countries. http://www3.who.int/whosis/country/compare.cfm?country=s&indicator=strPcTotEOHinIntD2000&language=english

14 This composite measure of overall health system attainment is based on a country's goals relating to health, responsiveness and fairness in financing. The measure varies widely across countries and is highly correlated with general levels of human development as captured in the human development index. Tandon A, Murray CLJ, Lauer JA, Evans DB. *Measuring Overall Health System Performance for 191 Countries*. GPE Discussion Paper Series: No. 30; WHO.

Chapter 14

Morocco

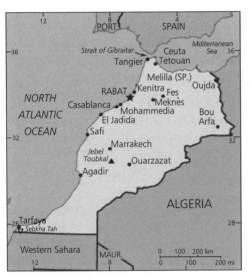

Morocco (population 32.21 million people) is a country in Northern Africa that covers an area of 446 550 km². Its boundaries border the North Atlantic Ocean and the Mediterranean Sea, between Algeria and Western Sahara. The capital of Morocco is Rabat.

According to the United Nations human development index (HDI), Morocco is ranked 125th out of 177 countries worldwide (value 0.620)[1] and sixth out of 45 in African countries for which an index is available. This places Morocco in the group of countries with medium human development.

Palliative care service provision

Current services

The Moroccan Society of Management of Pain and Palliative Care was created within the National Institute of Oncology in Rabat in 1995. This designated centre provides the only palliative care service in Morocco: a 10-bed hospital inpatient unit and an outpatient clinic (Table 14.1).

The Moroccan Society of Management of Pain and Palliative Care

The majority of patients seen at the centre are those with metastatic cancer pain. Occasionally the centre attends to those living with HIV and suffering from chronic non-cancer pain. Up to 50 000 new cases of cancer are registered each year in Morocco, yet treatment reaches only 10 000 of those, leaving many with no treatment and significant pain.[2]

The organization manages a biennial conference for up to 400 participants to expand interest in palliative care. Since April 2003, the need to manage pain has been endorsed by health authorities as a national priority. The Moroccan Society of Management of Pain and Palliative Care in Rabat is the first National Centre of Pain and Palliative Care

Table 14.1 Palliative care provision in Morocco, 2004

	Free-standing unit	Hospital unit	Hospital support team	Home care	Day care	Clinic/drop-in centre	Total
Moroccan Society of Management of Pain and Palliative Care, Rabat	1					1	2

in Morocco and is due to be formally inaugurated in early 2006. The aim of the Centre will be 3-fold: care, training and research in the field of pain.

Reimbursement and funding for services

The Global Fund approved US$9 238 754 on 29 January 2003 to be disbursed by the Ministry of Health of Morocco in Round 1 of a project aimed at support and implementation of the national strategic plan to fight HIV/AIDS. The proposal targets vulnerable at-risk groups and implements a social communication programme aimed at young people, women and the general population. It addresses provisions of diagnosis, support and treatment for people living with HIV/AIDS, but does not mention palliative care.

The National Centre of Pain and Palliative Care at the National Institute of Oncology in Rabat submitted a proposal to the Paris-based NGO Douleurs Sans Frontieres (DSF) to fund a broad-ranging strategy to relieve pain associated with varied conditions including AIDS and cancer. An amount of €146 377 was requested for a 2-year project from January 2004 to December 2005.

The objectives of the proposal are designed to assist the centre in its fight against pain by developing a day clinic, a mobile unit and guidelines for the treatment of pain. They also include the creation of a resource centre, training of pain specialists and the inclusion of pain control in medical and paramedical training. Significantly, the proposal prioritizes palliative care for patients living with a life-limiting condition, notably AIDS and cancer. At April 2005, DSF funds a 'training of trainers' curriculum at the centre.

The Ministry of Health provided US$1 million for the construction of the National Centre of Pain and Palliative Care.

Opioid availability and consumption

Mati Nejmi, founder of the Moroccan Society of Management of Pain and Palliative comments:

> Morphine consumption is increasing each year and is a thousand per cent more important now than in 1995. Few Moroccan doctors prescribe morphine because of barriers of ignorance and fear of side effects. But things are changing now, slowly but surely.[2]

The International Narcotics Control Board[3] has published the following figures for the consumption of narcotic drugs in Morocco: codeine 519 kg; morphine 4 kg; pholcodine 119 kg; dextropropoxyphene 943 kg; ethylmorphine 16 kg.

For the years 2000–2002, the average defined daily dose consumption of morphine for statistical purposes (S-DDD)[4] in Morocco was 3 (Appendix 1).

National and professional organizations

Douleurs Sans Frontières (DSF)

The French NGO DSF is based in Paris and has seven projects around the world. Mati Nejmi is the Director of its research programme in Morocco. The organization currently supports a 'training of trainers' programme at the National Institute of Oncology in Rabat.

There is no national cancer programme in Morocco, nor is there a national palliative care association.

Palliative care coverage

Up to 50 000 new cases of cancer are registered each year in Morocco. Approximately 10 000 of these receive some form of treatment although few receive palliative care. The Moroccan Society of Management of Pain and Palliative Care in Rabat provides the only palliative care in Morocco. Since opening the centre, 750 patients have been treated each year for post-operative pain, 800 patients are hospitalized each year for cancer pain and >4500 patients have attended pain consultations.[2]

Education and training

Initial palliative care training and education in Morocco has been undertaken by the Moroccan Society of Management of Pain and Palliative Care located in Rabat. In 1999, the 3rd Euro-Maghrêbin conference on Pain and Palliative Care was held in Marrakech for between 300 and 400 health professionals. This initiative is repeated every 2 years. This organization runs a training of trainers programme to disseminate palliative care skills around the country. Since 2003, a total of 40 Moroccan doctors have participated in this course. Nurses are also trained in palliative care by the organization.

In 2004, the 4th Europe–Maghreb conference was held in Tabarka, Tunisia and adopted the theme *Pain and Supportive Care: Current Advances*. (The Maghreb is a region that includes Algeria, Morocco and Tunisia.) Significantly, nurse educator Françoise Porchet and three European colleagues were invited to provide a full day's training. They report:

> This opportunity allowed us to provide our nursing colleagues in the Maghreb with up-to-date knowledge on palliative care according to our individual specialties, while enabling them to acquire the knowledge through a process of exchange and constructive learning. It is very gratifying to note that the spirit of palliative care can transcend borders, cultures and languages. It is also important to realise all the possibilities that can arise from a training initiative put together between colleagues from three European countries and the extent to which this is a unifying event.[5]

Palliative care workforce capacity

The Moroccan Society of Management of Pain and Palliative Care has a team of five doctors and 15 nurses.

History and development of hospice–palliative care in Morocco

Building on the establishment of the National Institute of Oncology in Rabat in 1985, the Moroccan Society of Management of Pain and Palliative Care was created a decade later. A designated 10-bed centre for the management of pain and palliative care was established in 1995 and formalized as a society in 1996. So began morphine use for cancer pain, post-operative pain and palliative care.

Life/oral histories

Mati Nejmi reports:

> My first interest in the field of pain began when I was designated to be the Head of Department of Anaesthesiology and Care at the National Institute of Oncology in Rabat. I was suddenly affected by the severe pain that the majority of them have. I asked a French friend of mine in Paris to come to Morocco and make a conference of how to manage their patients. The first survey was done at the end of 1994 and morphine use started in March 1995. I founded the Moroccan Society of Study of Pain in July 1996. Managing pain is now a national priority since April 2003. The Ministry of Health gave us one million dollars for building a new National Centre of Pain and Palliative Care to have more capacity to treat cancer pain but also HIV patients with pain and chronic pain in general.[6]

Public health context

Population

Morocco's population of around 32.21 million people is made up of the following ethnic groups: Arab-Berber 99.1 per cent, Jewish 0.2 per cent, and other 0.7 per cent.

Religious groups include: Muslim 98.7 per cent, Christian 1.1 per cent and Jewish 0.2 per cent.[7]

Epidemiology

In Morocco, the WHO World Health Report (2004) indicates an adult mortality[8] rate per 1000 population of 160 for males and 104 for females. Life expectancy for males is 68.8; for females 72.8. Healthy life expectancy is 59.5 for males; and 60.9 for females.[9]

Morocco has been affected by the HIV/AIDS epidemic in Northern Africa. Estimates suggest that in Morocco, between five and 30 000 people were living with HIV/AIDS at the end of 2003. There are no figures available for adults and children who are thought to have died from the disease (Table 14.2).

UNAIDS reports:

> Morocco's HIV prevalence rate remains at a relatively low level. However, the National AIDS Control Programme estimates that the number of persons living with HIV has now reached

Table 14.2 Morocco HIV and AIDS estimates, end 2003

Adults (15–49) HIV prevalence rate	0.1 per cent (range 0.0–0.2 per cent)
Adults (15–49) living with HIV	15 000 (range 5000–30 000)
Adults and children (0–49) living with HIV	15 000 (range 5000–30 000)
Women (15–49) living with HIV	No figures available
AIDS deaths (adults and children) in 2003	No figures available

Source: 2004 Report of the global AIDS epidemic.

approximately 15,000. While HIV prevalence remains less than 1%, even in the most affected areas of the country, an increase of AIDS cases and HIV prevalence has been observed in some provinces. The National AIDS Control Programme (NACP) has recently completed the various phases of a National Strategic Plan (NSP) with the main conclusions highlighting: a) increase from 4 to 5 regions infected; b) existence of behavioural, social and economic factors of vulnerability; c) impact of AIDS on certain sectors; and d) confirmation of the relatively high prevalence of STIs in the country. The NSP has also led to the identification of the national programme's strengths and weaknesses. As a result of this process, a plan of action was formulated for 2002–2004 with the guiding principle of undertaking essential activities focused on the most vulnerable groups in the most affected areas. Simultaneously, the NACP will strengthen multisectoral coordination to ensure national coverage of prevention efforts.[10]

Health care system

In 2001, the total per capita expenditure on health care was Intl $199; 5.1% of GDP[11] (Appendix 3).

The WHO overall health system performance score places Morocco 29th out of 191 countries.[12]

Political economy

A manifesto of the Istiqlal (Independence) Party in 1944 was one of the earliest public demands for independence.

Gradual political reforms in the 1990s resulted in the establishment of a bicameral legislature in 1997. Parliamentary elections were held for the second time in September 2002, and municipal elections were held in September 2003. Morocco faces the problems typical of developing countries—restraining government spending, reducing constraints on private activity and foreign trade, and achieving sustainable economic growth. Despite structural adjustment programmes supported by the IMF, the World Bank and the Paris Club, the dirham is only fully convertible for current account transactions. Reforms of the financial sector are being contemplated. Droughts depressed activity in the key agricultural sector and contributed to a stagnant economy in 2002. Morocco reported large foreign exchange inflows from the sale of a mobile telephone licence, and partial privatization of the state-owned telecommunications company and the state tobacco company. Favourable rainfall in 2003 led to a growth of 6 per cent. Formidable long-term challenges include: preparing the economy for freer trade with the EU and USA, improving education, and attracting foreign investment to boost living standards and job prospects for Morocco's youth.[7]

The Moroccan economy is becoming increasingly diversified. Morocco has the largest phosphate reserves in the world. Other mineral resources include copper, fluorine, lead, barite, iron and anthracite. It has a diverse agricultural (including fishing) sector, a large tourist industry, a growing manufacturing sector (especially clothing) and considerable inflows of funds from Moroccans working abroad. The export of phosphates and its derivatives accounts for more than a quarter of Moroccan exports. Morocco is increasing production of phosphoric acid and fertilizers. About one-third of the Moroccan manufacturing sector is related to phosphates and one-third to agriculture, with virtually all of the remaining third divided between textiles, clothing and metalworking. The clothing sector, in particular, has shown consistently strong growth over the last few years as foreign companies established large-scale operations geared toward exporting garments to Europe. Agriculture plays a leading role in the Moroccan economy, generating between 15 and 20 per cent of GDP (depending on the harvest) and employing about 40 per cent of the work force. Morocco is a net exporter of fruits and vegetables, and a net importer of cereals; > 90 per cent of agriculture is rain-fed. Fishing is also important to Morocco, employing > 100 000 people, including the canning and packing industries.[13]

GDP per capita is Intl $3887(Appendix 4).

References

1 Report of the United Nations Development Programme 2004 (HDI 2002). Launched by the United Nations in 1990, the Human Development Index measures a country's achievements in three aspects of human development: longevity, knowledge and a decent standard of living. It was created to re-emphasize that people and their lives should be the ultimate criteria for assessing the development of a country, not economic growth. Current values range from 0.956 (Norway, first of 177 countries) to 0.273 (Sierra Leone, 177th out of 177 countries). Countries fall into one of three groups: countries 1–55 = high development; 56–141 = medium development; 142–177 = low development. See: http://hdr.undp.org/statistics/data/indic/indic_8_1_1.html

2 Personal communication: Mati Nejmi—5 April 2005.

3 International Narcotics Control Board. *Narcotic Drugs: Estimated World Requirements for 2004. Statistics for 2002.* New York: United Nations, 2004.

4 'The term *defined daily doses for statistical purposes* (S-DDD) replaces the term *defined daily doses* previously used by the Board. The S-DDDs are technical units of measurement for the purposes of statistical analysis and are not recommended prescription doses. Certain narcotic drugs may be used in certain countries for different treatments or in accordance with different medical practices, and therefore a different daily dose could be more appropriate'. The S-DDD used by the INCB for morphine is 100 mg. International Narcotics Control Board. *Narcotic Drugs: Estimated World Requirements for 2004. Statistics for 2002.* New York: United Nations, 2004: 176–177.

5 Porchet F, Schaerer G, Larkin P, Leruth S. Intercultural experiences of training in the Maghreb. *European Journal of Palliative Care* 2005; **12(1)**: 35–37.

6 Personal communication: Mati Nejmi—19 April 2005.

7 See: http://www.cia.gov/cia/publications/factbook/geos/mo.html

8 This refers to adult mortality risk, which is defined as the probability of dying between 15 and 59 years.

9 See: WHO statistics for Morocco at: http://www.who.int/countries/mar/en/

10 http://www.unaids.org/en/geographical+area/by+country/morocco.asp

11 Total health expenditure per capita is the per capita amount of the sum of Public Health Expenditure (PHE) and Private Expenditure on Health (PvtHE). The international dollar is a common currency unit that takes into account differences in the relative purchasing power of various currencies. Figures expressed in international dollars are calculated using purchasing power parities (PPP), which are rates of currency conversion constructed to account for differences in price level between countries. http://www3.who.int/whosis/country/compare.cfm?country =s&indicator=strPcTotEOHinIntD2000&language=english

12 This composite measure of overall health system attainment is based on a country's goals relating to health, responsiveness and fairness in financing. The measure varies widely across countries and is highly correlated with general levels of human development as captured in the human development index. Tandon A, Murray CLJ, Lauer JA, Evans DB. *Measuring Overall Health System Performance for 191 Countries*. GPE Discussion Paper Series: No. 30; WHO.

13 United States Government. *Background Notes on Countries of the World*. Washington, DC: US Government, Bureau of Public Affairs/Office of Public Communication, 2003.

Chapter 15

Nigeria

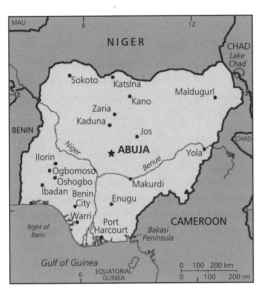

Nigeria (population 137.25 million) is a country in Western Africa that covers an area of 923 768 km². Its boundaries border the Gulf of Guinea, between Benin and Cameroon, Niger and Chad. The capital city of Nigeria is Abuja.

According to the United Nations human development index (HDI), Nigeria is ranked 151st out of 177 countries worldwide (0.466)[1] and 21st out of 45 in African countries for which an index is available. This places Nigeria in the group of countries with low human development.

Palliative care service provision

Current services

Palliative care services are provided by two organizations in Nigeria, the Palliative Care Initiative (Ibadan) and Hospice Nigeria (Lagos) (Table 15.1).

Palliative care services in Nigeria are undeveloped. There is continuing resistance to some palliative care concepts including opiate use, the multidisciplinary team approach to the management of medical problems and the inclusion of patient and family as the unit of care.

Table 15.1 Palliative care provision in Nigeria, 2004

	Free-standing unit	Hospital unit	Hospital support team	Home care	Day care	Clinic/drop-in centre	Total
Palliative Care Initiative, Ibadan		1				1	2
Hospice Nigeria, Lagos				1			1
Total services		1		1		1	3

Palliative Care Initiative, Nigeria (PCIN)

Palliative care is being introduced to Nigeria through the Palliative Care Initiative, Nigeria based at the College of Medicine, University of Ibadan. PCIN is a multidisciplinary group of medical specialists who implement the major objectives of training, service and research in this area of medical care. The group was formed in January 2003 and, in addition to sensitizing the public on the importance of palliative care, it has sponsored some of its members to attend palliative care courses and conferences in other countries. It operates a pain and palliative care clinic at the University College Hospital, Ibadan. This was commissioned in February 2005 to provide support for patients with chronic pain and for cancer patients.[2] The group is working towards including palliative care in the curriculum of medical and nursing students, based upon guidelines developed by Hospice Africa Uganda. Funding is being sought to develop home-based palliative care services. A train the trainers programme is expected to produce locally trained palliative care practitioners. Olaitan Soyannwo summarizes the current situation:

> So what we have in terms of palliative care right now is a lot of individuals—oncologists, surgeons, physicians—just managing patients as best as they can. But the holistic approach is missing. We've just introduced that using a small clinic in the radiotherapy unit and a group of us—two anaesthetists, one oncologist, one nurse and a psycho-oncologist (who does counselling)—run a clinic once a week. Patients with terminal illness on the ward are referred to us, but one major problem is the availability of opioids. We don't have oral morphine in the country: we have injectable opioids but even that was not available for about four years. We had to do a lot of advocacy because some years back there was a regulatory problem and opioids were banned because they were grouped with narcotics. So although it's on the National Drug Formulary, we don't have the oral form—even on the Formulary—so we are doing a lot of advocacy to get that in now for palliative care and management of ill patients.[3]

She envisages palliative care as a helpful approach in managing the HIV/AIDS epidemic in Nigeria.

> We had a group, an international group—a collaborative between my university, the Medical Women's Association from Lagos, and a group from Chicago, who were mainly alumni of the university and are interested in cancer care. Although we focused on cancer of the breast and cervix, which are the two commonest cancers, we want to use the template to do a lot of advocacy for patients with cancer and HIV/AIDS. And the good thing that I think we have in my institution is that we're already on the national programme in terms of ARV therapy and also prevention of mother to child transmission. Since that is already established, I am hoping that it will not be too difficult, with the support from APCA, for this new organization to be able to convince them back home that palliative care should be part of the AIDS programme in the country.[3]

PCIN organized a 1-day workshop on the art and science of palliative care and the management of terminally ill patients in Nigeria on 27 January 2005. Participants included the Provost and Principal Officers of the College of Medicine, The Chief Medical Director, Chairman, Medical Advisory Committee and Director of Administration of the University College Hospital, Ibadan. Also present were representatives of the Commissioner of Health (Oyo State), Permanent Secretary, Ministry of Health (Osun State), retired and serving members of the judiciary, clergy, health professionals, students, the public and the press. There were also representatives of Hospice Nigeria based in Lagos and the Palliative Care Association based in Abeokuta. International guests included Anne Merriman, Founder of Hospice Africa Uganda, and Jack Jagwe, a Senior Adviser on Drugs Policy in Uganda.[2] A primary focus for the workshop was to advocate for palliative care in Nigeria. The main outcomes of the workshop are as follows:

> . . . to promote a greater awareness of the benefits of palliative medicine in the population at large, and among all cadres of professional and traditional health care providers. The workshop also recommended a review of the existing restrictions on the availability of oral morphine and other opioids in recognized hospitals and clinics for the relief of severe pain, especially in terminal care situations. It recognizes palliative care as a specialty in itself and the need to train trainers in the field.
>
> The workshop recognizes the leadership roles of the Federal Ministry of Health (FMOH) and the National Agency for Food and Drug Administration and Control (NAFDAC) in these endeavours and urges the Palliative Care Initiative of Nigeria (PCIN) to seek the co-operation of these institutions in these matters.
>
> The workshop strongly recommends the formation of a National Committee or a National Association on Palliative Care to coordinate the activities of satellite groups nationwide, to establish the standards and ethics of terminal care, and to foster relations with similar organizations worldwide.[2]

Hospice Nigeria

This NGO in Lagos was registered in 1993 and provides home-based care to the terminally ill. It is most often utilized by patients returning home to Nigeria from abroad. The founder, Olusola Fatunmbi, explains the system:

> I had more patients referred to me from London at Lagos Hospitals than within Nigeria, but they knew I had drug problems, and on that basis they promised to see that the patients come with enough oral morphine and some other palliative drugs for their use. And my home care service with my husband and occasionally some of the members of the Trustees, was acquired, was free because we had no funding from anybody, and the counselling, the only thing is that the patients buy their own drugs.[4]

A cancer public awareness campaign has resulted in a few local patients benefiting from the organization's help although scarce supplies of oral morphine result in poor pain management.

Several other organizations and individuals may offer some elements of palliative care in clinics and support services for HIV/AIDS patients. Two doctors based at Federal Medical Centre, Abeokuta (Ogun State) and Zaria have formed a Palliative Care Association and are understood to be promoting palliative care.

Reimbursement and funding for services

The Diana, Princess of Wales Memorial Fund sponsored a visit by Olaitan Soyannwo and two of her colleagues to Hospice Africa Uganda. The aim of this visit was to develop a strategy towards training of trainers within Nigeria in order to build palliative care capacity. The visit of a third colleague was later sponsored by the College of Medicine, University of Ibadan.

A 1-day palliative care workshop in Ibadan in January 2005 was co-sponsored by Help the Hospices, UK and the African Palliative Care Association (APCA).

Initial funding is being sought by Hospice Africa Uganda to develop home-based care services by PCIN. This programme has not yet been established.

President's Emergency Plan for AIDS Relief (PEPFAR)

During the 2004 financial year (FY), funding of around US$55.49 million was enacted for country-managed programmes in Nigeria and US$15.43 million for central programmes. During FY2005, it is anticipated that a total of US$108.86 million will be enacted: US$84.36 million for country-managed programmes and US$24.50 million for central programmes[5] (Appendix 2).

The Diana, Princess of Wales Memorial Fund/Hospice Africa Uganda

In Central and East Africa, Hospice Africa Uganda became the Diana Fund's partner agency in a 3-year project which attracted funding of £300 000. It was expected that during this period, Hospice Africa Uganda would:

♦ Provide technical support and advice on the identification of countries with the capacity and political will to initiate palliative care services

♦ Provide guidance and training to such countries

♦ Set up and run a distance learning Diploma in Palliative care for African countries

♦ Set up a resource centre of palliative care materials for Africa, at Makindye, Kampala

♦ Improve services within Uganda so that a model can be developed that works for the poorest and that can be duplicated in other African countries.

Anne Merriman comments:

> In 2001, the Diana, Princess of Wales, Memorial Fund in London, invited Hospice Africa Uganda to be their technical experts in assisting other African countries to start or strengthen palliative care services using the public health approach and integrating with existing health systems. Working with World Health Organisation, this initiative has brought the Hospice training programmes to several other African countries.[6]

As part of this vision, Hospice Africa Uganda has assisted PCIN in its efforts to introduce palliative care into Nigeria.

The UK Forum for Hospice and Palliative Care Worldwide has awarded grants to

♦ PCIN—for a 2-day regional advocacy workshop involving health professionals, policy makers and others from the south west of Nigeria: £2000.

♦ Federal Medical Centre—support for Folaju Oyebola (Master's degree in Palliative Medicine): £1500.

Opioid availability and consumption

The International Narcotics Control Board[7] has published the following figures for the consumption of narcotic drugs in Nigeria: codeine 296 kg; Pholcodine 19 kg; and pethidine 5 kg.

For the years 2000–2002, the average defined daily dose consumption of morphine for statistical purposes (S-DDD)[8] in Nigeria was 0 (Appendix 1).

Olaitan Soyannwo confirms that opioid analgesics (parenteral and oral) are not available in government stores and health facilities.[2]

National and Professional Associations

There is no national association in the country. This has been identified as a priority by the participants of the palliative care workshop held in February 2005 in Ibadan.

Palliative care coverage

In January 2005, representatives of APCA presented papers at a workshop convened in Ibadan to promote advocacy for palliative care in Nigeria

Palliative Care Initiative, Nigeria

There are approximately 3000 patients per year who attend the radiotherapy unit at the University College Hospital in Ibadan either as inpatients or as outpatients. About 30 cancer patients admitted to the hospital each year are referred to the PCIN team.

Hospice Nigeria

The majority of patients seen by this home-based care programme are Nigerians recently returned home from abroad. Very few local Nigerians utilize the service.

Education and training

In the absence of formal palliative care policies, palliative care education has been undertaken by individuals.

Palliative Care Initiative, Nigeria

Olaitan Soyannwo uses her position as lecturer and senior academic to spread knowledge of palliative care.

> Right now at Ibadan we have a new group in the College of Medicine and we've introduced palliative care into the curriculum of medical students and nursing students. The proposal has been sent from the Faculty, it's now awaiting approval at the College level so that once that is passed it can go into the curriculum.[3]

From April 2005, an oncology nurse from PCIN will undertake an 8-week course at Hospice Africa Uganda.

Hospice Nigeria

This home-based care programme has identified the model of training used by Hospice Africa Uganda as appropriate for its training development. Nurse Olusola Fatunmbi comments:

> I now know that the Uganda model is much, much more relevant to us in Africa, I mean in terms of setting something up. The facilities are very limited here, and I'm thinking that it would be easier to incorporate palliative care training and teaching into the existing health care model that is within the country, so that everybody, even right up to the village health workers, are trained. Because in terms of malaria, for example, they are training people to give home care; so if people are trained at every level on palliative care, then even if the patients are discharged to distant places, you can have some contact point. And after training a few experts in palliative care—I mean doctors, nurses, social workers—they can now train the others locally. That's the way.[4]

History and development of hospice—palliative care in Nigeria

Palliative Care Initiative, Nigeria

As Professor of Anaesthesia and Dean of Clinical Sciences at the College of Medicine, Olaitan Soyannwo developed an interest in pain management, especially of patients undergoing acute surgery and trauma. Expanding her interest to cancer pain, she attended the World Pain Congress in 1996 and thereafter established a palliative care team in her home country. The Palliative Care Initiative, Nigeria is being registered as an NGO. Three members of the group have experience in palliative care.

Hospice Nigeria

Olusola Fatunmbi is a nurse and became aware of international hospice programmes during the 1990s. A combination of training courses at St Christopher's Hospice in the UK and a visit by Anne Merriman to Nigeria provided her with the confidence to establish a home-based care programme in Lagos for people living with terminal illness.

Life/oral histories

Professor Olaitan Soyannwo—*dean of clinical sciences, College of Medicine, University of Ibadan*: interviewed by David Clark, 4 June 2004. Length of interview (West Africa group): 40 min.

Professor Olaitan Soyannwo explains how her interest in pain management arose out of seeing the suffering of surgical and trauma patients. Realizing that cancer patients received no pain management at all, she attended the World Pain Congress of the International Association for the Study of Pain (IASP) in 1996 and returned to Nigeria inspired to establish a pain and palliative care team at the University Teaching Hospital. This led to inauguration of the Society for the Study of Pain which is now a chapter of IASP; the Palliative Care Initiative, Nigeria to be established by her team. She lists the fora through which she

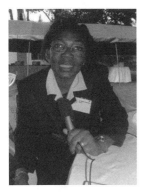

spreads the word of palliative care principles, including the West African College of Surgeons and the Faculty of Anaesthesia. Advocacy for palliative care and accessibility to oral morphine is a priority. Introduction of palliative care methods into the curriculum for medical and nursing students has been presented for ratification by the university authorities. Hospice Uganda has been the model for training health professionals. Without oral morphine in the country, health professionals do what they can with injectable morphine. Beginning with cancers of the breast and cervix, this group of professionals is developing a protocol of holistic care that can be applied to other conditions, including HIV/AIDS. The hospital is already registered for ARV therapy and prevention of mother to child transmission. She hopes that palliative care will be implemented by these programmes. Turning to the APCA and her role as board member, Olaitan Soyannwo reflects on Anne Merriman's efforts to introduce palliative care to Nigeria before moving to Kenya and Uganda. She hopes that APCA will give the necessary impetus to the implementation of palliative care by both the public health system and the private sector in Nigeria. She identifies the need to form a national palliative care association in the country in order to gain an accurate picture of the various services.

Olusola Fatunmbi—*nurse, founder of Hospice Nigeria*: interviewed by David Clark, 4 June 2004. Length of interview (West Africa group): 40 min.

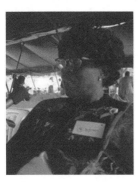

Olusola Fatunmbi attended the Sixth International Conference at St Christopher's Hospice in 1991 and was inspired to return to Nigeria to implement home-based palliative care. Having met Anne Merriman at the conference, she invited her to Nigeria in 1993 to advocate with the Ministry of Health for the necessary systems to be put in place for palliative care. Talks were held at the Lagos Teaching Hospital, but there was little political will at the time to embrace this medical speciality. Having attended further palliative care courses at St Christopher's Hospice, she began to network with an oncologist in the region who shared her vision of home-based care for the needy. Establishing a home-based care service with her husband and other interested professionals, she facilitates palliative care for many Nigerian patients referred from St Christopher's Hospice. She describes how oral morphine is unavailable in Nigeria, necessitating patients arriving from the UK with their own supply of palliative drugs. Referrals of patients from the diaspora continue to account for the majority of her patients. Olusola Fatunmbi gives a moving account of one of her patients whose symptoms were well controlled using locally available vegetables. She concludes by sharing her vision for palliative care education to be incorporated into existing health care systems in Africa in general and Nigeria in particular, using the model championed by Hospice Africa, Uganda.

Public health context

Population

Nigeria is Africa's most populous country (137.25 million), it is composed of >250 ethnic groups; the following are the most populous and politically influential: Hausa and Fulani 29 per cent, Yoruba 21 per cent, Igbo (Ibo) 18 per cent, Ijaw 10 per cent, Kanuri 4 per cent, Ibibio 3.5 per cent and Tiv 2.5 per cent

Religious groups include: Muslim 50 per cent, Christian 40 per cent and indigenous beliefs 10 per cent.[9]

Epidemiology

In Nigeria, the WHO World Health Report (2004) indicates an adult mortality[10] rate per 1000 population of 453 for males and 392 for females. Life expectancy for males is 48.0; for females 49.6. Healthy life expectancy is 41.3 for males; and 41.8 for females.[11]

Nigeria is one of the worst HIV/AIDS-affected countries in Western Africa. Estimates suggest that in Nigeria, between 2.4 and 5.4 million people were living with HIV/AIDS at the end of 2003. In the same year, up to 490 000 adults and children are thought to have died from the disease (Table 15.2).

UNAIDS reports:

> While Nigeria's infection rate is lower than those of neighbouring countries, it nonetheless represents higher number of infections, given the large population; the country now has the highest number of HIV/AIDS-infected adults in West Africa. HIV/AIDS was first reported in Nigeria in 1986. Since then, the epidemic has been growing rapidly. In 2002 alone, more than 200,000 AIDS-related deaths occurred, and it was estimated that Nigeria had more than one million children orphaned by AIDS. Many factors that favour a rapid spread of the virus are prevalent in Nigeria, including high mobility, trafficking of young girls, marginalization of women, poverty, social and economic inequality, and specific socio-cultural practices. The 'Next Wave of HIV/AIDS' report of the US National Intelligence Council predicts an estimated 10-15 million people living with HIV in the country by 2010.

Table 15.2 Nigeria HIV and AIDS estimates, end 2003

Adults (15–49) HIV prevalence rate	5.4 per cent (range: 3.6–8.0 per cent)
Adults (15–49) living with HIV	3 300 000 (range: 2 200 000–4 900 000)
Adults and children (0–49) living with HIV	3 600 000 (range: 2 400 000–5 400 000)
Women (15–49) living with HIV	1 900 000 (range: 1 200 000–2 700 000)
AIDS deaths (adults and children) in 2003	310 000 (range: 200 000–490 000)

Source: 2004 Report of the global AIDS epidemic.

Nigeria has put in place the necessary coordinating and decision-making bodies: the Presidential AIDS Council is chaired by the president of the country and includes the main line ministries. The federal coordination mechanism, the National Action Committee on AIDS (NACA), has been fully established with adequate infrastructure and capacity. Civil society participation in the fight against HIV/AIDS has been institutionalized through the establishment of coordination mechanisms such as the Network of People Living with HIV in Nigeria (NEPWAN), the Civil Society Consultative Group on HIV/AIDS in Nigeria (CiSCGHAN), the Faith-based Forum on HIV/AIDS, and the Nigeria Business Council on HIV/AIDS (NIBUCAA). The timeframe of the HIV/AIDS Emergency Action Plan (HEAP) 2000-2003 has elapsed and a review of the HEAP is being planned in the context of the participatory development of the new National HIV/AIDS Strategic Framework 2005-2009. Preparations for the drafting of the National Health Sector Strategic Plan and an advocacy strategy are well under way.[12]

Health care system

In 2001, the total per capita expenditure on health care was Intl $31; 3.4% of GDP[13] (Appendix 3).

The WHO overall health system performance score places Nigeria 187th out of 191 countries.[14]

Political economy

Before the colonial period, the area that comprises modern Nigeria had an eventful history. More than 2000 years ago, the Nok culture in the present Plateau state worked iron and produced sophisticated terra cotta sculpture. In the northern cities of Kano and Katsina, recorded history dates back to approximately 1000 AD. In the centuries that followed, these Hausa kingdoms and the Bomu empire near Lake Chad prospered as important terminals of north-south trade between North African Berbers and forest people who exchanged ivory and kola nuts for salt, glass beads, coral, cloth, weapons, brass rods, and cowrie shells used as currency. In the southwest, the Yoruba kingdom of Oyo was founded about 1400, and at its height from the seventeenth to nineteenth centuries attained a high level of political organization and extended as far as modern Togo. In the south central part of present-day Nigeria, as early as the fifteenth and sixteenth centuries, the kingdom of Benin had developed an efficient army; an elaborate ceremonial court; and artisans whose works in ivory, wood, bronze and brass are prized throughout the world today. In the early nineteenth century, the Fulani leader, Usman dan Fodio, launched an Islamic crusade that brought most of the Hausa states and other areas in the north under the loose control of an empire centred in Sokoto.[15]

Since independence, the economy has increasingly come under the influence of the oil industry which has moved the country away from its agricultural base. However, oil has affected the way in which successive military regimes have approached economic management as well as investment and consumption patterns.[16] The capital-intensive oil sector provides 20 per cent of GDP, 95 per cent of foreign exchange earnings and about 65 per cent of budgetary revenues. The largely subsistence agricultural sector has failed to keep up with rapid population growth—Nigeria is Africa's most populous country—and the country, once a large net exporter of food, now must import food. The IMF have proposed a number of market-oriented reforms, such as modernization of the banking system, the curbing of inflation by blocking excessive wage demands, and the resolution of regional disputes over the distribution of earnings from the oil industry.

During 2003, the government deregulated fuel prices and announced the privatization of the country's four oil refineries. GDP growth will probably rise marginally in the future, led by oil and natural gas exports. The country faces the daunting task of rebuilding a petroleum-based economy and institutionalizing democracy if it is to build a sound foundation for economic growth and political stability.[9]

There has been a long-term, halting diffusion of the liberal democratic state. Key contextual factors of transition include: international pressure for democratization, geopolitical dynamics of pro-democracy coalitions, and local and trans-local political economic relationships. Nigeria, under the military governments of Babangida and Abacha (1985–1998), was in a perpetual half-hearted state of transition to democracy. The country's status as a major oil exporter allowed it relative immunity from international pressure for democratization. Mobilization for state creation served to divide opposition to military government because it focused attention at the local scale, as new state movements competed for access to centrally controlled resources and political recognition of their ethno-regional group(s).[17] In 1999, following 15 years of military rule, a new constitution was adopted and a peaceful transition to civilian government was eventually completed; the first civilian transfer of power in Nigeria's history.

GDP per capita is Intl $915 (Appendix 4).

References

1 Report of the United Nations Development Programme 2004 (HDI 2002). Launched by the United Nations in 1990, the Human Development Index measures a country's achievements in three aspects of human development: longevity, knowledge and a decent standard of living. It was created to re-emphasize that people and their lives should be the ultimate criteria for assessing the development of a country, not economic growth. Current values range from 0.956 (Norway, first of 177 countries) to 0.273 (Sierra Leone, 177th out of 177 countries). Countries fall into one of three groups: countries 1–55 = high development; 56–141 = medium development; 142–177 = low development. See: http://hdr.undp.org/statistics/data/indic/indic_8_1_1.html

2 Personal communication: Olaitan Soyannwo—25 March 2005.

3 IOELC interview: Olaitan Soyannwo—4 June 2004.

4 IOELC interview: Olusola Fatunmbi—4 June 2004.

5 *Engendering Bold Leadership*. The President's Emergency Plan for AIDS Relief. First Annual Report to Congress, 2005: 115. http://www.state.gov/documents/organization/43885.pdf

6 Merriman A. Hospice Africa Uganda: 10th Anniversary (1993–2003). In: *Proceedings from Palliative Care: Completing the Circle of Care*, 16–17 September 2003.

7 International Narcotics Control Board. *Narcotic Drugs: Estimated World Requirements for 2004. Statistics for 2002*. New York: United Nations, 2004.

8 'The term *defined daily doses for statistical purposes* (S-DDD) replaces the term *defined daily doses* previously used by the Board. The S-DDDs are technical units of measurement for the purposes

of statistical analysis and are not recommended prescription doses. Certain narcotic drugs may be used in certain countries for different treatments or in accordance with different medical practices, and therefore a different daily dose could be more appropriate'. The S-DDD used by the INCB for morphine is 100 mg. International Narcotics Control Board. *Narcotic Drugs: Estimated World Requirements for 2004. Statistics for 2002*. New York: United Nations, 2004: 176–177.

9 See: http://www.cia.gov/cia/publications/factbook/geos/ni.html

10 This refers to adult mortality risk, which is defined as the probability of dying between 15 and 59 years.

11 See: WHO statistics for Nigeria at: http://www.who.int/countries/nga/en/

12 http://www.unaids.org/en/geographical+area/by+country/nigeria.asp

13 Total health expenditure per capita is the per capita amount of the sum of Public Health Expenditure (PHE) and Private Expenditure on Health (PvtHE). The international dollar is a common currency unit that takes into account differences in the relative purchasing power of various currencies. Figures expressed in international dollars are calculated using purchasing power parities (PPP), which are rates of currency conversion constructed to account for differences in price level between countries.http://www3.who.int/whosis/country/compare.cfm?country=s&indicator= strPcTotEOHinIntD2000&language+english

14 This composite measure of overall health system attainment is based on a country's goals relating to health, responsiveness and fairness in financing. The measure varies widely across countries and is highly correlated with general levels of human development as captured in the human development index. Tandon A, Murray CLJ, Lauer JA, Evans DB. *Measuring Overall Health System Performance for 191 Countries*. GPE Discussion Paper Series: No. 30; WHO.

15 US Department of State, Bureau of Public Affairs, Office of Public Communication. *Background Notes on Countries of the World 2003*. Washington, DC: US Department of State, Bureau of Public Affairs, Office of Public Communication, 2003.

16 World of Information Business Intelligence Report, 2001. Nigeria: Economy, Politics and Government. *Business Intelligence Report: Nigeria* 2001;**1**(1): 1–46.

17 **Kraxberger B.** Geo-historical trajectories of democratic transition: the case of Nigeria. *Geojournal* 2004; **60**(1): 81–92.

Chapter 16

Sierra Leone

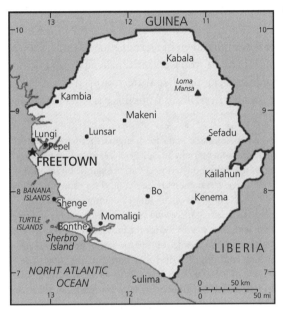

The Republic of Sierra Leone (population 5.88 million) is a country in Western Africa bordering the North Atlantic Ocean. It covers an area of 71 740 km^2 and its boundaries border the countries of Guinea and Liberia. The capital of the country is Freetown.

According to the United Nations human development index (HDI), Sierra Leone is ranked 177th out of 177 countries worldwide (value 0.273)[1] and 45th out of 45 in African countries for which an index is available. This means that Sierra Leone has the lowest measure for human development both in Africa and in the world.

Palliative care service provision

Current services

In Sierra Leone, palliative care services are provided by The Shepherd's Hospice (TSH), Freetown (Table 16.1).

Table 16.1 Palliative care provision in Sierra Leone

	Free-standing unit	Hospital unit	Hospital support team	Home care	Day care	Clinic/drop-in centre	Total
The Shepherd's Hospice	1			1		1	3

At TSH, the range of services includes:

- Home-based care
- Inpatient care (24 h symptom control)
- Outpatients clinics (twice a week)
- Education and training
- Orphans and Vulnerable Children's programme
- Women's Wellness Project (WWP)
- Advocacy.

During the 1990s, when palliative care was unknown in Sierra Leone, Gabriel Madiye became aware of the lack of provision for patients who were terminally ill. In an attempt to find a way forward, he set out to determine the disparate standpoints of those involved: health professionals, patients and relatives. It was from this base that the service developed:

Health caregivers in Freetown, the doctors and nurses, had a whole lot of stigma; they were discriminating against people living with HIV/AIDS and other terminal cases. Myths existed: that treating HIV-infected cases and admitting them together with non-terminal cases might be injurious or harmful to the non-HIV cases. So the health caregivers demonstrated the need for some sort of a place to isolate cases or, to be very informal, probably to say where they can dump terminal cases, and for somebody to be there as a governor to take care of those who could not be cared for within the mainstream of the health care delivery system. That was a need for the health caregivers.

For the people living with HIV/AIDS and cancer, they needed compassion; they needed acceptance and they needed information. How long will I live? If I die today how can my property be protected against uncles who might want to grab it and possess it and leave my children without property? How long do I need to live with HIV and AIDS? Does being HIV positive mean you are dying tomorrow? So their needs were principally centred on a need for compassion, for acceptance and information.

And for the family members, their needs centred on somebody to treat their relatives that were now sick; they wanted care at all costs, and they wanted professional medical care to be provided for their ill relatives.

Putting all these needs together we are able to plan and say, yes, if the Minister of Health and Sanitation is saying, 'Let us have inpatient palliative care', or the health caregivers want that to serve as a place where cases that are rejected within the main health care services could be accommodated: yes, fine—palliative care inpatient could be one service.[2]

Today, the hospice is housed in two adjacent three-storey buildings. Accommodation is as follows:

Building 1

- Ground floor: pharmacy, 4-bed female ward, 2-bed male ward
- First floor: administration offices, clinic office and resource centre/library
- Second floor: Training Hall

Building 2

- Ground floor: garage and store
- First floor: kitchen and dining room
- Second floor: smaller training hall/resource centre, also used for fundraising activity

The wards are currently unused because of a lack of privacy (outsiders can see through the windows) and aggressive reaction towards HIV/AIDS patients. Erection of a surrounding fence is seen as a priority.[3]

Ruth Cecil (clinical nurse specialist, palliative care) joined Sheila Hurton (Princess Alice Hospice) and Jacqui Boulton (SRN and midwife) on a visit to TSH in January 2004 and subsequently wrote:

> Driving through Freetown and along Kissy Road I saw the war damaged buildings and the offices of some of the 106 NGOs said to be helping re-build Sierra Leone following the war.
>
> Sierra Leone has few doctors and nurses as many leave to work in Europe/USA. Capacity building is a term used for the dissemination of knowledge, in this case of HIV/AIDS prevention and care and palliative care.
>
> What is happening in Sierra Leone is excruciatingly shocking. The battle against HIV/AIDS is taking place in a climate of denial and lack of basic resources. I have great admiration for the work of TSH and its staff. This work includes sensitisation to combat the stigma associated with HIV/AIDS. It is this stigma connected with job loss, family rejection, and social ostracism, which prevents people taking the AIDS test and seeking help. Education about HIV/AIDS and its prevention, and schooling for AIDS orphans, are also tasks undertaken by TSH.[4]

Jacqui Boulton comments:

> We continued to get a feel for the work of TSH by visiting the Women's Wellness Project at Tombo, a village outside Freetown. The project seeks to provide something positive for women who are diagnosed with HIV, integrating them with women from other vulnerable groups to provide literacy, numeracy, life skills and health education. In response, they agree to act as 'peer educators' in the community.
>
> I was fortunate to spend a morning at the United Methodist Church Maternity centre. This is one of the hospice partner institutions with staff seconded to TSH for training. I was shown around by Isata, a student midwife who had attended our training course and who was now responsible for counselling those pregnant mothers agreeing to be tested for HIV. On the morning of our visit 84 women were waiting in the antenatal clinic. These would be seen on a first come, first served basis and some were asleep having arrived from 6 a.m. As an incentive for attendance, the mothers received a helping of yoghurt eaten in the presence of a uniformed nurse![5]

Reimbursement and funding for services

As an NGO, TSH relies on fundraising and charitable donations to meet its costs.

The hospice building was twice destroyed (1998 and 1999) in the 11-year civil war that badly affected Sierra Leone during the 1990s. However, intermittent funding from the UK enabled the reactivation of the hospice's work and, with the additional help of Help the Hospices (HtH) and the World Bank, the main building (Building 1) was completed in mid-2002.

In 2001, designated funding from the Catholic Organization for Relief and Development (CORDAID) and Bread for the World supported education programmes focusing on HIV/AIDS prevention and care, while UK funds were still needed for drugs and general running costs.

Further funds, including those from the US Embassy and UNICEF, enabled construction of a second building (Building 2) to provide garage, storage and support services (kitchen, dining room and resource centre) for training. This building was completed in late 2003.

Funding has also been received from the US Embassy, Catholic Relief Services, Friends of The Shepherd's Hospice (UK), Christian Health Association of Sierra Leone and the Ministry of Health and Sanitation.[3] Additionally, British Executive Service Overseas (BESO) supported accounting training programmes in 2002 and 2004 with placement of their volunteers, and HtH funded a palliative care education and training course in 2002.

Opioid availability and consumption

The International Narcotics Control Board[6] has published the following figures for the consumption of principle narcotic drugs in Sierra Leone: morphine 2 kg.

For the years 2000–2002, the average defined daily dose consumption of morphine for statistical purposes (S-DDD)[7] in Sierra Leone was 8 (Appendix 1).

National and professional organizations

Christian Health Association of Sierra Leone (CHASL)[8]

This is a non-governmental, non-profit making, interdenominational health co-ordinating agency whose secretariat in Freetown serves > 30 (Christian-based) member health institutions in Sierra Leone.

Friends of The Shepherd's Hospice (UK)

This UK-based group supports the hospice in variety of ways, such as raising funds and providing training.

Palliative care coverage

TSH takes patients from Freetown and parts of the western area of Sierra Leone.

Education and training

Gabriel Madiye reflects on the first ever training course at TSH:

> In 1997, our first volunteer training was conducted whereby around 27 community volunteers were trained. The model we used was from the United States. Working with Catholic Relief Services, we contacted some hospices in the United States and we contacted WHO as they also have models on palliative care for people living with HIV/AIDS and other terminal diseases. And we used that to train our first batch of volunteers.[2]

In April 2002, a request for training in Sierra Leone was answered by Gilly Burn, Helen Passant and Dr Charles (Charlie) Bond. Gilly Burn and Helen Passant have wide-ranging teaching experience having previously worked in India; Charlie Bond—palliative care physician at the Sue Ryder Unit, Nettlebed (Henley on Thames, UK)—has experience of working in Uganda and Malawi. Gilly Burn:

> Prior to departure, I had been in touch with the airline to register excess baggage for books, and so we departed with 120 kg baggage between the three of us! I visited TALC (Teaching AIDS at Low Cost) before we left and we had also been in touch with pharmaceutical companies who generously supplied books and other educational materials. We flew overnight and arrived at Lungi, Freetown's rather primitive airport, very early in the morning, then took a helicopter to Lower Allen Town.
>
> We taught at the YMCA on the top floor. I had taken out slides—but they could only be used every other day! On the days when there *was* electricity, there were no blackout blinds! Appearances on national radio and TV also gave us valuable opportunities to talk about the reason for our visit, and we hope that these may have stimulated further support for the work of the hospice.
>
> There were 29 course participants from all over Sierra Leone. We were impressed by the eagerness to learn, by the openness and sharing of experiences, by the lack of embarrassment about not knowing and being prepared to ask questions repeatedly if there was misunderstanding. The days started with and ended with prayers and singing, and our work was interspersed with fun and humour. The teaching was:

◆ Symptom control

◆ Palliative care for people with AIDS

◆ Communication skills

◆ Maximizing care through touch

◆ Enhancing nursing care.[9]

Today, TSH is involved in a wide range of training programmes. These include:

◆ Capacity building in partnership with 23 health care institutions. These are ongoing partnerships whereby the hospice offers an ongoing training programme for health professionals and volunteers.

◆ Training health professionals and volunteers to work in their own communities, with training part preventative (i.e. safe sex) and also to help them identify people who are HIV positive or who have cancer.

◆ HIV/AIDS education outside of the hospice setting—for example, in the workplace and in schools (on request).

◆ In addition, a 2-day course was arranged in January 2004, facilitated by Sheila Hurton, Ruth Cecil, and Jacqui Boulton (Box 16.1). It included:

◆ Twenty-seven participants, including nurses, midwives, social workers and volunteers

◆ Content and structure according to the training needs assessed during the first session and in discussion with the Executive Director who stressed the need for documentation, WHO analgesic ladder and principles of palliative care.

Library facilities at TSH are increasing. Through the generosity of UK supporters, TSH has expanded its small library of medical reference books. These are generally available to institution partners/course participants visiting TSH. Photocopying facilities are also available.

Course programme

Day 1

1 Participants' expectations

2 Pain control—analgesic ladder adapted to medication available in Freetown.

3 Communications and role-play taking HIV/AIDS as the basic subject.

Day 2

1 Group work on four aspects of palliative care: physical, social, spiritual and psychological

2 First assessment and documentation of first assessment

3 Fundraising

4 Wound care/demonstration of charcoal dressing

5 Implementing change in the workplace

6 Evaluation

Palliative care workforce capacity

TSH is managed by a board of seven directors.

In 2004, hospice staff included: one executive director (a former public health officer), one senior nurse, one home care co-ordinator (nurse), one social worker/chaplain, one health education officer, one community health officer, one finance officer, one pharmacist (part time), administrative and domestic staff, and volunteers.

History and development of hospice–palliative care in Sierra Leone

The first hospice developments in Sierra Leone began in 1994 as a response to the needs of people living with a terminal illness. Gabriel Madiye, founder of TSH, contacted St Christopher's Hospice, London, and subsequently made contact with hospices in the USA. As the nascent movement developed, Sierra Leone was engulfed by a civil war and, during the hostilities, the hospice premises were destroyed twice.[10] The vision survived, however, and as the war came to an end, Gabriel Madiye began again and brought the vision to reality once more. He recalls:

> It all started with the recognition of the problem in a very genuine way and it continued with organizing a community effort; sensitizing people around the problem to see how they can rally around. It was essentially a volunteer movement and we started in 1994. By 1995, we were able to write the initial statement, write a strategic plan, and we were able to register with the government

of Sierra Leone as a non-governmental organization with a mandate to deliver a service that was basically palliative care.

My own role in the hospice has been management, planning and research; making sure that services are appropriate to the needs of the local community. And I try to make sure that our pro-grammes are based on sound research. Because of that, we have always maintained good donor relations—with donor confidence and donor interest in our work. We initially started from nowhere and today, over the last four years, we have been able to work with 11 international donors, including the World Bank, WHO, Bread for the World, Help the Hospices, and now we are doing some work with Comic Relief.

The project itself is capacity building, which implies that The Shepherd's Hospice itself is a facil-itating institution: we have patients referred to us; we train their family caregivers; we train volun-teers; the volunteers pay visits to the home once every week; and the family caregiver is almost always there in the home. The professional team is multidisciplinary, consisting of the social worker, a medical officer and the nurses; they stay at the hospice and they have a routine schedule to visit those patients. And you can call on the professional team at any time and we are mobile; we can go in.[2]

As plans for the hospice took shape, Gabriel Madiye contacted Sheila Hurton in the UK to join the *Voices for Hospices* event of 1997. At that time, she was unaware of develop-ments in Sierra Leone:

The whole *Voices for Hospices* idea just snowballed; so we went from the first event in 1991 when we had simultaneous concerts in all four countries in the UK—plus a late one in Malta—to 23 countries in 1994, by which time we had decided to make it a triennial event. In the next event in 1997, we had gone up to 35 countries. But by this time Gabriel in Sierra Leone had started an embryonic service in 1994; and he had read somewhere about Hospice Information, because nobody in Sierra Leone knew about palliative care; they didn't know about hospice. So he regis-tered with Hospice Information, got our leaflet and in 1996 he wrote and said, 'We could take part' and so from that point we've been in contact.

As in all *Voices* events, we send out information and, as we are a co-ordinating body, we ask for information back. So he was going to do his event in the national stadium, and had it all planned; then sudden silence. And after each event we always ask 'Can you tell us what the event did for you? How much it made, any benefits/spin offs and so on?' Nothing from Sierra Leone came back. And then it was a few months later, into 1998, that we suddenly got a heart breaking—I mean heart breaking—fax from Gabriel explaining that they'd been overtaken by the coup in May 1997; the hospice had been destroyed, and there was no way he could continue with his *Voices* event. And the incoming military president had found in former President Kabbah's drawer an invitation to go to the hospice event. 'Why hadn't Gabriel invited the new rebel president?' As a result, Gabriel was physically abused, his wife and children were physically abused and so on. Gabriel's fax was a real cry for help, 'There's no money in Sierra Leone, I want to get the hospice service restarted—can you help?'

Similar faxes went to Help the Hospices and Hospice Information. I talked to my own Voices for Hospices trustees, of which I'm one, and according to our Memorandum of Association we could not give money away. So I had permission from my own board members to go it alone on this one because it's the only way I could do it, and put out a plea and the money started to come in. I was aware, even at that stage, that every pound I raised here was worth ten pounds to them: money goes a long, long way in Sierra Leone. So I was sending money out as I received it and then one day I came home and my husband showed me a fax that had just come through that day, and he was in tears; and I was also in tears after I'd read it. The rebels had come again and destroyed what had been left.

Since the first destruction, they had been working under destroyed walls with just plastic sheeting for a roof and every time it rained, it soaked all the papers and everything in the office, a simple building. But the rebels had been again; they'd destroyed what was left, they'd destroyed the files and furniture; they'd stolen the truck—which was absolutely necessary to get about. They had burnt down Gabriel's house and abducted his wife and two young children, and had also burnt down another 150 buildings in the area. I mean, where do you start?

I went into Princess Alice Hospice the next day and spoke to the voluntary services co-ordinator, showed her the fax and she said 'we've got to do something' and we decided that we'd have a [special] Sierra Leone day. Within three weeks, we got the hospice volunteers, friends and staff on board, and on the day we sold goods on stalls, ran competitions, had a fashion show, served refreshments and many people were involved. By the end of the day we'd raised £3000. During the course of the day, someone came from the church just up the road and said they were just about to choose a charity for Lent, and he would like to propose to the church that it make The Shepherd's Hospice its Lent charity. And at the end of six weeks I was given a cheque for £2600. That's £26 000 to them. So I sent out the £3000, and then later £2600 so rebuilding could start, and I also started a newsletter for the growing number of supporters here. Just the fact that somebody, somewhere else was thinking of them seemed to give a huge morale boost. Gabriel said, 'You're thinking of us and the staff are just amazed that people somewhere else are thinking of them'.

And then it came to the point where they were coming up to the rainy season and they urgently needed to put a roof on the first floor. I needed to find almost £4000 and knew I just couldn't do it in time. So I wrote a letter to David Praill (Help the Hospices) and said 'I just don't know where else to turn and this matter is urgent'. And Help the Hospices generously made a one-off £3500 donation. At that stage, and we're talking about 1999, Help the Hospices had no international involvement so were brilliant to make an exception and meet a really urgent need. So the money was sent and the roof went on—and the rest is history.[11]

Hospice success stories

Sheila Hurton describes some successes of the hospice:

A major success of the service is: beginning to get the message across. The staff are now very much respected by other health care institutions in their part of the country.

Gabriel is a man with enormous knowledge and he's now acquiring skills in proposal writing which he is already passing on to others seeking funding. He has the respect of the director general of Ministry of Health and Sanitation, who has been to the hospice several times. Gabriel broadcasts regularly and we did a television broadcast while we were there last year, talking about palliative care and how beneficial it is, how cheap it is, how important it is; and they're beginning to get their volunteers to encourage people in the community to go and have the test if they feel that that person may be HIV positive.

There's a huge message to get across, but the hospice is succeeding—like a phoenix which has risen from the ashes of the most awful trauma that you could imagine; but they have the vision, they have the respect of local people. They also have the Women's Wellness project—a project to get women off the streets to stop them spreading HIV/AIDS. It was an 11 year civil war in which the rebels destroyed schools, hospitals, clinics, churches, whole villages, so some of these girls, who are now mums, never went to school.

The hospice has legal responsibility for about 67 orphans and vulnerable children and receives some international grants to pay for their school fees for a year, two sets of school uniform and some books and pencils. The children either live with foster parents or at home if they still have a parent who's living but dying of HIV/AIDS, but the hospice undertakes to look after them for a year and then tries to place them with a foster parent or in an orphanage; and we've seen one of the orphanages which was really impressive.[11]

Life/oral histories

Dr Gabriel Madiye—*founder and executive director, The Shepherd's Hospice, Freetown*: interviewed by David Clark, 4 June 2004. Length of interview: 24 min.

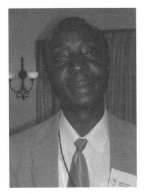

Gabriel Madiye has a background in public health and worked in Sierra Leone's Ministry of Health and Sanitation. In the 1990s, as the number of HIV/AIDS patients increased, he became aware of the lack of provision for people with a terminal illness. Eventually, he came into contact with St Christopher's Hospice, London, and contacted the USA for help with palliative care training. By 1994, he was raising awareness of palliative care in Freetown and, in 1995, registered the hospice as an NGO. Training for volunteers began in 1997 and premises were obtained in an old railway building. Then came the military coup and the hospice was destroyed in the ensuing hostilities; nevertheless, a service has been operational since 2000. Gabriel Madiye speaks of the challenges facing palliative care in Sierra Leone; of the stigmatization of patients and the isolation of the terminally ill; of the worries surrounding property and inheritance; of the need for counselling; of the training of volunteers and family members; and of the development of the multidisciplinary team.

Sheila Hurton—*board member, The Shepherd's Hospice, Sierra Leone; Princess Alice Hospice (UK) Council; management committee member, UK forum for hospice and palliative care worldwide*: interviewed by Michael Wright, 21 March 2005. Length of interview: 30 min.

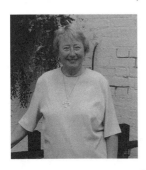

Sheila Hurton became involved with the Hospice movement in the UK in 1982 when she was invited to raise funds for what became the Princess Alice Hospice in Esher (opened 1985). By the 1990s, she had founded the *Voices for Hospices* initiative with its global simultaneous concerts held every 3 years, and it was this which prompted Gabriel Madiye to get in touch with her, asking to take part. The military coup and civil war (1997) intervened, but when Gabriel Madiye wrote asking for support to rebuild the hospice, Sheila Hurton responded with a range of fundraising activities. She has supported the hospice ever since and is now a member of The Shepherd's Hospice board. She speaks of the needs of the hospice; of the challenges faced by a service in one of the poorest countries in the world; of the stigmatization of patients; and the effects of civil war. She also tells of the remarkable resilience of those connected with the hospice movement in Sierra Leone, and how, despite all the difficulties, hospice care has become established.

Public health context

Population

Sierra Leone's population of around 5.88 million is made up of the following ethnic groups: 90 per cent native African tribes (30 per cent Temne, 30 per cent Mende and 30 per cent other); 10 per cent Creole (Krio)—descendants of freed Jamaican slaves who were settled in the Freetown area in the late eighteenth century—refugees from Liberia's recent civil war; and small numbers of Europeans, Lebanese, Pakistanis and Indians.

Religious groups include: Muslim 60 per cent, indigenous beliefs 30 per cent and Christian 10 per cent.[12]

Epidemiology

In Sierra Leone, the WHO World Health Report (2004) indicates an adult mortality[13] rate per 1000 population of 682 for males and 569 for females. Life expectancy for males is 32.4; for females 35.7. Healthy life expectancy is 27.2 for males; and 29.9 for females.[14]

Sierra Leone ranks bottom of the global World Bank Development Index based on multiple health and economic indices, and lacks the resources even to purchase HIV diagnostic kits.[15] Estimates of HIV/AIDS prevalence in Sierra Leone fluctuate significantly. The preliminary findings of a survey conducted by the Centers for Disease Control and Prevention in April 2002 suggest an overall national HIV prevalence rate of 4.9 per cent. HIV/AIDS awareness is generally low, even among medical staff, and hospitals do not have adequate testing facilities. Blood donors are tested, but, in general, are not informed if found to be HIV positive because of a lack of counselling capabilities and support networks. The government, previously criticized for its poor response to the epidemic, has now qualified for a World Bank Specific Investment Loan of US$15 million for HIV/AIDS.[16]

The 2004 Report of the global AIDS epidemic was unable to estimate the prevalence of HIV/AIDS in Sierra Leone as sufficient data for the previous 6 years were unavailable. However, in 2001, it was estimated that the prevalence rate of HIV/AIDS amongst the adult population (15–49 years) was approximately 7 per cent, the number of people living with HIV/AIDS was approximately 170 000, and the number of HIV/AIDS deaths per year was approximately 11 000.[12]

Available data regarding antenatal clinic attendees in Sierra Leone indicate a steadily worsening HIV epidemic. Nationally, < 1 per cent of pregnant women tested positive for the virus in 1989. By 1996, 7 per cent were infected with the virus. A 1995 sero-survey conducted among sex workers in Freetown found that 27 per cent tested positive for HIV-1. In an unspecified locale outside of major urban areas, 70 per cent of sex workers were HIV positive in 1997. Outside major urban areas, 9 per cent of police officers were HIV positive in 1996. In 1997, 12 per cent of security forces were infected.[17]

Health care system

In 2001, the total per capita expenditure on health care was Intl $26; 4.3% of GDP[18] (Appendix 3).

The WHO overall health system performance score places Sierra Leone 191st out of 191 countries.[19]

Political economy

The 1991–2002 war resulted in many deaths and the displacement of > 2 million people, many of whom are now refugees in neighbouring countries. The support of the UN peacekeeping force and contributions from the World Bank and the international community enabled national elections to be held in 2002, and the constitutionally elected democratic government has continued slowly to re-establish its authority. However, the gradual withdrawal of most UN Mission in Sierra Leone (UNAMSIL) peacekeepers in 2004 and 2005 represents a challenge to the continuation of Sierra Leone's stability. Sierra Leone is an extremely poor African nation with tremendous inequality in income distribution. It does have substantial mineral, agricultural and fishery resources, yet the social infrastructure is not well developed, and serious social disorders continue to hamper economic development following the 11-year civil war. The fate of the economy depends upon the maintenance of domestic peace and the continued receipt of substantial aid from abroad, which is essential to offset the severe trade imbalance and to balance government revenues.[12] The success or failure of Sierra Leone remains a test case for international engagement in Africa more broadly.[20] External agencies have played a critical role in the quest for peace—strong political leadership and substantial support by the international community are essential to manage the crisis and attain continuing peace.[21]

GDP per capita is Intl $606 (Appendix 4).

References

1 Report of the United Nations Development Programme 2004 (HDI 2002). Launched by the United Nations in 1990, the Human Development Index measures a country's achievements in three aspects of human development: longevity, knowledge and a decent standard of living. It was created to re-emphasize that people and their lives should be the ultimate criteria for assessing the development of a country, not economic growth. Current values range from 0.956 (Norway, first of 177 countries) to 0.273 (Sierra Leone, 177th out of 177 countries). Countries fall into one of three groups: countries 1–55 = high development; 56–141 = medium development; 142–177 = low development. See: http://hdr.undp.org/statistics/data/indic/indic_8_1_1.html

2 IOELC interview: Gabriel Madiye—4 June 2004.

3 Sheila Hurton. *Report from Visit to The Shepherd's Hospice, Sierra Leone: 23 January to 2 February 2004.*

4 Ruth Cecil writing in *News from The Shepherd's Hospice, Sierra Leone.* July 2004.

5 Jacqui Boulton writing in *News from The Shepherd's Hospice, Sierra Leone.* July 2004.

6 International Narcotics Control Board. *Narcotic Drugs: Estimated World Requirements for 2004. Statistics for 2002*. New York: United Nations, 2004.

7 'The term *defined daily doses for statistical purposes* (S-DDD) replaces the term *defined daily doses* previously used by the Board. The S-DDDs are technical units of measurement for the purposes of statistical analysis and are not recommended prescription doses. Certain narcotic drugs may be used in certain countries for different treatments or in accordance with different medical practices, and therefore a different daily dose could be more appropriate'. The S-DDD used by the INCB for morphine is 100 mg. International Narcotics Control Board. *Narcotic Drugs: Estimated World Requirements for 2004. Statistics for 2002*. New York: United Nations, 2004: 176–177.

8 See: http://www.daco-sl.org/encyclopedia2004/4_part/4_5chasl.htm

9 **Burn G.** Teaching in Sierra Leone. *Hospice Information Bulletin* 2002; **1**(4): 1–2.

10 See: Hurton S. The Shepherd's Hospice—Sierra Leone. *Hospice Information Service* 1999; **7**: 1.

11 IOELC interview: Sheila Hurton—21 March 2005.

12 See: http://www.cia.gov/cia/publications/factbook/geos/sl.html

13 This refers to adult mortality risk, which is defined as the probability of dying between 15 and 59 years.

14 See: WHO statistics for Sierra Leone at: http://www.who.int/countries/sle/en/

15 **Willoughby VR, Sahr F, Russell JB, Gbakima AA.** The usefulness of defined clinical features in the diagnosis of HIV/AIDS infection in Sierra Leone. *Cellular and Molecular Biology* 2001; **47**(7): 1163–1167.

16 **Bazergan R.** *HIV/AIDS and Peacekeeping: A Field Study of the Policies of the United Nations Mission in Sierra Leone*. London: Kings College London, 2002.

17 http://www.who.int/GlobalAtlas/PDFFactory/HIV/EFS_PDFs/EFS2004_SL.PDF

18 Total health expenditure per capita is the per capita amount of the sum of Public Health Expenditure (PHE) and Private Expenditure on Health (PvtHE). The international dollar is a common currency unit that takes into account differences in the relative purchasing power of various currencies. Figures expressed in international dollars are calculated using purchasing power parities (PPP), which are rates of currency conversion constructed to account for differences in price level between countries.
http://www3.who.int/whosis/country/compare.cfm?country=s&indicator=strPcTotEOHinIntD2000&language=english

19 This composite measure of overall health system attainment is based on a country's goals relating to health, responsiveness and fairness in financing. The measure varies widely across countries and is highly correlated with general levels of human development as captured in the human development index. Tandon A, Murray CLJ, Lauer JA, Evans DB. *Measuring Overall Health System Performance for 191 Countries*. GPE Discussion Paper Series: No. 30; WHO.

20 **Hirsch JL.** War in Sierra Leone. *Survival* 2001; **43**(3): 145–162.

21 **Davies V.** Sierra Leone: ironic tragedy. *Journal of African Economies* 2000; **9**(3): 349–369.

Chapter 17

Swaziland

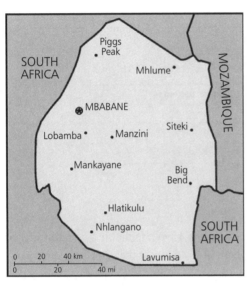

The Kingdom of Swaziland (population 1069 000) is a small landlocked country in Southern Africa covering an area of 17 364 km^2 between South Africa and Mozambique. The capital, Mbabane, is situated in north west Swaziland in the Mdzimba Mountains. Lobamba, the royal and legislative capital of Swaziland, lies about 20 km south of Mbabane.

Swaziland is governed by King Mswati III, a hereditary monarch. The prime minister is appointed by the king and thereafter recommends cabinet appointments for the monarch's approval. A former British protectorate, Swaziland became independent in 1968. Since 1973, Swaziland's system of government has been adapted to bring together both parliamentary and traditional systems. A constitutional review is ongoing.

According to the United Nations human development index (HDI), Swaziland is ranked 137th out of 177 countries worldwide (value 0.519)[1] and 12th out of 45 in African countries for which an index is available. This places Swaziland in the group of countries with medium human development.

Palliative care service provision

Current services

Four NGO provide six hospice–palliative care services in Swaziland: Hope House; Swaziland Hospice at Home; Parish Nursing; and the Salvation Army (Table 17.1).

In addition, several community-based church organizations provide supportive care to terminally ill patients.[2]

Table 17.1 Palliative care provision in Swaziland, 2003

	Free-standing unit	Hospital unit	Hospital support team	Home care	Day care	Clinic/drop-in centre	Total
Hope House	1						1
Parish Nursing				1			1
Swaziland Hospice at Home				1	1		2
Salvation Army				1	1		2
Total services	1			3	2		6

Table 17.2 Patients cared for by Hospice at Home 2001–2003

Year	No. of patients
2000–2001	522
2001–2002	683
2003	1144

Source: Thulie Msane.[4]

Swaziland Hospice at Home

Hospice at Home was registered as an NGO in July 1990. Stephanie Wyer, founder of Swaziland Hospice at Home, outlines the plight of the dying at that time:

> They were being taken into the government hospitals, with whatever their symptoms were, they were told in no—it just wasn't told gently, they were told that they were going to die, they were taking up a bed and they would just have to go home and wait to die. And there was nobody, *absolutely nobody*. If they had somebody at their home, that was their good fortune: if they didn't, they went back to their huts and they just lay there and waited to die. And that was it, there was just absolutely nothing available.[3]

The stated aim of the hospice is to improve the quality of life for terminally ill people and their families. This is achieved by providing:

◆ Counselling—for the patient and family members

◆ Pain management

◆ Control of distressing symptoms

◆ Day care

◆ Training and advice—for family and community carers

◆ Bereavement support.

Patients are referred to Hospice at Home by hospitals, relatives or friends. During the period 2000–2003, the number of patients cared for by Hospice at Home more than doubled (Table 17.2).

Salvation Army

The Swaziland Community Care Programme was established in Mbabane by the Salvation Army in 1985. Due to the ever-increasing number of HIV/AIDS patients, a palliative care programme was initiated in 2000. Provision includes:

- Home-based care
- HIV clinic—in the Mbuluzi district of Mbabane.
- Bereavement care
- Orphan care—currently 300 children.[4]

Around 180 clients are seen daily.

Hope House

Located in Manzini, Hope House is an inpatient unit modelled on the Swazi homestead which caters for the needs of AIDS patients at the end of life. The facility opened in 2000 and consists of a group of bungalows which provides accommodation for HIV patients and caregivers.

The Hope House concept was developed by World Vision International[6] in partnership with the Roman Catholic Church during the late 1990s. Funding was provided by the National Office of World Vision International: Austria, Germany, Ireland and Taiwan. Other support has come from The Italian Co-operation,[7] and Women and Law in Southern Africa (WILSA).[8]

Patients may be referred to Hope House by a number of organizations, including Swaziland Hospice at Home and the Swaziland AIDS Support Organization (SASO).[9]

Parish Nursing

This 3-year project began in 2000 supported by the 'Secure Future' programme of the Bristol Myers-Squibb Company.[10] Located in the Roman Catholic Diocese of Manzini, it is run in partnership with Maternal Life International (MLI).[11] The project is summarized as follows:

> Swaziland has under-developed health infrastructure and is predominately a rural area with a shortage of health care professionals specializing in HIV/AIDS care. By working through the Catholic Church, this program will demonstrate how countries can tap into existing infrastructure and draw the community into HIV/AIDS work. Community-Based Parish Nursing's project plan covers curriculum development, use of telecommunication for ongoing training, direct patient and family care, HIV testing and counselling, education and training of community volunteers.[12]

Thandiwe Dlamini, administrator of Parish Nursing, describes the care provided by parish nurses and outlines its underlying principles. She writes:

> Parish Nursing aims to integrate the practice of faith with the science of nursing. It links nurses with churches to focus on health related issues and to provide a holistic approach in the healing and caring process of a patient. The programme offers patients a holistic health approach which combines physical and spiritual dimensions. The Parish Nurses work part time and are assisted by

community members who have been trained in home-based care. Each nurse sees around five to eight patients per day and approximately 240 patients per month.[13]

Reimbursement and funding for services

All the hospice services are charities and rely heavily on donations for their income. Yet funds come from a variety of sources, as indicated below:

Hope House: each patient pays the equivalent of US$1 per day. Support has also come from the Catholic Bishop's Forum which agreed to pay administrative costs for a period of 6 months.

Swaziland Hospice at Home: is subvented by the government and also receives funds from its international partners including Friends of Swaziland Hospice at Home (UK).

Parish Nursing: is supported by a grant of US $273 000 over a 3-year period from inception by the Bristol Myers-Squibb Company.

Salvation Army: the Rotary Club of Mbabane has supported the salaries of the medical staff and continues to give periodic assistance. The clinic charges a fee for medicines and is self-funding in this respect. Nursing, counselling and home-based care are free of charge, supported by charitable donations. Two international donors provide support for orphans, and assistance also comes from the Southern African AIDS Training Programme (Canadian Public Health Association).

Opioid availability and consumption

The International Narcotics Control Board[14] has published the following figures for the consumption of narcotic drugs in Swaziland: dihydrocodeine 1 kg; pethidine 1 kg.

For the years 2000–2002, the average defined daily dose consumption of morphine for statistical purposes (S-DDD)[15] in Swaziland was 1 (Appendix 1).

Sibusiso Dlamini writes:

> Morphine syrup is not [generally] available in the country, but there are morphine tablets. These are prescribed by doctors only. I have personally been talking to the chief pharmacist asking them to avail morphine syrup as it's cheap and easy to use for clients, but until now this has not been attended to by the government.[2]

Thulie Msane describes how morphine and other drugs are prescribed and supplied to Swaziland Hospice at Home patients:

> Morphine syrup is only made available as needed per patient. It is not stocked in large volumes. This can be accessed by patients as indicated. Hospice is . . . the custodian of morphine as alluded to by the home based care manual for Swaziland.
>
> Morphine is prescribed with the assistance of a visiting doctor, after the patient has gone through the pain management protocol—a new nursing diagnosis to manage pain—and morphine is indicated. Other drugs are prescribed by nurses after they have made a physical assessment and come up with a nursing diagnosis. All prescribed medications are supplied to patients by hospice nurses.[16]

Parish nurses use analgesics such as Stilpayne, Painagon and Tylenol; they do not give morphine.

National and professional organizations

At a meeting of palliative care providers held in June 2003, a commitment was made to form a national palliative care association.

Palliative care coverage

Hospice at Home offers support to all Swaziland inhabitants with a terminal illness. Singer and Dlamini report:

> Swaziland is divided into four regions; each region is served by one nurse from SHAH. The nurse makes home visits to referred patients from his/her own region. The nurse determines the frequency of home visits. This depends on time available and the patient's condition. It is impossible to schedule more than 4–5 home visits a day because of distances and poor road conditions. The home visit is used to: follow up on the patient's condition, to change and modify treatment plans according to the patient's condition, to give psychological and spiritual counselling to the patient and to the caring family, to teach and support good patient care. Often, appropriate medications are dispensed at this time.[17]

Visits to remote homesteads can be hazardous, however, as Stephanie Wyer explains in this story about Patrick, a hospice nurse:

> Patrick was a very wonderful young man with fantastic knowledge of hospice and palliative care; a wonderful nurse; wonderful with his patients, very loved. And about two years ago, I went back to see them as I do most years—we went out for three weeks and did lots of lectures. Anyway, Patrick came to the airport when we were coming back and saw us off. And three days later, I had a called from Sibusiso who told me that I must sit down, he had the most *awful* news, Patrick had been out visiting his patient and he had—in between one patient and the other—he'd come to some road works and it said, 'Do not continue beyond this point' and it had an arrow pointing, and he obviously went the way of the arrow, and went straight over a mountain and was killed. So they lost their senior nurse and we lost a very dear friend. So that was a big setback, a very big setback.[3]

Parish Nursing: the programme covers 30 communities in the four regions of the country. In each case, the area covered is within walking distance from the home of the nurse.

Salvation Army: the clinic serves three local communities around Mbuluzi. at present three out of 10 nurses provide palliative care alongside 50 (volunteer) community/family carers.

Palliative care workforce capacity

Hospice at Home has five full-time nurses; one part-time nurse; one part-time doctor; five administrative staff and 150 volunteers. These volunteers play an important role within palliative care. Singer and Dlamini state:

> Swaziland Hospice At Home volunteers are called 'friends'. This is based on the love and friendship between our volunteers and the patients. They develop a friendship relationship with the terminally ill patient, thereby committing their time, money, and energy to help improve the quality of life of terminally ill Swaziland patients.[17]

Parish Nursing has 30 (retired) nurses in the programme. These nurses work part time with the support of community members trained in home-based care.

The Salvation Army has 10 nurses in the community care programme; three are palliative care trained; four are double qualified in nursing and midwifery; and three nursing assistants work in the clinic. In addition, there are a total of 50 trained community carers and family carers (volunteers) who give assistance.

Education and training

Driven by the impact of HIV and AIDS, a home care strategy was implemented nationally in 2000. This strategy included palliative care education for health professionals, together with a determined drive to raise public awareness of palliative care. Hospice providers played a key role, as Thulie Msane[18] indicates:

> As government initiated the strategy, there was a need for hospice to train caregivers (Rural Health Motivators), civic society, churches and schools in raising awareness of the home-based concept and palliative care concept.
>
> The schools of nursing invited hospice as facilitators on home-based palliative care and students have been trained in the following topics:

- Palliative care concept
- Symptom management
- Death, grief and bereavement
- Pain management
- Home-based palliative care
- Spiritual care
- HIV/AIDS symptom management.

As of June 2003, a total of 4316 people have been trained across a broad range of groups and services (Tables 17.3 and 17.4).

Table 17.3 Personnel trained under the national home-based care strategy 2000–2002

Year	Doctors	Nurses	Student nurses	Civic group	Community carers	Total
2000–2001	31	63	35	1217		1311
2001–2002	25	466	70	993	807	1941

Source: Thulie Msane.

Table 17.4 Personnel trained under the national home-based care strategy 2002–2003

Year	Health professionals	Defence force	Civic group	Correctional services	Total
2002–2003	500	40	474	150	1164

Source: Thulie Msane.

History and development of hospice–palliative care in Swaziland

Hope House

This inpatient unit is managed by Sarah Dlamini, a nurse and former director of the Co-ordinating Assembly of Non-Governmental Organizations (CANGO). The Hope House project involved a team of church and lay volunteers under the leadership of Fr Larry McDonnell. Journalist James Hall writes (2000):

> A team of church and lay volunteers under the leadership of a local Catholic priest and educator, Fr Larry McDonnell, have erected 15 units, with 10 more awaiting construction in an innovative community that combines traditional Swazi hospitality with the latest applied theories in AIDS treatment and prevention. The complex is noteworthy for another reason. While only able to offer accommodation to a mere fraction of AIDS sufferers in Swaziland, it presents a prototype for imitation elsewhere in the kingdom.
>
> Among the deeply-traditional Swazi people, the subject of AIDS is taboo. Sufferers do not acknowledge the cause of their illness, lest fearful family members refuse to attend their funerals. The health care and leadership vacuum has been filled by volunteers and social workers like Fr McDonnell, who has been ministering to Swazis for three decades, mostly as an educator.
>
> In March this year, the project called Hope House will receive its first tenants. Fifteen of 25 homes have been completed on the edge of Swaziland's commercial hub, Manzini, on land owned by the Catholic Archdiocese. Hope House is set on the rim of a beautiful green valley, and has the feel of a homestead.
>
> Patients are not warehoused to die, but live what remains of their lives in dignity as part of a community. 'Our residents will be men and women who are no longer allowed to stay in hospital', says Fr McDonnell. Swazi health facilities are unable to cope with the influx of AIDS patients, who are discharged when death is near. 'Swazis live in strong extended family units, but sometimes there is no one at a traditional homestead to tend to an AIDS sufferer. A father may be dead, a mother sick, and children incapable of the responsibility'.[19]

Swaziland Hospice at Home

Ingrid Watkins—chairperson of Friends of Swaziland Hospice, outlines the history of the hospice as follows:

> Mrs Stephanie Wyer MBE founded the Swaziland Hospice at Home. She went to live in Swaziland to join her husband who was working there. She arrived in Swaziland in March 1990. Her background was Macmillan nursing and in that spirit and experience the hospice work started almost immediately. She found a doctor who would work with her for prescribing medication, etc. She acquired THE 'yellow jeep', which soon became well known. She started to visit cancer patients at home and soon other patients and their families would ask for her help. Swazi nurses became interested in her work.
>
> A steering group was formed. The Hospice was registered as an NGO on 4 July 1990. A part-time nurse Judith Mamba (first member of staff) joined her and they worked together. People who started to work as volunteers, mainly for fundraising also offered help. In August 1990, the British High Commissioner gave a caravan to the Hospice. [In post was Mr Brian Watkins, who is now Patron of FOSH (Wales).] The Fire Station in Manzini offered a site on their land to put the caravan on. This caravan became the centre for courses in palliative care for nurses and other health professionals in Swaziland. During the same period of time, Stephanie asked her friends in Wales

to support the work she had started. At the end of 1990, we formed FOSH (Wales) UK (Friends of Swaziland Hospice). Up to date, this is a registered charity raising funds for SHAH (Swaziland Hospice at Home).

In 1991, Stephanie interviewed Mr Stuart Craig in London. He was appointed to become the first Administrator of SHAH through Skill Share Africa. In 1992, two part-time nurses were appointed to work with Stephanie and Judith. One nurse was from South Africa the other from Zimbabwe, both with palliative care experience. At the end of that year (1992), they left and two Swazi nurses joined the team; they were Ms Sweetness Masonga and Mr Sibusiso Dlamini. Both needed in-service training. In 1993, a lady called Ms Bunny Boyder with the help of Dr Samuel Hind donated land to the Hospice. When this lady died, she left more land and a house to Hospice. During 1994, the caravan was replaced by a one-storey building. Today this building facilitates the clinic where patients and families can come for treatment, help and advice.

In March 1994, Stephanie and her husband returned to Wales. She went back to Swaziland in August 1994 to assist the educator with a course she was running. She stayed for a month, in which time a new director was appointed called Gcebile. Stephanie officially handed her work over to her in September 1994. Stephanie returned again in December 1994 to give the new Director support that was needed. She was then able to hand over the full management of SHAH to the Swazi people.

A director was appointed. Specialist nurses delivered the hospice service in the community. Administration staff were employed. Through the years, FOSH (Wales) had enabled SHAH to get equipment for patient care (such as syringe drivers, special beds, etc.), books, magazines for education, and cars (including maintenance) for the nurses to visit patients.

In 1999, FOSH was successful in getting a community grant from the Lottery Board for Education for a period of three years. This project should have ended in September 2002, but will be finalized in January 2003. The project has enabled the hospice to grow into a centre for courses in palliative care in Africa. FOSH has been able to facilitate training in Britain for Swazi nurses in further education at St Christopher's Hospice. This is ongoing at present. In the same year, FOSH was able to raise monies for the appointment of a doctor. This proved to be complicated, but in April 2002 a doctor started to work for the Hospice. During the same year, a group of supporters in Swaziland formed FOSH (Swaziland).

In 2001, the American Embassy donated an extended two-storey building to the Hospice. This was opened in 2002 and used for administration, conferences and lecturing. The original building is now a centre for patients and families to walk into for advice, food, clothes and medical help. A doctor and a nurse are present to see those who come. Patients can rest before they go home again (often they walk a fair distance; also their illness makes them very tired).

Mr Sibusiso Dlamini, a trained nurse working with hospice, was prepared to pay a visit to Wales in 1997. FOSH (Wales) sponsored him and gave him a second home during this time. He stayed on and went to St Christopher's in London, gaining a degree from the Royal Marsden Hospital, London in palliative care in 2000. He returned to hospice in 2000. Small beginnings have developed into much needed and valued palliative care work.[20]

Sibusiso Dlamini has since moved from Swaziland Hospice at Home to take up a post with the National Emergency Response Committee on HIV/AIDS (NERCHA).

Parish Nursing: 'A New Robe' parish nurse programme

The parish nurse model for Africa was developed by Maternal Life International in collaboration with Dr Cynthia Gustafson, director of the Carroll College Parish Nurse Centre in Helena, Montana. It is based upon a Christian philosophy of care:

> The parish nurse role reclaims the historic roots of health and healing found in many religious traditions. Parish nurses live out the early work of monks, nuns, deacons and deaconesses, church

nurses, traditional healers and the nursing profession itself. The spiritual dimension is central to parish nursing practice. Personal spiritual formation is essential for the parish nurse. The practice holds that all persons are sacred and must be treated with respect and dignity. Compelled by these beliefs the parish nurse serves, advocating with compassion, mercy and justice. The parish nurse assists and supports individuals, families, and communities in becoming more active partners in the stewardship of personal and communal health resources. The parish nurse understands health to be a dynamic process, which embodies the spiritual, psychological, physical, and social dimensions of the person. Spiritual health is central to well being and influences a person's entire being. A sense of well being can exist in the presence of disease, and healing can exist in absence of cure.[21]

The administrator of the Parish Nurse programme is Thandiwe Dlamini—a former director of the Swaziland Red Cross and the founder of many health care and social service organizations in the country. She was appointed Counsellor for Distinguished Service of His Majesty King Mswati III in 1998. The Parish Nurse programme came about as follows:

In the summer of 2000, Maternal Life International (MLI) was awarded a grant for $272,900 from the Bristol Myers-Squibb 'Secure the Future' Foundation. The purpose of the award was to allow MLI to design and implement a parish nurse programme in twenty-five communities in Swaziland. The resulting programme, entitled 'A New Robe' is the first parish nurse programme to be implemented in Africa. It provides a range of services, including hospice home-based care for AIDS patients, HIV testing and counseling, and HIV/AIDS community education. Similar to programmes in the United States, the programme reflects a holistic approach to health care, inclusive of the spiritual and social dimensions of AIDS care.

The common thread that binds 'A New Robe' together is a profound respect for the life and dignity of the human person. Working with the Catholic Church of Swaziland and utilizing the start-up money provided by Bristol Myers-Squibb, MLI has hired and trained an in-country nursing director and 19 nurses. Ongoing support and education, as well as medicines and supplies are being provided through MLI's fundraising efforts.[22]

Hospice success stories

The successes of Swaziland Hospice at Home are described as follows:

The organization has managed to train health workers including nurses and doctors on palliative care and home-based palliative care. The transfer of skills to health caregivers has enabled the organization to roll out hospice service to eligible clients in the rural areas, the pro poor, and poor clients, providing access to quality of care. The organization has managed to alleviate pain and suffering of all terminal patients and advocate for care and support, reducing stigma and marginalization of such clients. We have succeeded in enlightening the nation on the concept of palliative care and the need to integrate this especially in the nursing circular. Student nurses are referred to hospice for skill development and practical experience of palliative care, especially pain management.[16]

Parish Nursing success stories are recounted thus:

Patients who have been discharged from hospital are visited regularly by the nurses and checked, and palliative treatment given. Professional guidance re medications is given to family carers. Some of our clients who had been bed-ridden after treatment have recovered and gone back to work. Successfully counselled people. Some of the terminally ill have never been to hospital and these visits are the only medical interventions they will ever have.[13]

Ethical issues

According to Sibusiso Dlamini, ethical issues relating to palliative care cluster around notions of acceptability and accessibility. He writes:

> Swaziland's health care system is basically divided into two. There is the modern western health system and the traditional indigenous system. Though this is not based on any research or survey in Swaziland, a majority of our terminally ill clients attend traditional healers either before or after attending the western or modern hospitals. In general, according to research, more than 70% of Swazis attend the traditional healers either before or after attending the modern western health system.
>
> The question could be: what role do our traditional healers play in palliative care? How is palliative care interpreted in the Swazi or African context? Does the Swazi traditional system have a palliative care concept?
>
> Most clients with terminal illnesses might believe they were bewitched or possibly believe they are being punished by their ancestors for some wrong doings. That challenges the acceptability of the palliative care concept in the country. Though the government is now fully accepting the concept, clients fight for their lives till the end. Swaziland is one of the leading countries in Africa who are holding on to culture and traditions.
>
> With approximately 200 000 HIV-positive people and 20 000 terminally ill due to AIDS in the country, the health system is now overstretched. The country has approximately 2000 hospital beds in total. Approximately 18 000 of these clients are discharged home, while the home-based care programme is very poor. Though a number of nurses have been trained in basic palliative care, most of them have left the country or are in the hospitals. Home-based palliative care is highly compromised. At the same time, those nurses who are trained on basic palliative care in the hospital have been allocated to other wards, e.g. maternity, hence their effect is questionable. In general only a few clients have access to palliative care.[23]

Life/oral histories

Stephanie Wyer—*founder, Swaziland Hospice at Home*: interviewed by Michael Wright, 1 July 2003. Length of interview: 1 h 15 min.

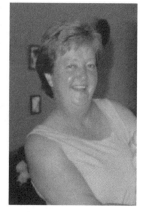

Stephanie Wyer speaks of her background in psychiatric nursing and her subsequent move into palliative care as a home care sister working for St David's Foundation in Gwent (Wales). When she accompanied her husband to Swaziland, she found little care for the dying and was encouraged to establish a local hospice. She recalls how her yellow jeep became the first hospice vehicle; how a nun helped her to form a steering committee; and how, despite bureaucratic difficulties, the hospice became a registered NGO in July 1990. She tells how early support came from the King's niece, a registered nurse, and from a South Africa-based physician who visited Swaziland weekly to provide medical expertise. She goes on to reflect upon how staff were recruited, educated and trained; how funds were raised and accommodation acquired; and the key roles played by individuals and groups both within Swaziland and internationally.

Public health context

Population

In 2004, Swaziland had an estimated population of around 1.07 million of which 97 per cent are African and 3 per cent European. Between 1991 and 2001, the annual population growth rate was 1.8 per cent. Around 55 per cent of the population are Protestant Christians; 10 per cent are Muslim; 5 per cent Roman Catholic Christians; and 30 per cent subscribe to indigenous beliefs.[24]

Epidemiology

In Swaziland, the WHO World Health report (2004) indicates an adult mortality[25] rate per 1000 population of 818 for males and 707 for females. This may be a conservative estimate. During 2002, around 15 000 deaths were recorded in Swaziland[23]—but as this figure takes no account of (unregistered) home deaths, the actual number is thought to be higher.

Life expectancy for males is 36.9; for females 40.4. Healthy life expectancy is 33.2 for males; and 35.2 for females.[26] Predictions suggest that life expectancy will fall to 27 by 2010—from a life expectancy of 61 in 1995.[27]

The disease profile of Swaziland is that of a developing country and reflects poor socio-economic conditions with some elements of epidemiological transition, typified by a rise in the prevalence of non-communicable diseases. Because it is a lower middle-income country, there is a reasonable level of infrastructure. According to Swaziland's Health Statistics Report 1999,[28] the four major causes of outpatient consultations were respiratory diseases (27.8 per cent), skin disorders (11.1 per cent), diarrhoeal diseases (11.1 per cent) and genital disorders (7.6 per cent).

Swaziland is one of the worst HIV/AIDS-affected countries in the world. The HIV prevalence in pregnant women grew from 3.9 per cent in 1992 to 34.2 per cent in 2000 and to 38.8 per cent in 2003.[29] Estimates suggest that between 210 000 and 230 000 people in Swaziland were living with HIV/AIDS at the end of 2003. In the same year, up to 23 000 adults and children are thought to have died from the disease (Table 17.5).

Table 17.5 Swaziland HIV and AIDS estimates, end 2003

Adult (15–49) HIV prevalence rate	38.8 per cent (range: 37.2–40.4 per cent)
Adults (15–49) living with HIV	200 000 (range: 190 000–210 000)
Adults and children (0–49) living with HIV	220 000 (range: 210 000–230 000)
Women (15–49) living with HIV	110 000 (range: 110 000–120 000)
AIDS deaths (adults and children) in 2003	17 000 (range: 13 000–23 000)

Source: 2004 Report in the global AIDS epidemic.

UNAIDS reports:

> Women of childbearing age make up 47.7% of women in Swaziland, or a quarter of the population (report of the 1997 Swaziland Population and Housing Census Vol. 4). This population is highly vulnerable to HIV infection, particularly the younger women. Periodic surveillance of antenatal clinics in the country has shown a consistent rise in the prevalence of HIV infection among women attending the clinics.
>
> The most recent surveillance report of 2002 gives an overall prevalence of 38.6%. The highest prevalence of 41.0% was among the younger age group of 15–29 years. The older women, 30 years and over, had a prevalence of 27.7% (Swaziland Ministry of Health Eighth HIV Sentinel Surveillance, 2002).
>
> It is also estimated that there are over 60,000 orphans, with approximately four children per household with an average age of 11 years. An estimated 15,000 households or more are headed by orphaned children, living on their own or with a sick parent or relative, with no resources or skills to provide for their basic needs.[30]

Health care system

Although Swaziland is classified as a lower middle-income country, the socio-economic indicators show widespread poverty and reflect huge inequities in access to services and opportunities vital to human life. An estimated 66 per cent of the population live below the poverty line, and rural–urban disparities are prominent. While 91 per cent of the urban population has access to safe water, this falls to 37 per cent for the rural population. Per capita expenditure on health for the urban population is three times that of the rural population.[31]

Sibusiso Dlamini explains how these conditions impact upon the delivery of palliative care:

> While we would like to ensure control of our clients' physical symptoms, starvation is the first symptom we face in Swaziland, and it is practically and professionally not possible to push a client to take a tablet or medication on an empty stomach. As a result, palliative caregivers are forced to scout for food to give to their clients as a first line of intervention.[32]

Prior to 1983, health care provision focused on curative measures provided by hospitals in urban areas. Access, therefore, was problematic for the rural dwellers who comprised 85 per cent of the population. This situation gave rise to the Primary Health Care Strategy of 1983, which sought better provision and increased accessibility within the country's rural areas. Health services have now been decentralized throughout the four regions of the country.

In 2001, the total per capita expenditure on health care was Intl $167; 3.3 per cent of GDP[33] (Appendix 3).

The WHO overall health system performance score places Swaziland 177th out of 191 countries.[34]

In 2001, there were six hospitals in Swaziland, five health centres and four public health units; 162 clinics and 187 outreach clinics. In 2003, around 600 nurses and 50 doctors were engaged in health care.

Political economy

The Kingdom of Swaziland is the second smallest country in Africa after Gambia.

Natural resources include asbestos, coal, clay, hydropower, forests, small gold and dia-mond deposits, quarry stone and talc. Environmental issues centre on the limited sup-plies of potable water; the depletion of wildlife populations due to excessive hunting; overgrazing; soil degradation; and soil erosion.

In this landlocked economy, subsistence agriculture occupies > 60 per cent of the pop-ulation. Manufacturing features a number of agroprocessing factories. Mining has declined in importance in recent years: diamond mines have shut down because of dwin-dling accessible reserves; iron ore deposits (high grade) were depleted by 1978; and health concerns have cut world demand for asbestos. Today, the main earners of hard currency are exports of soft drink concentrate, sugar and wood pulp.

Swaziland is heavily dependent on South Africa from which it receives four-fifths of its imports and to which it sends two-thirds of its exports. Remittances from the Southern African Customs Union and Swazi workers in South African mines substan-tially supplement domestically earned income. The government is trying to improve the atmosphere for foreign investment. Prospects for 2001 are strengthened by gov-ernment millennium projects, increased road building and factory construction plans.[24]

In 1997, a wide-ranging report[41] produced under the auspices of the United Nations commented as follows:

> Swaziland's achievements since independence are a justifiable source of pride in many areas, but a cause for complacency in none. Huge strides have been made in areas such as education and aver-age life expectancy, but little has been achieved in managing the consequences of population growth, and with:
>
> ◆ one of the highest national antenatal HIV rates on earth
>
> ◆ a high population growth rate of 2.7 per cent
>
> ◆ increasing civil disturbances
>
> ◆ serious unemployment
>
> ◆ serious or very serious soil erosion and other environmental degradation
>
> ◆ heavily skewed income distribution with much of the population living in absolute poverty
>
> ◆ indicators such as total fertility rates and under-five mortality being more in keeping with low human development nations than medium human development nations, and
>
> ◆ the recent slowing of growth both in formal employment and GDP.
>
> the challenges ahead appear to be even greater than those already overcome.

GDP per capita is Intl $5029 (Appendix 4).

References

1 Report of the United Nations Development Programme 2004 (HDI 2002). Launched by the United Nations in 1990, the Human Development Index measures a country's achievements in three aspects of human development: longevity, knowledge and a decent standard of living. It was created to

re-emphasize that people and their lives should be the ultimate criteria for assessing the development of a country, not economic growth. Current values range from 0.956 (Norway, first of 177 countries) to 0.273 (Sierra Leone, 177th out of 177 countries). Countries fall into one of three groups: countries 1–55 = high development; 56–141 = medium development; 142–177 = low development. See: http://hdr.undp.org/statistics/data/indic/indic_8_1_1.html

2 Personal communication: Sibusiso Dlamini—5 June 2003.

3 IOELC interview: Stephanie Wyer—1 July 2003.

4 Personal communication: Thulie Msane—16 June 2003.

5 IOELC interview: Major Brenda Greenidge—26 July 2003.

6 World Vision International is an international Christian aid agency which was established in 1950 and focuses particularly on the needs of children. In 2002, the charity was active in 96 countries, See: http://www.wvi.org/home.shtml

7 The Italian Co-operation is an initiative of the government of Italy. Established in 1987, it is intended to offer assistance to resource-poor areas of the world, and has focused particularly upon Africa. See: http://www.unccd.int/cop/reports/developed/2000/italy-summary-eng.pdf

8 Women and Law in Southern Africa is an educational and research trust which operates in seven countries in Southern Africa.

9 This is a country-wide AIDS support organization, founded in 1993. See: http://www.enda.sn/africaso.org/swazilandaidssupp.html

10 In 1999, Bristol Myers-Squibb Company, together with the Bristol Myers-Squibb Foundation, pledged US$100 million over a 5-year period to help South Africa, Botswana, Namibia, Lesotho and Swaziland find sustainable solutions for women, children and communities suffering from the HIV/AIDS epidemic in their countries. See: http://www.securethefuture.com/

11 Maternal Life International is a Roman Catholic organization which moves beyond contraceptive technology as a sole solution to the AIDS pandemic and attempts to address the broader needs of women in terms of obstetrical care, AIDS-specific interventions and education. See: http://www.maternallifeintl.com/locations.htm

12 Swaziland Community-based Parish Nursing: See: http://www.securethefuture.com

13 Personal communication: Thandiwe Dlamini—22 June 2003.

14 International Narcotics Control Board. *Narcotic Drugs: Estimated World Requirements for 2004. Statistics for 2002.* New York: United Nations, 2004.

15 'The term *defined daily doses for statistical purposes* (S-DDD) replaces the term *defined daily doses* previously used by the Board. The S-DDDs are technical units of measurement for the purposes of statistical analysis and are not recommended prescription doses. Certain narcotic drugs may be used in certain countries for different treatments or in accordance with different medical practices, and therefore a different daily dose could be more appropriate'. The S-DDD used by the INCB for morphine is 100 mg. International Narcotics Control Board. *Narcotic Drugs: Estimated World Requirements for 2004. Statistics for 2002.* New York: United Nations, 2004: 176–177.

16 Personal communication: Thulie Msane—18 December 2003.

17 **Singer Y, Dlamini S.** The role of the Swaziland Hospice at Home in the delivery of palliative care in the Kingdom of Swaziland. 1999. http://www.hospicecare.com/travelfellow/tf1999/swaziland.htm

18 Personal communication: Thulie Msane—18 June 2003.

19 **Hall J.** Swaziland: giving AIDS sufferers a loving bye. *Africanews* February 2000. http://www.peacelink.it/afrinews/47_issue/p7.html

20 Personal communication: Ingrid Watkins—11 November 2003 and 6 February 2004.

21 The parish nurse model of care. See http://ipnrc.parishnurses.org/forpn.phtml#philosophy

22 'A New Robe' parish nurse programme. See:
    http://apha.confex.com/apha/129am/techprogram/paper_22536.htm

23 Personal communication: Sibusiso Dlamini—18 June 2003.

24 See: http://www.cia.gov/cia/publications/factbook/geos/wz.html

25 This refers to adult mortality risk, which is defined as the probability of dying between 15 and 59 years.

26 See: WHO statistics for Swaziland at: http://www.who.int/countries/swz/en/

27 Fact sheet 2002: The USG response to Swaziland's HIV and AIDS epidemic February 1 2002 (US Embassy in the Kingdom of Swaziland). See: http://usembassy.state.gov/posts/wz1/wwwhhivfsheet.html

28 Published by Swaziland Ministry of Health and Social Welfare.

29 7th HIV Sentinel Surveillance Report, 2000.

30 See: http://www.unaids.org/en/geographical+area/by+country/swaziland.asp

31 WHO Country Co-operation Strategy 2002–2005.

32 **Dlamini S.** Palliative care in Swaziland. *Progress in Palliative Care* 2003; **11(4)**: 191–192.

33 Total health expenditure per capita is the per capita amount of the sum of Public Health Expenditure (PHE) and Private Expenditure on Health (PvtHE). The international dollar is a common currency unit that takes into account differences in the relative purchasing power of various currencies. Figures expressed in international dollars are calculated using purchasing power parities (PPP), which are rates of currency conversion constructed to account for differences in price level between countries. http://www3.who.int/whosis/country/compare.cfm?country= s&indicator=strPcTotEOHinIntD2000&language=english

34 This composite measure of overall health system attainment is based on a country's goals relating to health, responsiveness and fairness in financing. The measure varies widely across countries and is highly correlated with general levels of human development as captured in the human development index. Tandon A, Murray CLJ, Lauer JA, Evans DB. *Measuring Overall Health System Performance for 191 Countries.* GPE Discussion Paper Series: No. 30; WHO.

35 MacDermott MD. Common Country Assessment, Swaziland, 1997, published on the web at http://www.ecs.co.sz/cca/index.htm

Chapter 18

Tanzania

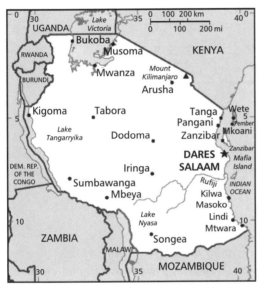

Tanzania (population 36.59 million) is a country in Eastern Africa, bordering the Indian Ocean, that covers an area of 945 087 km². Its boundaries border Kenya, Uganda, Rwanda, Burundi, Democratic Republic of Congo, Zambia, Malawi and Mozambique. The capital of Tanzania is Dar es Salaam.

According to the United Nations human development index (HDI), Tanzania is ranked 162nd out of 177 countries worldwide (value 0.407)[1] and 30th out of 45 in African countries for which an index is available.

This places Tanzania in the group of countries with low human development.

Palliative care service provision

Current services

In Tanzania, palliative care is provided by four organizations: Selian Hospital, Muheza Hospice Care, PASADA and Ocean Road Cancer Institute (Table 18.1).

Faith-based organizations, particularly the church-related hospitals, provide 50 per cent of the health care in the country.[2] Plans are in place to extend palliative care coverage into the Christian hospitals (~82) throughout Tanzania. The Evangelical Lutheran Church, which has its national headquarters in Arusha, is introducing palliative care into its 20 Lutheran hospitals. Health care is traditionally family and home based due to the low doctor to population ratio.

Selian Lutheran Hospital

This 100-bed hospital in Arusha services 55 000–60 000 patients annually.[2] The hospice programme is a response to the burden of AIDS in the area and consists of a small team that provides home-based care. The service is administered by the hospital. The team has

Table 18.1 Palliative care provision in Tanzania, 2004

	Free-standing unit	Hospital unit	Hospital support team	Home care	Day care	Clinic/drop-in centre	Total
Selian Hospital			1	1			2
Muheza Hospice Care	1	1		1	1	1	5
PASADA			1			1	2
Ocean Road Cancer Institute		1				1	2
Total services	1	3	3	1	3		11

Table 18.2 Muheza Hospice Care attendances, 2004

Facility	No. of attendances
Diana Centre/non-day hospice	5832
Day hospice	703

trained 120 volunteers that visit approximately 300 patients on a weekly basis to provide ongoing care after discharge from hospital. This includes spiritual care and symptom relief.

Muheza Hospice Care

This is a rural community-based palliative care programme based at Teule District Hospital. This district hospital is partly run by the Anglican United Society for the Propagation of the Gospel, and partly by the Tanzanian Government. The hospice service comprises a 5-bed palliative care ward within the hospital, a separate hospice building administering home-based care using village health workers and volunteers, a once weekly day hospice and a drop in centre open 5 days a week for medical examinations, voluntary counselling and testing (VCT) and counselling. A weekly STI clinic was opened in April 2004 and was attended to 225 patients by the end of 2004. The activity in 2004 is shown in Table 18.2.[3]

During 2004, the home care team made 253 visits to a total of 98 patients.[3]

Activity from 2002 is shown in Table 18.3.

A monthly 'Kids Club' provides support for around 40 HIV-affected children. Angela Kaiza explains:

> The aim of the club is to gather around all the children who are sick so that they have time together, so that they may enjoy that we may give them some food, we may talk with them, and we see, we try to see also their underlying problems, emotional problems, social problems which are facing them.[4]

This is achieved in a programme incorporating story telling, drawing, games, HIV education and hygiene.

Most palliative care activities operate from a separate hospice building known as The Diana Centre, at the entrance to the hospital. The centre is intended to be both an

Table 18.3 Muheza Hospice Care activity and patient diagnoses, 2002–2004

	2002	2003	2004
Inpatient referrals	372	571	618
Day hospice attendances	N/R	1731	2472
New patients seen in day hospice	119	467	703
Home visits	134	187	253
Patient diagnoses			
HIV	224	390	439
Cancer	119	171	147
Other	19	10	18

N/R = not recorded.

Source: Muheza Hospice Care Annual Report, 2004.

outpatients unit and a social venue. From an initial 12 patients, the numbers have grown dramatically, partly because food is provided. Karilyn Collins explains:

> We have a lot of starving patients who see day hospice as a day when they can get food, but they also see it as a day when they have to see the doctor . . .[5]

The hospice also attends to about 20–30 patients on other wards in the hospital. After discharge, patients are referred to the hospice for regular monitoring and home visits. Trained community volunteers and village health workers continue to visit the patients once they are home.

A well-established ARV programme provides free treatments for staff and patients. During 2004, 161 patients, 21 staff and 32 children received ARV therapy.[3]

Pastoral Activities and Services for People with AIDS Dar es Salaam Archdiocese (PASADA), Dar es Salaam

This home-based urban outreach programme specifically cares for patients with HIV and AIDS. PASADA collaborates with the Diocesan Community Health Education Programme (DCHEP) whose community volunteers are trained in basic nursing and counselling skills so as to be able to identify those people in need of care within their communities. The volunteers remain in contact with about 600 families under supervision from the PASADA team. The service by late 2004 was comprehensive: medical assistance and routine treatment of opportunistic infections; laboratory services; a pharmacy; counselling; home-based palliative care; support to orphans and vulnerable children; a programme for Prevention of Mother to Child Transmission (PMTCT); TB diagnosis and treatment; and training. The Orphans Department provides counselling for children whose parents have died. They also lobby the legal system to protect these children who are vulnerable to abuse, and have noticed an increase in the number of orphans who are prepared to talk of the sexual abuse they have suffered. By November 2004, there were 12 000 registered HIV-positive clients, including 600 children.

Ocean Road Cancer Institute (ORCI)

This is the only dedicated cancer hospital in Tanzania. Palliative care services are in their infancy but, with the support of the Hospital Director Twalib Ngoma, a palliative care unit has developed within the hospital. Its main function is that of a hospital support team. The unit operates an outpatient clinic as well as a hospital support team. Ward rounds and regular consultation with hospital medical staff ensure that patients are referred to the palliative care unit when appropriate. Patients are assessed each morning in the palliative care team office. Inpatients are visited three times a week. The team additionally accompanies members of staff on their ward rounds to be able to identify patients who could benefit from their input. The team links with already established home care providers in the city to provide continuity upon discharge. Due to financial constraints, there are no immediate plans to develop hospital home-based care. This is identified by the palliative care team as a gap in the provision of care. Another gap is follow-up of patients who live outside of Dar es Salaam. The existing home-based care providers are both NGO and government district hospital teams. They have limited training in providing support for the dying at home, and are not trained in pain control. While minimal support is therefore available in Dar es Salaam, this is entirely lacking when patients return to their rural homes. Mary Haule explains some of the problems:

> We have cancer patients who have AIDS also, but we know there are a lot of AIDS patients at home who are, have not cancer but they are suffering from severe pain, but this pain they are not attended to, but there is, they have no skill, the home care team, especial those by the government, they have no training in pain control . . . sometimes they can't appreciate that this patient will need some strong pain medication because there is still fear in many of these people that morphine is a dangerous drug, is a lethal drug.[6]

The palliative care team relies on family members to inform them of the patient's progress and collect medication. Only those patients who have access to home-based care support receive care at the end of life. Notification of a patient's death depends on the family's ability to come to the hospital.

Alongside these services, the William Jefferson Clinton Foundation has identified an HIV/AIDS care and treatment plan for Tanzania for 2003–2008:

> Goal one: to provide quality, continuing care and treatment to as many HIV + residents of the United Republic of Tanzania as possible, building on the careful planning already completed by the Ministry of Health and the Tanzania Commission for AIDS.
>
> Goal two: to contribute to strengthening the healthcare structure of Tanzania, through expansion of healthcare personnel, facilities and equipment and comprehensive training in the care and treatment of people living with HIV/AIDS (PLWHA).
>
> Goal three: to foster information, education and communication efforts focused on increasing public understanding of care and treatment alternatives, reducing the stigma associated with HIV/AIDS, and supporting ongoing prevention campaigns.
>
> Goal four: to contribute in strengthening social support for care and treatment of PLWHA in Tanzania, through home-based care, local support groups, and treatment partners.[7]

Reimbursement and funding for services

Selian Lutheran Hospital

Tanzania is an identified country for the USA's President's Emergency Programme for AIDS Relief (PEPFAR). The funding is divided into several tracks for ARV care, and orphan and vulnerable children care. Selian Lutheran Hospital hospice programme is eager to find an effective way to link the support it is receiving from PEPFAR with scaling up and making a difference to a much wider population. Other funding is primarily sourced internationally from churches. As the hospice service is administered by Selian Lutheran Hospital, any local fundraising activities focus on funding for the whole institution. Although the hospital charges for its services, these are heavily subsidized from other sources. Hospice patients do not pay for any services. Hospice staff salaries are funded entirely by the hospital.

Muheza Hospice Care

Initial funding to establish the 5-bed palliative care ward in Teule Hospital came from personal donations from well wishers in the UK. The Diana, Princess of Wales Memorial Fund provided money to build the free-standing hospice centre that accommodates offices, day centre, counselling and examination rooms, and an education centre. In 2004, funding from St Mary's Church in Oxford, UK was used to add a second consulting room/STI clinic, and a small office to the centre. Securing funds for building extensions is an ongoing problem, although Geneva Global donated US$50 000 to pay for an extension of six rooms in 2004. The rooms are expected to be in use in 2005. The Elton John AIDS Foundation contributed £35 900 in 2004 for running expenses of the hospice when The Diana Princess of Wales Memorial Fund monies were suspended due to internal problems at the end of 2003. This funding also covered the purchase of a vehicle and the implementation of the education programme.

Rapid Funding Envelope (RFE) is a funding initiative by 10 foreign embassies in Tanzania. Administered by Deloitte and Touche, it is dedicated to supporting comprehensive care for HIV-positive patients. In November 2003, RFE funded the purchase of a flow cytometer to measure CD4 counts. RFE also provided the hospice with a fluorescent microscope for use in STI diagnosis. AIDS Relief Consortium chose Muheza Hospice Care as one of their points of service to receive PEPFAR funding for ARVs. An increasing number of patients and hospital staff receive ARVs funded by sponsors in the UK. Cytotoxic drugs are funded by individual donors.

PEPFAR funding pays for the salaries of several staff members.

PASADA

Until mid-2003, the main donors of this service were Catholic Relief Services USA and the Diana, Princess of Wales Memorial Fund. Both organizations suffered internal problems during 2003 and had to withdraw their funding commitments, leaving PASADA in a serious financial situation. Realizing that dependence on a couple of donors was tenuous, the Executive Director, Mary Ash, developed links with several other funding agencies. The Stephen Lewis Foundation in Canada took over the home-based care funding for 2 years. The remaining programmes were divided into mini-projects, and applications were made to appropriate donors for each project. Catholic Relief Services have channelled funds from PEPFAR and the Clinton Foundation to support PASADA. With these additional funds, the organization is financially secure for the immediate future. In early 2003, the organization had a budget of US$350 000. By 2004, this had grown to >US$1 000 000.[8] The local archdiocese contributes the takings from their Sunday service collections to PASADA. The need to source funding for nutritional support for patients is ongoing.

Ocean Road Cancer Institute

This government hospital is funded entirely by state funds. The palliative care team salaries are paid by the hospital. Free chemotherapy is provided to paediatric patients, primarily for those diagnosed with Burkitts lymphoma.

President's Emergency Plan for AIDS Relief (PEPFAR)

During the 2004 financial year (FY), funding of around US$45.79 million was enacted for country-managed programmes in Tanzania and US$24.84 million for central programmes. During FY2005, it is anticipated that a total of US$104.93 million will be enacted: US$84.21 million for country-managed programmes and US$20.72 million for central programmes.[9]

Opioid availability and consumption

The International Narcotics Control Board[10] has published the following figures for the consumption of narcotic drugs in Tanzania: morphine 1 kg; pethidine 27 kg.

For the years 2000–2002, the average defined daily dose consumption of morphine for statistical purposes (S-DDD)[11] in Tanzania was 1 (Appendix 1).

Morphine is procured and supervised from government stores via Ocean Road Cancer Institute in Dar es Salaam. The pharmacist at the Institute advises that 100 mg of morphine powder is dispensed each month, making 10 l of strong solution of morphine. This is then diluted as required.

Selian Lutheran Hospital

The hospice at Selian Lutheran Hospital receives 10 l of diluted morphine every 3 months from ORCI. Morphine is prescribed by the medical team but administered by volunteers and family in the home. The volunteers alert the medical team when there is a change in the status of a patient. Patients or their family members source drugs directly from Selian Lutheran Hospital. The step 2 drugs on the WHO analgesic ladder are often used successfully to manage pain.

Muheza Hospice Care

This service receives 5 l of concentrated morphine solution every 3 months from ORCI and is the largest user of morphine in Tanzania outside of ORCI.

PASADA

PASADA has authorization from the Ministry of Health as the only non-hospital organization in Tanzania to use oral morphine for the control of pain. The morphine report for 2004 describes the history and development of opioid use at PASADA. It indicates that the first patient was given oral morphine on 27 May 2002 and, from then until the end of 2003, 14 patients with severe pain were treated with morphine with good results. In 2004, this number increased to 30 patients and included patients with severe diarrhoea and dyspnoea when other treatments had failed. No side effects have been reported from the use of oral morphine.

The small numbers of patients receiving morphine at PASADA is attributed to the fact that pain in HIV/AIDS patients is largely due to infection. When infection is treated, pain recedes and morphine is not required. However, the report acknowledges there may be additional reasons:[12]

♦ Lack of knowledge regarding pain assessment

♦ Patients do not report pain

♦ Reluctance to prescribe morphine

♦ Regulations regarding opioids prescription

♦ Fear of addiction.

Other drugs include other analgesics on the WHO analgesic ladder; non-steroidal anti-inflammatory drugs (NSAIDs); oral antifungals (ketaconazole, fluconazole, clotrimazole, miconazole oral gel and nystatin suspension), skin preparations; clotrimazole cream; steroids and locally made preparations. These include a steroidal aqueous cream and a mixture of 15 ml of nystatin suspension, 400 mg of acyclovir and 400 mg metronidazole/flagyl (NAF). Basic medications for opportunistic infections, TB treatments and ARVs are all provided by this service. Lessons have been learned from the antiretroviral pilot project undertaken in 2003. Ongoing negotiations surrounding funding and logistics for distribution of ARVs are taking place with the Clinton Foundation, Catholic Relief Services USA and the PEPFAR programme.

Ocean Road Cancer Institute

All morphine in Tanzania is distributed by ORCI after the regulatory pharmaceutical board approved it as the sole distributor in the country in 2001. The Medical Stores Department is responsible for importing the raw powder, mixing it into an oral solution and distributing the different strength solutions to other health care providers throughout Tanzania. There is continuing resistance to morphine among hospital doctors who fear its addictive qualities. However, in recent years, the palliative care team has been using the drug with great success, and has led training sessions for doctors. Outside of the hospital, however, resistance continues.

> They still think that they prefer pethidine than morphine, and pethidine is not very good for chronic pain. Sometimes they go for Tramadol, this is an expensive drug and mostly they get it injected.[13]

National and professional organizations

Tanzanian Palliative Care Association

A national association was formed in Arusha in June 2004 to provide a voice for palliative care in Tanzania. About 50 care providers in Tanzania were represented, mainly from the Lutheran hospitals and home-based care organizations.

Palliative care coverage

Selian Lutheran Hospital

The population in the district is about 1 million. Arusha town is estimated at about 300 000. The area surrounding the hospital itself is densely populated.

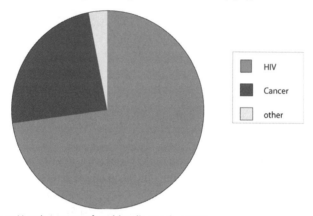

Fig. 18.2 Muheza Hospice care: referral by diagnosis, 2004

Table 18.4 Teule Hospital Ward Referrals to Muheza Hospice Care, 2004

Ward	Patient diagnosis			Total referrals
	HIV	Malignancy	Other	
Azimio				4
Bartlett	24	42	11	77
Chipukisi	32	3		35
Hills	22	20		42
ICU	3			3
Imani	169	18	4	191
Jenner	12	24		36
Mwenge	98	21	3	122
Nightingale	73	19		102
Wallace	2	4		6
Total	439	147	18	618

Source: Muheza Hospice Care Annual Report, 2004.

Muheza Hospice Care

The hospice services the whole of Muheza district. Based at Teule Hospital, most of its referrals come from the hospital. Figure 18.2 and and Tables 18.4 and 18.5 provide the 2004 referral details.

PASADA

The service covers the geographical area of the Archdiocese of Dar es Salaam. This includes all three districts of Dar es Salaam plus three districts of the coast region. Dispensaries are widespread, the furthest being 110 km from the PASADA headquarters. The catchment area population is about 800 000. The free service is available to people of all faiths and to everyone who can access it, including the very poor:

Table 18.5 Cancer referrals to Muheza Hospice Care, 2004

Myeloma	1
Prostate	1
Uterus	1
Leukaemia	1
Retinoblastoma	1
Oesophagus	2
Squamous cell	2
Bowel	2
Ovary	2
Chorion carcinoma	2
Lung	2
Osteosarcoma	3
Stomach	3
Breast	4
Melanoma	4
Rectum	8
Bladder	8
Unknown primary	10
Hepatoma	16
Kaposi sarcoma	16
Lymphoma	19
Cervix	25
Burkitts	43

Source: Muheza Hospice Care Annual Report, 2004.

the problems are very often they don't have the money for the bus fare or they don't have money for food or for other things. So . . . the idea of decentralization, taking the services as close to the community as possible, also makes it more accessible for people.[8]

Ocean Road Cancer Institute

Cancer patients are referred here from all over the country. Many patients simply arrive at the hospital without a referral. The hospital does not have the financial capacity to provide follow-up support for patients, and contact is often lost. The palliative care team acknowledges how emotionally difficult this is, having established relationships with many of the patients over several years.

Hussein Mtiro:

> So they come here, we know each other, we are friends . . . we get information, when they die some relative will inform us that the patient has died. Some will write, some will 'phone. We need to support them but we can't do that, we have no facilities, so we just pray for them.[13]

Education and training

Selian Lutheran Hospital

Volunteers in the local church community are trained in basic skills to care for the ill and dying in their villages. A week-long training course for health professionals is based upon the Hospice Uganda and Nairobi Hospice training modules. Kristopher Hartwig has been appointed to implement palliative care into 20 Lutheran Hospitals in the country. One of these is Kilimanjaro Christian Medical Centre, one of the five big zonal institutions in Tanzania that incorporates a medical school.

Muheza Hospice Care

Approximately 90 village health workers and 30 community volunteers have been trained in simple techniques to ensure a better quality of home-based care. They receive a small supplement from the hospice because '. . . they visit patients in their homes, they bring their books in, they look after their morphine, they look after their medication'.[5] The medical director has a diploma in palliative care. Mary Aloyce, a palliative care nurse, gained her diploma in palliative medicine from Makerere University in Uganda in 2004 and is one of the first nurses in Tanzania to achieve this qualification.

PASADA

Most staff members are trained in palliative care by Hospice Africa Uganda. PASADA designs and organizes a number of courses and workshops for health workers in Tanzania. The main courses include VCT and home-based care for nurses. Elements of palliative care are included in the home-based care training. The demand for workshops on how to establish HIV/AIDS services has pressurized the organization to consider creating a formal training unit. The model of care used here can be effectively replicated to other national HIV/AIDS bodies, but resources are minimal. Many of the social workers and counsellors involved in the Orphans Department have received training in psychosocial counselling and bereavement in Zimbabwe and Uganda.

Ocean Road Cancer Institute

Specialist palliative care training of staff is undertaken at Hospice Africa Uganda. The head of the palliative care team studied palliative care in South Africa in 2004. The palliative care team organizes weekly internal training sessions with the other doctors at the hospital. Various topics have been presented, including morphine use, holistic care and breaking bad news to the patient and family. Efforts are made to familiarize the four oncologists at the hospital with palliative care principles.

Palliative care workforce capacity

Selian Lutheran Hospital

The hospice team has six members: one nurse, two evangelists, one pastor, one social worker and one clinical officer. Kristopher Hartwig is a part-time doctor with the programme. The programme is largely volunteer based. The area served is largely Christian. Most of the volunteers are affiliated or linked to the many denominational congregations in the area.

Muheza Hospice Care

PEPFAR funding allowed for a significant increase in staffing in 2004. According to the Muheza Hospice Care Annual Report 2004,[3] the present hospice staff comprises:

Medical doctors: two (salaries paid by PEPFAR)
  Clinical officers: two. Bathlomew Bakari is seconded to the hospice from Teule hospital and is studying for the diploma in palliative medicine from Makere University Uganda through Hospice Africa Uganda. Christian Maembe is studying the distance learning diploma in palliative medicine from Oxford Brookes University through Nairobi Hospice (salary paid by RFE/PEPFAR).
  One ARV adherence officer (salary paid by PEPFAR)
  Nursing:

- ◆ Christopher Mnzava, district AIDS control co-ordinator (seconded from Teule Hospital)
- ◆ Mary Aloyce, palliative care nurse (seconded from Teule Hospital)
- ◆ Florence Koshuma (seconded from Teule Hospital)
- ◆ Ingehedi Mbago (seconded from Teule Hospital)
- ◆ Kijoi Mbwana (salary paid by PEPFAR)
- ◆ Peter Kilimahana (salary paid by PEPFAR)
- ◆ Omari Sempombe. Counsellor (seconded from Teule Hospital)
- ◆ Paulo Mwamgunda. Counsellor (seconded from Teule Hospital)
- ◆ Mr Rajabu Sige. Counsellor (salary paid by Tanga AIDS Working Group)

Nurse auxiliary: One
Project manager: One
Accounts: two (salaries paid by PEPFAR and RFE).
Information technology: two
Social worker: one (salary paid by PEPFAR)
Pharmacist: one (salary paid by PEPFAR)
Laboratory assistant: one (salary paid by PEPFAR)
Domestic: four (salaries paid by Elton John Aids Foundation)

PASADA

There are 82 employed members of staff. Twenty-four employees work in the dispensaries and the rest are based at the PASADA headquarters. Within the Medical Department, there are three doctors, two assistant medical officers, five clinical officers and 10 nurses. The Orphans' Department employs six social workers. There are six counsellors in the Counselling Department. Two part-time volunteers assist with computers and the Orphans' Department. There are 160 volunteers involved mostly in the home care programme. A proposal to Comic Relief (UK) for a partnership project between PASADA and DCHEP to increase the recruitment of volunteers to work in the community was approved in November 2004. This will result in 250 new volunteers being recruited and trained.

Ocean Road Cancer Institute

The palliative care team comprised six employees at the end of 2004:

- Two clinical officers
- Three nurses
- One social worker.

A doctor currently training in palliative care is expected to join the team on completion of their studies. Doctors leaving to study and obtaining lucrative employment elsewhere are some of the reasons for being understaffed. Hussein Mtiro explains:

> For the last two months things have changed a little because there was a shortage, some doctors left so the team was distributed . . . And then we are not working now as the team, palliative care team alone, but we are mixed in the departments so we see patients routinely. So we are lacking also some of what we've been doing before, we have a weekly training which we are not doing at the moment. Our routine round, three day times a week is, we are not doing it right now, but we see patients just on the ward round as now.[13]

History and development of hospice–palliative care in Tanzania

Selian Lutheran Hospital

Mark Jacobson describes how the approach of the Selian Lutheran Hospital hospice team integrates faith into home-based care. The addition of practical skills to the support already provided by the local church community provides holistic care to patients 'where people are coming together to pray with the patients who are unwell . . . we simply grafted onto that some skills, some training that enhances what they're able to do in the homes'.[2] The community immediately seemed to recognize this was something that they needed.

> There was this sense of Eureka moment of people coming together and talking with leadership in the community, talking with the religious community, and when we would begin to talk about what could be accomplished through hospice, or what the concept was in palliative care. It was striking because literally within a few minutes of starting our presentation . . . it was as though

there was this great need that people had not been able to articulate before, and when somebody put before them the idea of marrying together a medical model with a spiritual model of caring for people who were at home dying, people got very excited, and that gave rise to our whole [volunteer based] approach.[2]

Mark Jacobson then describes the beginnings of palliative care at this hospital:

About five years ago we had our first opportunity; we had a patient who actually asked us to come and care for him at home. He was dying from a lymphoma and he didn't want to be in hospital and he asked if, as his caregivers, we could provide him with some care at home and some pain relief for his disease. He wanted to go through this process of dying, and this really triggered for us kind of a Eureka moment . . .[2]

The epidemic of HIV/AIDS was a major impetus for scaling up home-based care as patients were unable to afford to be in hospital. Selian Lutheran Hospital was already involved in traditional community health and deeply involved in working with community health workers and other caregivers in the village. The church was known, accepted and appreciated in the villages through its work in HIV prevention, education and development work, so it was an easy transition to extend its involvement into home-based care for the dying. This coincided with the AIDS epidemic peaking in Tanzania at the turn of the millennium. The wish of Africans to die at home and be buried on their home property meant that when there was no medical cure the patient readily agreed to return home to die and relinquished the responsibilities of care from the hospital to the family. Mark Jacobson:

[There was] . . . an assumption that because there were centuries of tradition of dying at home, that there was also a tradition of knowing how to care for people at home, and sadly, as with most assumptions, that turned out to be incorrect . . . Often people were going home to die in a place where no-one knew how to care for them, where there was no-one to relieve their symptoms, there were great difficulties for families being able to talk to somebody who was dying, about their dying.[2]

Kristopher Hartwig became involved with the Selian Lutheran Hospital hospice team through his colleague Mark Jacobson. He hopes that the national hospice association established in 2004 will embrace the often unrecognized AIDS organizations who manage to provide good patient care without oral morphine. Concerned at the artificial divide between palliative care and AIDS service organizations, he partly blames donor funding that is often exclusively AIDS driven.[14]

I'm afraid that, as we organize Tanzania palliative care, we'll miss so many people who are doing it because they think they're just doing good work with AIDS—which they are—but we want to be linked, we want to be sharing the work and the expertise . . . And I think the divide is artificial; it's partly driven by the disease (which is AIDS) and the condition, and partly driven by the nature of the donor community, where funds that come for AIDS are just for AIDS. And if you develop cancer while you have AIDS, you can take care of that cancer. But in this part of Tanzania, every region has it's own very interesting epidemiological differences. So we don't see much cancer as part of HIV/AIDS here, now.[14]

He identifies economic hardship as one of the greatest challenges faced by patients, and emphasizes the need to be aware of the many cultural contexts in which palliative care is practised in Tanzania. He describes an exciting and effective 'Selian model' that has evolved specifically in response to their unique situation and goes on to expand on comments he made in a paper published in 2001.[15]

Muheza Hospice Care

Alison Hills was the medical superintendent at Teule Hospital in the early 1990s. She started a small palliative care team of one nurse who had been trained at a hospice in Hereford, UK and one nursing auxiliary. Karilyn Collins describes the conditions:

> This little team was going through the wards with a bucketful of equipment, looking at patients who were referred to them who were on the point of dying, and they were very much looking at the very terminally ill patients. There was also a Department of HIV that were running from a converted container: it was dreadful, the temperature went up to goodness knows what. There were just two rooms in this container: one where people sat and waited and one where people had their counselling. There were two counsellors and the District AIDS Co-ordinator and they were very much linked with Tanga's working group who were using herbal medicine for the treatment of HIV/AIDS and they'd been doing that since 1992.[5]

Karilyn Collins arrived at Teule hospital in September 2001 without a job description, but saw the need for palliative care in this setting to help cancer and AIDS patients. A meeting of interested parties formed Muheza Hospice Care as an independent NGO:

> We had our first meeting and we discussed what we should be called. I wanted to be called St Thomas's Hospice because I thought there were lots of doubts about what we were doing and also I trained at St Thomas's. That was voted out. Everything was done very democratically and they said 'We want to be Muheza Hospice Care'. So that was where the name came from.[5]

An already existing community AIDS home-based care system provided the structure for home-based palliative care. Funds were initially provided by well wishers in England to convert the hospital TB ward into a designated 5-bed palliative care ward in February 2002.

By late 2004, this hospice service had a comprehensive package of care. Patients on the wards in the hospital are assessed to provide a care plan on discharge, home support offers counselling and monitoring, and re-admissions are recommended as necessary. As further programmes are implemented, the rapid growth of this service creates increasing administrative demands for the staff. There is concern that HIV, the ARV therapy and the strict monitoring programmes that accompany the illness will undermine good palliative care for cancer patients.

PASADA

This organization was started as a self-help group in 1992 by a small group of people living with HIV. Motivated by the desire to do something for themselves and others living in similar situations, they applied to the Catholic Church who gave them a small building in Dar es Salaam. The number of members steadily increased until, in 1994, a small dispensary was opened to offer basic medical assistance and drugs for the treatment of opportunistic infections. At the end of 1994, there were 150 HIV-positive clients registered. By late 2004, >12 000 registered clients reflect the trend of the pandemic in this city and the success of this service. PASADA is now managed by a professional team of administrators and medical practitioners.

Ocean Road Cancer Institute

A hospital pain team comprising four doctors, a nurse and two social workers was brought together by Twalib Ngoma in July 1994. He attended a course on palliative care in the UK and returned to Tanzania committed to establishing a pain team. He initiated morphine use and organized palliative care training for his staff in 2000. As Director of ORCI, he no longer has the time to develop palliative care, but actively supports the palliative care team in its work.

Hospice success stories

Selian Lutheran Hospital

Kristopher Hartwig suggests 'what is very successful about Selian is . . . they've neither been able or not bothered to really copy anyone else, they've done their own things'.[14] This ability to chart their own way in providing a unique and effective service has been made possible by active leadership and a willingness to network with allied services to spread palliative care skills. Their plan to expand their training to many more hospitals in the country will increase coverage significantly.

Muheza Hospice Care

A combination of different hospice and palliative care models results in this hospice providing a comprehensive service to many patients. The sound relationship with the hospital means that continuity of palliative care is provided from time of admission to community-based support and follow-up. Successful community programmes, an active day centre, expansion of education and training programmes and the development of a children's programme attract sustained donor funding and encouragement to replicate this service elsewhere. Despite the many successes, the team identifies areas for development.

> There are areas that are not working well; for example, the bereavement programme. It's not yet tackled, and I see that we really need a lot of social workers. And then we are not also much trained on how to do palliative care. How to arrange programmes, so that these sick people may generate their own income; that also is another gap, because we just give them the money, just give then the food, things like that. So we just have the one step. But we need to move farther, to help them genererte their own income so that they may not depend too much.[4]

PASADA

Mary Ash:

> I think one of the things that I found in PASADA that impressed me immediately and obviously was due to who came before me, the motivation of the staff. It was obviously faith based. People who come to work in PASADA are people who believe in doing something for others, and that comes from their own personal faith. Without that staff motivation I think it would be very difficult to provide the quality of care that we do, and that is one of the successes of PASADA, the quality. And the compassionate care. I dare to use the word 'compassion' in the sense that everybody here cares about the clients and I think that's one of the most important things for people.

I think the success is the model itself. Also, the recognition that PASADA gave a long time ago—and a long, long while before the government did or anybody else did—to the importance of care and support [to those living with HIV/AIDS]. PASADA is the only organization in Dar es Salaam, probably in Tanzania, offering this kind of holistic service. So what does that mean? When people go to drop-in VCT centres and they unfortunately end up with a positive result, the question is, 'What do I do now? Where do I go?' So everybody says, 'Go to PASADA', because they know it's the only place where they will get this kind of help. So I think the success is also that recognizing that model so long ago—and in time developing it into what it is today; it was a very good intuition. And I hope we will be able to help other people to set up in their own environment, obviously modifying it to their own environments, but to set up services like this.[8]

She identifies areas for attention:

The kind of people, obviously who are now working, and including myself, are those who have been trained and have certain qualifications and experience to give to the organization. So that has also cut out a lot of people living with HIV/AIDS, because many of them don't have those qualifications, and that is something that I would like to work on more in PASADA. It's still a community-based organization, definitely, and that is another aspect of its success. But for example: the collaboration, or the participation, of people living with HIV/AIDS is, apart from being clients obviously, very limited. We have trained some in counselling. We've trained others in other things as well, and they are active within the sector, but it's not enough. We have monthly client meetings where we have 450 people at a time at the meetings and there's a lot going on there. But let's face it, if people were not HIV positive, we wouldn't be here. So why should we be here and them not be more involved in what's going on? And this is one of the things I see for the future that we need to look at.[8]

PASADA has been successful in forging good relationships with the Tanzanian government, including the Ministry of Health and the National AIDS Control Programme. Their collaboration is regularly sought in developing policies relating to AIDS. Proof of the respect in which PASADA is held came in the form of a certificate of recognition for their work presented by the President at a Global Fund ceremony in 2004.

Ocean Road Cancer Institute

ORCI is the sole distributor of oral morphine to other hospices in the country and succeeds in ensuring an uninterrupted supply. The number of staff who are receiving palliative care training is seen as a success, although AIDS home-based care providers still require training to improve end-of-life care for all patients. Mary Haule:

What they are doing is just visiting patients, talking with them, they don't even have pain medication. So we are trying to teach them to use morphine. But also to see cancer patients, not concentrate on AIDS just because they are visiting mainly AIDS patients. Now doctors are going for training, and nurses. So there is a change in knowledge and skills which are applied to patients—and they're teaching other staff. So this is one of the successes. Also we are getting more co-operation from colleagues.[6]

Hussein Mtiro shares his impressions of the success of his team:

There is a lot of difference, actually, because at least now we know our patient; those in the ward or those at home, those in difficulties, those in pain. They, at least, know where their problems can be solved. It was not easy before the palliative care team. Patients say it's nobody's business, who comes here. They don't know what to do. But after this training, people are more skilled in communication and knowledge of how to control symptoms. So we consider most of our patients are symptom-free, because of all the medication; and we can talk with them. There is really a difference in the ward and at home.[13]

He identifies areas for improvement:

We just feel that we have a long way to go. We are still lagging behind, we are missing a lot of service to some of these patients. We can give them medication, we can talk with them, we can counsel them, but really we are not open to the maximum because we can't follow them to their home. We can't see how they are dying, how the family is supported day after day. So we still think we need to do more.[13]

He identifies a need to network with other agencies, and to avoid an overemphasis on AIDS. Early diagnosis of cancer through screening would help to increase survival rates.

Ethical issues

There are close to 100 ethnic groups in Tanzania with distinct ways of caring for people who are dying. Not every community or group has high HIV prevalence, and some of the traditional herbalists have access to analgesics while others do not. Kristopher Hartwig describes the traditional medical approach:

[The traditional approach] . . . was not to tell people about their terminal condition, but rather prescribe something and do a referral, and that's still done to a large degree with cancers, which are very obviously cancer and very obviously incurable to anyone with a medical background. But it's very difficult and it's not within the training, still, to talk openly about the disease—except for HIV/AIDS. Where it is now, there is a prescribed avenue which I think we all understood, and in a way that has opened the door for a kind of truth-telling which has not been in the medical culture before.[14]

A reliance on both traditional and allopathic medical systems often results in late presentations for treatments. There are only three referral hospitals in the country that can diagnose cancer, and cancer patients from all over Tanzania have to travel to ORCI in Dar es Salaam for treatment. Biopsies taken at another centre can take up to 6 months for a result. The capacity for biopsies is around 2000 specimens per year, but >10 000 samples are received. Specimens sent to Europe are often diagnosed in 3 weeks. A biopsy can be 'fast tracked' at ORCI within 2 weeks but costs the equivalent of US$25, which many patients are unable to afford.

Life/oral histories

Mary Ash—*Executive Director, PASADA, Dar es Salaam, Tanzania*: interviewed by Jenny Hunt, 9 November 2004. Length of interview: 41 min.

Mary Ash describes the early development of Pastoral Activities and Services for People with AIDS, Dar es Salaam Archdiocese (PASADA) from 1992. Initiated by a small group of HIV-positive people, the organization grew rapidly. By 1994, there were 150 clients registered, and a small dispensary was established with funds from the Catholic Church to provide medications. She lists the current service: medical assistance and routine treatment of opportunistic infections for 12 000 registered HIV-positive clients, including

600 children; laboratory services; a pharmacy; counselling; home-based palliative care; support to orphans and vulnerable children; a programme for Prevention of Mother to Child Transmission (PMTCT); TB diagnosis and treatment; and training. Further details are given for the home-based care programme, and morphine and drug policies. Turning to future plans for her organization, Mary Ash discusses the challenge of providing a quality service to large numbers of patients. She sees the solution as decentralization, utilizing the 16 parishes within the archdiocese of Dar es Salaam that have dispensaries. She is keen to ensure that PASADA retains its holistic approach and to integrate the ARV programme as a complement to the other services. Staffing and volunteer details are discussed together with the training programmes required to implement this growing service. Concluding with a summary of PASADA's successes Mary acknowledges an ongoing need for major funding to support quality care, and the need to network with other service organizations to share the load.

Dr Karilyn Collins—*medical director, Muheza Hospice Care, Teule Hospital, Muheza*: interviewed by Jenny Hunt, 7 November 2004. Length of interview: 25 min.

Karilyn Collins was brought up in the UK in a family that had no medical background. She showed signs of wanting to be a doctor early in life and, although she had a strong interest in music, she remained focused on this achievement. While training at St Thomas's Hospital in London, she met her husband Richard Collins and they married as students. After graduating, they went into general practice and developed a successful family health practice over 25 years. Although they derived great satisfaction from this, they determined to give the end of their lives to tropical medicine in the developing world. In 1995, they went to Liverpool and studied for the Diploma in Tropical 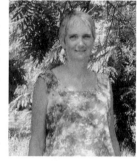 Medicine and Hygiene from Liverpool Tropical Medicine School. They then went to Tanzania because the hospital at Muheza had a link with Hereford. Enjoying the challenge of medicine in such a different context, the couple gave their notice in at their practice and returned to do a locum in Tanzania. Upon returning to the UK once more, Karilyn Collins realized that palliative care would be a useful addition to her medical skills if they were ever to return to Tanzania. She worked at a hospice in Hereford to gain palliative care experience and developed a passion for hospice work. During another short visit to Tanzania in 1999, she realized that her future lay in palliative care and applied to Cardiff University to do the Diploma in Palliative Medicine. Having completed that diploma, she arrived in Muheza in September 2001 along with her husband who had been employed as the medical superintendent of Teule Hospital. Having established Muheza Hospice Care since then, she now administers a comprehensive palliative care programme that attends to pain control, social, spiritual and emotional needs and offers continuity of care in the community. Palliative care enables her to use her wide experience in alternative therapies, including hypnosis and acupuncture, as well as the broad depth of experience gained from family medicine.

Dr Kristopher Hartwig—*physician, Selian Hospital, Arusha*: interviewed by Jenny Hunt, 4 November 2004.

Kristopher Hartwig tells the story of his early life in Tanzania with his teacher parents. The family left to live in the USA when he was about 8 years old and he did not return

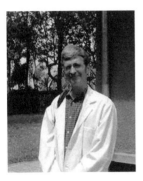

until many years later. After marrying a Tanzanian-born daughter of Lutheran missionaries, the couple determined to work in the country and did so at a faith-based hospital for several years. Upon reflection, he laments his ignorance of pain control at that time. They returned to the USA where he practised family medicine and later joined a hospice. His friend Mark Jacobson from Selian Lutheran Hospital asked him to visit Tanzania for 2 months and help to establish a hospice service at the hospital in Arusha. It seemed unlikely at that time, given the responsibilities of raising and educating their five children, that he would return full time. Yet in 2002, the couple did return for an indefinite period. He ascribes some of that decision to the inspirational staff members that were then working in the hospice programme. Kristopher Hartwig shares his sense of privilege at working with a hospice team but realizes that hospice in this setting can never hope to meet all the needs of the many dying patients in the area. Despite this frustration, he believes he will remain in this field and speaks of it passionately. Reflecting on how faith influences his work, he is surprised at the ease with which hospice workers integrate faith into their work in this setting. Drawing on his own beliefs keeps him motivated in seemingly impossible situations. He talks of his need for faith in a God who can achieve things that he feels he is unable to do. He shares his dream for palliative care to be widely and fully integrated into health- and faith-based services around Tanzania, and hopes to be part of that achievement.

Dr Mark Jacobson—*medical director, Selian Hospital, Arusha*: interviewed by David Clark, 4 June 2004. Length of interview: 57 min.

Mark Jacobson has been working in Tanzania as a physician for almost 20 years. His base is a 100-bed Lutheran Church Hospital that serves 55 000–60 000 patients annu-

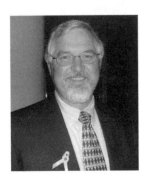

ally. He first began to become interested in palliative care in the late 1990s. He describes the African traditions associated with dying at home, but highlights the lack of skills and support available to families and communities in this situation. He also refers to the growing incidence of chronic disease among the local population, and also to the new epidemic of HIV/AIDS.

Our awareness of needing to care for end of life at home, or starting our hospice programme, really coincided with the timing of this epidemic, when it really began to peak here in Tanzania, which was in the late '90s and the early part of 2000–2001.

His group began to share ideas with the local community, and also to engage in discussions with others in Tanzania interested in the development of palliative care.

The programme at Selian consists of a team based at the hospital which gives the leadership as well as the medical back-up for the care provided at home. This team meets and trains volunteers in the local communities. Those volunteers then become the weekly visitors to the patients who are in the hospice–palliative care programme. Currently, at any given time, some 300 patients are in the programme. A small team of medical nursing staff support about 120 volunteers out in the surrounding communities, and work together with them to provide the ongoing care in the home. Oral morphine has been available for about the last one and a half years. All of the work is done in the homes of the patients. Some patients in hospital are introduced to and acquainted with the programme in hospital, but there is no inpatient component to the programme.

Turning to the wider development of palliative care in Tanzania, Mark Jacobson points out that it seems to have started more or less simultaneously in three or four parts of the country. He refers to plans to develop palliative care services in the 20 Lutheran hospitals in the country as well as in the hospitals of other denominations.

> It would be a tremendous scaling up and we're really excited by it . . . I think that the faith-based organizations, because of their existing infrastructure, are in an ideal place to do that, if we're able to identify models that are cost-effective and relatively inexpensive to graft onto existing services.

He concludes the interview by describing the creation of a Tanzanian national association for palliative care, coming together in discussions at Arusha in June 2004. He also outlines his involvement in the newly formed African Palliative Care Association (APCA).

Angela Kaiza—*social worker, Muheza Hospice Care, Teule Hospital, Muheza*: interviewed by Jenny Hunt, 8 November 2004. Length of interview: 18 min.

Angela Kaiza joined Muheza Hospice Care in October 2004, having obtained a degree in sociology. Although she had not previously heard of palliative care, her interest in helping disadvantaged people was stimulated by dreams as a 17 year old. She describes the programme at Muheza Hospice Care and provides detail on the main social and emotional problems experienced by the patients. She shares her ideas on how to reduce stigma amongst HIV-positive people and identifies groups in the community who need to be targeted to ensure that HIV-affected people are accepted in their villages. Turning to the specifics of the monthly 'Kids Club', Angela Kaiza provides details about the day's programme that encourages HIV-infected children and their families to socialize together, share food and learn about the illness. She identifies the gaps that she sees in the current provision of care and hopes to work towards developing a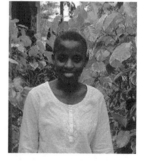

bereavement service. She also shares her commitment to increase the numbers of social workers actively involved in hospice programmes throughout Tanzania.

Paulina Natema—*public health nurse, Selian Lutheran Hospital, Arusha*: interviewed by Jenny Hunt, 5 November 2004. Length of interview: 48 min.

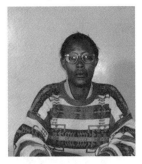

Paulina Natema is responsible for providing spiritual and emotional support and training as part of the holistic palliative care service provided by Selian Lutheran Hospital. She tells of becoming involved in this work at a time when her mother-in-law was dying from cancer. She discovered the benefits of writing a will and dying without pain, and was keen to introduce these concepts to her community. Paulina saw how home-based palliative care could reduce hospital costs for cancer and AIDS patients living in poverty, and recognized the value of families utilizing their own capacities for care and support. She highlights the benefits of families, including children, being informed and prepared for a death. She compares how differently the bereaved are handled nowadays, and sees her role as a hospice worker as finding ways for families to remember the deceased. Paulina Natema discusses specific difficulties experienced by families: not having a will; rights of widows and children; and not having enough time to prepare and counsel children. She highlights the impact that local Masaai culture has on implementing palliative care principles and notes some changing trends. Turning to her motivation to do this work, Paulina expresses her great love for her community and the poor and disadvantaged within it. That she was born nearby and has lived in this community all her life makes her feel totally accepted and respected by the people she helps. She gives a moving account of her personal family losses and acknowledges how difficult it can be to continue with hospice work when she herself is grieving.

Dr Hussein Mtiro—*acting head of the palliative care team, Ocean Road Cancer Institute, Dar es Salaam* and Mary Haule—*palliative care nurse, Ocean Road Cancer Institute, Dar es Salaam*: interviewed by Jenny Hunt, 10 November 2004. Length of interview: 52 min.

Hussein Mtiro summarizes the development of the palliative care team at this hospital. From the inception of a pain control team in July 1994 by Twalib Ngoma, now the

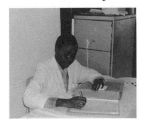

director of the hospital, its main emphasis was on pain control. Now that three members of staff are trained in palliative care, the more holistic approach warrants the label of palliative care team.

Hussein Mtiro and Mary Haule give details of the current programme that attends to both inpatients and outpatients.

In September 2004, staff shortages forced the palliative care team to spread itself among different wards, and its palliative care focus and development have been compromised. Hussein Mtiro expresses concern at the level of support provided by the home-based care organizations on whom they depend to provide continuity of care after the patient is discharged. He comments that these volunteers have no training in pain control and also comments on the continuing resistance of doctors to using morphine.

Mary Haule tells how regulations concerning the importation of morphine in Tanzania were relaxed after successful advocacy from Hospice Africa Uganda. Moving to issues of education and training, she gives details of the team's efforts to inform hospital doctors about morphine, breaking bad news and how to disclose a diagnosis in a culturally sensitive manner.

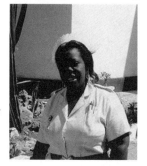

Expanding on cultural issues, Hussein Mtiro discusses the role of traditional healers, and links them and geographical distance with late cancer referrals. He paints a picture of severely limited diagnostic facilities countrywide, no follow-up service for patients outside of Dar es Salaam and expensive diagnostic systems that are beyond the reach of most ordinary Tanzanians. He suggests that a solution lies in expanding the number of government cancer hospitals around the country and developing a palliative care policy. Going on to list the most common cancers in different regions of Tanzania, he advises that cervical screening was only introduced at the hospital in 2002. None of the four oncologists at the Institute has palliative care training. Treatments available at the hospital are described.

Mary Haule shares her concern that cancer has been overshadowed by AIDS and, despite the presence of the WHO palliative care team in Tanzania, there is a lack of political will to prioritize it as a health need. Hussein Mtiro shares his dissatisfaction with the lack of co-ordination of palliative care. He also identifies gaps in the Ocean Road Cancer Institute service, primarily the lack of good home-based care for patients diagnosed with a life-threatening cancer.

In conclusion, they count their successes as introducing morphine, training staff in palliative care skills and co-operating well with their hospital colleagues. They acknowledge personal frustration at not being able to do more for late referrals and recognize the emotional burden they bear in this work.

Public health context

Population

Tanzania's population of around 36.59 million people is made up of the following ethnic groups: mainland—native African 99 per cent (of which 95 per cent are Bantu consisting of >130 tribes), other 1 per cent (consisting of Asian, European and Arab); Zanzibar—Arab, native African, mixed Arab and native African.

Religious groups include: mainland—Christian 30 per cent, Muslim 35 per cent, indigenous beliefs 35 per cent; Zanzibar—more than 99 per cent Muslim.[16]

Epidemiology

In Tanzania, the WHO World Health Report (2004) indicates an adult mortality[17] rate per 1000 population of 561 for males and 512 for females. Life expectancy for males is 45.5; for females 47.5. Healthy life expectancy is 40.0 for males; and 40.7 for females.[18]

There is a perceived epidemiological shift from acute and infectious diseases towards chronic diseases. Prior to the AIDS epidemic, Mark Jacobson saw that age cohorts were growing older. For the first time in his experience there were large numbers of cancers, congestive heart failure, chronic diseases, diabetes, hypertension and pulmonary artery disease. This shift away from acute illnesses and trauma towards an ageing population experiencing chronic illnesses created the need for palliative care.

There appear to be marked variations in cancer prevalence patterns in different parts of the country. In the Arusha region, 'probably the most common female cancer is cervical . . . then oesophageal cancer is quite common.'[14] Although liver cancer is common in the west of the country, it is less so around Arusha. AIDS-related TB is the number one opportunistic infection at Selian Lutheran Hospital in Arusha, yet this is rare around the Kilimanjaro region where cryptoccal meningitis is more common. Clinicians at Selian Lutheran Hospital have yet to diagnose one such case. A condition likely to be toxoplasmosis is common in both Arusha and Kilimanjaro. There are however, diagnostic limitations in this country, and clinical diagnoses are often all that are available.

ORCI reports that up to 70 per cent of their patients present with advanced cancer of the cervix. Cervical screening was only introduced in 2002. AIDS-related Kaposi's sarcoma is now the next most common cancer, closely followed by cancer of the breast. There are high prevalence rates of head and neck cancers, cancer of the oesophagus and stomach cancer. Types of cancer relating to geographical location have been noted here too. Burkitt's lymphoma is a common paediatric cancer.

Approximately 2500 cancer patients per year are attended to at ORCI. This is assumed to be only 20 per cent of the estimated people living with cancer in the country.

Tanzania is one of the worst HIV/AIDS-affected countries in Eastern Africa. Estimates suggest that in Tanzania, approximately 1 600 000 people were living with HIV/AIDS at the end of 2003. In the same year, up to 230 000 adults and children are thought to have died from the disease (Table 18.6).

UNAIDS reports:

> HIV prevalence is far higher in the mainland than in the island territory of Zanzibar, which has about 1 million inhabitants and a prevalence rate estimated at 0.6% in 2002. Women are significantly more affected than men; accounting for 60% of the new infections reported among youth aged 15–24 years. The net effect and impact of the epidemic on per capita GNP growth is substantial and increasingly being felt by many families. Although HIV/AIDS awareness among the population is high (above 80%), behaviour change is very slow with new infections being contracted.

Table 18.6 Tanzania HIV and AIDS estimates, end 2003

Adult (15–49) HIV prevalence rate 8.8 per cent	(range: 6.4–11.9 per cent)
Adults (15–49) living with HIV	1 500 000 (range: 1 100 000–2 000 000)
Adults and children (0–49) living with HIV	1 600 000 (range: 1 200 000–23 000 000)
Women (15–49) living with HIV	840 000 (range: 610 000–1 100 000)
AIDS deaths (adults and children)in 2003	160 000 (range: 110 000–230 000)

Source: 2004 Report of the global AIDS epidemic.

In 2000 the President of the United Republic of Tanzania declared HIV/AIDS a national disaster, which led to the establishment of the National AIDS Commission (TACAIDS) in Tanzania mainland and the Zanzibar AIDS Commission (ZAC) in Zanzibar. These multisectoral bodies are responsible for guiding national efforts to fight HIV/AIDS. Both commissions have successfully formulated a Multisectoral Strategic Framework to fight HIV/AIDS for the period 2003–2007. TACAIDS has developed its three-year Midterm Expenditure Framework (MTEF), action plan and budget. The prime minister launched the National AIDS Policy in November 2001 and the National Multisectoral Strategic Framework (2003–2007) was launched in May 2003. Zanzibar has not yet developed its AIDS policy and MTEF. In the mainland multisectoral HIV/AIDS committees have been set up at local government council level and at ward and village level. Zanzibar is adapting existing DACOMS and SHACOMS to assume a similar role, but extensive capacity building will be required to enable them to function more efficiently and effectively.[19]

Health care system

In 2001, the total per capita expenditure on health care was Intl $26; 4.4% of GDP[20] (Appendix 3).

The WHO overall health system performance score places Tanzania 156th out of 191 countries.[21]

The WHO palliative care project in Tanzania recognizes the following strengths and opportunities in the country:

◆ Home-based care is integrated in the health system

◆ Existing palliative care team at ORCI

◆ Palliative care provided at district level by some NGOs

◆ Support of the Ministry of Health, district health management and NGOs

◆ Government provides funds for palliative care treatments.[22]

◆ Concerns centre on:

◆ Training of home-based care providers

◆ Availability of manuals on home-based care

◆ Link between hospital-based services and home-based services

- Only medical doctors have a licence to prescribe opioid drugs
- Radiotherapy is only available at ORCI.

In Tanzania, there is some concern that the needs of cancer patients are overshadowed by the needs of people living with AIDS.

Currently, the AIDS Control Programme is in the process of establishing national policies for home-based care, but this lacks several components of palliative care. There is a cancer registry but no developed National Cancer Control programme.

Political economy

The coastal area first felt the impact of foreign influence as early as the eighth century, when Arab traders arrived; by the twelfth century, traders and immigrants came from as far away as Persia (now Iran) and India. They built a series of highly developed city and trading states along the coast, the principal one being Kibaha, a settlement of Persian origin that held ascendancy until the Portuguese destroyed it in the early 1500s. The Portuguese navigator Vasco da Gama explored the East African coast in 1498 on his voyage to India. By 1506, the Portuguese claimed control over the entire coast. This control was nominal, however, because the Portuguese did not colonize the area or explore the interior. Assisted by Omani Arabs, the indigenous coastal dwellers succeeded in driving the Portuguese from the area north of the Ruvuma River by the early eighteenth century. Claiming the coastal strip, Omani Sultan Seyyid Said (1804–56) moved his capital to Zanzibar in 1841.

European exploration of the interior began in the mid-nineteenth century. Two German missionaries reached Mount Kilimanjaro in the 1840s. British explorers Richard Burton and John Speke crossed the interior to Lake Tanganyika in 1857. David Livingstone, the Scottish missionary–explorer who crusaded against the slave trade, established his last mission at Ujiji, where he was 'found' by Henry Morton Stanley, an American journalist–explorer, who had been commissioned by the New York Herald to locate him. German colonial interests were first advanced in 1884. In 1886 and 1890, Anglo-German agreements were negotiated that delineated the British and German spheres of influence in the interior of East Africa and along the coastal strip previously claimed by the Omani sultan of Zanzibar. In 1891, the German Government took over direct administration of the territory from the German East Africa Company and appointed a governor with headquarters at Dar es Salaam. German colonial domination of the area ended after the First World War when control of most of the territory passed to the UK under a League of Nations mandate.

After the Second World War, the country became a UN trust territory under British control. Subsequent years witnessed Tanganyika moving gradually toward self-government and independence. In 1954, Julius K. Nyerere, a school teacher who was then one of only two Tanganyikans educated abroad at the university level, organized a political party— the Tanganyika African National Union (TANU). TANU-supported candidates were victorious in the Legislative Council elections of September 1958 and February 1959. In December 1959, the UK agreed to the establishment of internal self-government following general elections to be held in August 1960. Nyerere was named chief minister of the subsequent government.[23]

Tanzania gained independence in 1961. Since that time, it has been ruled by TANU and its subsequent incarnation Chama Cha Mapinduzi (CCM). In the 1960s, Tanzania adopted a single-party political system that generated much academic interest and was touted as a possible model for other parts of the developing world. Through elections, individuals participated in a national event, listened to campaigns in the national language, engaged with the symbols of nationalism and gained an impression that their votes made a difference. As a result, Tanzania was remarkably politically stable. Tanzania, which began liberalizing its polity in the 1990s, is currently regarded by donors as a promising case of political reform.[24]

One-party rule came to an end in 1995 with the first democratic elections held in the country since the 1970s. Zanzibar's semi-autonomous status and popular opposition have led to two elections since 1995, which the ruling party have won.

Tanzania is one of the poorest countries in the world. The economy depends heavily on agriculture, which accounts for about half of the GDP, provides 85 per cent of exports, and employs 80 per cent of the work force. Topography and climatic conditions, however, limit cultivated crops to only 4 per cent of the land area. Industry traditionally featured the processing of agricultural products and light consumer goods. The World Bank, the International Monetary Fund and bilateral donors have provided funds to rehabilitate Tanzania's economic infrastructure and to alleviate poverty. Growth in 1991–2002 featured a pick up in industrial production and a substantial increase in output of minerals, led by gold. Oil and gas exploration and development played an important role in this growth. Recent banking reforms have helped increase private sector growth and investment. Continued donor assistance and solid macroeconomic policies supported real GDP growth of >5.2 per cent in 2004.[16]

GDP per capita is Intl $599. This falls within the range of $8272 (Libya) and $346 (Democratic Republic of the Congo) in the countries of Africa (Appendix 4).

References

1 Report of the United Nations Development Programme 2004 (HDI 2002). Launched by the United Nations in 1990, the Human Development Index measures a country's achievements in three aspects of human development: longevity, knowledge and a decent standard of living. It was created to re-emphasize that people and their lives should be the ultimate criteria for assessing the development of a country, not economic growth. Current values range from 0.956 (Norway, first of 177 countries) to 0.273 (Sierra Leone, 177th out of 177 countries). Countries fall into one of three groups: countries 1–55 = high development; 56–141 = medium development; 142–177 = low development. See: http://hdr.undp.org/statistics/data/indic/indic_8_1_1.html

2 IOELC interview: Mark Jacobson—4 June 2004.

3 Muheza Hospice Care Annual Report 2004.

4 IOELC interview: Angela Kaiza—8 November 2004.

5 IOELC interview: Karilyn Collins—7 November 2004.

6 IOELC interview: Mary Haule—10 November 2004.

7 United Republic of Tanzania HIV/AIDS Care and Treatment Plan 2003–2008 (Draft Document: 19 April 2004). Business Plan 4.0, 1 September 2003: 2.

8 IOELC interview: Mary Ash—9 November 2004.

9 *Engendering Bold Leadership*. The President's Emergency Plan for AIDS Relief. First Annual Report to Congress, 2005: 115. http://www.state.gov/documents/organization/43885.pdf

10 International Narcotics Control Board. *Narcotic Drugs: Estimated World Requirements for 2004. Statistics for 2002*. New York: United Nations, 2004.

11 'The term *defined daily doses for statistical purposes* (S-DDD) replaces the term *defined daily doses* previously used by the Board. The S-DDDs are technical units of measurement for the purposes of statistical analysis and are not recommended prescription doses. Certain narcotic drugs may be used in certain countries for different treatments or in accordance with different medical practices, and therefore a different daily dose could be more appropriate'. The S-DDD used by the INCB for morphine is 100 mg. International Narcotics Control Board. *Narcotic Drugs: Estimated World Requirements for 2004. Statistics for 2002*. New York: United Nations, 2004: 176–177.

12 PASADA Morphine Report 2004.

13 IOELC interview: Hussein Mtiro—10 November 2004.

14 IOELC interview: Kristopher Hartwig—4 November 2004.

15 **Hartwig K.** The development of hospice care in Arusha, Tanzania: lessons from the neighbouring states of Kenya and Uganda. *Journal of Palliative Care* 2001; **17**(2): 121–125.

16 See: http://www.cia.gov/cia/publications/factbook/geos/tz.html

17 This refers to adult mortality risk, which is defined as the probability of dying between 15 and 59 years.

18 See: WHO statistics for Tanzania at: http://www.who.int/countries/tza/en/

19 http://www.unaids.org/en/geographical+area/by+country/united+republic+of+tanzania.asp

20 Total health expenditure per capita is the per capita amount of the sum of Public Health Expenditure (PHE) and Private Expenditure on Health (PvtHE). The international dollar is a common currency unit that takes into account differences in the relative purchasing power of various currencies. Figures expressed in international dollars are calculated using purchasing power parities (PPP), which are rates of currency conversion constructed to account for differences in price level between countries.http://www3.who.int/whosis/country/compare.cfm?country=s&indicator=strPcTotEOHinIntD2000&language=english

21 This composite measure of overall health system attainment is based on a country's goals relating to health, responsiveness, and fairness in financing. The measure varies widely across countries and is highly correlated with general levels of human development as captured in the human development index. Tandon A, Murray CLJ, Lauer JA, Evans DB. *Measuring Overall Health System Performance for 191 Countries*. GPE Discussion Paper Series: No. 30; WHO.

22 WHO report: Community Health Approach to Palliative Care for HIV/AIDS Patients, 2004: 21. Available to download at: http://whqlibdoc.who.int/publications/2004/9241591498.pdf

23 US Department of State, Office of East African Affairs, Bureau of African Affairs. *United Republic of Tanzania: Background Notes on Countries of the World 2003*. Washington, DC: US Department of State, Office of East African Affairs, Bureau of African Affairs, 2003.

24 **Kelsall T.** Governance, democracy and recent political struggles in mainland Tanzania. *Commonwealth and Comparative Politics* 2003; **41**(2): 55–82.

Chapter 19

The Gambia

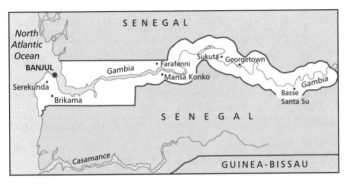 Gambia (population 1.55 million people) is a country in Western Africa that covers an area of 11 300 km². Its boundaries border the North Atlantic Ocean and Senegal. The capital of Gambia is Banjul.

According to the United Nations human development index (HDI), Gambia is ranked 155th out of 177 countries worldwide (value 0.452)[1] and 24th out of 45 in African countries for which an index is available. This places Gambia in the group of countries with low human development.

Palliative care service provision

Current services

Just one organization provides palliative care services in Gambia, Future Care Hospice (Table 19.1).

Future Care Hospice was officially registered as a charitable organization in October 2004.[2]

In April 2005, Abel Iqbe (hospice co-ordinator) reported that the hospice provides home care and day care services. Since the hospice opened, around 200 patients have

Table 19.1 Palliative care provision in The Gambia, 2005

	Free-standing unit	Hospital unit	Hospital support team	Home care	Day care	Clinic/drop-in centre	Total
Future Care Hospice				1		1	2

been cared for. About 25 patients attend day care. Plans for the future include the establishment of a clinic.[3]

The programme includes symptom control, domiciliary care and prevention advice for all sectors of society who have advanced disease. Objectives of the programme are to embark on training nurses to be highly professional and to support the Government effort in the provision of vital preventive and curative drugs for incurable conditions.[2]

Reimbursement and funding for services

Future Hospice Care is a charity and relies on fundraising and voluntary donations for its income. Financial pressures are severe and, since the service began, two nurses have left because of financial constraints. Future Care Hospice needs financial assistance to train personnel, expand their services and improve the availability of drugs.[3]

The Global Fund has committed significant funding to HIV/AIDS programmes in the Republic of the Gambia in Round 3 of an extensive strategy to combat the effects of the AIDS pandemic[4]. The agreement was signed on 31 August 2004 with the National AIDS Secretariat of the Republic of the Gambia.

The project aims to provide the highest standard of available treatment, care and support to people living with and/or affected by HIV/AIDS. US$6 241 743.00 has been approved to implement the project over two years. Although palliative care is not mentioned in the proposal, the project goal includes some elements of holistic care. The provision of antiretroviral therapies is part of a continuum of care that includes compassion, support and the alleviation of stigma.

Opioid availability and consumption

No figures were available from the International Narcotics Control Board[5] regarding the consumption of narcotic drugs in Gambia.

For the years 2000–2002, the average defined daily dose consumption of morphine for statistical purposes (S-DDD)[6] in Gambia was 0 (Appendix 1).

Palliative care coverage

Patients within travelling distance of Future Care Hospice are covered.

Palliative care workforce capacity

In 2004, Future Care Hospice opened with four nurses, one chaplain, five auxiliary nurses and three voluntary workers.[3]

Public health context

Population

The Gambia's population of around 1.55 million people is made up of the following ethnic groups: African 99 per cent (Mandinka 42 per cent, Fula 18 per cent, Wolof 16 per cent, Jola 10 per cent, Serahuli 9 per cent and other 4 per cent) and non-African 1 per cent.

Table 19.2 The Gambia HIV and AIDS estimates, end 2003

Adults (15–49) HIV prevalence rate	1.2 per cent (range 0.3–4.2 per cent)
Adults (15–49) living with HIV	6300 (range 1700–23 000)
Adults and children (0–49) living with HIV	6800 (range 1800–24 000)
Women (15–49) living with HIV	3600 (range 970–13 000)
AIDS deaths (adults and children) in 2003	600 (range 200–1500)

Source: 2004 Report of the global AIDS epidemic.

Religious groups include: Muslim 90 per cent, Christian 9 per cent and indigenous beliefs 1 per cent.[7]

Epidemiology

In the Gambia, the WHO World Health Report (2004) indicates an adult mortality[8] rate per 1000 population of 330 for males and 265 for females. Life expectancy for males is 55.4; for females 58.9. Healthy life expectancy is 48.5 for males; and 50.5 for females.[8]

Gambia is a country in Western Africa that has been affected by the HIV/AIDS crisis. Estimates suggest that in Gambia, between 1800 and 24 000 people were living with HIV/AIDS at the end of 2003. In the same year, up to 1500 adults and children are thought to have died from the disease (Table 19.2)

UNAIDS reports:

Tuberculosis and malaria are major health problems in Gambia; in 2000, the malaria prevalence rate was 17,340 per 100,000, while TB affected 283 per 100,000 in 2001. The government has acknowledged the necessity of a multicultural/multisectoral response to the HIV/AIDS epidemic for successful containment. A National AIDS Control Programme (NACP) was formed in 1987, followed in 1995 by a National AIDS Committee, which developed a National AIDS Policy. The National AIDS Secretariat (NAS) was formed in 2000, supported by the National AIDS Council (NAC) as a policy building body. At present there are five Divisional AIDS Committees (DACs) throughout the Gambia supporting national initiatives and monitoring local needs.

The UNAIDS Theme Group TWG has provided technical assistance in the review of the national socio-cultural survey, which is intended for use in the various HIV/AIDS related planning and intervention activities. The UNAIDS Theme Group TWG participated in the formulation, development and revision of a five-year National Strategic Plan on HIV/AIDS and contributed toward its successful formulation. UNAIDS participated in the development and revision of the Global Fund Project Proposal, with the assistance of international and national consultants. The Theme Group was involved in the analysis of the situation of people living with HIV in the Gambia.

The situation analysis is expected to identify the existing support groups for people living with HIV; assess the needs of people living with HIV; assess the capacity and gaps of existing organizations; and identify the way forward to strengthen their capacity. UNAIDS, in collaboration with the NAS, coordinated the Department of State for Youth and Sports and the National Youth Council to mobilize Gambian youth to attend the Pan-African Youth Forum in Dakar (22–26

March 2004). The National Youth Council established a task force and facilitated coordination, and 15 youths were able to attend the forum.[10]

Health care system

In 2001, the total per capita expenditure on health care was Intl $78; 6.4 of GDP[11] (Appendix 3).

The WHO overall health system performance score places Gambia 146th out of 191 countries.[12]

Political economy

The Gambia gained its independence from the UK in 1965; it formed a short-lived federation of Senegambia with Senegal between 1982 and 1989. In 1991, the two nations signed a friendship and co-operation treaty. A military coup in 1994 overthrew the president and banned political activity, but a 1996 constitution and presidential elections, followed by parliamentary balloting in 1997, completed a nominal return to civilian rule. The country undertook another round of presidential and legislative elections in late 2001 and early 2002. Yahya A. J. J. Jammeh, the leader of the coup, has been elected president in all subsequent elections.

The Gambia has no important mineral or other natural resources and has a limited agricultural base. About 75 per cent of the population depends on crops and livestock for its livelihood. Small-scale manufacturing activity features the processing of peanuts, fish and hides. Re-export trade normally constitutes a major segment of economic activity, but a 1999 government-imposed pre-shipment inspection plan, and instability of the Gambian dalasi (currency) have drawn some of the re-export trade away from Gambia. The government's 1998 seizure of the private peanut firm Alimenta eliminated the largest purchaser of Gambian peanuts; the following two marketing seasons have seen substantially lower prices and sales. A decline in tourism in 2000 has also held back growth. Unemployment and underemployment rates are extremely high. Short run economic progress remains highly dependent on sustained bilateral and multilateral aid, on responsible government economic management as forwarded by IMF technical help and advice, and on expected growth in the construction sector.[7]

GDP per capita is Intl $1214 (Appendix 4).

References

1 Report of the United Nations Development Programme 2004 (HDI 2002). Launched by the United Nations in 1990, the Human Development Index measures a country's achievements in three aspects of human development: longevity, knowledge and a decent standard of living. It was created to re-emphasize that people and their lives should be the ultimate criteria for assessing the development of a country, not economic growth. Current values range from 0.956 (Norway, first of 177 countries) to 0.273 (Sierra Leone, 177th out of 177 countries). Countries fall into one of three groups: countries 1–55 = high development; 56–141 = medium development; 142–177 = low development. See: http://hdr.undp.org/statistics/data/indic/indic_8_1_1.html

2 IAHPC news online: 2005, 6(3). See: http://www.hospicecare.com/newsletter2005/mar05/editor.html

3 Personal communication: Abel Igbe—21 April 2005.

4 http://www.theglobalfund.org/search/portfolio.aspx?countryID=GMB#HIV/AIDS#HIV/AIDS

5 International Narcotics Control Board. *Narcotic Drugs: Estimated World Requirements for 2004. Statistics for 2002.* New York: United Nations, 2004.

6 The term *defined daily doses for statistical purposes* (S-DDD) replaces the term *defined daily doses* previously used by the Board. The S-DDDs are technical units of measurement for the purposes of statistical analysis and are not recommended prescription doses. Certain narcotic drugs may be used in certain countries for different treatments or in accordance with different medical practices, and therefore a different daily dose could be more appropriate'. The S-DDD used by the INCB for morphine is 100 mg. International Narcotics Control Board. *Narcotic Drugs: Estimated World Requirements for 2004. Statistics for 2002.* New York: United Nations, 2004: 176–177.

7 See: http://www.cia.gov/cia/publications/factbook/geos/ga.html

8 This refers to adult mortality risk, which is defined as the probability of dying between 15 and 59 years.

9 See: WHO statistics for Gambia at: http://www.who.int/countries/gmb/en/

10 http://www.unaids.org/en/geographical+area/by+country/gambia.asp

11 Total health expenditure per capita is the per capita amount of the sum of Public Health Expenditure (PHE) and Private Expenditure on Health (PvtHE). The international dollar is a common currency unit that takes into account differences in the relative purchasing power of various currencies. Figures expressed in international dollars are calculated using purchasing power parities (PPP), which are rates of currency conversion constructed to account for differences in price level between countries.
http://www3.who.int/whosis/country/compare.cfm?country=s&indicator=strPcTotEOHinInt D2000&language=english

Chapter 20

Zambia

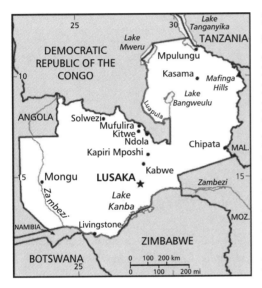

Zambia (population 10.7 million)[1] is a landlocked country in Southern Africa that covers an area of 5664 km². Its boundaries border Angola, Democratic Republic of the Congo, Malawi, Mozambique, Namibia, Tanzania and Zimbabwe. Formerly known as Northern Rhodesia, the territory was administered by the South Africa Company from 1891 until it was taken over by the UK in 1923. The name was changed to Zambia upon independence in 1964.

According to the United Nations human development index (HDI), Zambia is ranked 164th out of 175 countries worldwide (value 0.389)[2] and 32nd out of 45 in African countries for which an index is available. This places Zambia in the low development group.

Palliative care service provision

Current services

In Zambia, palliative care is provided by six organizations delivering a total of 20 services (Table 20.1).

A feature of Zambian palliative care services is the prominence of the inpatient unit. Following a visit to Zambia (2004) on behalf of the Diana, Princess of Wales Memorial Fund (Diana Fund), Dr Anne Merriman commented:

Hospices have sprung up to meet needs where caring people have been inspired to set up alternative provision for those dying or critically ill within an inpatient setting. Most have an additional home care service which is mainly support care, covering patients from diagnosis to end of life . . . [There was] the presumption throughout all we met in hospices in Zambia that for everyone there came a time when they were too sick to stay at home. We found this rather sad, when we have witnessed dying at home to bring so much more peace for patient and family in other parts of Africa.[3]

Table 20.1 Palliative care provision in Zambia, 2004

	Free-standing unit	Hospital unit	Hospital support team	Home care	Day care	Clinic/drop-in centre	Total
Mother of Mercy Hospice, Chilanga	1			1		1	3
Jon Hospice, Lusaka	1			1	1	1	4
Ranchhod Hospice, Kabwe	1			1	1	1	4
Our Lady's Hospice, Lusaka	1			1		1	3
Martin Hospice, Choma	1			1	1		3
Cicetekelo Hospice, Ndola	1			1		1	3
Total services	6			6	3	5	20

She went on to list the following reasons for the growth of inpatient units in Zambia:

1 Death certification is done in the hospital and police have to be notified of a death at home and order the body to be taken to hospital for certification which costs a lot of money.

2 The history of the men being employed in the copper mines means that 20 per cent of the population are urban and have not the network support from local communities seen in other African countries. Thus families reject the dying and orphans. This is also given as a reason for the many orphanages.

3 Powdered morphine only available for cancer and only at the University Teaching Hospital (UTH). Thus patient has to have injectable [morphine] unless there are tablets available from donors. This is only possible in an inpatient facility.

4 Morphine: laws regulating morphine are very strict, leading to imprisonment. Law enforcement is separate to the police and is a group of clinical officers with a mandate to imprison without asking questions if the drugs are found on health worker or patient!

Mother of Mercy Hospice[4]

The programme was established in 1992 to provide care for terminally ill patients in the community of Chilanga, approximately 16 km south of Lusaka. Most patients are HIV positive. The original home-based care programme grew rapidly to meet the growing need for medical care and palliative support. It now operates a home-based care programme for 520 patients, a 22-bed inpatient hospice, an outpatient clinic and a school for children affected by HIV/AIDS. The small day centre that was built 3 years ago has been converted into a large community school (Guardian Angel School) for about 130 pupils ranging from 6 to 16 years old. There are four teachers. Up to 60 patients at a time are attended to at the outpatient clinic, and 280 patients from the home-based care programme receive food from the UN World Food Programme.

There is an active ARV programme in place, with 80 patients (50 children and 30 adults) currently enrolled on the programme. Fewer than 10 per cent of inpatients are on ARV therapy. A local doctor who has specialized in ARV treatments allocates 2–4 h per week to this programme. The acting director, Alison Hill, connects a donor (either international or local) with a patient, whereupon the donor agrees to pay for treatment during the patient's life. She then conducts the basic examinations, management of opportunistic infections, the preliminary laboratory work, CD4 counts and liver function. The doctor then has a consultation with the patient and prescribes any necessary medication. Patients are counselled and monitored. The adherence rate is very good due to the close monitoring on site. For the first six–eight weeks, the children live in close proximity to the director, and she directly observes their treatment. During this time, they spend 15 min or more with the counsellor every day to discuss the importance of taking medication and what their medications look like.

Up to 100 patients are visited in their homes each month by the home care team. The average occupancy at the hospice is between 95 and 100 per cent; many inpatients are registered home-based care patients requiring intensive care. The hospice additionally provides physiotherapy and extensive laboratory testing. All inpatients are screened for HIV, have a full blood count, and urine and stool analysis. The laboratory has the capacity to do most STI screenings, pregnancy testing, cryptoccocal meningitis and sputum testing for TB. The hospice approaches palliative care for HIV/AIDS patients with a combination of symptom management, aggressive therapy, public health work in local communities, counselling and nutritional support. The hospice has a refrigerated three-body mortuary unit on site. The deceased are kept here until such time as funeral arrangements have been made by the family.

Jon Hospice

This service is one of several programmes run by Kara Counselling. The hospice was founded in 1999 to cater for the needs of those dying from AIDS. Apart from a 26-bed hospice unit, Jon Hospice operates a mobile hospice service to cater for the needs of patients, primarily children, in the community, as well as a day care centre for children. In 2003, there were approximately 500 admissions to Jon Hospice, and approximately 40 per cent of those patients died at the unit. In April 2004, there were 56 admissions. There are 130 children registered at the day centre although 30 children attend regularly. Many receive education here as well, although some attend for medical care only. The multidisciplinary mobile hospice team works closely with other home-based care programmes to complement rather than duplicate services, and travels twice weekly into the surrounding community. A three-body mortuary is on site and operates as a transit facility for the removal of the body from the ward prior to removal to a government health facility.

Other Kara Counselling programmes include Hope House (life skills training and VCT), Umoyo training (skills training and literacy classes for orphaned girls), Martin Hospice and Ranchhod House, Kabwe.

Ranchhod House[5]

This service was established in late 2003. A town office in Kabwe doubles as a drop-in centre for HIV counselling and testing. From July to December 2003, 182 VCT sessions were held. For the same period, 21 people received general counselling. Numbers have increased dramatically since then. From January to May 2004, a total of 551 received VCT counselling while 31 people were counselled on other issues. Ranchhod House (named after the Asian businessman who donated the house) incorporates a 15-bed adult hospice unit that opened on 9 October 2003. It has expanded to provide a children's day centre for 40 children aged up to 7 years. A street children's programme is also being established as a preventative measure for vulnerable children. There were 127 admissions and 29 deaths from October 2003 to May 2004.

Our Lady's Hospice

This establishment began operating its training and outreach programme in 2001, and the custom-designed 22-bed inpatient unit opened in August 2003. The facility is designed to serve patients with any terminal condition, but most have HIV-related cancers. The hospice comprises four houses, each with three rooms that are furnished with two beds. There is also an 8-bed special care/observation unit where acute day patients are stabilized before transfer to the wards.

The organization trains its volunteers who then visit patients in their homes. The outreach programme is thought to be the most important aspect of the service. Relatives are encouraged to look after patients at home with support from hospice staff who provide medical care and training, together with advice and encouragement. An outpatient clinic operates twice weekly and provides a mobile service—also twice a week. A comprehensive ARV programme has been implemented by the doctors on the board. This links into an agreement between the Zambian and US governments and the University of Alabama. All inpatients receive these treatments. School fees for 30 children in the surrounding community are paid by the hospice as a sustainable effort to help families cope with poverty and illness.

Martin Hospice

Based in Choma, about 5 h drive from Lusaka, this programme offers a 12-bed inpatient unit, a day care centre for 25 children, and an outreach programme using already existing diocesan home-based care programmes.

Cicetekelo Hospice (Ndola Hospice)

Anne Merriman notes in her report to the Diana Fund:

> At the entrance to the Ndola Hospice Compound there is a notice: *Ecumenical Hospice Association, Ndola.* However it is known popularly as Ndola Hospice.[3]

Robert Sihubwa visited the hospice in October 2004 as part of a national survey of hospices in Zambia (on behalf of the Power of Love Foundation) and comments:

> Cicetekelo Hospice is about 30 minutes drive from the main town of Ndola in Lubutu Community . . . The hospice is built on a plot of land measuring approximately 30 × 100 metres. The hospice also owns and manages a grocery shop and grinding hammer mill that are used as income generating activities for the hospice.[6]

There is a 25-bed inpatient unit for cancer patients and HIV patients. This can be extended to 30 beds if necessary. The majority of patients are terminally ill with HIV-related illnesses. There is also home-based care for 200 registered patients and 1200 orphans. Provision of food through the World Food Programme is a central part of the organization's services.[7]

Alongside these services, the Power of Love Foundation, an NGO based in San Diego, seeks to minimize the impact of HIV/AIDS through a new initiative. It conducted a survey of hospices in Zambia in October 2004, each one visited in person by Robert Sihubwa. The organization is involved in a number of projects in Zambia and intends to open a new, low-cost hospice in association with the Anglican Children's Project.

> Land for the hospice has been donated by the community and zoned for construction. The hospice will be built on lessons learned from a study of best practices among hospices. The focus will be on leveraging technology and lessons learned to hit our target capital and operating costs. The hospice will operate an OPC (outpatient clinic) on site. The hospice will operate a mobile-clinic to specific areas within the target communities to: Provide neighbourhood-based medical response to the sick children; Support the community health workers; Follow up with cases discharged from the care.[8]

Reimbursement and funding for services

Mother of Mercy Hospice

This organization is primarily funded by the Archdiocese of Lusaka. Other donations in cash or kind are made by the local community, international donors, individual benefactors and local companies. International and local donors provide funds to purchase school uniforms and materials.

All services including medications are provided free to patients. Drugs are donated or purchased through donations. ARV therapies are sponsored by local and international donors who commit to providing the drugs for the patient's life. Basic antibiotics, antidiarrhoeals and other medications are provided monthly by the Archdiocese.

Quarterly, the hospice receives large shipments of medications from the church in Austria. There is no financial input from the Zambian government. The volunteer caregivers receive monthly food rations and health care; often they too are HIV positive. Zone leaders in each compound travel by hospice bicycle.

Jon Hospice

Initial funds for the establishment of Jon Hospice were provided by a Dutch benefactor, Pola van der Donck. A combination of donors now sustains this organization. The day care for children is funded by Firelight Foundation (USA)[9] and AIDS Alliance.[10] The hospice itself receives operating funds from the Diana, Princess of Wales Memorial Fund. Local donations include 25 kg of beef to contribute towards food costs.

Ranchhod House

These services are financially managed by Kara Counselling in Lusaka although local and international donations are sourced by Kabwe directly. Funding has come from such diverse quarters as Irish Aid (water system), Abbot Pharmaceuticals (HIV test kits), local farmers and businesses (foodstuffs) and the Zambian NGO—Community Response to HIV and AIDS (extension of the women's ward).

Our Lady's Hospice

The main funding for this service comes from the Catholic Church. An initial payment of US$10 000 from Franciscans in the USA paid for the pilot study to determine the appropriate hospice model. Free ARVs from the University Teaching Hospital (UTH) are available through the hospice board doctors. Funds from the Catholic Church in the USA will support the building of a laboratory for HIV testing.

Cicetekelo Hospice (Ndola Hospice)

Funding comes from donors, both local and international. International donors include: the Nuffield Foundation; the Diana Fund; Irish GPs (who raised €27 000 following the recording of a Band Aid-type *Song in my Heart* CD)[11] and the Irish Government's Joint Committee on Foreign Affairs. A report of the Joint Committee's delegation to Zambia in 2003 notes:

> Cicetekelo Hospice, which is run by Sr Eileen Keane of the Holy Rosary Sisters, provides palliative care for those chronically ill HIV/AIDS patients who are not able to care for themselves or have no one to do so. The hospice currently caters for 25 patients at any given time with at least one patient dying a day. However because of the growing demand the hospice recently requested 25,000 Euro to assist them construct a compound, St Theresa's Village, which would cater for many more patients.[12]

President's Emergency Plan for AIDS Relief (PEPFAR)

During the 2004 financial year (FY), funding of around US$57.93 million was enacted for country-managed programmes in Zambia and US$23.85 million for central programmes. During FY2005, it is anticipated that a total of US$114.92 million will be enacted: US$84.75 million for country-managed programmes and US$30.17 million for central programmes.[13]

Opioid availability and consumption

Data from the International Narcotics Control Board[14] show the following figures for narcotic consumption in Zambia, 2002 unless stated: codeine 17 kg (2000); morphine 2 kg (2000); dihydrocodeine 4 kg (2000); pholcodine 9 kg (2000); dextropropoxyphene 25 kg; tilidine 2 kg (2000); pethidine 2 kg; and diphenoxylate 2 kg.

For the years 2000–2002, the average defined daily dose consumption of morphine for statistical purposes (S-DDD)[15] in Zambia was 3 (Appendix 1).

Zambia has strict importation rules pertaining to medication. Jon Hospice has taken the lead in lobbying the Medical Council of Zambia for the import of morphine and relaxing the restrictive legislation of the Narcotics Control Board of Zambia. While progress has been made, research may yet be needed to convince the state of the need for easily accessible morphine. There is little understanding amongst health professionals as to the benefits of morphine, and myths surrounding its effects persist. Consequently, assessment and management of pain is underdeveloped.

Mother of Mercy Hospice uses the basic analgesics, non-steroidals and lower opiates (pethidine). Injectable morphine is inexpensive and available through UTH, although oral morphine is extremely difficult to obtain. The hospice nurses and clinical officer assess pain and are able to recommend morphine use. The prescription is signed by the hospice doctor and the drug administered by the nurse. Home-based patients requiring morphine are visited daily by a nurse, although logistically it is simpler for such patients to be admitted to the hospice. No syringe drivers are available.

Jon Hospice continues to campaign actively for easy access to morphine for palliative care. Only injectable morphine is easily accessed, and there are legislative obstacles to providing a range of pain medications. Morphine is underprescribed and this hospice acknowledges that many patients die in pain. Cromwell Shalunga: 'Sometimes we have no option but to use pethidine'.[16] Jon Hospice uses the WHO pain ladder, and most drugs are available but expensive.

Ranchhod House nurses administer pain medications as necessary. These include paracetamol, analgesics and ibuprofen, diazepam and septrin when necessary. As there is no doctor attached to the hospice, injectable morphine is not used although it is easily accessed. Morphine tablets are donated occasionally by a US-based donor, and these are used when required. Mary Chidgey:

> I think we are controlling pain. The Zambians are not used to taking medications at every turn.
> I think their pain tolerance is quite high, so they respond quite well to what we give.[17]

Our Lady's Hospice does not utilize the injectable morphine available in Zambia as they do not have a doctor on site to source it. They receive donated morphine (oral and tablets) from external donors but this is used sparingly due to erratic supply, preferring not to start it if they cannot continue. Sr Crucis:

> The concept of pain is different here too. Pain is something to be endured. Most people have only had access to simple remedies like aspirin, so their belief is that pain just happens and is part of the illness and part of suffering.[18]

Cicetekelo Hospice (Ndola Hospice). Accessing morphine is extremely difficult, and palliative care in this setting is often challenged to achieve pain control without either Step two or Step three of the WHO analgesic ladder. Morphine is rarely available at Ndola Central Hospital.[19]

National and professional organizations

Catholic Archdiocese of Lusaka

The Catholic Archdiocese of Lusaka is the managing agent of the Mother of Mercy Hospice in Chilanga. There are 52 home-based care services managed under this organization but little interaction between them and other organizations.

Zambian Palliative Care Association

An informal national association was developed some years ago mainly linking Mother of Mercy Hospice and Jon Hospice. A palliative care conference and inaugural meeting of the association was held in June 2004 with the aim of improving networking and interaction between the various hospices around the country.

Hospice of Illinois (USA) is twinned with Ranchhod House, Kabwe.

Palliative care coverage

A visit by palliative care development consultant Anne Lloyd-Williams to Zambia in 2001[20] and the collation of country information by Faith Mwangi-Powell[21] have highlighted the challenges faced by palliative care activists in Zambia. At this time, despite the hospice programmes currently operational, specialist knowledge of palliative care seemed sparse. Crucially, there was a lack of enthusiasm from government, which appeared sceptical of the benefits of hospice care. In this scenario, the Diana Fund turned to Hospice Africa Uganda as an appropriate organization which could assist with advocacy and training. Issues related to the adoption of a palliative care policy; access to pain-relieving drugs—including morphine—and an improved standard of palliative care in health referrals. A team from Hospice Africa Uganda visited Zambia in February 2004 and, in its report to the Diana Fund, included key recommendations in the areas of education, drugs availability and government policy against a 3-year time scale.

Mother of Mercy Hospice

The hospice services eight villages, the closest being 0.5 km away and the furthest about 25 km from the hospice. Although there are government clinics in the area, this is the only residential facility for the care of the critically ill and dying. The total population of the catchment area is unknown, but a 2002 census estimated the population of one of the eight compounds as 20 000 with 63 per cent of the population under 13 years old.

Jon Hospice

This service covers greater Lusaka with a population of 1.3 million. The five neighbouring townships (population 500 000) are well served by faith-based home-based care teams whose referrals to the hospice constitute the majority of patients.

Ranchhod House

The hospice services the whole of greater Kabwe with its many townships. The population is estimated at 300 000.

Our Lady's Hospice

Patients are drawn from the surrounding three large compounds comprising many sections. The population is officially estimated at 100 000 but considered by the hospice to be closer to 250 000.

Cicetekelo Hospice (Ndola Hospice)

This hospice serves both urban and rural Ndola and is one of only two hospices on the Copperbelt (the other being Ranchhod House, Kabwe).

Education and training

Mother of Mercy Hospice maintains an active training programme for its staff and uses medical and caregiver meetings to present cases and discuss problems. Improving counselling skills is addressed at least bi-annually by Kara Counselling, while nursing and laboratory workshops with a focus on HIV/AIDS, TB and STIs are held with the Zambian National AIDS committee and/or the Ministry of Health.

Volunteer home-based caregivers are trained by the Archdiocese in pastoral services, basic assessing skills, basic medical skills and counselling. Monthly meetings have been held with the informal Zambian Hospice Association to discuss experiences and hospice issues.

The Guardian Angel School is in the process of establishing an Open Community School Association with the aim of sharing ideas and resources. It has also initiated a creative learning workshop with help from visiting teachers from the UK.

Two counsellors have received VCT and child counselling training by Kara Counselling. Two social workers have undergone courses at the University of Zambia and Social Welfare. The director, Alison Hill, is certified in HIV/AIDS counselling, STI counselling and reproductive health. In-house training on monitoring ARV treatments is informal.

Jon Hospice comes under the Kara Counselling umbrella and benefits from the many counselling training programmes. There are five trained counsellors/social workers at the hospice. The clinical officer is the only palliative care-trained member of staff. All hospice staff are trained by Kara Counselling, as are most of the home-based care groups in the area. The home-based care groups are not trained in any palliative care skills, however, and tend to focus on faith support rather than attending to the physical needs of the patient.[16] Increasingly, the hospice staff are relied upon to provide palliative care training within the Kara Counselling courses. A training course is planned at Jon Hospice to cater for the demand in palliative care training.

Ranchhod House

All counsellors are trained by Kara Counselling. Kabwe Hospice plans to implement basic skills training, including drip monitoring, for caregivers of patients.

Our Lady's Hospice

At the time of establishing this service, three nurses were sent for palliative care training at a hospice in Dublin run by the Sisters of Charity. Those nurses currently hold positions as matron, clinic nurse and home-based care nurse. Training of primary care-givers was conducted by one of these nurses. The training of volunteers for the outreach programme is AIDS focused, with information on hygiene, nursing care, bereavement, simple communication skills and opportunistic infections.

Palliative care workforce capacity

Mother of Mercy Hospice

The services here are provided by: one administrative director (usually Sisters of St Charles); two part-time doctors; one full-time clinical officer; two full-time nurses; one part-time nurse; 17 paid caregivers; 56 volunteer caregivers; and two counsellors who provide VCT and couples counselling, ARV, nutritional and grief counselling.

In the last year, a team of four social workers has been encouraged to address public health issues, monitor patient wellness, monitor circumstances of orphans, and create education and awareness programmes for patients, staff and communities.

Other staff include a receptionist, three programme co-ordinators, four teachers, ground staff, watchmen and cooks.

Jon Hospice

Staff include: one part-time volunteer doctor; and one part-time chaplain. All other staff are full time: one palliative care-trained clinical officer; three nurses; six auxiliary nurses; one social worker; three counsellors; one administrative assistant; one co-ordinator (care and support); one manager; one driver; one international volunteer nurse; and 10 volunteers trained by the diocese from the local community who do cleaning and provide spiritual care

Staffing at the day care/school: one teacher full time; one teacher part time; one social worker; one coordinator; one international volunteer music therapist; and one cook.

Ranchhod House

Staff include: one manager (for both drop-in and in-patient unit); four nurses working in rotation; one clinical officer; two counsellors; one cook; seven volunteers work in the hospice; and three volunteers work in the day care facility. All staff and volunteers work full time (40 h week). Volunteers are remunerated with food, a monthly allowance, uniform, bicycle, washing powder and health care.

Our Lady's Hospice

Two doctors sit on the board and are available for consultations; one managing director/religious nursing sister; two clinical officers; one matron; one senior nurse; one community senior nurse; one pharmacist; two social workers/counsellors; one administrator; one administrative assistant; and one accountant. There are seven general maintenance staff and 58 volunteer caregivers who receive a stipend

Cicetekelo Hospice (Ndola Hospice)

There are 35 paid staff, including a doctor, nurses and caregivers, financial support staff and drivers. There are 37 volunteer caregivers and 38 community volunteers; all volunteers are trained by the hospice.

History and development of hospice–palliative care in Zambia

Mother of Mercy Hospice

Alison Hill, the acting director, describes how the hospice became established:

> Twelve years ago a Polish nun, Sr Leonia Kournas, came here as a registered nurse. She recognized there was a need for palliation in terms of home based care within the communities. At that time HIV was just becoming noticeable in terms of symptomatic patients. So she started the home based care programme. About six years ago it had grown to a point where she needed more staff, more people working and really just a point to work from, where patients could come in if they were acutely ill and receive care.[22]

Sr Kournas[23] has written a brief history of Mother of Mercy Hospice from which these extracts are taken:

> Six years ago the first of the hospice buildings was erected and Mother of Mercy Hospice began admitting patients for around the clock medical care and palliative support.
>
> Through a network of community care-givers, we receive updates on patient conditions and daily, send a group of care-givers and medical staff to our out-stations to assess the situations and provide medical care to those who are unable to come into the hospice. The hospice additionally provides extensive counselling services, physiotherapy and a wide variety of laboratory testing.
>
> The UN-WFP food aid consists of monthly rations of maize meal, cooking oil, high protein porridge and occasionally dried beans. This food is given to more than 300 of the patients in our home-based care program, to the hospice for preparing daily meals as well as to our school. Local farmers and other donors bring in surplus vegetable crops and an Irish donor has organized a ration of meat given weekly for the hospice inpatients.
>
> A combination of poverty and drought has created widespread starvation and malnutrition in our communities. Although HIV positive, a significant number of the illnesses we treat and deaths we suffer are a direct result of, or exacerbated by, issues of nutritional deficiencies. Food has become one of the most important treatments we offer at the hospice. The hospice prepares three main meals a day, consisting of the local staple, nshima made from maize meal, vegetables and a source of protein, either beans, meat or fish. We also provide high protein porridge in the morning and smaller snacks between meals. The school prepares at least one meal per day for the students.
>
> Three years ago the hospice built a small day centre for the children of our clients to offer some education, activities, and food during the daytime. As time went by, the number grew and the day centre was not big enough to accommodate the need. In March of 2002 construction on a larger open community school was started and on September 9, 2002 the doors of this school were opened to approximately 80 children. Since that time, the numbers continue to increase. Although governmental schools are now considered free to attend, affording the required supplies, uniforms and shoes exclude many children from attending. We offer morning classes including mathematics, science, English, reading and history as well as afternoon classes involving music, art, sports and drama. The open community school implements a reduced curriculum from approximate grade 1–7.
>
> Poverty, disease and starvation are a daily reality here, as they are in many countries across the globe. The world can no longer turn a blind eye to the issues surrounding HIV/AIDS as its devastation is felt across all boundaries; geographically, economically, and socially. Addressing our present situation involves focusing on supportive treatments for opportunistic infections, anti-retroviral treatment for extending life, emotional and spiritual support for the patients and their families, and social support for food security and basic welfare. Addressing issues of the future involve providing a safe place for our children to grow up and ensuring the education they need to create change.

Alison Hill came to work in Zambia from the USA in 2001 and was attached to this hospice as a medical intern. Sr Kournas asked her to stand in as Director while she went on sabbatical. Alison considers this organization to be more of an HIV care rather than a hospice:

> We do have the hospice itself which functions a whole lot like a hospital, dealing with an opportunistic infection, monitoring it and aggressively treating a bacterial infection or TB, getting them up and running and getting them back home. We stretch the definition to incorporate more aggressive therapy.[22]

Jon Hospice

Jon Hospice was opened in 1999, fully funded by a Dutch national Pola van der Donck whose musician brother died of HIV disease. His dying wish was to provide funds to help HIV-positive people in developing countries. Pola had no prior vision about how to begin, but came to Zambia to offer care and support. She met Father Kelly, the founder of Kara Counselling (the name is derived from 'friend' in Irish), who suggested building a hospice. This was perceived as a gap in the other Kara programmes, and the idea of a hospice was born. The same donor provided funds for the building of Mother of Mercy Hospice, Chilanga, and for Martin Hospice in Choma.

Sr Leonie Kornas, Zambia's first hospice pioneer and a Polish nun, transferred the inpatient Polish hospice model to Zambia. Cromwell Shalunga, a clinical officer working at the hospice says:

> What we are coming to understand now is that institutionalized type of care actually is not the ideal one, though we are left with no options, because the structures are already in existence. The mobile type of hospice would have done more work compared with what we have done because we are taking care of a limited number of patients.[6]

Our Lady's Hospice

The story of Our Lady's is told by Sr Crucis, the managing director:

> The thinking came from my experience teaching at the University Teaching Hospital (UTH) where there is officially something like 1500 beds but unofficially more like 2000 patients, many of those patients on the floor. One came to the conclusion that with the advent of AIDS, it has created a huge crisis in the health service here which was totally unprepared. UTH was then being used as a hospital for the terminally ill without being designed as such and nobody was prepared for that.[18]

Sr Crucis describes how initially people came to a health centre, received treatment and went away. Now there is chronic sickness, families are being decimated, the extended family system has collapsed, and neither family nor the medical profession is prepared for dealing with long term illness. She continues:

> So with that in mind we tried to look at a new model of care for chronically ill people. We [that is, another nurse, a senior nursing office at UTH, religious congregations and Sr Crucis] formed a small committee and actually got ten thousand dollars from the USA, from the Franciscans, and we decided to do a pilot study. So we visited Uganda, Kenya, Zimbabwe, Chikankata here to see

how they were managing the problem. We thought Uganda was a good choice because they had come out before others about the AIDS issue. We pooled all the information together to see what suited us best. We found that in the rural places in Uganda, especially in the mission hospitals, they had a good outreach programme, but when we got to Kenyatta Hospital, it was another UTH; total confusion. In fact in Kenya we were told that AIDS had been kept quiet for so long because they were worried about their tourism.

So we came to the conclusion that there was no way we could build a structure that could cater for all the patients. Whatever model of care you had, it had to be community based. We decided on an inpatient unit because we found that the patients in the community could not be cared for by their relatives if there was some kind of crisis with opportunistic infections. This was made worse by poverty and the resulting malnutrition, anaemia, so you have to sort those things out to some degree. So we decided we also needed a clinic because patients would need to come for review, new patients identified. At the time we started ARVs were not available or affordable, so all we could do was treat the opportunistic infections and symptomatic care, including the spiritual aspect, grief, death and dying.

Cicetekelo Hospice (Ndola Hospice)

Sr Keane was the Acting Head of the Medical Department at Ndola Central Hospital in 1992 when she became increasingly concerned at the levels of HIV infection in her department. By 1998, she estimated 70 per cent of the patients were HIV positive, and there were 2000 deaths alone that year at the hospital. She heard many stories of family caregivers feeling unable to cope with the burden of illness. There had been suggestions by some nurses that a hospice was necessary, but it took a meeting of religious leaders in 1999 to create the Ecumenical Hospice Association to oversee the development of this interdenominational hospice. The hospice is registered with the newly formed national palliative care association.

Hospice success stories

Mother of Mercy Hospice

The hospice is proud of its ability to provide not just basic health care but a quality of health care usually unavailable in impoverished communities. Working in communities that are challenged economically as well as by disease and starvation, the supportive care provided by this hospice attends to all the patients' needs. The integrated approach fostered by this organization expands the meaning of hospice work to include aggressive therapies, public health work and nutritional support. The director believes that the majority of their patients die pain free and, although resources are limited and the demand so high, they try to respond to every call they receive. This hospice also feels that they recognize and support people living with AIDS in what is still a stigmatizing environment.

The ARV programme that started in February 2003 is regarded as a success. Alison Hill:

> We had a child come in who hadn't walked for two years, with a CD4 count of 11. We started her on ARVs and her count is at about 300 now.[17]

Jon Hospice

The de-stigmatization of hospice being associated with AIDS and with dying is a big achievement for this service. Patients are often discharged and continue to live normal lives, and increasingly the hospice is viewed as providing a much needed service. Margaret Chirwa:

> We have been able to rehabilitate people and get them back home. Initially people believed that when they came to hospice they would die. Now we see people even after a year and it is very nice for us.[24]

Kabwe Kara Counselling/Ranchhod House

Mary Chidgey, who has been instrumental in establishing these, attributes the vibrancy and rapid growth of the services to the dynamic personality of the manager who has successfully created a true community service. The central location of the drop-in ensures high accessibility and acceptance. The energetic volunteers and staff at the hospice are committed to providing a service that meets the needs of the local community.

Our Lady's Hospice

Sr Crucis considers they have succeeded in their core business of providing clinical support and knowledge to international standards. They would like to share this knowledge with other organizations doing similar work and hope to improve the standard of care. There is little formal training in palliative care in this country, and this hospice has concerns about the quality of care provided and would like to improve it.

Cicetekelo Hospice (Ndola Hospice)

A major success of the hospice is the establishment of St Theresa's village approximately 7 km away. Patients who are discharged from the hospice and who have nowhere to stay can live here and continue to receive supportive care from 25 caregivers employed by the hospice.

Public health context

Population

Zambia has an estimated population of 10.70 million of which around 99 per cent are African and 1 per cent European. The major religions are Christian, Hindu and Muslim.

Epidemiology

The WHO World Health Report (2003) indicates an adult mortality[25] rate per 1000 population of 700 for males and 654 for females. Life expectancy for males is 39.1; for females 40.2. Healthy life expectancy is 34.8 for males; and 35.0 for females.[26]

Zambia is one of the worst HIV/AIDS-affected countries in Southern Africa. Estimates suggest that between 730 000 and 1.1 million people were living with HIV/AIDS in Zambia at the end of 2003; AIDS-related deaths were thought to be as high as 130 000 (Table 20.2).

Table 20.2 Zambia HIV and AIDS estimates, end 2003

Adult (15–49) HIV prevalence rate	16.5 per cent (range: 13.5–20.0 per cent)
Adults (15–49) living with HIV	830 000 (range: 680 000–1 000 000)
Adults and children (0–49) living with HIV	920 000 (range: 730 000–1 100 000)
Women (15–49) living with HIV	470 000 (range: 380 000–570 000)
AIDS deaths (adults and children) in 2003	89 000 (range: 63 000–130 000)

Source: 2004 Report on the global AIDS epidemic.

UNAIDS reports:

Zambia's most critical developmental and humanitarian crisis today is HIV/AIDS. The projected life expectancy has reduced from 60 years at birth (without HIV/AIDS) to 45 years due to the scourge (2002 ZDHS figures). The high mortality rate among adults has increased the number of orphans to about one million as at 2002.

Zambia's government established the National AIDS Council (NAC), and in 2002 a National Strategic Framework was developed. The National HIV/AIDS/STI/TB Interventions Strategic Plan, with a budget of US$558,702,000 for four years (2002–2005), pursues the following objectives: promotion of behaviour change, prevention of mother-to-child transmission, safe blood transfusion, voluntary counselling and testing, care and support for people living with HIV and orphans and vulnerable children, development of an information system database, and coordination of multisectoral interventions at district, provincial and national levels.

The government has made a commitment to provide antiretroviral drugs to 100,000 people infected with HIV by the end of 2005 under the WHO/UNAIDS '3 by 5' Initiative.[27]

Health care system

In its World Health Report, 2004, WHO noted that the total per capita expenditure on health care in Zambia was Intl $52; 5.7% of GDP[28] (Appendix 3).

The WHO overall health system performance score places Zambia 182nd out of 191 countries.[29]

Political economy

Despite progress in privatization and budgetary reform, Zambia's economic growth remains below the 5–7 per cent necessary to reduce poverty significantly. Privatization of government-owned copper mines relieved the government from covering mammoth losses generated by the industry and greatly improved the chances for copper mining to return to profitability and spur economic growth. Copper output increased in 2003 and is expected to increase again in 2004, due to higher copper prices. The maize harvest doubled in 2003, helping boost GDP by 4.0 per cent. Co-operation continues with international bodies on programmes to reduce poverty, including a new lending arrangement with the IMF expected in the second quarter of 2004. A tighter monetary policy will help cut inflation, but Zambia still has a serious problem with fiscal discipline.[30]

Zambia's GDP per capita is Intl $906 (Appendix 4).

References

1 WHO statistics 2000–2002.

2 Report of the United Nations Development Programme 2004 (HDI 2002). Launched by the United Nations in 1990, the Human Development Index measures a country's achievements in three aspects of human development: longevity, knowledge and a decent standard of living. It was created to re-emphasize that people and their lives should be the ultimate criteria for assessing the development of a country, not economic growth. Current values range from 0.956 (Norway, first of 177 countries) to 0.273 (Sierra Leone, 177th out of 177 countries). Countries fall into one of three groups: countries 1–55 = high development; 56–141 = medium development; 142–177 = low development. See: http://hdr.undp.org/statistics/data/indic/indic_8_1_1.html

3 **Anne Merriman**. *Report of Visit to Zambia to Assess, Share and Assist with Advice re Palliative Care Provision*. 21 Feb–1 March 2004: 9.

4 See: http://www.helfen-wir.org/English/Projekte/Zambia/hospice_chilanga.htm

5 See: www.karacounsellingkabwe.com

6 See: http://www.poweroflove.org/Reports/Report%20National%20Zambia%20Hospice%20Survey,%20October%202004.pdf

7 Personal communication:**Sr Stephanie** —31 January 2005.

8 See: http://www.poweroflove.org/pages/care_centres.htm

9 See: http://www.firelightfoundation.org/ourstory.htm

10 See: http://www.aidsalliance.org/eng/

11 See: http://www.globalfamilydoctor.com/publications/news/june/member_3.htm

12 See: http://66.102.9.104/search?q = cache:ogwYXa6ZhR8J:www.irlgov.ie/oireachtas/Committees-29th-D%C3%A1il/jcfa-debates/JCFA%2520Report%2520Oct27Nov103.doc +Cicetekelo+Hospice&hl = en

13 *Engendering Bold Leadership*. The President's Emergency Plan for AIDS Relief. First Annual Report to Congress, 2005: 115. http://www.state.gov/documents/organization/43885.pdf

14 International Narcotics Control Board. *Narcotic Drugs: Estimated World Requirements for 2004. Statistics for 2002*. New York: United Nations, 2004.

15 'The term *defined daily doses for statistical purposes* (S-DDD) replaces the term *defined daily doses* previously used by the Board. The S-DDDs are technical units of measurement for the purposes of statistical analysis and are not recommended prescription doses. Certain narcotic drugs may be used in certain countries for different treatments or in accordance with different medical practices, and therefore a different daily dose could be more appropriate'. The S-DDD used by the INCB for morphine is 100 mg. International Narcotics Control Board. *Narcotic Drugs: Estimated World Requirements for 2004. Statistics for 2002*. New York: United Nations, 2004: 176–177.

16 Personal communication: Cromwell Shalunga—13 May 2004.

17 Personal communication: Mary Chidgey—11 May 2004.

18 Personal communication: Sr Crucis–14 May 2004.

19 Personal communication: Sr Stephanie and Sr Keane—31 January 05.

20 **Anne Lloyd Williams**. *Visit to Zambia in April 2001*. Report to the Diana, Princess of Wales Memorial Fund, 15 May 2001.

21 **Faith Mwangi-Powell**. Country Summary—Zambia. (undated).

22 Personal communication: **Alison Hill**—10 May 2004.

23 **Sr Leonia Kournas**. Mother of Mercy Hospice: A Brief History. (undated).

24 Personal communication: Margaret Chirwa—13 May 2004.

25 This refers to adult mortality risk, which is defined as the probability of dying between 15 and 59 years.

26 See: WHO statistics for Uganda at: http://www.who.int/countries/uga/en

27 See http://www.unaids.org/en/geographical+area/by+country/zambia.asp

28 Total health expenditure per capita is the per capita amount of the sum of Public Health Expenditure (PHE) and Private Expenditure on Health (PvtHE). The international dollar is a common currency unit that takes into account differences in the relative purchasing power of various currencies. Figures expressed in international dollars are calculated using purchasing power parities (PPP), which are rates of currency conversion constructed to account for differences in price level between countries.http://www3.who.int/whosis/country/compare.cfm?country = s&indicator = strPcTotEOHinIntD2000&language = english

29 This composite measure of overall health system attainment is based on a country's goals relating to health, responsiveness and fairness in financing. The measure varies widely across countries and is highly correlated with general levels of human development as captured in the human development index. Tandon A, Murray CLJ, Lauer JA, Evans DB. *Measuring Overall Health System Performance for 191 Countries*. GPE Discussion Paper Series: No. 30; WHO.

30 See: http://www.cia.gov/cia/publications/factbook/geos/za.html

Part 5

Hospice-palliative care service development in Africa: countries with capacity building activity

We identified 11 countries in which there is evidence that steps are being taken to create the organizational, workforce and policy capacity for hospice–palliative care services to develop, though currently no operational services exist (Fig. 1). Countries in this category are characterized by: the presence of sensitized personnel; expressions of interest with key hospice–palliative care organizations such as APCA, HAU, IAHPC and Hospice Information; the establishment of international links with service providers; conference participation; visits to hospice–palliative care organizations; education and training provided by visiting teams; the preparation of a strategy for service development; and lobbying of policymakers/health ministries

This group of 11 countries comprises: Algeria, Cameroon, Cote d'Ivoire, Democratic Republic of the Congo (Congo-Kinshasa), Ethiopia, Ghana, Lesotho, Mozambique, Namibia, Rwanda and Tunisia.

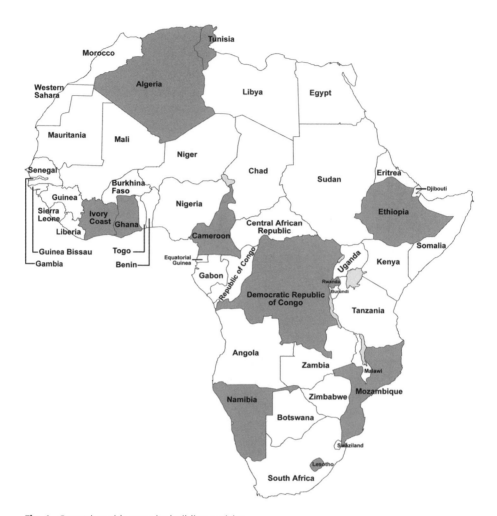

Fig. 1. Countries with capacity building activity

Chapter 21

Algeria

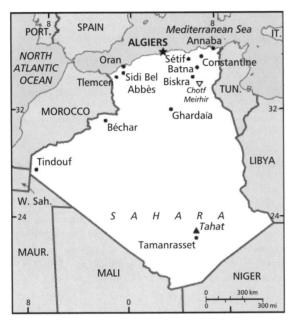

Algeria (population 32.13 million people) is a country in Northern Africa, bordering the Mediterranean Sea that covers an area of 2 381 740 km². Its boundaries border Tunisia, Libya, Niger, Mali, Mauritania, Western Sahara and Morocco. The capital of Algeria is Algiers.

According to the United Nations human development index (HDI), Algeria is ranked 108th out of 177 countries worldwide (value 0.704)[1] and fourth out of 45 in African countries for which an index is available. This places Algeria in the group of countries with medium human development.

Palliative care service provision

Current services

As yet, palliative care services have not been identified in Algeria, but there is evidence of growing interest. In September 2004, the 4th Europe–Maghreb conference was held in Tabarka, Tunisia, and adopted the theme *Pain and Supportive Care: Current Advances*. (The Maghreb is a region that includes Algeria, Morocco and Tunisia.)

Significantly, nurse educator Françoise Porchet (Switzerland) and three European colleagues, Gisele Schaerer (Switzerland), Philip Larkin (Ireland) and Sophie Leruth (Belgium), were invited to provide a full day of training. With the exception of Philip Larkin, all had been speakers at the previous conference in 2002.

A report on the conference in 2005, addressing the issue of palliative care accessibility in the Maghreb stated:

> Home care does not exist in the Maghreb; it is the family and/or community that provides any care. A huge distance has to be covered, sometimes as much as 1000 km, to visit the specialized

oncology centres—the few places where consultations on dealing with the treatment of pain are available.[2]

Opioid availability and consumption

Françoise Porchet and her colleagues write:

> [In the Maghreb], the distribution of opioids is subject to the 'seven day law'; in other words, doctors are not allowed to issue prescriptions for periods in excess of one week. Therefore, patients or their families have to return to the physician regularly to obtain a new prescription. Morphine is very expensive and only available in sustained-release form.[2]

The International Narcotics Control Board[3] has published the following figures for the consumption of narcotic drugs in Algeria (2002): codeine 93 kg; pholcodine 699 kg; dextropropoxyphene 135 kg; and pethidine 2 kg.

For the years 2000–2002, the average defined daily dose consumption of morphine for statistical purposes (S-DDD)[4] in Algeria was 0 (Appendix 1).

Education and training

Nurse educator Françoise Porchet and her colleagues report on the training they gave in the Maghreb, 2004:

> This opportunity allowed us to provide our nursing colleagues in the Maghreb with up-to-date knowledge on palliative care according to our individual specialties, while enabling them to acquire the knowledge through a process of exchange and constructive learning. It is very gratifying to note that the spirit of palliative care can transcend borders, cultures and languages. It is also important to realise all the possibilities that can arise from a training initiative put together between colleagues from three European countries and the extent to which this is a unifying event.[2]

Public health context

Population

Algeria's population of around 32.13 million people is made up of the following ethnic groups: Arab-Berber 99 per cent and European <1 per cent.

Almost all Algerians are Berber in origin, not Arab; the minority who identify themselves as Berber live mostly in the mountainous region of Kabylie east of Algiers; the Berbers are also Muslim but identify with their Berber rather than Arab cultural heritage; Berbers have long agitated for autonomy; the government is unlikely to grant autonomy but has offered to begin sponsoring teaching the Berber language in schools.

Religious groups include: Sunni Muslim (state religion) 99 per cent, and Christian and Jewish 1 per cent.[5]

Epidemiology

In Algeria, the WHO World Health Report (2004) indicates an adult mortality[6] rate per 1000 population of 170 for males and 128 for females. Life expectancy for males is 67.5; for females 71.2. Healthy life expectancy is 59.7 for males; and 61.6 for females.[7]

Algeria is a country in Northern Africa that has been affected by the HIV/AIDS epidemic. Estimates suggest that in Algeria, approximately 0.1 per cent of the population were living with HIV/AIDS at the end of 2003.

UNAIDS reports:

> UNAIDS supports the national response to HIV/AIDS in Algeria through the UN Theme Group, composed of the UNAIDS Cosponsors present in the country, and through the Expanded Theme Group on HIV/AIDS, which also includes other international partners, national and NGO representatives. These efforts are supported by a recently established Technical Working Group, comprising the HIV/AIDS Focal Points of Cosponsors, government representatives, NGOs, and other partners. The Theme Group on HIV/AIDS has promoted a multisectoral response to the epidemic, actively supporting the development of sectoral plans, awareness raising, efforts towards the establishment of second-generation surveillance, and resource mobilization. The Theme Group will develop the UN Joint Action Plan on HIV/AIDS as part of collective support for the national strategic plan on HIV/AIDS. The UNAIDS Focal Point is assisting Theme Group efforts aiming to coordinate and enhance support to the national HIV/AIDS response. This also includes technical support to national partners, NGOs and international agencies on different priority areas of the response. UNAIDS, through Programme Acceleration Funds and other means, has supported the development of the National Strategic Plan on HIV/AIDS 2002–2006 at both national and sectoral levels. Other activities include strengthening NGOs' capacity, building partnership with religious leaders, as well as initiating innovative HIV/AIDS prevention activities among police forces and prisoners.
>
> HIV prevalence remains low in Algeria, but the existence of risk and behaviour among vulnerable groups, diversity in prevalence rates across regions and other determinants require immediate action to prevent further spread of the epidemic. Existing information, though limited, indicates a prevalence of 0.1% among the general population, with higher rates in the south of the country.
>
> The national serosurveillance survey implemented in five sites in 2000 yielded 1% prevalence among pregnant women in the southern most part of the country, and 20% among sex workers in two sites (Oran and Tamanrasset). These rates, coupled with the socio-economic environment, mobility and a high level of unemployment, may serve to drive the epidemic in a country where young people represent 70% of its 30 million total population, and where HIV transmission is mainly through heterosexual contacts. Since 2001, the level of political commitment to fight HIV/AIDS has increased substantially, in particular following the commitment expressed by the President of Algeria during the Abuja Summit. An HIV/AIDS project proposal of Algeria was approved by the Global Fund to Fight AIDS, TB, and Malaria (GFATM), providing US$10 million for a three year period to support the implemention of HIV/AIDS prevention and care services, as well as strengthening capacities of public and civil society organizations.[8]

Health care system

In 2001, the total per capita expenditure on health care was Intl $169; 4.1% of GDP[9] (Appendix 3).

The WHO overall health system performance score places Algeria 81st out of 191 countries.[10]

Political economy

After more than a century of rule by France, Algerians fought through much of the 1950s to achieve independence, which was granted in 1962. Algeria's primary political party, the

National Liberation Front (FLN), has dominated politics ever since. Many Algerians in the subsequent generation were not satisfied, however, and moved to counter the FLN's centrality in Algerian politics. The surprising first round success of the Islamic Salvation Front (FIS) in the December 1991 balloting spurred the Algerian army to intervene and postpone the second round of elections to prevent what the secular elite feared would be an extremist-led government from assuming power. The government gained the upper hand by the late 1990s, and FIS's armed wing, the Islamic Salvation Army, disbanded in January 2000. The army placed Abdelaziz Bouteflika in the presidency in 1999 but claimed neutrality in his 2004 landslide re-election victory. A number of longstanding problems continue to face Bouteflika in his second term, including the ethnic minority Berbers' ongoing autonomy campaign, large-scale unemployment, a shortage of housing, unreliable electrical and water supplies, and government inefficiencies. Algeria must also diversify its petroleum-based economy, which has yielded a large cash reserve but which has not been used to redress Algeria's many social and infrastructure problems. Algeria assumed a 2 year seat on the UN Security Council in January 2004.[5]

Algeria's political and geographical divisions are reflected by the respective economic outputs—and problems—of the different regions. The north is densely populated, with high levels of unemployment. The centre of the country has relatively low levels of industrial, services and manufacturing output. The south is rich in oil and natural gas, the exploitation of which is dominated by the state-owned company, Sonatrach; for decades this has been the foremost generator of government revenue.[11]

GDP per capita is Intl $4104 (Appendix 4).

References

1 Report of the United Nations Development Programme 2004 (HDI 2002). Launched by the United Nations in 1990, the Human Development Index measures a country's achievements in three aspects of human development: longevity, knowledge and a decent standard of living. It was created to re-emphasize that people and their lives should be the ultimate criteria for assessing the development of a country, not economic growth. Current values range from 0.956 (Norway, first of 177 countries) to 0.273 (Sierra Leone, 177th out of 177 countries). Countries fall into one of three groups: countries 1–55 = high development; 56–141 = medium development; 142–177 = low development. See: http://hdr.undp.org/statistics/data/indic/indic_8_1_1.html

2 **Porchet F, Schaerer G, Larkin P, Leruth S.** Intercultural experiences of training in the Maghreb. *European Journal of Palliative Care* 2005; **12(1)**: 37.

3 International Narcotics Control Board. *Narcotic Drugs: Estimated World Requirements for 2004. Statistics for 2002.* New York: United Nations, 2004.

4 'The term *defined daily doses for statistical purposes* (S-DDD) replaces the term *defined daily doses* previously used by the Board. The S-DDDs are technical units of measurement for the purposes of statistical analysis and are not recommended prescription doses. Certain narcotic drugs may be used in certain countries for different treatments or in accordance with different medical practices, and therefore a different daily dose could be more appropriate'. The S-DDD used by the INCB for morphine is 100 mg. International Narcotics Control Board. *Narcotic Drugs: Estimated World Requirements for 2004. Statistics for 2002.* New York: United Nations, 2004: 176–177.

5 See: http://www.cia.gov/cia/publications/factbook/geos/ag.html

6 This refers to adult mortality risk, which is defined as the probability of dying between 15 and 59 years.

7 See: WHO statistics for Algeria at: http://www.who.int/countries/dza/en/

8 http://www.unaids.org/en/geographical+area/by+country/algeria.asp

9 Total health expenditure per capita is the per capita amount of the sum of Public Health Expenditure (PHE) and Private Expenditure on Health (PvtHE). The international dollar is a common currency unit that takes into account differences in the relative purchasing power of various currencies. Figures expressed in international dollars are calculated using purchasing power parities (PPP), which are rates of currency conversion constructed to account for differences in price level between countries.
http://www3.who.int/whosis/country/compare.cfm?country=s&indicator=strPcTotEOHinInt D2000&language=english

10 This composite measure of overall health system attainment is based on a country's goals relating to health, responsiveness and fairness in financing. The measure varies widely across countries and is highly correlated with general levels of human development as captured in the human development index. Tandon A, Murray CLJ, Lauer JA, Evans DB. *Measuring Overall Health System Performance for 191 Countries*. GPE Discussion Paper Series: No. 30; WHO.

11 World of Information, Business Intelligence Report. Algeria: Economy, Politics, and Government. *Business Intelligence Report* 2001; **1(1)**: 1–37.

Chapter 22

Cameroon

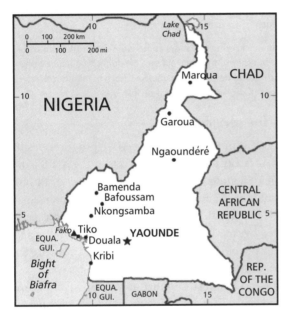

Cameroon (population 16.06 million people) is a country in Western Africa bordering the Bight of Biafra that covers an area of 475 440 km². Its boundaries border Nigeria, Chad, Central African Republic, Congo, Gabon and Equatorial Guinea. The capital of Cameroon is Yaoundé.

According to the United Nations human development index (HDI), Cameroon is ranked 141st out of 177 countries worldwide (value 0.501)[1] and 13th out of 45 in African countries for which an index is available. This places Cameroon in the group of countries with medium human development.

Palliative care service provision

Current services

In resource-poor areas, the blending of supportive care with hospice–palliative care is frequently linked to the development of previously established services, particularly home-based care. Family Health International (FHI) defines home and community-based care as 'the provision of care and support that endeavours to meet the nursing and psychosocial needs of persons with chronic illnesses and their family members in their home environment'.[2]

While HCBC delivers patient care in the home environment, palliative care is an approach that attends to the needs of patients and families affected by a life-threatening illness in a variety of settings including the home, hospice, hospital, clinic and community.

The health repercussions of the AIDS epidemic have been the impetus for introducing care to the chronically ill in Cameroon. Palliative care in the country is almost non-existent.

Cameroo Baptist Convention Health Board

Several HIV/AIDS programmes, including Prevention of Mother-to-Child-Transmission, are in place at this rural hospital to provide support to those living with HIV/AIDS. Raising awareness of the epidemic has been prioritized, along with co-ordinating with other support organizations. The need for the development of palliative care in Cameroon was given a boost by the attendance of two delegates at the African Palliative Care Association conference in Arusha in June 2004.

Some support for the chronically ill is provided by several other organizations in the country. George Mbeng describes the situation in his country:

> We have many people in Cameroon who are carrying out support activities. Some of them will have not heard much about palliative care but they think that what they are doing is palliative care. I just thing that going back to tell them the good news about palliative care, what it all involves, will only strengthen their views about support, care and support for people.[3]

Reimbursement and funding for services

The Global Fund[4] has committed significant funding to HIV/AIDS programmes in Cameroon in Round 3 of an extensive strategy to combat the effects of the AIDS pandemic. The agreement was signed on 10 September 2004 for the Ministry of Public Health of the Government of the Republic of Cameroon to manage a project aimed at scaling up treatment and care of people living with HIV/AIDS. US$14 641 407 has been approved to implement the project over 2 years. The goal is to improve accessibility and quality of overall case management for people living with HIV/AIDS and support for orphans and vulnerable children by December 2008.

Cameroon proposes to use Global Fund financial support to improve overall case management in order to complete the range of services available to people affected by AIDS, including 10 000 orphans and vulnerable children. The objectives of the project include making laboratory tests and antiretroviral therapies available to >36 000 people living with AIDS. Although palliative care is not mentioned in the proposal, home-based care, free treatment of opportunistic infections and adherence support are identified as priorities. Furthermore, economic, psycho-social and medical support will be covered by the Global Fund programme. Expected results include upgraded professional training of doctors, social workers, nurses and other health personnel. Community-based agents will receive training on comprehensive home-based care.

In Round 4 of a related project, the Global Fund approved US$6 347 296 on 17 December 2004 for CARE International to mobilize civil society for the fight against AIDS.[5]

Opioid availability and consumption

The International Narcotics Control Board[6] has no published figures for the consumption of narcotic drugs in Cameroon.

For the years 2000–2002, the average defined daily dose consumption of morphine for statistical purposes (S-DDD)[7] in Cameroon was 0 (Appendix 1).

Education and training

Cameroon Baptist Convention Health Board

George Mbeng studied for the Diploma in Palliative Care at Hospice Africa Uganda in 2004.

Life/oral histories

George Mbeng—*nurse, HIV/AIDS counsellor/trainer, Cameroon Baptist Convention Health Board*: interviewed by David Clark, 4 June 2004. Length of interview (West Africa group): 40 min.

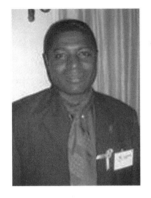 George Mbeng refers to the current early development of services for those living with HIV/AIDS in Cameroon. His background as a nurse counsellor and trainer equips him for his role as supervisor on the Prevention of Mother-to-Child Transmission programme that is one of several AIDS control programmes administered by the Ministry of Health. Much of the current focus of the government approach is aimed at supporting mothers to prevent transmission to their infants. Raising awareness of these issues and co-ordinating the work of related NGOs is pivotal to the AIDS programme. The next priority is to provide care for those living with HIV/AIDS, hence the decision to incorporate palliative care into the health system. George Mbeng is studying for the Palliative Care Diploma at Hospice Africa Uganda and hopes to share his skills with colleagues in Cameroon. He feels that being a member of the African Palliative Care Association will strengthen the ability of his organization to lobby his government to develop palliative care support for those living with cancer and AIDS. He identifies the need for further training and for funds to be sourced to support their work. He concludes by highlighting the importance of collaborating with other African countries. He describes current services in Cameroon as mainly support based with no established palliative care provision.

Jam Devine—*Physician, Cameroon Baptist Convention Health Board*: interviewed by David Clark, 4 June 2004. Length of interview: (West Africa group): 40 min.

Jam Devine briefly explains his hospital role as assessing patients who would benefit from antiretroviral therapies. He explains the value of attending the APCA conference as enabling him to develop strategies to implement palliative care in the Cameroon health system.

Public health context

Population

Cameroon's population of around 16.06 million people is made up of Cameroon Highlanders 31 per cent, Equatorial Bantu 19 per cent, Kirdi 11 per cent, Fulani 10 per cent, Northwestern Bantu 8 per cent, Eastern Nigritic 7 per cent, other African 13 per cent and non-African <1 per cent.

Table 22.1 Cameroon HIV and AIDS estimates, end 2003

Adults (15–49) HIV prevalence rate	6.9 per cents (range 4.8–9.8 per cent)
Adults (15–49) living with HIV	520 000 (range 360 000–740 000)
Adults and children (0–49) living with HIV	560 000 (range 390 000–810 000)
Women (15–49) living with HIV	290 000 (range 200 000–420 000)
AIDS deaths (adults and children) in 2003	49 000 (range 32 000–74 000)

Source: 2004 Report of the global AIDS epidemic.

Religious groups include: indigenous beliefs 40 per cent, Christian 40 per cent and Muslim 20 per cent.[8]

Epidemiology

In Cameroon, the WHO World Health Report (2004) indicates an adult mortality[9] rate per 1000 population of 519 for males and 454 for females. Life expectancy for males is 47.2; for females 49.0. Healthy life expectancy is 41.1 for males; and 41.8 for females.[10]

Cameroon is a country in Western Africa that has been severely affected by the HIV/AIDS epidemic. Estimates suggest that in Cameroon, between 390 000 and 810 000 people were living with HIV/AIDS at the end of 2003. In the same year, up to 74 000 adults and children are thought to have died from the disease (Table 22.1).

UNAIDS reports:

> Coordination of AIDS control in Cameroon is the responsibility of the National AIDS Control Committee (CNLS) which is chaired by the Minister of Health. The Committee's Central Technical Group coordinates implementation of activities throughout the country, with the assistance of 10 provincial technical groups run by 10 provincial coordinators.CNLS is made up of 13 representatives of the public sector, including the offices of the President of the Republic and the Prime Minister, representatives of the private sector (an employers' organization and a trade union), national and international nongovernmental organizations, the representatives of the two networks of associations of people living with HIV, the representatives of donors, and in particular la Coopération Française, GTZ, the European Union, the members of the Theme Group, including the UNAIDS country coordinator and representatives of parliament. CNLS holds two statutory meetings per year, convened by its chair.
>
> The action of CNLS is supervised by its joint monitoring Committee. This is an audit and control body which also serves as an advisory body to CNLS. It is chaired by the Ministry of Territorial Administration and Decentralization and meets four times a year. It approves the annual and quarterly plans of action and the annual activities report. The Theme Group takes part in its work. The Country Coordinating Mechanism has just taken its place in this organization, specifically in connection with the follow-up of activities funded by the Global Fund. The Country Coordinating Mechanism has 30 members and is chaired by the Chairman of CNLS. National initiatives such as agreements signed between the government and the private sector

are subject to a further level of coordination, determined by their specifications and at the proposal of the private sector.[11]

Health care system

In 2001, the total per capita expenditure on health care was Intl $42; 3.3% of GDP[12] (Appendix 3).

The WHO overall health system performance score places Cameroon 164th out of 191 countries.[13]

Political economy

The earliest inhabitants probably were the Pygmies, who still inhabit the southern forests. Bantu speakers were among the first groups that invaded Cameroon from equatorial Africa, settling in the south and later in the west. The Muslim Fulani from the Niger basin arrived in the eleventh and nineteenth centuries and settled in the north. Contact with Europeans began in the 1500s. During the next three centuries, Spanish, Dutch and British traders visited the area, and there was costar slave trading. Christian missions appeared in the mid-1800s and still are active.

In July 1884, Germany, the UK and France each attempted to annex the area. In a treaty with local chiefs, the German Consul of Tunis, Tunisia, extended a protectorate over Cameroon. Germany strengthened its claim and expanded its territory by treaties with the UK and France, but British and French armies invaded the German colony in 1914. A 1919 declaration divided Cameroon between the UK and France, with the larger, eastern area under France. A 1922 League of Nations mandate sanctioned the division; in 1946, the United Nations converted the mandates to trusteeships. In December 1958, the French trusteeship was ended.[14] The post-colonial state in Cameroon began in 1961, under Ahidjo's leadership, as a federal union of UN trusteeships that were administered by Britain and France. In the drive to consolidate power, multiparty politics was supplanted by single-party politics in 1966, and in 1972 the federal republic was constitutionally replaced by a unitary state. Ahidjo voluntarily resigned the state presidency in 1982 and was replaced by Paul Biya, his Prime Minister since 1975.[15]

Cameroon has generally enjoyed stability since that time, which has permitted the development of agriculture, roads and railways, as well as a petroleum industry. Because of its oil resources and favourable agricultural conditions, Cameroon has one of the best endowed primary commodity economies in sub-Saharan Africa. Still, it faces many of the serious problems facing other underdeveloped countries, such as a top-heavy civil service and a generally unfavourable climate for business enterprise.

Since 1990, the government has embarked on various IMF and World Bank programmes designed to spur business investment, increase efficiency in agriculture, improve trade and recapitalize the nation's banks. In June 2000, the government completed an IMF-sponsored, 3-year structural adjustment programmes; however, the IMF is pressing for more reforms, including increased budget transparency, privatization and poverty reduction programmes. International oil and cocoa prices have considerable impact on the economy.[8] Although the Cameroonian economy remains in a relatively promising position, a higher rate of economic growth could very well be within its potential were it to utilize all its natural resources. The government must continue to implement IMF-led economic reform measures to realize quickly its goal of social and economic regeneration aimed at raising the living standards of its 14 million people.

Despite occasional tensions, Cameroon still continues to enjoy a political and social stability lacking in many African countries. This has enabled the government to concentrate on developing social and economic infrastructures. In addition, Cameroon's abundant supply of oil and its favourable agricultural conditions have created one of the most solid foundations for economic development on the continent.[16]

GDP per capita is Intl $1269 (Appendix 4).

References

1 Report of the United Nations Development Programme 2004 (HDI 2002). Launched by the United Nations in 1990, the Human Development Index measures a country's achievements in three aspects of human development: longevity, knowledge and a decent standard of living. It was created to re-emphasize that people and their lives should be the ultimate criteria for assessing the development of a country, not economic growth. Current values range from 0.956 (Norway, first of 177 countries) to 0.273 (Sierra Leone, 177th out of 177 countries). Countries fall into one of three groups: countries 1–55 = high development; 56–141 = medium development; 142–177 = low development. See: http://hdr.undp.org/statistics/data/indic/indic_8_1_1.html

2 Family Health International, Comprehensive Care and Support Framework.

3 IOELC interview: George Mbeng—4 June 2004.

4 See: http://www.theglobalfund.org/search/contact.aspx?countryID=CMR&contactType=PR&round=3&component=HIV/AIDS

5 CARE International in Cameroon: http://www.theglobalfund.org/search/contact.aspx?countryID=CMR&contactType=PR&round=4&component=HIV/AIDS

6 International Narcotics Control Board. *Narcotic Drugs: Estimated World Requirements for 2004. Statistics for 2002.* New York: United Nations, 2004.

7 'The term *defined daily doses for statistical purposes* (S-DDD) replaces the term *defined daily doses* previously used by the Board. The S-DDDs are technical units of measurement for the purposes of statistical analysis and are not recommended prescription doses. Certain narcotic drugs may be used in certain countries for different treatments or in accordance with different medical practices, and therefore a different daily dose could be more appropriate'. The S-DDD used by the INCB for morphine is 100 mg. International Narcotics Control Board. *Narcotic Drugs: Estimated World Requirements for 2004. Statistics for 2002.* New York: United Nations, 2004: 176–177.

8 See: http://www.cia.gov/cia/publications/factbook/geos/cm.html

9 This refers to adult mortality risk, which is defined as the probability of dying between 15 and 59 years.

10 See: WHO statistics for Cameroon at: http://www.who.int/countries/cmr/en/

11 http://www.unaids.org/en/geographical+area/by+country/cameroon.asp

12 Total health expenditure per capita is the per capita amount of the sum of Public Health Expenditure (PHE) and Private Expenditure on Health (PvtHE). The international dollar is a common currency unit that takes into account differences in the relative purchasing power of various currencies. Figures expressed in international dollars are calculated using purchasing power parities (PPP), which are rates of currency conversion constructed to account for differences in price level

between countries. http://www3.who.int/whosis/country/compare.cfm?country =s&indicator=strPcTotEO HinIntD2000&language=english

13 This composite measure of overall health system attainment is based on a country's goals relating to health, responsiveness and fairness in financing. The measure varies widely across countries and is highly correlated with general levels of human development as captured in the human development index. Tandon A, Murray CLJ, Lauer JA, Evans DB. *Measuring Overall Health System Performance for 191 Countries*. GPE Discussion Paper Series: No. 30; WHO.

14 United States Government. *Background Notes on Countries of the World*. Washington, DC: United States Department of State, Bureau of Public Affairs/Office of Public Communication, 2003.

15 Dickson E. Through the prism of a local tragedy: political liberalisation, regionalism and elite struggles for power in Cameroon. *Africa* 1998; 68(3): 338–359.

16 World of Information Business Intelligence Report. Cameroon: Economy, Politics and Government. *Business Intelligence Report* 2001; 1(1): 1–36.

Chapter 23

Cote d'Ivoire

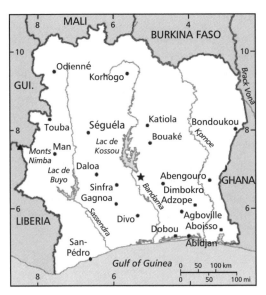

Cote d'Ivoire (population 17.33 million) is a country in Western Africa that covers an area of 322 460 km². Its boundaries border the North Atlantic Ocean between Liberia, Guinea, Mali, Burkina Faso and Ghana. The capital city of Cote d'Ivoire is Yamoussoukro

According to the United Nations human development index (HDI), Cote d'Ivoire is ranked 163rd out of 177 countries worldwide (0.399)1 and 31st out of 45 in African countries for which an index is available. This places Cote d'Ivoire in the group of countries with low human development.

Palliative care service provision

Current services

There are no established palliative care services in Cote d'Ivoire. The HIV/AIDS epidemic has brought to the fore the need for a comprehensive and sustainable health package for terminally ill patients at community level. Although some health professionals in Cote d'Ivoire are familiar with the use of morphine for cancer and neurological pain, there has yet to be a co-ordinated and structured plan to incorporate managed pain control into the public health system. Joseph Essombo explains the current situation:

> There are already health professionals who use drugs such as morphine for pain management with cancer patients, with patients suffering from neurological diseases, with patients who suffer from rheumatology problems, but it is really not yet well structured and implemented and especially it is not yet working with the community's involvement.[2]

Reimbursement and funding for services

President's Emergency Plan for AIDS Relief (PEPFAR)

During the 2004 financial year (FY), funding of around US$13.04 million was enacted for country-managed programmes in Cote d'Ivoire and US$11.29 million for central programmes. During FY2005, it is anticipated that a total of US$39.34 million will be enacted: US$26.16 million for country-managed programmes and US$13.18 million for central programmes.[3]

The US-funded Centres for Disease Control provide technical support to the Ministry of Health to develop a strategy to combat the HIV/AIDS epidemic. It also acts as the conduit for funds from PEPFAR to several government departments involved in the prevention and treatment of AIDS.

Opioid availability and consumption

For the years 2000–2002, the average defined daily dose consumption of morphine for statistical purposes (S-DDD)[4] in Cote d'Ivoire was 0 (Appendix 1).

While it is reported that limited supplies of opioids are available in the main cities, they are not accessible to rural communities in Cote d'Ivoire.[5]

Education and training

No palliative care training has been implemented in Cote d'Ivoire. A comprehensive approach has been identified for future implementation, that would include training of health professionals and community-based organizations. This training would best be delivered in combination with the lobbying of government to ensure that structures are in place to provide sustainable and effective palliative care at all levels throughout the country.[5]

History and development of hospice–palliative care in Cote d'Ivoire

Narrative history of palliative care

The inaugural conference of the African Palliative Care Association in June 2004 was crucial for the two health professionals who attended from Cote d'Ivoire to plan a strategy for palliative care development in their country. The experiences of other practitioners on the continent provided guidance for the creation of programmes that will target people living with cancer, HIV/AIDS and other conditions. Joseph Essombo summarizes the value of the conference for Cote d'Ivoire:

> I think that this is the beginning of the reflection and to participate to this conference is highly important for us. It gives us the opportunity to reconsider the question of palliative care as a central question for the management and care of persons living with AIDS, but also for those ones suffering other chronic diseases, with pain as a central point. It comforts us in our vision and we think that we can bring all the support that the health ministry will need. I think of mobilizing human resources . . . in Africa and that we met here, of relating to experiences that have worked out well and that we heard about here, to really help the health ministry of Côte d'Ivoire to set up a palliative care programme and to integrate it not only for patients living with AIDS but also for all patients suffering and who have a problem of pain management.[2]

Life/oral histories

Dr Joseph Essombo——*co-ordinator, Centers for Disease Control Project Retroci, Abidjan*: interviewed by David Clark, 4 June 2004. Length of interview (West Africa group): 40 min.

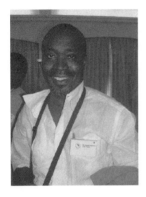

Joseph Essombo, a physician interested in HIV/AIDS and public health, describes the dual role played by the US Centers for Disease Control (CDC) in Cote d'Ivoire with regards to HIV/AIDS. Technical support is provided to the Ministry of Health to establish a strategy to combat the epidemic. Secondly, funds from the President's Emergency Plan For AIDS Relief (PEPFAR) are channelled through CDC to several government departments involved in the prevention and treatment of AIDS. He suggests that palliative care is only now being considered as a way to tackle the AIDS problem. Although health professionals in Cote d'Ivoire are familiar with the use of morphine for cancer and neurological pain, there has yet to be a co-ordinated and structured plan to incorporate managed pain control into the health system. He reflects on the value of the inaugural African Palliative Care Association conference as an opportunity to learn from palliative care practitioners and organizations all over the continent. This gives him the confidence to advocate for palliative care development in Cote d'Ivoire. He prioritizes supporting and advising the Ministry of Health in order to implement palliative care not only for those with AIDS, but for all patients requiring pain management.

Professor Beugre Kouassi—*neurologist, University of Abidjan-Cocody/Ministry of Health*: interviewed by David Clark, 4 June 2004. Length of interview (Wet Africa group): 40 min.

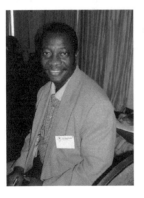

Beugre Kouassi, a neurologist, has a particular interest in the neurological manifestations of AIDS. He informs that 10 per cent of the population of Cote d'Ivoire is HIV positive. For several years, his government has attempted to mobilize resources to combat the effects of the epidemic. He identifies a gap in the holistic care and treatment of such patients. He highlights the value of palliative care as providing more than merely symptom control and pain management. While opioids are available in the main cities, pain-relieving drugs are harder to source in rural parts of the country and consequently accessibility is compromised. He shares his vision for palliative care being integrated into a complete health care package for all people living with AIDS within 3 years. This will require training health professionals and community organizations in palliative care, and the lobbying of government to ensure that structures are in place to provide sustainable and effective palliative care at all levels throughout the country.

Public health context

Population

Cote d'Ivoire's population of around 17.33 million is made up of the following ethnic groups: Akan 42.1 per cent, Voltaiques or Gur 17.6 per cent, Northern Mandes 16.5 per cent, Krous 11 per cent, Southern Mandes 10 per cent and other 2.8 per cent.

Religious groups include: Christian 20–30 per cent, Muslim 35–40 per cent and indigenous 25–40 per cent.[6]

Epidemiology

In Cote d'Ivoire, the WHO World Health Report (2004) indicates an adult mortality[7] rate per 1000 population of 577 for males and 502 for females. Life expectancy for males is 43.1; for females 48.0. Healthy life expectancy is 37.6 for males; and 41.3 for females.[8]

Cote d'Ivoire is one of the worst HIV/AIDS-affected countries in Western Africa. Estimates suggest that in Cote d'Ivoire, between 370 000 and 750 000 people were living with HIV/AIDS at the end of 2003. In the same year, up to 72 000 adults and children are thought to have died from the disease (Table 23.1).

UNAIDS reports:

> The political and military instability in the recent history of Côte d'Ivoire has had major social and health impacts on the population. HIV prevalence in Côte d'Ivoire, already high before the conflict that began in 2002, is likely to increase as a result of the massive displacement of local populations, both within and across the country's borders. Overall, the functioning of health services has been severely affected by the crisis, resulting in limited access to health care and medication, particularly in the conflict zone. 2003 was principally marked by an upheaval in AIDS control activities following the political crisis. Although measures were taken to reduce the humanitarian consequences at the start of the conflict, HIV/AIDS-related aspects were not immediately integrated within priority-rated measures to deal with the effects of the crisis. An emergency team was therefore set up on the initiative of the UNAIDS Office in Côte d'Ivoire in order to address the lack of actions and organization, and to coordinate the immediate response to HIV/AIDS. Under the chair of the Ministry for AIDS Control, this team brought together, in addition to government representatives,

Table 23.1 Cote d'Ivoire HIV and AIDS estimates, end 2003

Adult (15–49) HIV prevalence rate	7.0 per cent (range: 4.9–10.0 per cent)
Adults (15–49) living with HIV	530 000 (range: 370 000–750 000)
Adults and children (0–49) living with HIV	570 000 (range: 390 000–820 000)
Women (15–49) living with HIV	300 000 (range: 210 000–420 000)
AIDS deaths (adults and children) in 2003	47 000 (range: 30 000–72 000)

Source: 2004 Report on the global AIDS epidemic.

the UN Theme Group on HIV/AIDS, development partners, national and international NGOs, and organizations and associations for AIDS control.[9]

Health care system

In 2001, the total per capita expenditure on health care was Intl $127; 6.2% of GDP[10] (Appendix 3).

The WHO overall health system performance score places Cote d'Ivoire 137th out of 191 countries.[11]

Political economy

France made its initial contact with Cote d'Ivoire in 1637, when missionaries landed at Assinie near the Gold Coast (now Ghana) border; Cote d'Ivoire officially became a French colony in 1893. From 1904 to 1958, Cote d'Ivoire was a constituent unit of the Federation of French West Africa. It was a colony and an overseas territory under the Third Republic. Until the period following the Second World War, governmental affairs in French West Africa were administered from Paris. In 1946, French citizenship was granted to all African 'subjects', the right to organize politically was recognized, and various forms of forced labour were abolished. In December 1958, as a result of a referendum, Cote d'Ivoire became an autonomous republic within the French community and then gained independence on 7 August 1960. In a region whose political systems have otherwise been noted for a lack of stability (e.g. those countries undergoing repeated military coups), Cote d'Ivoire showed remarkable political stability after its independence from France in 1960. Cote d'Ivoire evolved from a single-party state, beginning in 1990, and opposition parties, independent newspapers and independent trades unions were all made legal.[12]

Although there has been an element of political and military instability in the recent history of the country, Cote d'Ivoire remains one of Africa's most diversified economies. Its location geographically and economically at the hub of Francophone West Africa leaves it ideally placed to capitalize on the economic development of the region.[13] Close ties to France since independence in 1960, the development of cocoa production for export, and foreign investment has made Cote d'Ivoire one of the most prosperous of the tropical African states. Cote d'Ivoire is among the world's largest producers and exporters of coffee, cocoa beans and palm oil. Consequently, the economy is highly sensitive to fluctuations in international prices for these products and to weather conditions. The economy is still heavily dependent on agriculture and related activities, which engage roughly 68 per cent of the population. The Ivorian economy began a comeback in 1994, due to the 50 per cent devaluation of the CFA franc and improved prices for cocoa and coffee, growth in non-traditional primary exports such as pineapples and rubber, limited trade and banking liberalization, offshore oil and gas discoveries, and generous external finance and debt rescheduling by multilateral lenders and France. The rising world prices for cocoa will help both the current account and the government balances.[6]

GDP per capita is Intl $2045 (Appendix 4).

References

1 Report of the United Nations Development Programme 2004 (HDI 2002). Launched by the United Nations in 1990, the Human Development Index measures a country's achievements in three aspects of human development: longevity, knowledge and a decent standard of living. It was created to re-emphasize that people and their lives should be the ultimate criteria for assessing the development of a country, not economic growth. Current values range from 0.956 (Norway, first of 177 countries) to 0.273 (Sierra Leone, 177th out of 177 countries). Countries fall into one of three groups: countries 1–55 = high development; 56–141 = medium development; 142–177 = low development. See: http://hdr.undp.org/statistics/data/indic/indic_8_1_1.html

2 IOELC interview: Joseph Essombo—4 June 2004.

3 *Engendering Bold Leadership*. The President's Emergency Plan for AIDS Relief. First Annual Report to Congress, 2005: 115. http://www.state.gov/documents/organization/43885.pdf

4 The term *defined daily doses for statistical purposes* (S-DDD) replaces the term *defined daily doses* previously used by the Board. The S-DDDs are technical units of measurement for the purposes of statistical analysis and are not recommended prescription doses. Certain narcotic drugs may be used in certain countries for different treatments or in accordance with different medical practices, and therefore a different daily dose could be more appropriate'. The S-DDD used by the INCB for morphine is 100 mg. International Narcotics Control Board. *Narcotic Drugs: Estimated World Requirements for 2004. Statistics for 2002*. New York: United Nations, 2004: 176–177.

5 IOELC interview: Beugre Kouassi—4 June 2004.

6 See: http://www.cia.gov/cia/publications/factbook/geos/iv.html

7 This refers to adult mortality risk, which is defined as the probability of dying between 15 and 59 years.

8 See: WHO statistics for Cote d'Ivoire at: http://www.who.int/countries/civ/en/

9 http://www.unaids.org/en/geographical+area/by+country/côte+d'ivoire+.asp

10 Total health expenditure per capita is the per capita amount of the sum of Public Health Expenditure (PHE) and Private Expenditure on Health (PvtHE). The international dollar is a common currency unit that takes into account differences in the relative purchasing power of various currencies. Figures expressed in international dollars are calculated using purchasing power parities (PPP), which are rates of currency conversion constructed to account for differences in price level between countries.
http://www3.who.int/whosis/country/compare.cfm?country=s&indicator=strPcTotEOHinIntD 2000&language=english

11 This composite measure of overall health system attainment is based on a country's goals relating to health, responsiveness and fairness in financing. The measure varies widely across countries and is highly correlated with general levels of human development as captured in the human development index. Tandon A, Murray CLJ, Lauer JA, Evans DB. *Measuring Overall Health System Performance for 191 Countries*. GPE Discussion Paper Series: No. 30; WHO.

12 US Department of State, Office of Francophone West African Affairs, Bureau of African Affairs, 2003. *Background Notes on Countries of the World 2003*. Washington, DC: US Department of State, Office of Francophone West African Affairs, Bureau of African Affairs.

13 World of Information Business Intelligence Report, 2001. Cote d'Ivoire: Economy, Politics and Government. *Business Intelligence Report*, **1(1)**: 1–42.

Chapter 24

Democratic Republic of the Congo (Congo-Kinshasa)

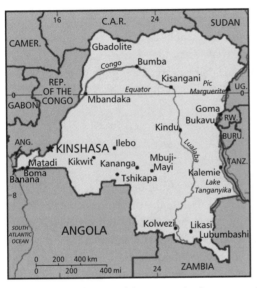

Democratic Republic of the Congo (population 58.32 million people) is a country in Central Africa that covers an area of 2 345 410 km². Its boundaries border Angola, Zambia, Tanzania, Burundi, Rwanda, Uganda, Sudan, Central African Republic and Republic of the Congo. The capital of Democratic Republic of the Congo is Kinshasa.

According to the United Nations human development index (HDI), Democratic Republic of the Congo is ranked 168th out of 177 countries worldwide (value 0.365)[1] and 36th out of 45 in African countries for which an index is available. This places Democratic Republic of the Congo in the group of countries with low human development.

Palliative care service provision

Current services

Interest in palliative care has come to light in the Democratic Republic of the Congo where a group based in Kinshasa is introducing a broader form of care at the general hospital and at the Clinique Universitaire. A nascent home care service is also being pioneered.

At the European Association of Palliative Care conference in Aachen (2005), nurse Anselme Kananga, currently studying in Belgium, represented the International Youth Association for Development. This NGO is linked with the international cultural organization *Tout-Age*.[2] He states:

> There has been palliative care in a small hospital in Kinshasa for four years. Our organization has 100 patients with cancers in palliative care. Some patients are cared for in the hospital but the condition is not good. Our organization provides student nurses and doctors to help volunteers in Kinshasa; about 80 patients are being cared for at home.
>
> We would like a clinic. If we have a clinic it would be easier for the patient. We would like to have autos for transport for the nurse volunteers, we want to have computers; and also education.

We would like to give medicine for the patient at home, but we would like to have more experience with palliative care. There is a need for education for nurses and for doctors.

And now we would like [integration] for palliative care in Kinshasa because we have a different culture from Europe and we must take account of the culture of Congo too.[3]

Reimbursement and funding for services

The International Youth Association for Development and its partner organization, Tout-Age are NGOs and rely on charitable donations

Opioid availability and consumption

The International Narcotics Control Board[4] has published the following figures for the consumption of narcotic drugs in the Democratic Republic of the Congo: codeine 13 kg; morphine 1 kg; pethidine 1 kg; and diphenoxylate 7 kg.

For the years 2000–2002, the average defined daily dose consumption of morphine for statistical purposes (S-DDD)[5] in Democratic Republic of the Congo was 0 (Appendix 1).

Life/oral histories

Anselme Kananga—*nurse, International Youth Association for Development*: interviewed by Michael Wright, 8 April 2005. Length of interview: 21 min.

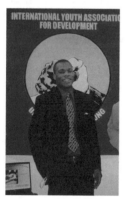

Anselme Kananga speaks of the beginnings of a palliative care service in Kinshasa despite the difficulties experienced in the country. The service is linked to two European NGOs and relies heavily on volunteer support, particularly from young people. He speaks of the resilience of those involved but of the need for enhanced facilities: computer technology, a day clinic, transport, materials and medication—all underpinned by education and training.

Public health context

Population

Democratic Republic of the Congo has a population of around 58.32 million people and is made up of >200 African ethnic groups of which the majority are Bantu; the four largest tribes—Mongo, Luba, Kongo (all Bantu) and the Mangbetu-Azande (Hamitic)—make up about 45 per cent of the population.

Religious groups include: Roman Catholic 50 per cent, Protestant 20 per cent, Kimbanguist 10 per cent, Muslim 10 per cent and other indigenous beliefs 10 per cent.[6]

Epidemiology

In Democratic Republic of the Congo, the WHO World Health Report (2004) indicates an adult mortality[7] rate per 1000 population of 585 for males and 449 for females. Life

Table 24.1 Democratic Republic of the Congo HIV and AIDS estimates, end 2003

Adult (15–49) HIV prevalence rate	4.2 per cent (range: 1.7–9.9 per cent)
Adults (15–49) living with HIV	1 000 000 (range: 410 000–2 400 000)
Adults and children (0–49) living with HIV	1 100 000 (range: 450 000–2 600 000)
Women (15–49) living with HIV	570 000 (range: 230 000–1 300 000)
AIDS deaths (adults and children) in 2003	100 000 (range: 50 000–220 000)

Source: 2004 Report of the global AIDS epidemic.

expectancy for males is 41.0; for females 46.1. Healthy life expectancy is 35.0 for males; and 39.1 for females.[8]

Democratic Republic of the Congo is a country in Central Africa that has been seriously affected by the HIV/AIDS epidemic. Estimates suggest that in Democratic Republic of the Congo, between 450 000 and 2.6 million people were living with HIV/AIDS at the end of 2003. In the same year, up to 220 000 adults and children are thought to have died from the disease (Table 24.1).

UNAIDS reports:

> The Democratic Republic of the Congo (DRC) is in a post-conflict period following five years of devastating war. The 2003 peace agreement brought a decisive turning point, with the adoption of a transitional constitution and government bodies. With support from the international community, backed by the UN peacekeeping mission (MONUC), the country is now engaged in the reunification of the army and the organization of democratic elections, the first in 30 years. The HIV/AIDS epidemic is among several major challenges confronting the DRC. Improved security conditions have, at least, enabled increased access to vulnerable populations and greater possibilities for humanitarian intervention. Available data from the isolated surveillance activities conducted in eastern DRC suggest that the prevalence rate may be much higher compared to that observed in the western part of the country, where prevalence among young people points to a growing epidemic. A multisectoral programme and a committee under the leadership of the president have been set up by a presidential decree.
>
> UNAIDS has provided continual support to the DRC, which helped sustain the national response during the most difficult period. The DRC is among UNAIDS priority countries for an intensified effort in support of the national response. UNAIDS gave technical support to develop Global Fund proposals that were approved for US$112 million. Similarly, it supported the development of the MAP proposal that was also granted. The political advocacy effort has included several high-level visits to the DRC, including visits by the UN Secretary-General and the UNAIDS Executive Director. During the past three years, UNAIDS successfully assisted the formulation of the National Strategic Plan. UNAIDS is supporting HIV/AIDS prevention and care activities in the military base of Kamina, which has received limited support because of its remote location and difficult access. An outstanding effort has been made in the area of political advocacy for a stronger leadership at the highest level and the adoption of a multisectoral approach. As a result, the head of state has been increasingly speaking out both nationally and internationally.[9]

Health care system

In 2001, the total per capita expenditure on health care was Intl $12; 3.5% of GDP[10] (Appendix 3).

The WHO overall health system performance score places Democratic Republic of the Congo 188th out of 191 countries.[11]

Political economy

Since 1997, the Democratic Republic of the Congo (formerly called Zaire) has been affected by ethnic strife and civil war, touched off by a massive inflow in 1994 of refugees from the fighting in Rwanda and Burundi. The government of former president Mobutu Sese Seko was toppled by a rebellion led by Laurent Kabila in May 1997; his regime was subsequently challenged by a Rwanda- and Uganda-backed rebellion in August 1998. A cease-fire was signed on 10 July 1999 by the DROC, Kabila was assassinated on 16 January 2001 and his son Joseph Kabila was named head of state 10 days later. In October 2002, the new president was successful in getting occupying Rwandan forces to withdraw from eastern Congo; 2 months later, the Pretoria Accord was signed by all remaining warring parties to end the fighting and set up a government of national unity. A transitional government was set up in July 2003; Joseph Kabila remains as president and is joined by four vice presidents from the former government, former rebel camps and the political opposition.

The economy of the Democratic Republic of the Congo—a nation endowed with vast potential wealth—has declined drastically since the mid-1980s. The war, which began in August 1998, has dramatically reduced national output and government revenue, and has increased external debt. Foreign businesses have curtailed operations due to uncertainty about the outcome of the conflict, lack of infrastructure and the difficult operating environment. Conditions improved in late 2002 with the withdrawal of a large portion of the invading foreign troops. Several IMF and World Bank missions have met with the government to help it develop a coherent economic plan, and President Kabila has begun implementing reforms. Much economic activity lies outside the GDP data. Economic stability, aided by international donors, improved in 2003. New mining contracts have been approved, which—combined with high mineral and metal prices—could improve Kinshasa's fiscal position and GDP growth.[6] In recent times, Democratic Republic of the Congo has been confronted with the most severe crisis since its independence. Confronted with this acute political emergency, the international community, which has a responsibility in promoting peace and security, has given an ambiguous message.[12]

GDP per capita is Intl $346 (Appendix 4).

References

1 Report of the United Nations Development Programme 2004 (HDI 2002). Launched by the United Nations in 1990, the Human Development Index measures a country's achievements in three aspects of human development: longevity, knowledge and a decent standard of living. It was created to re-emphasize that people and their lives should be the ultimate criteria for assessing the

development of a country, not economic growth. Current values range from 0.956 (Norway, first of 177 countries) to 0.273 (Sierra Leone, 177th out of 177 countries). Countries fall into one of three groups: countries 1–55 = high development; 56–141 = medium development; 142–177 = low development. See: http://hdr.undp.org/statistics/data/indic/indic_8_1_1.html

2 Personal communication: Anselme Kananga and Avril Jackso—21 April 2005.

3 Personal communication: Anselme Kananga—8 April 2005.

4 International Narcotics Control Board. *Narcotic Drugs: Estimated World Requirements for 2004. Statistics for 2002.* New York: United Nations, 2004.

5 'The term *defined daily doses for statistical purposes* (S-DDD) replaces the term *defined daily doses* previously used by the Board. The S-DDDs are technical units of measurement for the purposes of statistical analysis and are not recommended prescription doses. Certain narcotic drugs may be used in certain countries for different treatments or in accordance with different medical practices, and therefore a different daily dose could be more appropriate'. The S-DDD used by the INCB for morphine is 100 mg. International Narcotics Control Board. *Narcotic Drugs: Estimated World Requirements for 2004. Statistics for 2002.* New York: United Nations, 2004: 176–177.

6 See: http://www.cia.gov/cia/publications/factbook/geos/cg.html

7 This refers to adult mortality risk, which is defined as the probability of dying between 15 and 59 years.

8 See: WHO statistics for Democratic Republic of the Congo at: http://www.who.int/countries/cod/en/

9 http://www.unaids.org/en/geographical+area/by+country/democratic+republic+of+congo.asp

10 Total health expenditure per capita is the per capita amount of the sum of Public Health Expenditure (PHE) and Private Expenditure on Health (PvtHE). The international dollar is a common currency unit that takes into account differences in the relative purchasing power of various currencies. Figures expressed in international dollars are calculated using purchasing power parities (PPP), which are rates of currency conversion constructed to account for differences in price level between countries. http://www3.who.int/whosis/country/compare.cfm?country= s&indicator=strPcTotEOHinIntD2000&language=english

11 This composite measure of overall health system attainment is based on a country's goals relating to health, responsiveness and fairness in financing. The measure varies widely across countries and is highly correlated with general levels of human development as captured in the human development index. Tandon A, Murray CLJ, Lauer JA, Evans DB. *Measuring Overall Health System Performance for 191 Countries.* GPE Discussion Paper Series: No. 30; WHO.

12 **Smis S, Oyatambwe W.** Complex political emergencies, the international community and the Congo conflict. *Review of African Political Economy* 2002; **29**(93–94): 411–430.

Chapter 25

Ethiopia

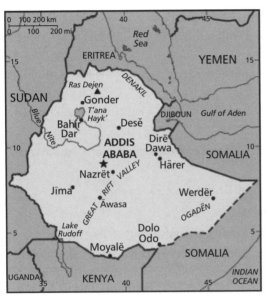

Ethiopia (population 67.85 million people) is a country in Eastern Africa that covers an area of 1 127 km². Its boundaries border Eritrea, Djibouti, Somalia, Kenya and Sudan. The capital of Ethiopia is Addis Ababa.

According to the United Nations human development index (HDI), Ethiopia is ranked 170th out of 177 countries worldwide (value 0.359)[1] and 38th out of 45 in African countries for which an index is available.

This places Ethiopia in the group of countries with low human development.

Palliative care service provision

Current services

Family Health International (FHI) defines home and community-based care (HCBC) as 'the provision of care and support that endeavours to meet the nursing and psychosocial needs of persons with chronic illnesses and their family members in their home environment'.[2] While HCBC delivers patient care in the home environment, palliative care is an approach that attends to the needs of patients and families affected by a life-threatening illness in a variety of settings including the home, hospice, hospital, clinic and community.

The concept of home-based care is relatively new in Ethiopia and has evolved as a response to the HIV/AIDS epidemic. Three non-governmental humanitarian organizations provide this care: the Medical Missionaries of Mary, Mekdem and Mary Joy.[2] According to a WHO (2002) Progress Report on the status of palliative care in Ethiopia, data indicated that most patients prefer to be treated and cared for in health facilities rather than at home.[3]

Addis Ababa was selected as the target area for a palliative care demonstration project by the WHO Ethiopia Palliative Care Team in 2001[3]. The WHO (2002) Progress Report for the project reports that no information is available on cancer incidence, prevalence or mortality within Ethiopia. However, the three most common cancers referred to the Radiotherapy Centre were cancers of the cervix, breast and head/neck. Most patients were diagnosed at the late stages of the disease. There is no cancer control programme or palliative care programme for advanced disease. The report further estimates that 13 per cent of the population of Addis Ababa are HIV infected, although antiretroviral drugs are neither available nor affordable for much of the population.

There is no palliative care component within the HIV/AIDS control programme in Addis Adaba.

The WHO palliative care project acknowledges the formidable difficulties confronting Ethiopia:

> Ethiopia, the largest country, was identified as having the greatest number of unmet needs and requiring the most support to improve its situation.[4]

Nevertheless, WHO considers that certain strengths and opportunities are recognizable in Ethiopia. These include:

- Strong political commitment for HIV/AIDS prevention and control
- Community support and commitment
- International organizations, local NGOs and government partnership
- Networking with other participating countries in the palliative care project
- Availability of national drug project.

Concerns centre on:

- Lack of trained health workers in palliative care
- Inadequate capacity to train for palliative care
- Social stigma (especially attached to AIDS)
- Poor behavioural change
- Cancer not adequately addressed
- Shortage of human and material resources.[4]

Reimbursement and funding for services

President's Emergency Plan for AIDS Relief (PEPFAR)[5]

During the 2004 financial year (FY), funding of around US$40.99 million was enacted for country-managed programmes in Ethiopia and US$7 million for central programmes. During FY2005, it is anticipated that a total of US$70.02 million will be enacted: US$61.36 million for country-managed programmes and US$8.66 million for central programmes.[6]

The Global Fund

The Global Fund has approved significant funding for HIV/AIDS prevention and control programmes in Ethiopia. An agreement was signed on 9 October 2003 for over US$55 million to be disbursed over 2 years through the HIV/AIDS Prevention and Control Office. The objectives of the proposal are to scale up and expand:

- Voluntary Counselling and Testing
- Clinical management of HIV (excluding antiretrovirals)
- Home-based care
- Clinical management of Prevention of Mother-to-Child Transmission
- Blood safety
- Prevention of nosocomial infections
- Information, Education and Communication, 'Behaviour change communication' and promotion of condoms
- Capacity building
- Surveillance and operational research
- Monitoring and evaluation mechanisms.[7]

An agreement for a further US$41 million for Round 4 of the project was signed on 11 February 2005. Palliative care is not mentioned in the proposals.

Opioid availability and consumption

The International Narcotics Control Board[8] has published the following figures for the consumption of narcotic drugs in Ethiopia: codeine 11 kg (2000); and Tilidine 3 kg (2002).

For the years 2000–2002, the average defined daily dose consumption of morphine for statistical purposes (S-DDD)[9] in Ethiopia was 0 (Appendix 1).

Palliative care coverage

There are no governmental programmes and only three NGOs that provide support for chronically ill patients in a home setting. Meeting the palliative care needs of cancer and HIV/AIDS patients is not considered a public health priority.

Ethical issues

According to the WHO (2002) Progress Report, there is a fusion of traditional and modern medicine that may affect the uptake of palliative care in Ethiopia.

> The practice of modern medicine, traditional medicine, and holy water treatment run side-by-side in Addis Ababa. Both HIV/AIDS and cancer patients tend to go first to modern health facilities, but these diseases are often not effectively managed at these centres. When there is not a satisfactory solution to the medical problem, patients consider seeking out assistance from traditional medicine or holy water treatment to fill the gap.[3]

Public health context

Population

Ethiopia's population of around 67.85 million people is made up of the following ethnic groups: Oromo 40 per cent, Amhara and Tigre 32 per cent, Sidamo 9 per cent, Shankella 6 per cent, Somali 6 per cent, Afar 4 per cent, Gurage 2 per cent and other 1 per cent.

Religious groups include: Muslim 45–50 per cent, Ethiopian Orthodox 35–40 per cent, animist 12 per cent and other 3–8 per cent.[10]

Epidemiology

In Ethiopia, the WHO World Health Report (2004) indicates an adult mortality[11] rate per 1000 population of 487 for males and 422 for females. Life expectancy for males is 46.8; for females 49.4. Healthy life expectancy is 40.7 for males; and 41.7 for females.[12]

Ethiopia has been severely affected by the HIV/AIDS epidemic. Estimates suggest that in Ethiopia, between 950 000 and 2.3million people were living with HIV/AIDS at the end of 2003. In the same year, up to 190 000 adults and children are thought to have died from the disease (Table 25.1).

UNAIDS reports:

> Ethiopia has a total population of 67 million people and is one of the poorest countries in the world. Antiretroviral therapy is accessible on payment in most regions. Guidelines for preventing mother-to-child transmission have been developed, and the implementation is underway. The National Monitoring and Evaluation Framework, Communication Guidelines and HIV/AIDS Behavioural Surveillance Survey have been developed. The National AIDS Council (NAC) is chaired by the president of the country and includes all stakeholders; the HIV/AIDS Prevention and Control Office (HAPCO) was legally established in 2002, both at federal and regional levels; and district (woreda) and lower district (kebele/community level) coordination mechanisms were established in 262 woredas (44% of the total districts). The National Strategic Framework (NSF) for 2000–2004 is now being updated after the joint midterm review of the National Response. The Country Coordinating Mechanism (CCM) Ethiopia has submitted the fourth round proposal to

Table 25.1 Ethiopia HIV and AIDS estimates, end 2003

Adults (15–49) HIV prevalence rate	4.4 per cent (range 0.9–7.3 per cent).
Adults (15–49) living with HIV	1 400 000 (range 890 000–2 100 000).
Adults and children (0–49) living with HIV	1 500 000 (range 950 000–2 300 000).
Women (15–49) living with HIV	770 000 (range 500 000–1 200 000).
AIDS deaths (adults and children) in 2003	120 000 (range 74 000–190 000).

Source: 2004 Report of the global AIDS epidemic.

the Global Fund for US$139 million over two years, of which the HIV/AIDS component of US$ 108 million focuses on treatment and care.[13]

The WHO report on palliative care in five African countries draws attention to the severity of problems caused by stigmatization:

> No prominent Ethiopian is willing to stand up, acknowledge infection and urge others to discuss the issue on a personal and public basis. Health professionals emphasize the unwillingness of Ethiopians to come forward for voluntary testing, even when kits are available. Because HIV/AIDS is correlated with promiscuity, many believe that only immoral people get AIDS. Death certificates, even when AIDS is highly suspected, routinely cite other causes of death, such as TB. When testing proves that AIDS was the cause of death, friends and relatives are usually not told. In fact, Ethiopian doctors are usually reluctant to pass along bad news to patients on any health matter, especially now with AIDS. When donated blood is found to be HIV+ the blood is destroyed and the donor not told. People with or suspected of having HIV are afraid they will be turned away from health care services, employment, or refused entry to a foreign country. Fear of discrimination often prevents many Ethiopians from seeking treatment for AIDS. In numerous cases, those with AIDS have been evicted from their homes by their families and rejected by their friends and colleagues. Infected children, and those who have parents infected by HIV, are often orphaned or abandoned. In Ethiopia, HIV/AIDS related stigma, characterised by silence, fear, ignorance, intolerance, discrimination and denial are fuelling the spread of HIV/AIDS and creating immense barriers to effective responses to the epidemic.[4]

Health care system

In 2001, the total per capita expenditure on health care was Intl $14; 3.6% of GDP)[14] (Appendix 3).

The WHO overall health system performance score places Ethiopia 180th out of 191 countries.[15]

Political economy

Unique among African countries, the ancient Ethiopian monarchy maintained its freedom from colonial rule, one exception being the Italian occupation of 1936–1941. In 1974, a military junta, the Derg, deposed Emperor Haile Selassie (who had ruled since 1930) and established a socialist state.[10] In spite of the rapid expansion of primary care, community participation was hampered by the protracted war and centralized, urban-based, bureaucratic approaches and attitudes that failed to promote an enabling environment for community participation. The socialist government, although implementing various community programmes and expanding the rural health services, did not succeed in revolutionizing the health services.[16] During the 1980s, Ethiopia experienced the effects of conflict, drought and famine on a scale far greater than many other complex political emergencies (CPEs)—a major humanitarian, political, social and economic crisis, with war and poverty as fundamental components. Its root causes were linked to political marginalization, socio-economic stress, and to ethnic identity and grievances, with the basic lesson that failure to address these would ensure the recurrence of conflict. In May 1991, after the decisive defeat of the military dictatorship of Mengistu Haile

Mariam by the Ethiopian Peoples' Revolutionary Democratic Front (EPRDF) and after decades of civil war, drought and famine, Ethiopia faced the prospects of peace and of much needed development.[17]

In the face of dramatically changed international circumstances, the EPRDF moderates embraced the free market, achieved a measure of economic progress, and took large steps towards state decentralization and smaller ones towards democratization.[18] A constitution was adopted in 1994 and Ethiopia's first multiparty elections were held in 1995. A two and a half year border war with Eritrea ended with a peace treaty on 12 December 2000.

Ethiopia's poverty-stricken economy is based on agriculture, which accounts for half of GDP, 60 per cent of exports and 80 per cent of total employment. The agricultural sector suffers from frequent drought and poor cultivation practices. Coffee is critical to the Ethiopian economy with exports of some US$156 million in 2002, but historically low prices have seen many farmers switching to qat to supplement income. The war with Eritrea in 1998–2000 and recurrent drought have buffeted the economy, in particular coffee production. In November 2001, Ethiopia qualified for debt relief from the Highly Indebted Poor Countries (HIPC) initiative. Under Ethiopia's land tenure system, the government owns all land and provides long-term leases to the tenants; the system continues to hamper growth in the industrial sector as entrepreneurs are unable to use land as collateral for loans. Drought struck again late in 2002, leading to a 2 per cent decline in GDP in 2003. Return to normal weather patterns late in 2003 helped agricultural and GDP growth recover in 2004. The government estimates that annual growth of 7 per cent is needed to reduce poverty.[10]

GDP per capita is Intl $382 (Appendix 4).

References

1 Report of the United Nations Development Programme 2004 (HDI 2002). Launched by the United Nations in 1990, the Human Development Index measures a country's achievements in three aspects of human development: longevity, knowledge and a decent standard of living. It was created to re-emphasize that people and their lives should be the ultimate criteria for assessing the development of a country, not economic growth. Current values range from 0.956 (Norway, first of 177 countries) to 0.273 (Sierra Leone, 177th out of 177 countries). Countries fall into one of three groups: countries 1–55 = high development; 56–141 = medium development; 142–177 = low development. See: http://hdr.undp.org/statistics/data/indic/indic_8_1_1.html

2 Family Health International, Comprehensive Care and Support Framework.

3 WHO Progress Report. Community Health Approach to Palliative Care for HIV/AIDS and Cancer Patients in Africa. 2002. See: http://www.who.int/cancer/palliative/africanproject/en/

4 WHO Report. Community Health Approach to Palliative Care for HIV/AIDS Patients, 2004:28. Available to download at: http://whqlibdoc.who.int/publications/2004/9241591498.pdf

5 See: http://www.usaid.gov/our_work/global_health/aids/pepfarfact.html

6 Engendering Bold Leadership. The President's Emergency Plan for AIDS Relief. First Annual Report to Congress, 2005: 115. http://www.state.gov/documents/organization/43885.pdf

7 Global Fund Portfolio of Grants.

8 International Narcotics Control Board. Narcotic Drugs: Estimated World Requirements for 2004. Statistics for 2002. New York: United Nations, 2004.

9 'The term *defined daily doses for statistical purposes* (S-DDD) replaces the term *defined daily doses* previously used by the Board. The S-DDDs are technical units of measurement for the purposes of statistical analysis and are not recommended prescription doses. Certain narcotic drugs may be used in certain countries for different treatments or in accordance with different medical practices, and therefore a different daily dose could be more appropriate'. The S-DDD used by the INCB for morphine is 100 mg. International Narcotics Control Board. *Narcotic Drugs: Estimated World Requirements for 2004. Statistics for 2002.* New York: United Nations, 2004: 176–177.

10 See: http://www.cia.gov/cia/publications/factbook/geos/et.html

11 This refers to adult mortality risk, which is defined as the probability of dying between 15 and 59 years.

12 See WHO statistics for Ethiopia: http://www.who.int/countries/eth/eth/en/index.html

13 http://www.unaids.org/en/geographical+area/by+country/ethiopia.asp

14 Total health expenditure per capita is the per capita amount of the sum of Public Health Expenditure (PHE) and Private Expenditure on Health (PvtHE). The international dollar is a common currency unit that takes into account differences in the relative purchasing power of various currencies. Figures expressed in international dollars are calculated using purchasing power parities (PPP), which are rates of currency conversion constructed to account for differences in price level between countries.http://www3.who.int/whosis/country/compare.cfm?country= s&indicator=strPcTotEOHinIntD2000&language=english

15 This composite measure of overall health system attainment is based on a country's goals relating to health, responsiveness and fairness in financing. The measure varies widely across countries and is highly correlated with general levels of human development as captured in the human development index. Tandon A, Murray CLJ, Lauer JA, Evans DB. *Measuring Overall Health System Performance for 191 Countries.* GPE Discussion Paper Series: No. 30; WHO.

16 **Kloos H.** Primary health care in Ethiopia under three political systems: community participation in a war-torn society. *Social Science and Medicine* 1998; **46(4–5)**: 505–522.

17 **Milas S, Latif JA.** The political economy of complex emergency and recovery in northern Ethiopia. *Disasters* 2000; **24(4)**: 363–379.

18 **Tadesse M, Young J.** TPLF: reform or decline? *Review of African Political Economy* 2003; **30(97)**: 389–404.

Chapter 26

Ghana

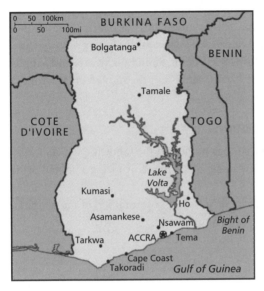

Ghana (population 20.76 million) is a country in Western Africa that covers an area of 239 460 km². Its boundaries border the Gulf of Guinea, between Cote d'Ivoire, Togo and Burkina Faso. The capital of the country is Accra.

According to the United Nations human development index (HDI), Ghana is ranked 131th out of 177 countries worldwide (value 0.568)[1] and ninth out of 45 in African countries for which an index is available. This places Ghana in the group of countries with medium human development.

Palliative care service provision

Current services

There are no established palliative care services in Ghana. In the absence of formal structures, individuals in Ghana have begun to incorporate palliative care principles into home-based care projects with AIDS and cancer patients.[2]

Terry Magee, director of education at Myland Hall Education Centre (St Helena Hospice, UK), has been involved in education initiatives in Ghana for the last 2 years. She notes:

> There are a number of initiatives that are a mixture of outreach and social and health support for people who are living in communities—rural communities mostly—who have HIV; and AIDS and there are services developing within the hospitals in Kumasi and Accra, to try to produce more information and more awareness for patients about issues like pain and symptom control and family support.
>
> As yet, there isn't a hospice as such, but the idea of hospice is very much alive in the practice. This time we did a series of story-telling workshops with the students where we talked to them

about what exquisite holistic care was all about, and we outlined the principles of hospice care, and we asked them to tell us stories of where they felt that was happening in their own practice, and how they were making that happen, and we heard some wonderful examples—it's not got a label 'hospice' over it, but it's hospice care nonetheless. Some lovely stories of where the care was delivered to a person, or the actions taken by health care professional, or a social care professional had resulted in some very, very fine holistic care and good quality of life in dying people, and some very fine examples of very appropriate after death care and support.[3]

Reimbursement and funding for services

The Global Fund signed an agreement on 12 December 2002 for nearly US$5 million. The project will increase access and generate greater demand for both prevention and care services for the groups vulnerable to HIV infection, and improve care and support for those already living with the virus.[4] Palliative care is not mentioned in the proposal agreement.

Opioid availability and consumption

The International Narcotics Control Board[5] has published the following figures for the consumption of narcotic drugs in Ghana: codeine 20 kg; dihydrocodeine 5 kg; and pethidine 50 kg (2001).

For the years 2000–2002, the average defined daily dose consumption of morphine for statistical purposes (S-DDD)[6] in Ghana was 0 (Appendix 1).

A restrictive policy limits the use of opiate drugs in Ghana.[7]

Education and training

Hospice Africa Uganda has been instrumental in disseminating information on palliative care to health officials and professionals. Further training is likely to come from experienced palliative care practitioners from other African countries, notably Uganda. An initial 'training of trainers' session in April 2004 was led by Hospice Africa Uganda. Plans are in place to extend the training programme. Vinolia Tonugble, a physician and trustee of the Cancer Society of Ghana:

> In the near future, we will initiate training, proper training of trainers, and then we'll spread it at three levels. We want to train the professional; we want to train the community staff; at the grass roots level we have the community's health centres; and then we want to train Red Cross and volunteers and go into full-scale palliative care.[7]

Terry Magee tells of the training courses she has helped to deliver in Ghana:

> We were first contacted two years ago by the African Medical Trust to talk about the development of palliative care services for people with cancer and AIDS in the nine regions of Ghana; and as a result of that, we started off by offering hospice placements, education and support to interested professionals who could get to England; experience life in a hospice and working alongside hospice staff.
> Following that, we worked together with the cancer society of Ghana in developing a national education programme for Ghana about palliative care, really an awareness-raising programme

aimed at health and social care professionals, to tell them a little bit about hospice care and hospice services and to try to help them to think about how that service might develop within the cultural imperative that exists in Ghana.

So we wrote a course and we collaborated with Hospice Uganda and we went to Ghana for the first time two years ago; and we carried out, with our Ugandan colleagues, an introduction to hospice and palliative care services course in the capital of Ghana—Accra. We had 190-odd people on that, and that was a week, full time; and during that time I also visited the students in the hospitals and outreach programmes where they worked, to see the situations that they were practising in.

That was a great success and so the Cancer Society of Ghana asked us if we would be willing to come back and take that programme, in a shorter form, out to the nine regions of Ghana. So this year—we obviously had to trim down the course, and we had to trim down the number of people that were going out there because this was a very big financial commitment for them to put a programme on in the nine regions so we had to slim it all down—we went back out in January and we travelled to another two regions of Ghana and carried out the programme again there; a region in the upper area of Ghana called Bolgatanga and we had about—I think we had about 80 or 90 people in Bolgatanga who took the course; and we also carried the course out in another region of Ghana which is called the Cape Coast region, and there we had again, about 90 health and social care professionals, and in Bolgatanga, we also had representatives from cultural healers and spiritual healers. Imams and Chaplains also did the course; and we have plans with the cancer society of Ghana to return as and when funding is available and we're available to do it—and to continue to do that until we've covered the nine regions of Ghana—so that hopefully, everybody, you know, who has an interest in Ghana has come along and heard a bit about hospice and palliative care services and the theory which underpins this work; and has an opportunity to think that one through and look for ways in which some of what we're doing in the west might influence some of what they will do in Africa.[3]

Colleagues from Hospice Africa Uganda, Dr Henry Ddungu and nurse Berna Basemera, comment on the course in May 2004:

The opening ceremony took place at the Ghana International Trade Fair. It was attended by many dignitaries including executive members of the Ghana Cancer society, government representatives and all the course participants. It was a very colourful occasion. The Keynote address was given by Dr Ken Sagoe, Director of Human resources, Ghana Health Services. He emphasized government's position towards palliative care in Ghana and their (Government) willingness to incorporate it into policy and advocacy. The opening ceremony was on the headlines for the evening news on TV3—a private TV company in Accra with a very wide coverage.

The training began on Tuesday 11th May 2004 with the first lecture given by Dr Henry Ddungu, on the hospice concept. It was made clear that even with minimal funding one can care for a dying patient in need of palliative care, as long as there was commitment. Examples of locally available remedies that have been tried and found to be working were given and emphasized. Dr Jack Jagwe discussed the laws governing use of Narcotics as well as 'Myths and Fears' on use of morphine to such a degree that all the fears they (participants) had waned away. Berna and John took the group through spirituality in the hospice context and the discussion groups never wanted to stop! It was such a good experience for the groups discussing various issues and sharing the various experiences.

Grief and bereavement in Ghana was another interesting topic. The group agreed to divide into the different ethnic groups—the Gas, the Akans, the Ewes, the Dogombas and Mamprusis, and the

Dagarees and Sissalas (Northern). Each of these groups gave their cultural beliefs towards grief and bereavement. It was so amazing to realize that even in the same country, different groups have differing cultures and beliefs when it comes to death and dying. It emphasized the importance of cultural considerations—Cultural Pain—and palliative Care.

The course ended well and it was explained to participants how they were to write a reflective diary to be submitted to the Cancer Society of Ghana before they could receive their certificates in June 2004. They were all ready and willing to do this and to-date, many have received their certificates.

As far as availability of oral morphine was concerned, this did not seem a very big problem because the Department of Health is already aware and willing to support the importation of oral morphine into the country. However we will see how this goodwill develops! It was however, emphasized that potential prescribers need to be sensitized on the use of morphine.[8]

History and development of hospice–palliative care in Ghana

In 2003, Mary Callaway (OSI) noted a significant development in Ghana. She writes, 'I had to share this news clip (undated) from Ghana':

Palliative care needed for terminal ill health—MOH

Dr Kwaku Afriyie, Minister of Health, on Monday asked donors and founders of palliative care and hospice to consider funding and to expand their activities in developing countries to enable patients bound to die to do so bravely through consolation. He said: 'The development of palliative and hospice care is essential to look after people suffering from HIV/AIDS and cancer and those terminally ill'.

Dr Afriyie was speaking at a two-day workshop, organized by the Hospice Ghana, a non-governmental organisation (NGO) that aims to train professional medical, health and social workers in giving palliative care, which was on the theme: *Providing Palliative Care For The Terminally-Ill*. He said with the absence of such a care 'many of such patients die, needlessly without proper dignity or preparation'. He said palliative care has been a traditional way of looking after patients whose disease did not respond to curative treatment and were then consoled, to face death in dignity in many developed countries.

Dr Afriyie said the Government recognized the private sector as the engine of growth and would, therefore, encourage private sector participation in health care delivery. He said the World Health Organization (WHO) recommended three measures if sustainable and appropriate palliative care services were to meet the needs of the poorest. The three measures are: Formally adopting a national policy on palliative care; outlining how services would develop in line with the health service and promoting standards of care with a commitment to train all health workers in managing pain while informing and educating the public on pain control.

The other policy measure is to ensure that the necessary drugs for pain control are available and for instance appropriately trained professionals prescribing drugs such as morphine. Dr Averil Fountain, Representative of the British Executive Services Overseas (BESO), said the UK forum for hospice and palliative care and BESO were currently working together on a partnership capacity-building project to develop palliative care in West Africa, especially Ghana, Nigeria, Gambia, Cameroon and Sierra Leone. BESO is a development agency that offers professional advice to organizations that could not afford commercial consultants.

Dr Fountain, who is also a resource person at the workshop, said the programme would provide opportunities for health professionals to network with each other and share knowledge and expertise between themselves to develop capacity of organizations to provide palliative care.

Mr Isaac Dweber Friph, Director of Hospice Ghana, said the collapse of the extended family system and the influence of western cultures on the lives of Ghanaians have resulted in retirees living alone and many aged people have little or no care at all. He said Hospice Ghana was interested in bringing back to life the practice of palliative care and to further develop people's knowledge and exploration of aspects of care and support required by those who were terminally-ill.[9]

Ethical issues

Terry Magee:

> Well the ethical issues are pretty utilitarian. It's about doing what one can. It's balancing out the quality with cost-effectiveness because they are about doing the greatest good for the greatest number of people. The other ethical issues are around issues such as consent to care which you know, can pose problems because there may be embargos upon people knowing what's wrong with them, so there are some tricky practitioner issues in terms of ethics there. Disclosure of diagnosis, that's another one; and then the whole business of finances of this care. I mean—Ghana's struggling at the moment to provide people with antiretroviral therapy and again it's about the fair use of resources, Antiretroviral therapy is a great, a very important thing in Ghana—and that's going to be a very big challenge for the Ghanaian Government before they even begin to think of, you now. 'Now we've actually done what we can to help this person who's dying—what can we do when they are actually dying?[3]

Life/oral histories

Terry Magee—*director of Education, Myland Hall Education Centre, St Helena Hospice, Colchester, UK*: interviewed by Michael Wright, 25 March 2005. Length of interview: 47 min.

Terry Magee tells how she became involved in palliative care education in Ghana after the African Medical Trust approached St Helena Hospice regarding the development of palliative care education in the country. Collaboration followed between the Myland Centre, Hospice Africa Uganda and interested parties in Ghana and, eventually, a national education programme was developed. The initial courses were so successful that a shorter version was adapted for the nine regions of Africa. Consequently, hospice philosophy is beginning to permeate practice in Ghana, and a number of initiatives have sought to incorporate the hospice ideal. Terry Magee speaks of the challenges facing palliative care development in Ghana: an underfunded health care system; diverse traditions around death and dying; widow inheritance in a context of polygamy; lack of national statistics or a cancer registry; large distances covered by health care staff; and endemic poverty. Yet she detects discernible successes: a clear implementation of theory into practice; better care for the sick; an increasing flow of Ghanaian health professionals training in the UK; the beneficial effects of advocacy;

the keeping of records and construction of databases—all of which will contribute to the development of palliative care in Ghana.

Dr Vinolia Tonugble—*physician, trustee of the Cancer Society of Ghana*: interviewed by David Clark, 4 June 2004. Length of interview (West Africa group): 40 min.

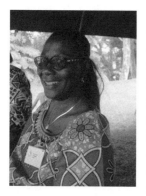

Vinolia Tonugble tells of her interest and involvement in charity work throughout West Africa, and details the process of registering the Cancer Society in Ghana. She describes the involvement of Hospice Africa Uganda in disseminating information about palliative care in Ghana. Current HIV programmes in the country do not incorporate palliative care. She identifies advocacy for morphine accessibility in the health system as a priority, along with palliative care training of health professionals, community health staff and volunteer community groups. To achieve this, funding and commitment from the state are required. She shares her belief that the experiences of other African countries should be built upon for developing Ghanaian services. Moving on to the role of opioids, she confirms the existence of a restrictive draft policy that limits use of opiate drugs. She emphasizes the need to convince government about the need for pain control in order to relax these laws. She is confident that government will be sympathetic to scaling up palliative care in Ghana. When policy structures are in place, she predicts a rapid rise in palliative care provision in Ghana.

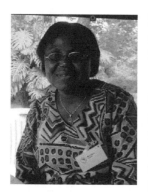

Mary Opare—*acting dean of the School of Nursing, University of Ghana, Legon, Accra*: interviewed by David Clark, 4 June 2004. Length of interview (West African group): 40 min.

Mary Opare describes how, in the absence of formal structures, individuals in Ghana have taken the initiative to incorporate palliative care principles into home-based care projects with AIDS and cancer patients. She highlights the need now to engage all levels of the health sector, including hospitals, with the needs of terminally ill patients. In her capacity as Head of Nursing at the university, she hopes to introduce practical palliative care into the nurse curriculum.

Public health context

Population

Ghana's population of around 20.76 million is made up of the following ethnic groups: black African 98.5 per cent (major tribes Akan 44 per cent, Moshi-Dagomba 16 per cent, Ewe 13 per cent, Ga 8 per cent, Gurma 3 per cent and Yoruba 1 per cent), and European and other 1.5 per cent.

Table 26.1 Ghana HIV and AIDS estimates, end 2003

Adult (15–49) HIV prevalence rate	3.1 per cent (range: 1.9–5.0 per cent)
Adults (15–49) living with HIV	320 000 (range: 200 000–520 000)
Adults and children (0–49) living with HIV	350 000 (range: 210 000–560 000)
Women (15–49) living with HIV	180 000 (range: 110 000–300 000)
AIDS deaths (adults and children) in 2003	30 000 (range: 18 000–49 000)

Source: 2004 Report on the global AIDS epidemic.

Religious groups include: Christian 63 per cent, Muslim 16 per cent and indigenous beliefs 21 per cent.[10]

Epidemiology

In Ghana, the WHO World Health Report (2004) indicates an adult mortality[11] rate per 1000 population of 354 for males and 303 for females. Life expectancy for males is 56.3; for females 58.8. Healthy life expectancy is 49.2 for males; and 50.3 for females.[12]

Ghana is severely affected by the HIV/AIDS epidemic. Estimates suggest that in Ghana, between 210 000 and 560 000 people were living with HIV/AIDS at the end of 2003. In the same year, up to 49 000 adults and children are thought to have died from the disease (Table 26.1).

UNAIDS reports:

Ghana's population of over 18 million has an HIV/AIDS prevalence rate currently estimated to be below the 5% threshold. While awareness of the epidemic is thought to be over 95%, this awareness has yet to translate into widespread behavioural change. The National Strategic Framework for HIV/AIDS (NSFW) was adopted in 2001 and constitutes one direction of the national response.

Ghana's HIV/AIDS strategic plan focuses on five thematic areas: prevention of new infection; care and support for people living with HIV; creating an enabling environment for the national response; decentralizing implementation through institutional arrangements; and research, monitoring and evaluation.

Multilateral and bilateral partners, NGOs and civil society organisations actively participate in the national response under government leadership. There are more than 2,500 community-based organisations and NGOs implementing HIV/AIDS interventions in the country. There has been substantial funding from bilateral and multilateral partners for the national HIV/AIDS response.[13]

Health care system

In 2001, the total per capita expenditure on health care was Intl $60; 4.7% of GDP[14] (Appendix 3).

The WHO overall health system performance score places Ghana 135th out of 191 countries.[15]

Political economy

Since the early 1990s, pressure for democratization in Ghana resulted in the return of a multiparty spolitical system. The victories of the ruling party in the 1992 and 1996 national elections legitimized the liberal economic reform sponsored by international donors; democratization in Ghana may suggest a model of political economy replicable in other African countries.[16] The country is developing a pro-democracy political culture and, although Ghana's political legacy was not seen as particularly conducive to democratization, the country's chances were buoyed not only by encouragement from external aid donors, but also by domestic demands for the end of authoritarian rule. Several developments suggest that there is progress towards democratic consolidation in Ghana, and many procedural criteria for democracy are respected, including multiple political parties and independent interest associations. All of Ghana's competing parties have stressed a common nationality rather than a divisive ethnic orientation, whilst the judiciary, civil society and independent media—institutions crucial to the success of democracy—have all grown in strength and autonomy.[17]

Compared with other countries in Africa, Ghana has been highly praised as the most successful example of Word Bank/IMF-sponsored structural adjustment programmes by Western donors, and there has been discussion about how Ghana's economic development model could be applied to other countries that face economic declines—Ghana has become one of the pioneering countries that have implemented adjustment programmes.[18] Well endowed with natural resources, Ghana has roughly twice the per capita output of poorer countries in Western Africa. Gold, timber and cocoa production are major sources of foreign exchange. Receipts from the gold sector should help sustain GDP growth in the future.[10] Subsistence agriculture carried out via kin-based production regimes is the primary mode of livelihood. Small-scale trade is equally an imperative of rural economic life. For example, one commodity—an oilseed known as shea (*Butyrospermun parkii*)—is at the centre of these efforts. Procured, processed and traded predominantly by women, this wild tree crop is a staple of the West African economy. The primary source of edible oil in Ghana, as elsewhere in the sub-African Sahara region, shea serves as an important source of food for all and a crucial source of revenue for rural women in particular.[19]

GDP per capita is Intl $1272 (Appendix 4).

References

1 Report of the United Nations Development Programme 2004 (HDI 2002). Launched by the United Nations in 1990, the Human Development Index measures a country's achievements in three aspects of human development: longevity, knowledge and a decent standard of living. It was created to re-emphasize that people and their lives should be the ultimate criteria for assessing the development of a country, not economic growth. Current values range from 0.956 (Norway, first of 177 countries) to 0.273 (Sierra Leone, 177th out of 177 countries). Countries fall into one of three

groups: countries 1–55 = high development; 56–141 = medium development; 142–177 = low development. See: http://hdr.undp.org/statistics/data/indic/indic_8_1_1.html

2 IOELC interview: Mary Opare—4 June 2004.

3 IOELC interview: Terry Magee—24 March 2005.

4 Global Fund portfolio of grants.

5 International Narcotics Control Board. *Narcotic Drugs: Estimated World Requirements for 2004. Statistics for 2002*. New York: United Nations, 2004.

6 'The term *defined daily doses for statistical purposes* (S-DDD) replaces the term *defined daily doses* previously used by the Board. The S-DDDs are technical units of measurement for the purposes of statistical analysis and are not recommended prescription doses. Certain narcotic drugs may be used in certain countries for different treatments or in accordance with different medical practices, and therefore a different daily dose could be more appropriate'. The S-DDD used by the INCB for morphine is 100 mg. International Narcotics Control Board. *Narcotic Drugs: Estimated World Requirements for 2004. Statistics for 2002*. New York: United Nations, 2004: 176–177.

7 IOELC interview: Vinolia Tonugble—4 June 2004.

8 See AIHPC report at: http://www.hospicecare.com/travelfellow/tf2004/ghana.htm

9 Personal communication: Mary Callaway—25 November 2003.

10 See: http://www.cia.gov/cia/publications/factbook/geos/gh.html

11 This refers to adult mortality risk, which is defined as the probability of dying between 15 and 59 years.

12 See: WHO statistics for Ghana at: http://www.who.int/countries/gha/en/

13 http://www.unaids.org/en/geographical+area/by+country/ghana.asp

14 Total health expenditure per capita is the per capita amount of the sum of Public Health Expenditure (PHE) and Private Expenditure on Health (PvtHE). The international dollar is a common currency unit that takes into account differences in the relative purchasing power of various currencies. Figures expressed in international dollars are calculated using purchasing power parities (PPP), which are rates of currency conversion constructed to account for differences in price level between countries. http://www3.who.int/whosis/country/compare.cfm?country=s& indicator=strPcTotEOHinIntD2000&language=english

15 This composite measure of overall health system attainment is based on a country's goals relating to health, responsiveness and fairness in financing. The measure varies widely across countries and is highly correlated with general levels of human development as captured in the human development index. Tandon A, Murray CLJ, Lauer JA, Evans DB. *Measuring Overall Health System Performance for 191 Countries*. GPE Discussion Paper Series: No. 30; WHO.

16 **Jeong HW.** Economic reform and democratic transition in Ghana. *World Affairs* 1998; **160 (4)**: 218.

17 **Haynes J.** Democratic consolidation in Africa: the problematic case of Ghana. *Commonwealth and Comparative Politics* 2003; **41(1)**: 48.

18 **Jeong HW.** Ghana: lurching toward economic rationality. *World Affairs* 1996; **159(2)**: 64.

19 **Chalfin B.** Risky business: economic uncertainty, market reforms and female livelihoods in northeast Ghana. *Development and Change* 2000; **31(5)**: 987–1008.

Chapter 27

Lesotho

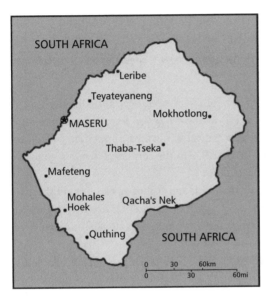

The Kingdom of Lesotho (population 1.8 million) is a mountainous, land-locked country completely surrounded by South Africa, which covers an area of 30 355 km². Formerly known as Bosutoland, the country was renamed when it gained independence from Britain in 1966. Maseru is the capital, and the country is divided into 10 districts for administrative purposes. Constitutional reforms preceded peaceful parliamentary elections in 2002.

According to the United Nations human development index (HDI), Lesotho is ranked 145th out of 177 countries worldwide (value 0.493)[1] and 17th out of 45 in African countries for which an index is available. This places Lesotho in the group of countries with low human development.

Palliative care service provision

Current services

The international Christian NGO, Beautiful Gate Ministries, aims to provide a range of services for disadvantaged children that includes hospice care for babies. The organization states:

> The care centre for abandoned and HIV/AIDS-affected children in Maseru, Lesotho, opened its doors in 2001 to provide care for abandoned or orphaned babies around Maseru. Initially we started out as Little Feet Ministry, but later joined forces with Beautiful Gate Ministries.
>
> As of November 2002, we have cared for a total of 46 babies, facilitated ten adoptions, 3 in foster-care pending adoption, returned 7 babies to families and 4 have passed away from HIV/AIDS related illnesses. Currently we have 25 babies in our care, five of whom are HIV+. We work closely with hospitals in the area and the police, who often discover abandoned children, as well as the departments of Social Welfare and Health. We also have the support of the Director of Social Welfare in Lesotho.

Beautiful Gate, Lesotho has two programmes: residential and hospice care, and an outreach programme. Through these programmes, we aim to:

- Provide loving care for abandoned and HIV+/AIDS babies between 0–5 years of age
- Give loving, dignified hospice care for those babies who are not placed with families, and who require specialised medical treatment
- Train and support our staff and the community in practical care-giving to HIV+/Aids and abandoned children
- Establish a foster-care/adoption programme in the community for abandoned and HIV+ children through networking with other organisations in Lesotho
- Provide biblical counselling for those in the community (especially children) affected by or infected with HIV/Aids.[2]

In Lesotho, HIV/AIDS has been the impetus for a perceived need for palliative care. A draft US Government Rapid Appraisal for HIV/AIDS Program Expansion in Lesotho[3] (Rapid Appraisal) identifies palliative care as a critical important component of an integrated health plan to combat the effects of HIV/AIDS in the country. However, palliative care is in reality, not at all developed.

Clinical and medical comprehensive palliative care and palliative care for children are nearly non-existent. Given the lack of progress in palliative care, service delivery in this regard primarily consists of fragmented social, spiritual and psychological support (with limited bereavement support).[3]

The National AIDS Strategic Plan 2002/2003–2004/2005 makes no reference to palliative care, and there are no palliative care policies or guidelines for pain control, and these have not been integrated into general health policies for dealing with cancer and other illnesses. Advocacy for palliative care is minimal, and it appears only on a limited basis in the nurses' training curriculum.

Suggestions for development in palliative care are highlighted in the short-term recommendations offered by the Rapid Appraisal.[3]

Palliative Care and Home and Community Based Care (HCBC):

- (OGAC) and the African Palliative Care Association (APCA), conduct a palliative care assessment as a first step in mobilizing the national response for palliative care.
- Provide technical assistance to form a National Palliative Care Association.
- Assist with a national participatory mapping and rapid assessment in collaboration with the US Office of the Global AIDS Coordinator exercise to identify current HCBC coverage and efforts, levels of HCBC being provided, gaps (geographic and provision of services), and to review the effectiveness of HCBC.
- Support training at the district and community levels in key technical areas: palliative care, children with HIV, psychological and emotional support, dealing with mental health issues, orphans and vulnerable children, communication skills, etc.

Family Health International (FHI) defines HCBC as 'the provision of care and support that endeavours to meet the nursing and psychosocial needs of persons with chronic illnesses and their family members in their home environment'.[4] While HCBC delivers patient care in the home environment, palliative care is an approach that attends to the needs of patients and families affected by a life-threatening illness in a variety of settings including the home, hospice, hospital, clinic and community.

A strong sense of community may be Lesotho's greatest strength in embracing palliative care to cope with the AIDS pandemic. Caring for others in the community is a traditional value. Community-based prevention and care activities, including peer education, are characteristics of the country's response to HIV/AIDS. Training in home-based care has been provided to 6000 community health workers. Home-based care and support groups for people living with HIV/AIDS and other illnesses are traditionally rooted and have been a spontaneous response to the health crisis. These include burial societies, traditional savings groups and womens' church groups who visit households with ill family members. The Rapid Appraisal recommends that these community-based initiatives be capitalized upon, but notes that there is no co-ordinating body or strategy to standardize or monitor HCBC provision. National training manuals provide some guidance but are limited in scope. HCBC workers in Lesotho described their work to the Rapid Appraisal team as set out in Table 27.1.[3]

Some plans have been developed for the creation of the Tsepong Community Hospice, to serve the areas of Tebellong, Qabane, Linakeng and Thabana-Tsooana. The objectives of the project are: to alleviate the effects of the HIV/AIDS crisis; to facilitate the development of a culture of community; to involve home-based care; and to develop an effective network of stakeholders such as churches, traditional healers and medical centres[6]. This initiative is being promoted by Sister Virginia Moorosi of the the Machaberg Hospital at Qacha's nek and would seek to raise funds through agricultural and horticultural projects. A needs assessment for HIV/AIDS was conducted in the district in 2003.[7] The report states that the hospice committee involves a large number of local people from several villages as well as a number of key individuals in the District of Qacha. A field has been donated for a building plot; rocks have been gathered and some fruit trees planted; there is potential for further land to be used for agricultural purposes. The vision in the community is to build a facility for respite care, and to offer training courses to the long-term sick. However, plans for the building will require significant capital investment beyond that available in the district.

Sister Moorosi describes the situation:

> I'm a social worker, so my work is to see the welfare of people, to see that people are having the higher standard of living, understanding how they can be infected or affected by HIV and AIDS and other terminal diseases, so while I was doing the research going on making the assemblies in the societies, I realized that there was a need to build a hospice where people can get counselling, where people, when they are neglected by their families, maybe two to three days they can come to the hospice to get counselling, even to get moral support, spiritual support, counselling, and other things, maybe washing, this can maybe raise their spirits up and go back to their families . . . After

Table 27.1 Lesotho HCBC workers' description of their work to the Rapid Appraisal team

Activity	Description
Respite care, e.g. house keeping and washing of clothes, blankets and linen.	This is often done on a daily basis for bedridden clients who are living on their own. For clients with other household members, it is done approximately on an as needed basis
Cooking	Daily basis for bedridden clients if food is available; as needed for those with other household members
Bathing client	Daily basis for bedridden clients who are living alone and as needed for those with other members in household
General assessment	Per visit, but there is no checklist, monitoring tool for clients or guide for consistency.
Monitoring of medication	Inconsistent observation for clients on medication—HCBC workers not trained in any aspect of medication use
Provision of panadol, paracetamol, nystatin	As needed per opinion of client and HCBC worker. Panadol and paracetamol are given for just about any symptom. Use of nystatin not clearly articulated
Counselling and prayer	Much of the support is in the area of counselling and prayer. Clients as well as HCBC workers often belong to different churches. An interdenominational approach is most commonly used
Referrals primarily to clinic and other care and support services	As needed, yet no clear guidelines or resource guide. Clinic relationships vary according to staff. HCBC workers reportedly try to accompany client to clinic and at times will use own money to pay for the visit and/or medications
Provision of traditional remedies	Basotho commonly uses traditional remedies. The most often cited is Soso, a drink made from boiling a mixture of peach tree branch, pine tree bark, grape leaf, African potato (moli), algae (bolele), aloe (moriri oa matlpa) and mofifi[5] which is sipped throughout the day. Soso is believed to clean ones blood, provide strength and to help with ulcers, but is *not* believed to cure AIDS or other illnesses. Other types of traditional remedies were also cited
Pain management	No access to pain medication or systematic way of assessing/managing pain. Heavy reliance on panadol and paracetamol without clear understanding of the difference
Material support	HCBC workers provide as much as they can from their own homes. Some HCBC groups have started their own gardens to provide fresh vegetables to clients and a few are starting IGA activities with the hope of raising money to support clients
Nutritional support	Donations from HCBC workers. Inconsistent and loosely targeted food assistance from WFP and UNICEF. Monitoring of food intake—including asking client what they will eat that day and checking in the home to see if the food is there

the research I got 3000 orphans in that place, it's where I was thinking that I can build a hospice for alleviation of those people living there, to give them education and to see how they can come to a better knowledge of how to understand how to take care of themselves, even these affected orphans. Up to now I have made a training of support groups, these are volunteers, people in the villages, and I did ask the government but the government also it's helping very little by supporting as well the workshops, to support the sick people and to those orphans by distributing the kits, and the paracetamols and small medicines to take care of the sick people . . . Because out of the research I made I have realized that many are dying alone in their families because of the neglect they get, because of the poverty, they don't get food nutrition and their cleanliness hygienically, they are not given by the carers because financially people in Lesotho are very poor and many are not working so they cannot tolerate with the sick people for a long time.[8]

Reimbursement and funding for services

As at March 2005, funding sources for palliative care in Lesotho were minimal. Lesotho is a non-focus country for the President's Emergency Plan for AIDS Relief (PEPFAR). However, the US government has pledged to provide technical support to the Government of Lesotho in key technical areas across the continuum of HIV-related health care. This will range from prevention to treatment and palliative care for adults and children.[3]

The Global Fund to Fight AIDS, Tuberculosis, and Malaria (GFATM) Round 2 HIV/AIDS grant[9] is for US$29 million over 5 years. The aim is to strengthen prevention and control of HIV/AIDS in Lesotho and to reduce HIV prevalence by 15 per cent. The funds, once released, are to be distributed through the Ministry of Finance and Development Planning. The World Bank approved US$5 million over 4 years from early 2005 to increase the capacity of the Lesotho government and community-based organizations to implement Global Fund activities, including provision of antiretroviral therapies and the training of 100 HCBC workers per district per year for 5 years. Palliative care is not mentioned in the GFATM grant.

Limited funding for HCBC comes from charities, small donors, faith-based organizations and mission hospitals. A characteristic of HCBC in this country is the willingness of workers to use their own limited resources to assist the ill and needy in their communities. The Rapid Appraisal states:

> HCBC workers do not receive any remuneration, payment, incentive or subsidies in cash or kind; instead, they use their own resources to help the families they are working with. This is viewed as a major challenge for the workers as they find it very difficult to 'go to someone's home that is hungry, sick and has nothing and not give something to help them'. Many instances are cited of giving food from their own gardens or supplies, blankets, transport money for the clinic, soap, etc. In extreme cases, this has caused problems for the workers with their spouses who become upset that 'the little they have is being given away'. The workers expressed a strong desire that even if they are not paid for what they do that they are given assistance to find ways of providing for the families they work with. Despite the HCBC workers' limited resources, they collectively provide HCBC to large numbers of people and use their own very limited resources to care for, feed and support ill people in their communities.[3]

Opioid availability and consumption

According to the International Narcotics Control Board,[10] the average defined daily dose consumption of morphine for statistical purposes (S-DDD)[11] in Lesotho (2000–2002) was 8 (Appendix 1).

According to the Rapid Appraisal, drug access in Lesotho for symptom control and pain management is limited. Pain management in health facilities and households primarily consists of aspirin, paracetamol, ibuprofen and Indocid. There is limited availability of morphine, especially oral morphine. The Rapid Appraisal prioritizes the need for greater accessibility to morphine, as part of a holistic approach to palliative care:

> While pain management, specifically access to opioids including morphine, is a priority for quality palliative care, comprehensive programs should address a wide range of needs including non-pharmaceutical pain management skills, management of chronic diarrhoea, cough and skin disorders, oral health, increasing ability to carry out activities of daily living, spiritual and emotional support and palliative care for infants and children.[3]

National and professional organizations

There is no national palliative care association in Lesotho. The need to form a national body is recognized in order significantly to promote the development of palliative care in the country. This development is identified as a priority in the Rapid Appraisal draft report.

Education and training

Minimal community-level home-based care training for volunteers is provided through the National HCBC training guide. The Ministry of Health and Social Welfare has developed a strong network of >6000 trained community health workers. Neither community health workers nor HCBC workers are trained in palliative care. There is a severe shortage of professional human resources in the country, and notably of nurses and social workers. This means there is no skilled help for families having to cope with the personal and interpersonal complications brought about by a life-threatening illness, and HIV/AIDS in particular. The Rapid Appraisal recommends that HCBC training should include the key technical areas of palliative care, HIV-positive children, psychological and emotional support, communication skills and identifying orphans and vulnerable children.[3]

Palliative care workforce capacity

There are no palliative care workers in Lesotho. The organizations currently delivering HIV counselling and testing are, however, well placed to integrate palliative care skills into their work. There are seven free-standing service points for HIV counselling and testing (HCT). Additional HCT services within health facilities are available in all 17 health service areas around the country.

History and development of hospice–palliative care in Lesotho

If recommendations to the US government made by the Rapid Appraisal team are acted upon, palliative care in Lesotho could begin to develop using already existing community groups and linking closely with HIV/AIDS programmes. The US government is urged to consider supporting the following recommendations in the report:[3]

Short term:

In collaboration with the US Office of the Global AIDS Coordinator (OGAC) and the African Palliative Care Association (APCA), conduct a palliative care assessment as a first step in mobilizing the national response for palliative care. It is recommended that the team be comprised of local stakeholders including People Living with HIV/AIDS (PLWHA) and traditional healers.

Provide technical assistance to form a National Palliative Care Association.

Medium and long term:

Provide technical assistance in the following key areas:

- Inclusion of palliative care in the soon-to-be-revised National AIDS Strategic Plan;
- Development of national palliative care policy, guidelines, standards and protocols including palliative care for children;
- Development of a national M&E system for palliative care; and
- Inclusion of pain and symptom management and other critical elements of palliative care in HCBC assessments.

Provide technical and programmatic assistance for:

- Pre- and in-service training of health professionals and training of community-based health workers
- Non Governmental Organisations, Community Based Organisations and Faith Based Organisations including those working in HCBC to increase their palliative care skills and program coverage.
- Provide support to strengthen and advocate for community-level palliative care for the spectrum of the population from infants to the elderly (using a family-centred approach). Some of this support can include the adaptation of the up-coming southern Africa Palliative Care Training Guide for Children Living with HIV and other Life-Threatening Illnesses.

Life/oral histories

Sr Virginia Moorosi—*Social Worker*: interviewed by David Clark, 2 June 2004. Length of interview: 22 min.

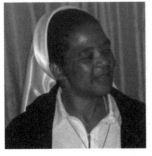

Sister Virginia Moorosi, of the Charity of the Sacred Heart of Jesus, is a social worker based in the government hospital of a remote rural area—Qacha's District, in Lesotho. She describes the problems of local people who are migrant workers in South Africa. They return infected with HIV and other diseases, which are then transmitted to their families. Thousands of people are dying with AIDS and, in a study undertaken by Sister Moorosi, some 3000 orphans were identified. She would like to build a hospice in her community and knows of another similar plan elsewhere in Lesotho.

Sr Moorosi was born in Lesotho in 1960. She joined her religious order in 1979 having been sponsored by the government of Lesotho to attend the University of Dar es Salaam in Tanzania to study for an Advanced Diploma in Social Work.

Ethical issues

The Rapid Appraisal:

> Basotho have a long tradition of caring for one another with the aim of relieving suffering and dying with dignity. Basotho will not directly say that someone is dying, they know when death is coming, and will express it through words such as '*bophelo bo hae bo felile*' (his or her life is finished). When these words are spoken, it is expected that the person will soon die. Basotho will try, by all means, to be with a person who is ill, to provide physical, spiritual and emotional comfort and to be there at the time of death. If someone is left alone during the time of suffering and death, it is considered to be a very sad affair. What may seem to be simple words, actions or desires are actually critical to the provision of palliative care and are indications that although formal palliative care is not provided, there is a strong traditional foundation that must be built upon to provide comprehensive care at the facility, community and household levels. Although the provision of formal comprehensive palliative care is nearly non-existent in Lesotho, it is clear that the tradition of care-giving among Basotho will provide a strong foundation for the implementation and scaling-up of palliative care.[3]

Public health context

Population

Lesotho's population of around 1.8 million is made up of the following ethnic groups: Sotho 99.7 per cent, and Europeans, Asians and other 0.3 per cent.

Religious groups include: Christian 80 per cent and indigenous beliefs 20 per cent.[12]

Epidemiology

In Lesotho, the WHO World Health Report (2003) indicates an adult mortality[13] rate per 1000 population of 902 for males and 742 for females. Life expectancy for males is 32.9; for females 38.2. Healthy life expectancy is 29.6 for males; and 33.2 for females.[14]

Lesotho is one of the worst HIV/AIDS-affected countries in Southern Africa and is facing a crisis of tremendous proportions. Estimates suggest that in this country of <2 million people, between 290 000 and 360 000 people were living with HIV/AIDS at the end of 2003. In the same year, up to 39 000 adults and children are thought to have died from the disease (Table 27.1). UNAIDS estimates that 31 per cent of the population are infected with HIV.

UNAIDS reports:

> AIDS constitutes an alarming threat to Lesotho and its people. HIV/AIDS, moreover, is not the only barrier to Lesotho's recovery from crisis. Land degradation, capacity depletion and economic decline are major obstacles to short- and long-term responses to humanitarian and development needs.
>
> The government has taken concrete actions to address the epidemic through the declaration of HIV/AIDS as a national disaster, the development of a National AIDS Strategic Plan (NASP) and

Table 27.2 Lesotho HIV and AIDS estimates, end 2003

Adult (15–49) HIV prevalence rate	28.9 per cent (range: 26.3–31.7 per cent)
Adults (15–49) living with HIV	300 000 (range: 270 000–330 000)
Adults and children (0–49) living with HIV	320 000 (range: 290 000–360 000)
Women (15–49) living with HIV	170 000 (range: 150 000–190 000)
AIDS deaths (adults and children) in 2003	29 000 (range: 22 000–39 000)

Source: 2004 Report of the global AIDS epidemic.

the establishment of the Lesotho AIDS Programme Coordinating Authority (LAPCA) under the Prime Minister's Office. The LAPCA was set up in 2001 to coordinate the multisectoral response to HIV/AIDS, but several factors have hindered the LAPCA in fulfilling its strategic role.

Lack of technical staff and the weak state of this coordinating body have undermined its effectiveness and adversely affected the national response. Most of the key posts remain unfilled, including that of the chief executive, which has been vacant since March 2003.

The move to establish a semi-autonomous national commission on HIV/AIDS is a timely and a corrective measure.

NGOs and community-based organizations have provided the mainstay of the response to HIV/AIDS in the country, especially in the area of community mobilization. Most of these operations are small and localized to specific geographical areas in urban centres. People living with HIV have formed support groups and are making a contribution to the fight against HIV/AIDS.

The biggest challenge lies in the establishment of national networks and civil society organizations on HIV/AIDS, most importantly among people living with HIV/AIDS and the NGO network.[15]

Health care system

In 2001, the total per capita expenditure on health care was Intl $101; 5.5% of GDP[16] (Appendix 3).

The WHO overall health system performance score places Lesotho 183rd out of 191 countries.[17]

Political economy

Small, landlocked and mountainous, Lesotho relies on remittances from miners employed in South Africa and customs duties from the Southern Africa Customs Union for the majority of government revenue, but the government has strengthened its tax system to reduce dependency on customs duties. Completion of a major hydropower facility in January 1998 now permits the sale of water to South Africa, also generating royalties for Lesotho. As the number of mineworkers has declined steadily over the past several years, a small manufacturing base has developed based on farm products that support the milling, canning, leather and jute industries, and a rapidly growing apparel-assembly sector. The economy is still primarily based on subsistence agriculture, especially livestock, although drought has decreased agricultural activity. The extreme inequality in the distribution of income remains a major drawback. Lesotho has signed an Interim Poverty Reduction and Growth Facility with the IMF.[12]

GDP per capita is Intl $1844 (Appendix 4).

References

1 Report of the United Nations Development Programme 2004 (HDI 2002). Launched by the United Nations in 1990, the Human Development Index measures a country's achievements in three aspects of human development: longevity, knowledge and a decent standard of living. It was created to re-emphasize that people and their lives should be the ultimate criteria for assessing the development of a country, not economic growth. Current values range from 0.956 (Norway, first of 177 countries) to 0.273 (Sierra Leone, 177th out of 177 countries). Countries fall into one of three groups: countries 1–55 = high development; 56–141 = medium development; 142–177 = low development. See: http://hdr.undp.org/statistics/data/indic/indic_8_1_1.html

2 See: http://www.beautifulgate.org/lesover.php

3 Draft report of US Government Rapid Appraisal for HIV/AIDS Program Expansion. Lesotho. September 5–13 2004. USAID and CDC.

4 Family Health International, Comprehensive Care and Support Framework.

5 No translation is available for mofifi.

6 Information provided by Sr Virginia Moorosi.

7 Dr Graham Thomas. *Wales Lesotho Link, HIV Health Needs Assessment 2003: Tebelong Community, Qacha's District, Lesotho.*

8 IOELC interview: Sr Virginia Moorosi—2 June 2004.

9 Global Fund to Fight Tuberculosis, AIDS and Malaria.

10 International Narcotics Control Board. *Narcotic Drugs: Estimated World Requirements for 2004. Statistics for 2002.* New York: United Nations, 2004.

11 'The term *defined daily doses for statistical purposes* (S-DDD) replaces the term *defined daily doses* previously used by the Board. The S-DDDs are technical units of measurement for the purposes of statistical analysis and are not recommended prescription doses. Certain narcotic drugs may be used in certain countries for different treatments or in accordance with different medical practices, and therefore a different daily dose could be more appropriate'. The S-DDD used by the INCB for morphine is 100 mg. International Narcotics Control Board. *Narcotic Drugs: Estimated World Requirements for 2004. Statistics for 2002.* New York: United Nations, 2004: 176–177.

12 See: http://www.cia.gov/cia/publications/factbook/geos/lt.html

13 This refers to adult mortality risk, which is defined as the probability of dying between 15 and 59 years.

14 See: WHO statistics for Lesotho at: http://www.who.int/countries/lso/en/

15 http://www.unaids.org/en/geographical+area/by+country/lesotho.asp

16 Total health expenditure per capita is the per capita amount of the sum of Public Health Expenditure (PHE) and Private Expenditure on Health (PvtHE). The international dollar is a common currency unit that takes into account differences in the relative purchasing power of various currencies. Figures expressed in international dollars are calculated using purchasing power parities

(PPP), which are rates of currency conversion constructed to account for differences in price level between countries.
http://www3.who.int/whosis/country/compare.cfm?country=s&indicator=strPcTotEOHinInt D2000&language=english

17 This composite measure of overall health system attainment is based on a country's goals relating to health, responsiveness and fairness in financing. The measure varies widely across countries and is highly correlated with general levels of human development as captured in the human development index. Tandon A, Murray CLJ, Lauer JA, Evans DB. *Measuring Overall Health System Performance for 191 Countries*. GPE Discussion Paper Series: No. 30; WHO.

Chapter 28

Mozambique

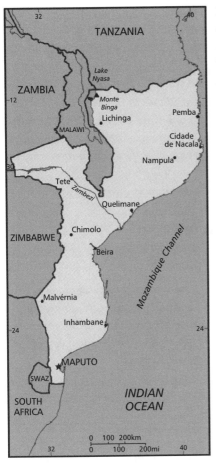

Mozambique (population 18.54 million) is a country in south eastern Africa that covers an area of 801 590 km². Its boundaries border Tanzania, Malawi, Zambia, Zimbabwe, South Africa and the Mozambique Channel. Almost five centuries as a Portuguese colony came to a close with independence in 1975. The following years were marked by economic dependence on South Africa, severe drought, and a prolonged civil war which hindered the country's development. Maputo, with its population of 1.1 million, is the capital city. For administrative purposes, the country is divided into 10 provinces.

According to the United Nations human development index (HDI), Mozambique is ranked 171st out of 177 countries worldwide (value 0.354)[1] and 39th out of 45 in African countries for which an index is available.

This places Mozambique in the group of countries with low human development.

Palliative care service provision

Current services

As at March 2005 palliative care in the country was non-existent.

The health repercussions of the AIDS epidemic have been the impetus for introducing care to the chronically ill in Mozambique. The Ministry of Health introduced regulations in 2002 to standardize and monitor home-based care for people living with HIV/AIDS and other chronic illnesses. Although the Ministry of Health does not implement or finance this care, policies have been established to guide practice and to supervise and co-ordinate implementing partners. Education, patient care and counselling are prioritized in the programme, and a palliative care component is included. The home-based care policies form part of an integrated approach to a national expansion in health care.[2]

Family Health International (FHI) defines home and community-based care (HCBC) as 'the provision of care and support that endeavours to meet the nursing and psychosocial needs of persons with chronic illnesses and their family members in their home environment'.[3] While HCBC delivers patient care in the home environment, palliative care is an approach that attends to the needs of patients and families affected by a life-threatening illness in a variety of settings including the home, hospice, hospital, clinic and community.

During 2004, there were 47 home-based care programmes operating in all but one of the provinces in the country, serving 17 790 people. All home-based care programmes are run by NGOs or community-based organizations (CBOs).

In a 5-year programme supported by the Global Fund from 2004, HIV/AIDS-related programmes are to be scaled up. Palliative care is not mentioned in the agreement although the provision of antiretroviral therapy forms part of the continuum of care for people living with HIV/AIDS. Salient points include the following:

◆ The proposal aims to reduce the spread of HIV/AIDS in Mozambique and mitigate the impact of HIV/AIDS among those already infected through the provision of a comprehensive programme of prevention, care and support

◆ The proposal builds on existing community, government and non-governmental organisation activities

◆ Targeted interventions include community and school based programmes, peer education, establishment of youth friendly services, training of health care workers, institutional and technical support to youth associations, community, condom promotion/distribution, support to PLWA and orphans, non-governmental organization strengthening, increased access to home care based services

◆ Fifty voluntary counselling and testing (VCT) centres are to be established within 5 years

◆ Fifty-six day clinics are to be established to treat 56 000 HIV-infected patients for opportunistic infections

◆ Antiretroviral therapies will be provided in 22 clinics to 20 000 patients

◆ Treatment for sexually transmitted infections will be implemented

◆ Interventions to prevent mother to child transmission (PMTCT) will include administering 20 000 newborns with nevirapine.[4]

Reimbursement and funding for services

Home-based care is primarily provided by donor-funded NGOs and CBOs whose volunteers are paid a stipend.

President's Emergency Plan for AIDS Relief (PEPFAR)[5]

During the 2004 financial year (FY), funding of around US$25.53 million was enacted for country-managed programmes in Mozambique and US$11.86 million for central programmes. During FY2005, it is anticipated that a total of US$54.68 million will be enacted: US$48.22 million for country-managed programmes and US$6.46 million for central programmes.[6]

The Global Fund

The Global Fund signed an agreement on 2 April 2004 for US$7.5 million over a 2-year period. Round 2 of this programme will focus on prevention and mitigation of the social impact of HIV/AIDS. Funds will be disbursed through the National AIDS Council (CNCS) of Mozambique and the Ministry of Health of the Government of Mozambique.

Opioid availability and consumption

The International Narcotics Control Board[7] has published the following figures for the consumption of narcotic drugs in Mozambique: codeine 2 kg; and pethidine 4 kg.

For the years 2000–2002, there was no reported average defined daily dose consumption of morphine for statistical purposes (S-DDD)[8] in Mozambique (Appendix 1).

Palliative care coverage

Palliative care has yet to be established in Mozambique. Home-based care provision is primarily targeted at people with HIV identified as Stage 3 and 4 according to the WHO staging protocol. Others living with chronic and debilitating illnesses are also included.

Education and training

The Ministry of Health runs an accredited 'training of trainers' programme for trainers working with home-based care-implementing organizations. There are 53 accredited trainers in the country. Of these, 75 per cent have some health training. The Ministry of Health also trains health personnel in opportunistic infection treatment with a home-based care component and a separate module on palliative care. These are minimum standards, and organizations are encouraged to provide additional training. An annual task force meeting provides a forum for organizations to discuss their work.[2]

Palliative care workforce capacity

The Ministry of Health has the following employees in the home-based care programme:

+ Central level: one technical advisor seconded from Centers for Disease Control (CDC), one co-ordinator, two trainers
+ Provincial level: one focal point in each of the 11 provinces. They are not exclusively dedicated to the home-based care programme due to a severe shortage of human resources.

- Technical support: health personnel at 79 health centres and CBO staff are trained in treating opportunistic infections. They provide technical support to home-based care programme volunteers and are based at the health centres. They do not undertake home visits.

- NGOs/CBOs: implement home-based care at the community level. Most volunteers are chosen according to their standing in the community and desire to help rather than through a selection process, due to the severe shortage of qualified personnel.

Public health context

Population

Mozambique's population of around 18.54 million is made up of the following ethnic groups: indigenous groups 99.66 per cent (Makhuwa, Tsonga, Lomwe, Sena and others), Europeans 0.06 per cent, Euro-Africans 0.2 per cent and Indians 0.08 per cent.

Religious groups include: indigenous beliefs 50 per cent, Christian 30 per cent and Muslim 20 per cent.[9]

Epidemiology

In Mozambique, the WHO World Health Report (2004) indicates an adult mortality[10] rate per 1000 population of 613 for males and 519 for females. Life expectancy for males is 41.2; for females 43.9. Healthy life expectancy is 36.3 for males; and 37.5 for females.[11]

Mozambique has a high HIV prevalence, with the majority of new infections occurring among those under 29 years old. Estimates suggest that in Mozambique, between 980 000 and 1.7 million people were living with HIV/AIDS at the end of 2003. In the same year, up to 160 000 adults and children are thought to have died from the disease (Table 28.1).

UNAIDS reports:

> Without an aggressive response to HIV/AIDS, life expectancy is projected to drop from 50.3 to 36 years by 2010. Underscoring the seriousness of the epidemic, major political leaders consistently refer to HIV/AIDS as a major threat to the nation's development.

Table 28.1 Mozambique HIV and AIDS estimates, end 2003

Adult (15–49) HIV prevalence rate	12.2 per cent (range: 9.4–15.7 per cent)
Adults (15–49) living with HIV	1 200 000 (range: 910 000–1 500 000)
Adults and children (0–49) living with HIV	1 300 000 (range: 980 000–1 700 000)
Women (15–49) living with HIV	670 000 (range: 520 000–860 000)
AIDS deaths (adults and children) in 2003	110 000 (range: 74 000–160 000)

Source: 2004 Report of the global AIDS epidemic.

A National AIDS Council (NAC), chaired by the prime minister, was established in May 2000. A National Strategic Plan (2001–2003) was launched the same year. The plan for 2004–2009 is expected to be revised by June 2004. The NAC established a Partners' Forum in 2003. Civil society's weak institutional and technical capacities, as well as lack of financial resources, have limited their effective involvement.

The World Bank has allocated US$5 million to develop the capacity of civil society organizations and an additional US$25 million to support their initiatives. The private sector will be mobilized and the Business Against AIDS network will be better supported with the World Bank grant and UN support.

More than US$500 million have been pledged or committed by the Global Fund, the Clinton Foundation and the World Bank MAP for the next five years. Mozambique will also benefit from the US Emergency Plan for AIDS Relief (PEPFAR), enabling a significant scale-up.[12]

Health care system

In 2001, the total per capita expenditure on health care was Intl $47; 5.9% of GDP[13] (Appendix 3).

The WHO overall health system performance score places Mozambique 184th out of 191 countries.[14]

Political economy

At independence in 1975, Mozambique was one of the world's poorest countries, exacerbated by a long civil war from 1977 to 1992. In 1987, the government embarked on a series of macroeconomic reforms designed to stabilize the economy. These steps, combined with donor assistance and with political stability since the multiparty elections in 1994, have led to dramatic improvements in the country's growth rate. Inflation was reduced to single digits during the late 1990s although it returned to double digits in 2000–2003. Fiscal reforms, including the introduction of a value-added tax and reform of the customs service, have improved the government's revenue collection abilities. In spite of these gains, Mozambique remains dependent upon foreign assistance for much of its annual budget, and the majority of the population remains below the poverty line. Subsistence agriculture continues to employ the vast majority of the country's workforce. A substantial trade imbalance persists, although the opening of the MOZAL aluminum smelter, the country's largest foreign investment project to date, has increased export earnings. Additional investment projects in titanium extraction and processing, and garment manufacturing should further close the import/export gap. Mozambique's once substantial foreign debt has been reduced under the IMF's Heavily Indebted Poor Countries (HIPC) and Enhanced HIPC initiatives, and is now at a manageable level.[9]

GDP per capita is Intl $805 (Appendix 4).

References

1 Report of the United Nations Development Programme 2004 (HDI 2002). Launched by the United Nations in 1990, the Human Development Index measures a country's achievements in three aspects of human development: longevity, knowledge and a decent standard of living. It was created to

re-emphasize that people and their lives should be the ultimate criteria for assessing the development of a country, not economic growth. Current values range from 0.956 (Norway, first of 177 countries) to 0.273 (Sierra Leone, 177th out of 177 countries). Countries fall into one of three groups: countries 1–55 = high development; 56–141 = medium development; 142–177 = low development. See: http://hdr.undp.org/statistics/data/indic/indic_8_1_1.html

2 Personal communication: Sandy McGunegill—18 February 2005.

3 Family Health International, Comprehensive Care and Support Framework.

4 Global Fund for Tuberculosis, AIDS and Malaria. Portfolio of Grants in Mozambique.

5 See: http://www.usaid.gov/our_work/global_health/aids/pepfarfact.html

6 *Engendering Bold Leadership*. The President's Emergency Plan for AIDS Relief. First Annual Report to Congress, 2005: 115. http://www.state.gov/documents/organization/43885.pdf

7 International Narcotics Control Board. *Narcotic Drugs: Estimated World Requirements for 2004. Statistics for 2002*. New York: United Nations, 2004.

8 'The term *defined daily doses for statistical purposes* (S-DDD) replaces the term *defined daily doses* previously used by the Board. The S-DDDs are technical units of measurement for the purposes of statistical analysis and are not recommended prescription doses. Certain narcotic drugs may be used in certain countries for different treatments or in accordance with different medical practices, and therefore a different daily dose could be more appropriate'. The S-DDD used by the INCB for morphine is 100 mg. International Narcotics Control Board. *Narcotic Drugs: Estimated World Requirements for 2004. Statistics for 2002*. New York: United Nations, 2004: 176–177.

9 See: http://www.cia.gov/cia/publications/factbook/geos/mz.html

10 This refers to adult mortality risk, which is defined as the probability of dying between 15 and 59 years.

11 See: WHO statistics for Mozambique at: http://www.who.int/countries/moz/en/

12 http://www.unaids.org/en/geographical+area/by+country/mozambique.asp

13 Total health expenditure per capita is the per capita amount of the sum of Public Health Expenditure (PHE) and Private Expenditure on Health (PvtHE). The international dollar is a common currency unit that takes into account differences in the relative purchasing power of various currencies. Figures expressed in international dollars are calculated using purchasing power parities (PPP), which are rates of currency conversion constructed to account for differences in price level between countries.
http://www3.who.int/whosis/country/compare.cfm?country=s&indicator=strPcTotEOHinIntD2000&language=english

14 This composite measure of overall health system attainment is based on a country's goals relating to health, responsiveness and fairness in financing. The measure varies widely across countries and is highly correlated with general levels of human development as captured in the human development index. Tandon A, Murray CLJ, Lauer JA, Evans DB. *Measuring Overall Health System Performance for 191 Countries*. GPE Discussion Paper Series: No. 30; WHO.

Chapter 29

Namibia

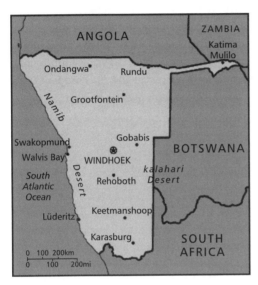

Namibia (population 1.95 million) is a country in Southern Africa bordering the South Atlantic Ocean that covers an area of 825 418 km^2. Its boundaries border Angola, Zambia, Botswana and South Africa. The capital of Namibia is Windhoek.

According to the United Nations human development index (HDI), Namibia is ranked 126th out of 177 countries worldwide (value 0.607)[1] and seventh out of 45 in African countries for which an index is available. This places Namibia in the group of countries with medium human development.

Palliative care service provision

Current services

In Namibia, home-based care provides the only service approximating to palliative care. The impetus for the development of these services has been the AIDS epidemic. It is estimated that 22.3 per cent of all pregnant women in Namibia are HIV positive and that 16 per cent of all children under the age of 15 have lost one or both parents.[2] There are an estimated 18 000 registered orphans and vulnerable children (OVCs) in Namibia. In response to the AIDS prevalence in the country, the US-funded Population Services International (PSI) opened two New Start Voluntary Counselling and Testing (VCT) centres in 2003, with more planned for 2004.

> What we have as palliative care so far in Namibia is really home-based care—it is most often without a true end-of-life specialty. Oral morphine is rarely provided outside the hospital setting, and that is what must be changed for this specialty to really take hold in this country. The good news is that oral morphine is schedule one drug and can move out of health facility into the community very easily.[3]

Catholic Aids Action (CAA)

This faith-based organization was established in 1998 and operates 14 offices nationally. It provides home-based care, HIV prevention education, VCT, support for OVCs, and community mobilization.[2]

The team networks widely with local agencies. Patients are referred to local clinics and district hospitals for treatment of opportunistic infections and ARV therapies. Referrals are made to government social workers for social welfare grants, while local pastors and churches are drawn on for spiritual support. Local NGOs provide material support. CAA advocates on behalf of its patients for school attendance, human rights and inheritance rights. Food remains the most significant issue to manage, and soup kitchens are run by this organization. CAA provides limited material support (such as school uniforms), advocacy for access to education, and experiential learning camps and Art Days for OVCs.

CAA reported the following service provision as at the third quarter of 2004:

- 313 VCT tests
- 6009 HIV-positive clients registered
- 2554 OVC material assistance
- 1727 OVC registered for activities
- 35 906 contacts for information, education and referral
- 17 085 meals to HIV-affected people
- 2836 participants in Stepping Stones (HIV education programme)
- Adventures Unlimited (Christian programme)[2]

Reimbursement and funding for services

Global Fund[4]

A portfolio of Global Fund Round 2 grants to Namibia includes specific funding for HIV/AIDS: Scaling up the Fight Against HIV/AIDS in Namibia. Signed on 23 November 2004, the 2-year agreement provides US$26 082 802 to be disbursed through the Ministry of Health and Social Services. The agreement is part of a 5-year proposal covering prevention, care and support. Youth education, condom promotion and distribution, increased access to VCT and prevention of mother-to-child transmission intervention, as well as ARV treatment and prophylaxis, and treatment of opportunistic infections are proposed.

President's Emergency Plan for AIDS Relief (PEPFAR)[5]

During the 2004 financial year (FY), funding of around US$21.19 million was enacted for country-managed programmes in Namibia and $3.09 million for central programmes. During FY2005, it is anticipated that a total of US$39.71 million will be enacted: US$36.01 million for country-managed programmes and US$3.70 million for central programmes.[6]

Opioid availability and consumption

The International Narcotics Control Board[7] has published the following figures for the consumption of narcotic drugs in Namibia: morphine 2 kg; and pethidine 4 kg.

For the years 2000–2002, the average defined daily dose consumption of morphine for statistical purposes (S-DDD)[8] in Namibia was 73 (Appendix 1).

National and professional organizations

In order for palliative care to develop and be effectively co-ordinated in Namibia, it will be necessary to create a national palliative care association. It is anticipated this may happen in August 2005, with CAA taking a leading role in its development.[3]

Palliative care coverage

Approximately 50 000 people living with advanced HIV infection in Namibia received either home-based or health facility-based care in 2004. This is provided by the public sector and NGOs.[3]

Catholic Aids Action

This organization registered 6009 HIV-positive patients by the third quarter of 2004.

Education and training

There is no formal training in palliative care in Namibia. Doctors and nurses are exposed to the Ministry of Health and Social Services guidelines for clinical management of HIV/AIDS and other chronic diseases.

Home-based care volunteers are trained by their organizations. Over 1700 trained and active CAA volunteers each received 64 h of training by the end of 2004. They are supported by monthly visits by staff, and receive limited incentives and supplies for their time. The volunteers' home care curriculum briefly covers psycho-social support of children and paediatric HIV.[2]

Palliative care workforce capacity

Catholic Aids Action

Approximately 1903 active volunteers work with people living with HIV/AIDS. By the end of 2004, the organization employed 90 staff as well as the volunteers.

Population

Namibia's population of around 1.95 million is made up of the following ethnic groups: about 50 per cent of the population belong to the Ovambo tribe and 9 per cent to the Kavangos tribe; other ethnic groups include Herero 7 per cent, Damara 7 per cent, Nama 5 per cent, Caprivian 4 per cent, Bushmen 3 per cent, Baster 2 per cent and Tswana 0.5 per cent.

Table 29.1 Namibia HIV and AIDS estimates, end 2003

Adult (15–49) HIV prevalence rate	21.3 per cent (range: 18.2–24.7 per cent)
Adults (15–49) living with HIV	200 000 (range: 170 000–230 000)
Adults and children (0–49) living with HIV	210 000 (range: 180 000–250 000)
Women (15–49) living with HIV	110 000 (range: 94 000–130 000)
AIDS deaths (adults and children) in 2003	16 000 (range: 11 000–22 000)

Source: 2004 Report of the global AIDS epidemic.

Religious groups include: Christian 80–90 per cent (Lutheran 50 per cent at least) and indigenous beliefs 10–20 per cent.[9]

Epidemiology

In Namibia, the WHO World Health Report (2004) indicates an adult mortality[10] rate per 1000 population of 605 for males and 529 for females. Life expectancy for males is 48.1; for females 50.5. Healthy life expectancy is 42.9 for males; and 43.8 for females.[11]

Namibia is severely affected by the HIV/AIDS crisis affecting countries in Southern Africa. Estimates suggest that in Namibia, between 180 000 and 250 000 people were living with HIV/AIDS at the end of 2003. In the same year, up to 22 000 adults and children are thought to have died from the disease (Table 29.1).

UNAIDS reports:

> Existing and anticipated poverty levels have significant implications for the spread of HIV and other diseases. Poverty is associated with food insecurity; parents of about 30% of all children are unable to provide nutritious food of adequate quality and required frequency. Based on the report of the 2002 National HIV Sentinel Survey published by the Ministry of Health and Social Services (MHSS), the HIV/AIDS prevalence rate among pregnant women attending antenatal care was estimated at 22%. Half of Namibia's population survives on approximately 10% of the average income. The national unemployment rate is 35%, and there is a significant disparity in income distribution across the population.
>
> The greater burden of the epidemic falls on women. HIV infection amongst young women accounts for 50% of all reported HIV infections. Current estimates put the number of orphans at 82,000, expected to rise to 120,000 by 2006. Namibia's proposal to the Global Fund to Fight AIDS, Tuberculosis and Malaria second round was approved in January 2003. The government has responded to the request for revision of some components of the proposal. The total amount for the three components for five years is US$113,157,021, of which US$105,319,841 is for HIV/AIDS. Namibia is one of the priority countries to benefit from the US Presidential Plan for AIDS Relief (PEPFAR).[12]

Health care system

In 2001, the total per capita expenditure on health care was Intl $342; 7.0% of GDP[13] (Appendix 3).

The WHO overall health system performance score places Namibia 168th out of 191 countries.[14]

Political economy

The economy is heavily dependent on the extraction and processing of minerals for export. Mining accounts for 20 per cent of GDP. Rich alluvial diamond deposits make Namibia a primary source for gem-quality diamonds. Namibia is the fourth largest exporter of non-fuel minerals in Africa, the world's fifth largest producer of uranium, and the producer of large quantities of lead, zinc, tin, silver and tungsten. The mining sector employs only about 3 per cent of the population, while about half of the population depends on subsistence agriculture for its livelihood. Namibia normally imports about 50 per cent of its cereal requirements; in drought years, food shortages are a major problem in rural areas. A high per capita GDP, relative to the region, hides the great inequality of income distribution; nearly one-third of Namibians had annual incomes of less than $1400 in constant 1994 dollars, according to a 1993 study. The Namibian economy is closely linked to South Africa, with the Namibian dollar pegged to the South African rand. Privatization of several enterprises in coming years may stimulate long-run foreign investment. Mining of zinc, copper and silver, and increased fish production led to growth in 2003.

South Africa occupied the German colony of South-West Africa during the First World War and administered it as a mandate until after the Second World War, when it annexed the territory. In 1966, the South-West Africa People's Organization (SWAPO) group launched a war of independence for the area that was soon named Namibia, but it was not until 1988 that South Africa agreed to end its administration in accordance with a UN peace plan for the entire region. Namibia won its independence in 1990 and has been governed by SWAPO since. Hifikepunye Pohamba was elected president in November 2004 in a landslide victory, replacing Sam Nujoma who led the country during its first 14 years of self-rule.[9] A factor that favoured the transition to democracy in Namibia was the singular nature of the pre-transition regime and the fact that Namibia's transition was one from decades of colonial rule to political independence, rather than from decades of independent neo-patrimonial rule to, hopefully, independent democratic rule. Many see strong and autonomous organizations of civil society as critical to the successful consolidation of democracy, and, in Namibia, a significant feature of the post-independence period has been a growing visibility and apparent influence of organizations of civil society throughout the country to meet a plethora of needs. Despite the many challenges, there is evidence of a growing influence on the part of civic organizations and the media in Namibia, and other circumstances related to Namibia's unique transition to democracy in the 1990s also potentially bode well for the future; indeed, it is widely cited as one of Africa's most successful new democracies.[15]

GDP per capita is Intl $4918 (Appendix 4).

References

1 Report of the United Nations Development Programme 2004 (HDI 2002). Launched by the United Nations in 1990, the Human Development Index measures a country's achievements in three aspects of human development: longevity, knowledge and a decent standard of living. It was created to re-emphasize that people and their lives should be the ultimate criteria for assessing the development of a country, not economic growth. Current values range from 0.956 (Norway, first of 177 countries) to 0.273 (Sierra Leone, 177th out of 177 countries). Countries fall into one of three groups: countries 1–55 = high development; 56–141 = medium development; 142–177 = low development. See: http://hdr.undp.org/statistics/data/indic/indic_8_1_1.html

2 UNICEF/WHO Consultative Meeting on Strengthening Paediatric and Adult Care in Community Home Based Care in Africa, Cape Town: Richard Bauer, November 22–25, 2004.

3 Personal communication: Lahya Shiimi—18 January 2005.

4 Global Fund portfolio of grants Round 2.

5 See: http://www.usaid.gov/our_work/global_health/aids/pepfarfact.html

6 *Engendering Bold Leadership*. The President's Emergency Plan for AIDS Relief. First Annual Report to Congress, 2005: 115. http://www.state.gov/documents/organization/43885.pdf

7 International Narcotics Control Board. *Narcotic Drugs: Estimated World Requirements for 2004. Statistics for 2002.* New York: United Nations, 2004.

8 The term *defined daily doses for statistical purposes* (S-DDD) replaces the term *defined daily doses* previously used by the Board. The S-DDDs are technical units of measurement for the purposes of statistical analysis and are not recommended prescription doses. Certain narcotic drugs may be used in certain countries for different treatments or in accordance with different medical practices, and therefore a different daily dose could be more appropriate'. The S-DDD used by the INCB for morphine is 100 mg. International Narcotics Control Board. *Narcotic Drugs: Estimated World Requirements for 2004. Statistics for 2002.* New York: United Nations, 2004: 176–177.

9 See: http://www.cia.gov/cia/publications/factbook/geos/wa.html

10 This refers to adult mortality risk, which is defined as the probability of dying between 15 and 59 years.

11 See: WHO statistics for Namibia at: http://www.who.int/countries/nam/en/

12 http://www.unaids.org/en/geographical+area/by+country/namibia.asp

13 Total health expenditure per capita is the per capita amount of the sum of Public Health Expenditure (PHE) and Private Expenditure on Health (PvtHE). The international dollar is a common currency unit that takes into account differences in the relative purchasing power of various currencies. Figures expressed in international dollars are calculated using purchasing power parities (PPP), which are rates of currency conversion constructed to account for differences in price level between countries.
http://www3.who.int/whosis/country/compare.cfm?country = s&indicator = strPcTotEO HinIntD2000&language = english

14 This composite measure of overall health system attainment is based on a country's goals relating to health, responsiveness and fairness in financing. The measure varies widely across countries and is highly correlated with general levels of human development as captured in the human development index. Tandon A, Murray CLJ, Lauer JA, Evans DB. *Measuring Overall Health System Performance for 191 Countries.* GPE Discussion Paper Series: No. 30; WHO.

15 **Bauer G.** Namibia in the first decade of independence: how democratic? *Journal of Southern African Studies* 2001; **27(1)**: 33–55.

Chapter 30

Rwanda

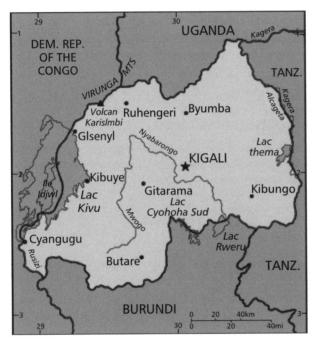

Rwanda (population 7.95 million people) is a country in Central Africa that covers an area of 26 338 km². Its boundaries border Democratic Republic of the Congo, Uganda, Tanzania and Burundi. The capital of Rwanda is Kigali.

According to the United Nations human development index (HDI), Rwanda is ranked 159th out of 177 countries worldwide (value 0.431)[1] and 27th out of 45 in African countries for which an index is available. This places Rwanda in the group of countries with low human development.

Palliative care service provision

Current services

In resource-poor areas, the blending of supportive care with hospice–palliative care is frequently linked to the development of previously established services, particularly home-based care. Family Health International (FHI) defines home- and community-based care (HCBC) as 'the provision of care and support that endeavours to meet the nursing and psychosocial needs of persons with chronic illnesses and their family members in their home environment'.[2]

While HCBC delivers patient care in the home environment, palliative care is an approach that attends to the needs of patients and families affected by a life-threatening illness in a variety of settings including the home, hospice, hospital, clinic and community. Ruth Wooldridge describes the situation in Rwanda:

> They said, 'Yes, we do home care'. So I said, 'That's great. What do you do?' And one group made denim backpacks and they took out Omo, plastic sheeting, soap and a towel. But actually nobody knew the word palliative care . . . The HIV rate's very high there. Go into hospital: there'll be beds full of people who need palliation even if they get antiretrovirals. They need some extra care: symptom control, to talk to someone and to understand what's happening to them.[3]

The Global Fund[4] has signed agreements to extend and improve services to people living with HIV/AIDS. While palliative care is not mentioned in the summary proposals, some elements of palliative care are included. In particular, Rwandan family structure is considered as paramount in the strategy to expand prevention messages within communities. The proposal aims to improve the quality and life expectancy of people with HIV/AIDS while strengthening prevention by a family approach. By decentralizing patient monitoring and health delivery, the project will centre around 30 health centres and five district hospitals. The proposal includes the following points:

> An initial investment in health structures and human resources will prepare the decentralised management phase: this initial phase will be validated by an approval process of district hospitals based on a minimum package of activities to be achieved . . . a total of 19,350 people on ARVs and 50,000 people on prophylaxis and treated for their opportunist infections.
> This management is supported by strengthening psychosocial and nutritional monitoring (6,000 families) via 40 local associations under the new National Network of People Living With HIV and via sponsoring and support groups.[4]

Expected results include the establishment of 117 voluntary counselling and testing sites, prevention of mother-to-child transmission clinics, and increased medical and psycho-social services, including antiretroviral therapies, across the country's health outlets.

Meanwhile, CARE International[5] in Rwanda supports collaboration and partnership across all programming sectors with the Ministries of Agriculture, Rehabilitation, Health, Public Works, Environment and Tourism, and Family and Promotion of Women, local authorities at prefecture and commune levels, and registered local and international NGOs.

From 1984 to 1994, CARE International implemented a range of development projects, including maternal health care. As a result of the civil war in Rwanda—which claimed an estimated 1 million lives—CARE International closed its Kigali office from April to July 1994. Emergency operations included the distribution of shelter, food, water, seeds and tools. At the height of the emergency in 1994, CARE International helped an estimated 1.5 million internally displaced people, returning refugees and impoverished local people.

Since that time, CARE International has built up a significant rehabilitation and development programme in Rwanda. Projects now include STD/AIDS prevention amongst other non-health-oriented projects. CARE International is currently working in six prefectures in response to expressed needs and requests of relevant government ministries.

The organization sponsored two nurses to attend the African Palliative Care Association (APCA) conference in Arusha in June 2004, indicating support for incorporating palliative care into its health projects.

Reimbursement and funding for services

Individuals committed to establishing palliative care services in Rwanda have sourced initial funding for specific projects. Ruth Wooldridge successfully campaigned for financial support to send two Rwandan nurses to Nairobi Hospice for training. The British government paid for the same nurses to attend the APCA conference in Arusha in June 2004. An application has been submitted to the UK Forum for Hospice and Palliative Care Worldwide for further training in May 2005. A US-based hospice linked with a Tanzanian hospice has also shown interest in financial support for palliative care development in Rwanda.

Global Fund

Furthermore, the Global Fund has committed significant funding to HIV/AIDS programmes in Rwanda in Round 3 of an extensive strategy. The agreement was signed on 30 June 2004 for the Ministry of Health of the Government of Rwanda to manage a project aimed at decentralizing the care and treatment for people living with HIV/AIDS. US$14 860 735 has been approved to implement the project over 2 years. A further US$8.5 million has been approved for expanding the number of voluntary counselling and testing centres.

President's Emergency Plan for AIDS Relief (PEPFAR)[6]

During the 2004 financial year (FY), funding of around US$27.97 million was enacted for country-managed programmes in Rwanda and US$11.33 million for central programmes. During FY2005, it is anticipated that a total of US$51.30 million will be enacted: US$41.07 million for country-managed programmes and US$10.22 million for central programmes.[7]

Opioid availability and consumption

The International Narcotics Control Board[8] has published the following figures for the consumption of narcotic drugs in Rwanda: pethidine 1 kg.

For the years 2000–2002, no report has been submitted to the International Narcotics Control Board regarding the average defined daily dose[9] consumption of morphine (Appendix 1).

Education and training

Two nurses from the school of nursing have received palliative care training at Nairobi Hospice in Kenya.

History and development of hospice–palliative care in Rwanda

Ruth Wooldridge speaks of some of the difficulties in Rwanda: of identifying individuals as palliative care pioneers and assuring people they are not forgotten.

> I thought, actually you are just the right person. And when I said 'what about homecare?' and explained about palliative care, she knew what I was talking about—and that she needed to be doing it. And she took me out on a home visit to a family who were HIV positive. We took some plastic sheeting for their house and a bit of food. The mother wasn't there and the kids were looking after themselves. The cupboard was bare—I mean they had not a grain of food in the house—and I just thought Grace was terrific.
>
> Then I went around other places and we met some women in the south. They'd got nothing. They took us to a room where there were about a hundred bodies that hadn't been moved since the genocide. It was so shocking and so sad and we said to them, 'We are shocked by this—what can we do for you?' Obviously we gave what money we'd got but that wasn't what they wanted. They said, 'Just tell the world what it's like here and not to forget us'.[3]

Knowing that the APCA conference in June 2004 would be a good networking opportunity—and for Rwandans to hear of palliative care experiences in other African countries—Ruth Wooldridge sourced funding for two nurses to attend. CARE International funded another two participants. Ruth Wooldridge:

> It was a good conference because it was a starter conference for people who hadn't any knowledge of palliative care. People were talking about pain and how it could be relieved, how you can introduce things and about models of care. So they came back very excited.[3]

Life/oral histories

Ruth Wooldridge—*co-founder, the Nairobi Hospice Kenya*: interviewed by Michael Wright, 23 January 2005. Length of interview: 1 h 3 min.

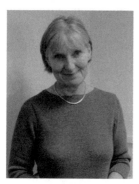

Ruth Wooldridge trained as a nurse at St Thomas's Hospital (London) and in her early career became concerned about the care of cancer patients and their families. She worked as a volunteer in Uganda (VSO) during the 1970s and returned to Africa in 1982 to take up a nursing post in Kenya. It was during this time that she met Nancy, a young teacher with cancer whose painful death made a deep impression on her. As she advocated for hospice, she persuaded Robert Twycross to visit Kenya on his way to South Africa. The effect was overwhelming and resulted in a grass roots movement towards a hospice service. With Jane Moore, she wrote a proposal for the Kenyan government and, with local support from Professor Kasilli, a piece of land was acquired in the grounds of Kenyatta Hospital (Nairobi). The Tudor Trust funded the erection of premises, an education project began and the hospice opened for patients in 1990. Ruth Wooldridge speaks of the challenges facing hospice development in resource-poor countries, of the need for communication and policy change, of the place of spirituality and care for family members. She then turns to her work in

South Africa, India and, more recently, in Rwanda. Ten years after the genocide in Rwanda, she was shocked to find how much needed to be done to support impoverished communities. She was heartened, however, by the presence of visionary people who, with appropriate training, could help to establish palliative care services.

Public health context

Population

Rwanda's population of around 7.95 million people is made up of the following ethnic groups: Hutu 84 per cent, Tutsi 15 per cent and Twa (Pygmoid) 1 per cent.

Religious groups include: Roman Catholic 56.5 per cent, Protestant 26 per cent, Adventist 11.1 per cent, Muslim 4.6 per cent, indigenous beliefs 0.1 per cent and none 1.7 per cent (2001).[10]

Epidemiology

In Rwanda, the WHO World Health Report (2004) indicates an adult mortality[11] rate per 1000 population of 605 for males and 474 for females. Life expectancy for males is 41.9; for females 46.8. Healthy life expectancy is 36.4 for males; and 40.2 for females.[12]

Rwanda is a country in Central Africa that has been severely affected by the HIV/AIDS epidemic. Estimates suggest that in Rwanda, between 170 000 and 380 000 people were living with HIV/AIDS at the end of 2003. In the same year, up to 36 000 adults and children are thought to have died from the disease (Table 30.1).

UNAIDS reports:

> In the 2002 antenatal clinic sentinel survey, median HIV prevalence rates were 6.9% and 3.0% in urban and rural sites, respectively. Political commitment regarding HIV/AIDS is high, with the personal involvement of the President and the First Lady. A Ministry of State in charge of HIV/AIDS, TB and related diseases has been created within the Ministry of Health. The National AIDS Control Programme was changed to the National AIDS Commission (NAC) in March 2001 and moved from the Ministry of Health to the Office of the President. The Treatment and Research AIDS Centre (TRAC) was also created to define treatment and care standards, as well as

Table 30.1 Rwanda HIV and AIDS estimates, end 2003

Adult (15–49) HIV prevalence rate	5.1 per cent (range: 3.4–7.6 per cent)
Adults (15–49) living with HIV	230 000 (range: 150 000–350 000)
Adults and children (0–49) living with HIV	250 000 (range: 170 000–380 000)
Women (15–49) living with HIV	130 000 (range: 86 000–200 000)
AIDS deaths (adults and children) in 2003	22 000 (range: 14 000–36 000)

Source: 2004 Report of the global AIDS epidemic.

to provide training and certification in HIV/AIDS care provision. The National Strategic Framework (2002–2006) is being implemented, and the Ministries of Youth and Sports, Defence, and Education have developed HIV/AIDS programmes. Six coordinating bodies have been created; they are the NGO Forum, National Network of People Living with HIV, the faith-based organizations, the private sector umbrella organization, APELAS (public sector bodies concerned with HIV/AIDS) and HIV/AIDS donor organizations. The current goal for the Government of Rwanda is to stabilize the spread of HIV/AIDS during the period 2002–2006.[13]

Health care system

In 2001, the total per capita expenditure on health care was Intl $44; 5.5% of GDP[14] (Appendix 3).

The WHO overall health system performance score places Rwanda 172nd out of 191 countries.[15]

Political economy

Rwanda is a poor rural country with about 90 per cent of the population engaged in (mainly subsistence) agriculture. It is the most densely populated country in Africa; landlocked with few natural resources and minimal industry. Primary foreign exchange earners are coffee and tea. GDP has rebounded, and inflation has been curbed. Export earnings, however, have been hindered by low beverage prices, depriving the country of much needed hard currency. Attempts to diversify into non-traditional agriculture exports such as flowers and vegetables have been stymied by a lack of adequate transportation infrastructure. Despite Rwanda's fertile ecosystem, food production often does not keep pace with population growth, requiring food to be imported. Rwanda continues to receive substantial aid money and was approved for IMF/World Bank Heavily Indebted Poor Country (HIPC) initiative debt relief in late 2000.[10]

There has been a strong trend toward democratization and openness in many civil matters, and the state has managed to create a base of legitimate state institutions. Rwanda has established a number of institutions (e.g. the National Human Rights Commission, the Unity and reconciliation commission, and the auditor-general) aimed at creating checks and balances as part of government policy, correlating as they do with the conditionalities imposed by external multilateral and bilateral funders. Positive growth shown in the economy in recent years has also contributed to the process of reform. The Rwandan economy has realized positive economic growth since the mid-1990s, and the IMF teams that have periodically visited the country have expressed their satisfaction with the economy's achievement of macroeconomic stability. The international community has committed significant funds to the process of democratization, good governance and poverty reduction. These have helped Rwanda to make progress in opening up and creating a relatively secure and stable environment for its people.[16]

GDP per capita is Intl $799 (Appendix 4).

References

1 Report of the United Nations Development Programme 2004 (HDI 2002). Launched by the United Nations in 1990, the Human Development Index measures a country's achievements in three aspects of human development: longevity, knowledge and a decent standard of living. It was created to re-emphasize that people and their lives should be the ultimate criteria for assessing the development of a country, not economic growth. Current values range from 0.956 (Norway, first of 177 countries) to 0.273 (Sierra Leone, 177th out of 177 countries). Countries fall into one of three groups: countries 1–55 = high development; 56–141 = medium development; 142–177 = low development. See: http://hdr.undp.org/statistics/data/indic/indic_8_1_1.html

2 Family Health International, Comprehensive Care and Support Framework.

3 IOELC interview: Ruth Wooldridge—27 January 2005.

4 Global Fund Portfolio of Grants.

5 http://www.careinternational.org.uk/cares_work/where/rwanda/projects/index.htm

6 See: http://www.usaid.gov/our_work/global_health/aids/pepfarfact.html

7 *Engendering Bold Leadership*. The President's Emergency Plan for AIDS Relief. First Annual Report to Congress, 2005: 115. http://www.state.gov/documents/organization/43885.pdf

8 International Narcotics Control Board. *Narcotic Drugs: Estimated World Requirements for 2004. Statistics for 2002*. New York: United Nations, 2004.

9 'The term *defined daily doses for statistical purposes* (S-DDD) replaces the term *defined daily doses* previously used by the Board. The S-DDDs are technical units of measurement for the purposes of statistical analysis and are not recommended prescription doses. Certain narcotic drugs may be used in certain countries for different treatments or in accordance with different medical practices, and therefore a different daily dose could be more appropriate'. The S-DDD used by the INCB for morphine is 100 mg. International Narcotics Control Board. *Narcotic Drugs: Estimated World Requirements for 2004. Statistics for 2002*. New York: United Nations, 2004: 176–177.

10 See: http://www.cia.gov/cia/publications/factbook/geos/rw.html

11 This refers to adult mortality risk, which is defined as the probability of dying between 15 and 59 years.

12 See: WHO statistics for Rwanda at: http://www.who.int/countries/rwa/en/

13 http://www.unaids.org/en/geographical+area/by+country/rwanda.asp

14 Total health expenditure per capita is the per capita amount of the sum of Public Health Expenditure (PHE) and Private Expenditure on Health (PvtHE). The international dollar is a common currency unit that takes into account differences in the relative purchasing power of various currencies. Figures expressed in international dollars are calculated using purchasing power parities (PPP), which are rates of currency conversion constructed to account for differences in price level between countries.
http://www3.who.int/whosis/country/compare.cfm?country=s&indicator=strPcTotEO HinIntD2000&language=english

15 This composite measure of overall health system attainment is based on a country's goals relating to health, responsiveness and fairness in financing. The measure varies widely across countries and is highly correlated with general levels of human development as captured in the human development index. Tandon A, Murray CLJ, Lauer JA, Evans DB. *Measuring Overall Health System Performance for 191 Countries*. GPE Discussion Paper Series: No. 30; WHO.

16 **Siridopoulos E**. Democratisation and militarisation in Rwanda. *African Security Review* 2002; **11(3)**: 77.

Chapter 31

Tunisia

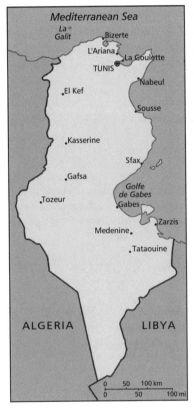

Tunisia (population 9.97 million people) is a country in Northern Africa, bordering the Mediterranean Sea, between Tunisia and Libya that covers an area of 163 610 km². The capital of Tunisia is Tunis.

According to the United Nations human development index (HDI), Tunisia is ranked 92nd out of 177 countries worldwide (value 0.745)[1] and second out of 45 in African countries for which an index is available. This places Tunisia in the group of countries with medium human development.

Palliative care service provision

Current services

As yet, palliative care services have not been identified in Tunisia, but there is evidence of growing interest. In September 2004, the 4th Europe–Maghreb conference was held in Tabarka (Tunisia) and adopted the theme *Pain and Supportive Care: Current Advances*. (The Maghreb is a region that includes Tunisia, Morocco and Algeria.)

Significantly, nurse educator Françoise Porchet (Switzerland) and three European colleagues, Gisele Schaerer (Switzerland), Philip Larkin (Ireland) and Sophie Leruth (Belgium), were invited to provide a full day of training. With the exception of Philip Larkin, all had been speakers at the previous conference in 2002.

Reporting on the conference in 2005, they address the issue of palliative care accessibility in the Maghreb and write:

> Home care does not exist in the Maghreb; it is the family and/or community that provides any care. A huge distance has to be covered, sometimes as much as 1000 km, to visit the specialised oncology centres—the few places where consultations on dealing with the treatment of pain are available.[2]

Opioid availability and consumption

Françoise Porchet and her colleagues write:

> [In the Maghreb], the distribution of opioids is subject to the 'seven day law'; in other words, doctors are not allowed to issue prescriptions for periods in excess of one week. Therefore, patients or their families have to return to the physician regularly to obtain a new prescription. Morphine is very expensive and only available in sustained-release form.[2]

The International Narcotics Control Board[3] has published the following figures for the consumption of narcotic drugs in Tunisia (2002): codeine 272 kg; morphine 16 kg; pholcodine 15 kg; ethylmorphine 66; dextropropoxyphene 1087 kg; and pethidine 5 kg.

For the years 2000–2002, the average defined daily dose consumption of morphine for statistical purposes (S-DDD)[4] in Tunisia was 37 (Appendix 1).

Education and training

Nurse educator Françoise Porchet and her colleagues report on the training they gave in the Maghreb, 2004:

> This opportunity allowed us to provide our nursing colleagues in the Maghreb with up-to-date knowledge on palliative care according to our individual specialties, while enabling them to acquire the knowledge through a process of exchange and constructive learning. It is very gratifying to note that the spirit of palliative care can transcend borders, cultures and languages. It is also important to realise all the possibilities that can arise from a training initiative put together between colleagues from three European countries and the extent to which this is a unifying event.[2]

Public health context

Population

Tunisia's population of around 9.97 million people is made up of the following ethnic groups: Arab 98 per cent, European 1 per cent, Jewish and other 1 per cent.

Religious groups include: Muslim 98 per cent, Christian 1 per cent, Jewish and other 1 per cent.[5]

Epidemiology

In Tunisia, the WHO World Health Report (2004) indicates an adult mortality[6] rate per 1000 population of 167 for males and 115 for females. Life expectancy for males is 69.5 for females 73.9. Healthy life expectancy is 61.3 for males; and 63.6 for females.[7]

Tunisia is a country in Northern Africa that has been affected by the HIV/AIDS epidemic. Estimates suggest that in Tunisia, between 400 and 2400 adults were living with HIV/AIDS at the end of 2003. In the same year, up to 400 adults and children are thought to have died from the disease (Table 31.1).

UNAIDS reports:

> No evidence of HIV infection was found among women attending prenatal clinics tested for HIV during 1989–1992, or in 1999. In 2001, however, one of 458 pregnant women (0.2%) was infected. HIV seroprevalence among blood donors has been relatively stable from 1989; for the past 3 years around 0.003%. Rates among high risk groups are low. In 1989 and 1992, a group of bar girls

Table 31.1 Tunisia HIV and AIDS estimates, end 2003

Adult (15–49) HIV prevalence rate	<0.1 per cent (range: <0.2 per cent)
Adults (15–49) living with HIV	1000 (range: 400–2300)
Adults and children (0–49) living with HIV	1000 (range: 400–2400)
Women (15–49) living with HIV	<500 (range: <1000)
AIDS deaths (adults and children) in 2003	<200 (range: <400)

Source: 2004 Report of the global AIDS epidemic.

tested revealed HIV prevalence rates of 1.3% and 2.3% respectively. Men who have sex with men were screened in 1989; there were no HIV positive cases among 72 individuals tested. Although about one-third of reported AIDS cases have been among injection drug users (IDUs), it is believed that the majority acquired their infection outside of Tunisia. However, the prevalence of HIV infection among IDUs was 1.6% in 1992 and 0.3% in 1997 indicating that, no matter where the infection was acquired, the risk for transmission within the country exists. In 1993, 0.4% of TB patients were HIV positive and 0.25% in 1996. Surveillance for STI patients is sporadic. The rate of HIV infection among this group was 2.3%, 0.8% and 0.0% in 1991, 1992 and 1999, respectively. The seroprevalence for syphilis among blood donors has been consistently less than 1%.[8]

Health care system

In 2001, the total per capita expenditure on health care was Intl $463; 6.4% of GDP[9] (Appendix 3).

The WHO overall health system performance score places Tunisia 52nd out of 191 countries.[10]

Political economy

Following independence from France in 1956, President Habib Bourguiba established a strict one-party state. In recent years, Tunisia has taken a moderate, non-aligned stance in its foreign relations. Domestically, it has sought to defuse rising pressure for a more open political society.

Tunisia has a diverse economy, with important agricultural, mining, energy, tourism and manufacturing sectors. Governmental control of economic affairs, while still heavy, has gradually lessened over the past decade with increasing privatization, simplification of the tax structure and a prudent approach to debt. Real growth, averaging 5 per cent for the latter half of the last decade, slowed to a 15 year low of 1.9 per cent in 2002 because of agricultural drought, slow investment and lacklustre tourism. Better rains in 2003, however, pushed GDP growth up to an estimated 6 per cent. GDP growth remained at 6 per cent in 2004. Tunisia has agreed to remove barriers to trade with the European Union gradually over the next decade. Broader privatization, further liberalization of the investment code to increase foreign investment, improvements in government efficiency and reduction of the trade deficit are among the challenges for the future.[5] However, with its track record on structural adjustment and moves towards a free market economy, Tunisia remains a friend of the West.

Economic growth in the 1990s was largely based on phosphate mining, oil and gas, the development of the textile industry and the development of the tourism industry. The government is oriented toward a free market policy through reducing fiscal deficits, liberalizing prices, trade and investment controls and decreasing the emphasis on the public sector to free up resources for the private sector.[11]

GDP per capita is Intl $7183 (Appendix 4).

References

1 Report of the United Nations Development Programme 2004 (HDI 2002). Launched by the United Nations in 1990, the Human Development Index measures a country's achievements in three aspects of human development: longevity, knowledge and a decent standard of living. It was created to re-emphasize that people and their lives should be the ultimate criteria for assessing the development of a country, not economic growth. Current values range from 0.956 (Norway, first of 177 countries) to 0.273 (Sierra Leone, 177th out of 177 countries). Countries fall into one of three groups: countries 1–55 = high development; 56–141 = medium development; 142–177 = low development. See: http://hdr.undp.org/statistics/data/indic/indic_8_1_1.html

2 Porchet F, Schaerer G, Larkin P, Leruth S. Intercultural experiences of training in the Maghreb. *European Journal of Palliative Care* 2005; 12(1): 37.

3 International Narcotics Control Board. *Narcotic Drugs: Estimated World Requirements for 2004. Statistics for 2002.* New York: United Nations, 2004.

4 'The term *defined daily doses for statistical purposes* (S-DDD) replaces the term *defined daily doses* previously used by the Board. The S-DDDs are technical units of measurement for the purposes of statistical analysis and are not recommended prescription doses. Certain narcotic drugs may be used in certain countries for different treatments or in accordance with different medical practices, and therefore a different daily dose could be more appropriate'. The S-DDD used by the INCB for morphine is 100 mg. International Narcotics Control Board. *Narcotic Drugs: Estimated World Requirements for 2004. Statistics for 2002.* New York: United Nations, 2004: 176–177.

5 See: http://www.cia.gov/cia/publications/factbook/geos/ts.html

6 This refers to adult mortality risk, which is defined as the probability of dying between 15 and 59 years.

7 See: WHO statistics for Tunisia at: http://www.who.int/countries/tun/en/

8 http://www.unaids.org/en/geographical+area/by+country/tunisia.asp

9 Total health expenditure per capita is the per capita amount of the sum of Public Health Expenditure (PHE) and Private Expenditure on Health (PvtHE). The international dollar is a common currency unit that takes into account differences in the relative purchasing power of various currencies. Figures expressed in international dollars are calculated using purchasing power parities (PPP), which are rates of currency conversion constructed to account for differences in price level between countries.
http://www3.who.int/whosis/country/compare.cfm?country = s&indicator = strPcTotEO HinIntD2000&language = english

10 This composite measure of overall health system attainment is based on a country's goals relating to health, responsiveness and fairness in financing. The measure varies widely across countries and is highly correlated with general levels of human development as captured in the human development index. Tandon A, Murray CLJ, Lauer JA, Evans DB. *Measuring Overall Health System Performance for 191 Countries*. GPE Discussion Paper Series: No. 30; WHO.

11 World of Information, Business Intelligence Report. Tunisia: economy, politics and government. *Business Intelligence Report* 2001; 1(1): 1–42.

Average daily consumption of defined daily doses (for statistical purposes) of morphine per million inhabitants, 2000–2002: countries of Africa

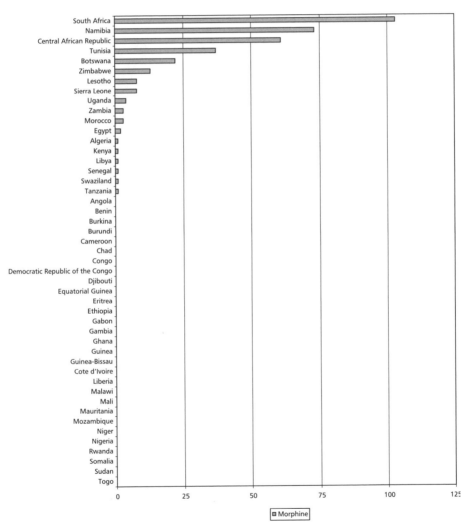

Source: International Narcotics Control Board. *Narcotic Drugs: Estimated World Requirements for 2004. Statistics for 2002.* New York: United Nations, 2004.

Appendix 2

Countries of Africa involved in PEPFAR, the Diana, Princess of Wales Memorial Fund (Diana Fund) and WHO projects

PEPFAR	Diana Fund	WHO
Botswana		Botswana
Cote d'Ivoire		
Ethiopia	Ethiopia	Ethiopia
Kenya	Kenya	
	Malawi	
Mozambique		
Namibia		
Nigeria		
Rwanda	Rwanda	
South Africa	South Africa	
Tanzania	Tanzania	Tanzania
Uganda	Uganda	Uganda
Zambia	Zambia	
	Zimbabwe	Zimbabwe

Total health expenditure (Intl $) per capita and as a percentage of GDP: countries of Africa, 2001

Health expenditure (Intl $) per capita: Africa		Health expenditure (Intl $) as a percentage of GDP: Africa	
South Africa	652	South Africa	8.6
Tunisia	463	Kenya	7.8
Botswana	381	Malawi	7.8
Namibia	342	Djibouti	7.0
Libya	239	Namibia	7.0
Morocco	199	Botswana	6.6
Gabon	197	Gambia	6.4
Algeria	169	Tunisia	6.4
Swaziland	167	Cote d'Ivoire	6.2
Egypt	153	Zimbabwe	6.2
Zimbabwe	142	Guinea-Bissau	5.9
Cote d'Ivoire	127	Mozambique	5.9
Liberia	127	Uganda	5.9
Kenya	114	Eritrea	5.7
Equatorial Guinea	106	Zambia	5.7
Lesotho	101	Lesotho	5.5
Djibouti	90	Rwanda	5.5
Gambia	78	Morocco	5.1
Angola	70	Senegal	4.8
Senegal	63	Ghana	4.7
Guinea	61	Central African Republic	4.5
Ghana	60	Sudan	4.5
Central African Republic	58	Angola	4.4
Uganda	57	Benin	4.4
Zambia	52	United Republic of Tanzania	4.4
Mozambique	47	Liberia	4.3
Mauritania	45	Mali	4.3

(Contd.)

Health expenditure (Intl $) per capita: Africa		Health expenditure (Intl $) as a percentage of GDP: Africa	
Togo	45	Sierra Leone	4.3
Rwanda	44	Algeria	4.1
Cameroon	42	Egypt	3.9
Benin	39	Niger	3.7
Malawi	39	Burundi	3.6
Sudan	39	Ethiopia	3.6
Guinea-Bissau	37	Gabon	3.6
Eritrea	36	Mauritania	3.6
Nigeria	31	Democratic Republic of the Congo	3.5
Mali	30	Guinea	0.5
Burkina Faso	27	Nigeria	3.4
Sierra Leone	26	Cameroon	3.3
United Republic of Tanzania	26	Swaziland	3.3
Congo	22	Burkina Faso	3.0
Niger	22	Libya	2.9
Burundi	19	Togo	2.8
Chad	17	Chad	2.6
Ethiopia	14	Somalia	2.6
Democratic Republic of the Congo	12	Congo	2.1
Somalia		Equatorial Guinea	2.0

Source: WHO World Health Report 2004.

GDP per capita (Intl $): countries of Africa, 2001

Country	GDP per capita (Int $)
Libya	8272
South Africa	7538
Tunisia	7138
Botswana	5747
Gabon	5514
Equatorial Guinea	5239
Swaziland	5029
Namibia	4918
Algeria	4104
Egypt	3901
Morocco	3887
Liberia	2965
Zimbabwe	2271
Cote d'Ivoire	2045
Lesotho	1844
Guinea	1752
Togo	1608
Angola	1578
Kenya	1452
Senegal	1323
Central African Republic	1289
Djibouti	1288
Ghana	1272
Cameroon	1269
Mauritania	1257
Gambia	1214
Sudan	1112
Congo	1036

(Contd.)

Country	GDP per capita (Int $)
Uganda	964
Nigeria	915
Zambia	906
Benin	888
Burkina Faso	886
Mozambique	805
Rwanda	799
Mali	700
Chad	656
Guinea-Bissau	630
Eritrea	629
Sierra Leone	606
Niger	604
United Republic of Tanzania	599
Burundi	529
Malawi	501
Ethiopia	382
Democratic Republic of the Congo	346
Somalia	

Source: WHO.

Appendix 5

Further reading

General further reading

Ahn MJ, Grimwood A, Schwarzwald H, Herman A. Ethics and the AIDS pandemic in the developing world. *Journal of the International Association of Physicians in AIDS Care* 2003; **2(2)**: 81–87.

Amado LE. Sexual and bodily rights as human rights in the Middle East and North Africa. *Reproductive Health Matters* 2004; **12(23)**: 125–131.

Clemens KE, Klaschik E. Palliative care delivery in Southern Africa. *European Journal of Palliative Care* 2004; **11(4)**: 164.

Defilippi K, Downing J, Merriman A, Clark D. A palliative care association for the whole of Africa. *Palliative Medicine* 2004; **18**: 583–584.

Duza MB. Development and human resources in the Islamic world: a study of selected countries. *Population Science* 1987; **7**: 1–30.

Gronemeyer R. *Living and Dying with AIDS in Africa.* Frankfurt: Brandes and Apsel, 2005.

Harding R, Higginson IR. *Palliative Care in Sub-Saharan Africa: An Appraisal. London: Diana,* Princess of Wales Memorial Fund, 2004. See: www.theworkcontinues.org/pressroon/6_3.publications.htm

Harding R, Stewart K, Marconi K, O'Neill JF, Higginson IJ. Current HIV/AIDS end-of-life care in sub-Saharan Africa: a survey of models, services, challenges and priorities. *BMC Public Health* October 2003; **3**: 33. See: http://www.biomedcentral.com/1471–2458/3/33

Hunter S. *Black Death: AIDS in Africa.* Basingstoke: Palgrave Macmillan, 2003.

Mpanga Sebuyira L, More J. Palliative care in the 21st century. *Health Exchange* 2003.

Norval D, Marcus C. AIDS. In: Bruera E, De Lima L, Wenk R, Farr W (ed.), *Palliative Care in the Developing World: Principles and Practice.* Houston: IAHPC Press, 2004: 143–185.

Selwyn P, Rivard M. Palliative care and AIDS: challenges and opportunities on the era of highly active anti-retroviral therapy. *Journal of Palliative Medicine* 2003; **6(3)**: 475–478.

Sepulveda C, Habiyambere V, Amandua J, Borok M, Kikule E, Mudanga B, Ngoma T, Solomon B. Quality care at the end of life in Africa. *British Medical Journal* 2003; **327(7408)**: 209.

Singer Y, Dlamini S, Fernandez C. Worldwide hospice & palliative care: focus on Africa. *American Journal of Hospice and Palliative Care* 2000; **17**: 298–299.

Stjernswärd J, Clark D. Palliative medicine—a global perspective. In: Doyle D, Hanks G, Cherny N, Calman K (ed.), *Oxford Textbook of Palliative Medicine.* Oxford: Oxford University Press, 2003: 1199–1224.

Country-specific further reading

Countries approaching integration

Kenya

Amuyunzu-Nyamongo, M. HIV/AIDS in Kenya: moving beyond policy and rhetoric. *African Sociological Review* 2001; **5(2)**: 86–101.

Mbatia PN, Bradshaw YW. Responding to crisis: patterns of health care utilization in Central Kenya amid economic decline. *African Studies Review* 2003; **46(1)**: 69–92.

Quaye RK. Paying for health services in East Africa: a research note. *Social Theory and Health* 2004; **2**(1): 94–105.

Spronk R. Female sexuality in Nairobi: flawed or favoured? *Culture, Health and Sexuality* 2005; **7**(3): 267–277.

South Africa

Bhana D. What matters to girls and boys in a black primary school in South Africa. *Early Child Development and Care* 2005; **175**(2): 99–111.

Edginton ME, Wong ML, Phofa R, Mahlaba D, Hodkinson HJ. Tuberculosis at Chris Hani Baragwanath Hospital: numbers of patients diagnosed and outcomes of referrals to district clinics *International Journal of Tuberculosis and Lung Disease* 2005; **9**(4): 398–402.

Parry CD. South Africa: alcohol today. *Addiction* 2005; **100**(4): 426–429.

Scott VE, Chopra M, Conrad L, Ntuli A. How equitable is the scaling up of HIV service provision in South Africa? *South African Medical Journal* 2005; **95**(2): 109–113.

Van Niekerk JP. Founder's syndrome—a serious corporate malady. *South African Medical Journal* 2005; **95**(2): 69.

Uganda

Blum RW. Uganda AIDS prevention: A, B, C and politics. *Journal of Adolescent Health* 2004; **34**: 428–432.

Dicklitch S, Furley O. The elusive promise of NGOs in Africa: lessons from Uganda. *Journal of Contemporary African Studies* 2003; **21**(1): 131–134.

Gladwin J, Dixon RA, Wilson TD. Implementing a new health management information system in Uganda. *Health Policy and Planning* 2003; **18**(2): 214–224.

Jagwe JGM. The introduction of palliative care in Uganda. *Journal of Palliative Medicine* 2002; **5**(1): 160–163.

Wendo C. Uganda begins distributing free antiretrovirals. If the plan succeeds, Uganda will be on track to meet WHO's 3 by 5 target for antiretroviral treatment. *Lancet* 2004; **363**: 2062.

Zimbabwe

Ball DE, Mazarurwi P. HIV/AIDS knowledge and attitudes amongst pharmacists in Zimbabwe. *Central Africa Journal of Medicine* 2003; **49**: 27–31.

Buchan T, Page T. Teaching the management of terminal illness in Zimbabwe. *Central Africa Journal of Medicine* 2003; **31**(4): 82–85.

Meekers D. Patterns of condom use in urban males in Zimbabwe: evidence from 4600 sexual contacts. *AIDS Care* 2003; **15**: 291–301.

Nazerali H, Hogerzeil HV. The quality and stability of essential drugs in rural Zimbabwe: controlled longitudinal study. *British Medical Journal* 1998; **22317**: 512–513.

Reynolds P, Whisson M. Traditional healers and childhood in Zimbabwe. *Journal of Contemporary African Studies* 1997; (**1**): 150–151.

Sutherland L. Island of strength. *Nursing Times* 1992; **88**: 44–45.

Countries with localized provision

Botswana

Berkhof F. HIV/AIDS and education in Botswana: the stay alive programme. *Perspectives in Education* 2003; **21**(2): 167–174.

Campbell EK, Rakgoasi SD. Condom use among youths in Botswana in the era of HIV and AIDS. *Social Development Issues* 2002; **24(1)**: 56–67.

Durham D, Klaits F. Funerals and the public space of sentiment in Botswana. *Journal of Southern African Studies* 2002; **28(4)**: 777–796.

Livingston J. Reconfiguring old age: elderly women and concerns over care in south eastern Botswana. *Medical Anthropology* 2003; **22(3)**: 205–232.

Norr KF, Norr JL, McElmurry BJ, Tlou S, Moeti MR. Impact of peer group education on HIV prevention among women in Botswana. *Health Care for Women International* 2004; **25**: 210–226.

Republic of the Congo (Congo-Brazzaville)

HIV/AIDS Profile: Congo (Brazzaville). http://www.census.gov/ipc/hiv/congo.pdf

Le-Couer S, Khlat M, Halembokaka G, Augereau-Vacher C, Batala-MPondo G, Baty, G, Ronsmans C. HIV and the magnitude of pregnancy-related mortality in Pointe Noire, Congo. *AIDS* 2005; **19(1)**: 69–76.

Tati G. Public–private partnership (PPP) and water-supply provision in urban Africa: the experience of Congo-Brazzaville. *Development in Practice* 2005; **15(3–4)**: 316–324.

Egypt

Amado LE. Sexual and bodily rights as human rights in the Middle East and North Africa. *Reproductive Health Matters* 2004; **12(23)**: 125–131.

Duza MB. Development and human resources in the Islamic world: a study of selected countries. *Population Science* 1987; **7**: 1–30.

Okasha A. Egyptian contribution to the concept of mental health. *Journal of East Mediterranean Health* 2001; **7(3)**: 377–380.

Soliman HA. Proactive solution to the drug problem in Egypt: an evaluation of a drug-training program. *Social Development Issues* 2004; **26(1)**: 95–107.

Tawfik MO. Egypt: status of cancer pain and palliative care. *Journal of Pain and Symptom Management* 1993; **8(6)**: 409–411.

Yount KM, Agree EM, Rebellon C. Gender and use of health care among older adults in Egypt and Tunisia. *Social Science and Medicine* 2004; **59(12)**: 2479–2497.

Malawi

Ellis F, Kutengule M, Nyasulu A. Livelihoods and rural poverty reduction in Malawi. *World Development* 2003; **31(9)**: 1495–1510.

Kaler A. AIDS-talk in everyday life: the presence of HIV/AIDS in men's informal conversation in Southern Malawi. *Social Science and Medicine* 2004; **59(2)**; 285–297.

Kishindo P. Community development in Malawi: experiences at the grassroots. *Development in Practice* 2003; **13(4)**: 380–387.

Sindima HJ. *Malawi's First Republic: An Economic and Political Analysis.* University Press of America, 2002.

Morocco

Ababou M. The impact of age, generation and sex variables on religious beliefs and practices in Morocco. *Social Compass* 2005; **52(1)**: 31–44.

Elharti E, Alami M, Khattabi H, Bennani A, Zidouh A, Benjouad A, El Aouad R. Some characteristics of the HIV epidemic in Morocco. *East Mediterranean Health Journal* 2002; **8(6)**: 819–825.

Nigeria

Adesoji FA, Moronkola OA. Changing social and cultural practices in the face of HIV/AIDS in Nigeria. *Africa Quarterly* 2003; **43**(3): 55–60.

Gruber J, Caffrey M. HIV/AIDS and community conflict in Nigeria: implications and challenges. *Social Science and Medicine* 2005; **60**(6): 1209–1218.

Imobighe TA (ed.). *Civil Society and Ethnic Conflict Management in Nigeria.* Ibadan: Spectrum Books, 2003.

Sierra Leone

Baker B, May R. Reconstructing Sierra Leone. *Commonwealth and Comparative Politics* 2004; **42**(1): 35–60.

Chonghaile CN. World Bank allocates funds to help war-torn Sierra Leone fight HIV/AIDS. *Lancet* 2002; **359**(9313): 1219.

Sillinger B (ed.). *Sierra Leone: Current Issues and Background.* New York: Nova Science, 2003.

Swaziland

Daly AD, Nxumalo MP, Biellik RJ. Missed opportunities for vaccination in health facilities in Swaziland. *African Medical Journal* 2003; **93**(8): 606–610.

Marquette CM, Pichón F. Survival strategies among rural Swazi households: historical, ecological and social dimensions. *Forum for Development Studies* 1997; **2**: 307–320.

Miles M. Urbanisation in Swaziland: a post-independence assessment of its implications on the changing role of women. *Urban Forum* 2000; **1**(1): 103.

Nxumalo SS. Government in Swaziland: a unique approach to democracy *Parliamentarian* 1998; LXXIX **2**: 146–150.

Singer Y, Dlamini S, Fernandez C. Worldwide hospice & palliative care: focus on Africa. *American Journal of Hospice and Palliative Care* 2000; **17**: 298–299.

Tanzania

Beegle K. Labor effects of adult mortality in Tanzanian households. *Economic Development and Cultural Change* 2005; **53**(3): 655–684.

Dilger H. Sexuality, AIDS, and the lures of modernity: reflexivity and morality among young people in rural Tanzania. *Medical Anthropology* 2003; **22**(1): 23–52.

Hartwig KA, Eng E, Daniel M, Ricketts T, Crouse Quinn S. Aids and 'shared sovereignty' in Tanzania from 1987 to 2000: a case study. *Social Science and Medicine* 2005; **60**(7): 1613.

Mella PP. Major factors that impact on women's health in Tanzania: the way forward. *Health Care for Women International* 2003; **24**(8): 712.

The Gambia

Cham M, Sundby J, Vangen S. Maternal mortality in the rural Gambia, a qualitative study on access to emergency obstetric care. *Reproductive Health* 2005; **2**: 3.

Touray OA, Nugent P. The Gambia and the world: a history of the foreign policy of Africa's smallest state, 1965–1995. *Africa* 2004; **74**(2): 312–313.

Semega-Janneh IJ, Bohler E, Holm H, Matheson I, Holmboe-Ottesen G. Promoting breastfeeding in rural Gambia: combining traditional and modern knowledge. *Health Policy and Planning* 2001; **16**(2): 199–205.

Van der Loeff MFS, Sarge-Njie R, Ceesay S, Awasana AA, Jaye P, Sam O, Jaiteh KO, Cubitt D, Milligan P, Whittle HC. Regional differences in HIV trends in The Gambia: results from sentinel surveillance among pregnant women. *AIDS* 2003; **17**(12): 1841–1846.

Zambia

Baskind R, Birbeck G. Epilepsy care in Zambia: a study of traditional healers. *Epilepsia* 2005; **46**: 1121–1126.

Saasa OS, Carlsson Jerker. *Aid and Poverty Reduction in Zambia: Mission Unaccomplished.* London: Nordic Africa Institute Global, 2002.

Slonim-Nevo V, Mukuka L. AIDS-related knowledge, attitudes and behaviour among adolescents in Zambia. *AIDS Behaviour* 2005; **9**: 223–231.

Stekelenburg J, Jager BE, Kolk PR, Westen EHMN, van der Kwaak A, Wolffers IN. Health care seeking behaviour and utilisation of traditional healers in Kalabo, Zambia. *Health Policy* 2005; **71**(1): 67–81.

Countries with capacity building activity

Algeria

Fargues P. Women in Arab countries: challenging the patriarchal system? *Reproductive Health Matters* 2005; **13**(25): 43–48.

Hadefri R. AIDS in Algeria: the disease and the shame. *AIDS Analysis Africa* 1995; **5**(2): 5.

Cameroon

Amoaku E. Voluntary screening for HIV: 1997 World AIDS Day experience in a rural mission hospital in Cameroon. *Tropical Doctor* 1998; **28**(4): 248–249.

Gros J-G (ed.). *Cameroon: Politics and Society in Critical Perspectives.* Lanham, MD: University Press of America, 2003.

Jean-Robert RM. The woman's status and condom use in Cameroon. *African Journal of Reproductive Health* 2003; **7**(2): 74–88.

Notermans C. Sharing home, food, and bed: paths of grandmotherhood in East Cameroon. *Africa* 2004; **74**(1): 6–27.

Cote d'Ivoire

Akribi HAD, Desgrees Du Lou A, Msellati P, Dossou R. Issues surrounding reproductive choice for women living with HIV in Abidjan, Cote d'Ivoire. *Reproductive Health Matters* 1999; **7**(13): 20.

Aye M, Champagne F, Contandriopoulos AP. Economic role of solidarity and social capital in accessing modern health care services in the Ivory Coast. *Social Science and Medicine* 2002; **55**(11): 1929–1946.

Zellner S L. Condom use and the accuracy of AIDS knowledge in Cote d'Ivoire. *International Family Planning Perspective* 2003; **29**(1): 41–47.

Democratic Republic of the Congo (Congo-Kinshasa)

Denolf D, Musongela J P, Nzila N, Tahiri M, Colebunders R. The HIV epidemic in Kinshasa, Democratic Republic of Congo. *International Journal of STD and AIDS* 2001; **12**(12): 832–833.

Mulanga C, Bazepeo SE, Mwamba JK, Butel C, Tshimpaka JW, Kashi M, Lepira F, Caravel M, Peeters M, Delaporte E. Political and socioeconomic instability: how does it affect HIV? A case study in the Democratic Republic of Congo. *AIDS* 2004; **18**(5): 832–833.

Dijkzeul D. Healing governance? Four health NGOs in war-torn Eastern Congo. *Journal of International Affairs* 2003; **57**(1): 183–199.

Ethiopia

Hodes R. Visiting Solomon: AIDS in Ethiopia. *AIDS* 2002; **16**(1): 1–3.

Mengesha B, Ergete W. Staple Ethiopian diet and cancer of the oesophagus. *East African Medical Journal* 2005; **82**(7): 353–356.

Okubaghzi G, Singh S. Establishing an HIV/AIDS programme in developing countries: the Ethiopian experience. *AIDS* 2002; **16(12)**: 1575–1586.

Ghana

Ahorlu CK, Koram KA, Ahorlu C, de Savigny D, Weiss MG. Community concepts of malaria-related illness with and without convulsions in southern Ghana. *Malaria Journal* 27 2005; **4**: 47.

Boadi KO, Kuitunen M. Environment, wealth, inequality and the burden of disease in the Accra metropolitan area, Ghana. *International Journal of Environmental Health Research* 2005; **15**: 193–206.

Mill JE. Shrouded in secrecy: breaking the news of HIV infection to Ghanaian women. *Journal of Transcultural Nursing* 2003; **14(1)**: 6.

Van der Geest S.'I want to go!' How older people in Ghana look forward to death. *Ageing and Society* 2002; **22**: 7–28.

Lesotho

Fletcher M. Helping Lesotho with HIV/AIDS crisis. *Cancer Nurse* 2004; **100**: 11

Modo IVO. Migrant culture and changing face of family structure in Lesotho. *Journal of Comparative Family Studies* 2001; XXXII(3): 443–452.

Mturi AJ, Moerane W. Premarital childbearing among adolescents in Lesotho. *Journal of Southern African Studies* 2001; **27(2)**: 259–276.

Mozambique

Agadjanian V. Gender, religious involvement, and HIV/AIDS prevention in Mozambique. *Social Science and Medicine* 2005; **61**: 1529–1539.

Cabrita JM. *Mozambique: The Tortuous Road to Democracy*. New York: St Martin's Press, 2000.

Sheldon KE, Zimba B. Pounders of grain: a history of women, work, and politics in Mozambique. *Journal of African History* 2004; **45(1)**: 166–168.

Namibia

O'Hara MJ, Dohrn J. A midwife's day in Namibia and South Africa. *Journal of Midwifery and Womens Health* 2005; **50**: 283–285.

Ojo K, Delaney M. Economic and demographic consequences of AIDS in Namibia: rapid assessment of the costs. *International Journal of Health Planning Monthly* 1997; **12(4)**: 315–326.

LeBeau D, Collett C. Dealing with disorder: traditional and western medicine in Katatura (Namibia). *African Studies Review.* 2004; **47(3)**: 201–202.

Rwanda

Hilsum L. Rwandan genocide survivors denied AIDS treatment. *British Medical Journal* 2004; **328(7445)**: 913.

Kalk A, Mayindo JK, Musango L, Foulon G. Paying for health in two Rwandan provinces: financial flows and flaws. *Tropical Medicine and International Health* 2005; **10(9)**: 872–888.

Pavlish C. Refugee women's health: collaborative inquiry with refugee women in Rwanda. *Health Care for Women International* 2005; **26(10)**: 880–896.

Rahlenbeck SI. Knowledge, attitude, and practice about AIDS and condom utilization among health workers in Rwanda. *Journal of the Association of Nurses in AIDS Care* 2004; **15(3)**: 56–61.

Tunisia

Kallel H, Bahoul M, Ksibi H, Dammak H, Chelly H, Hamida CB, Chaari A, Rekik N, Bouaziz M. Prevalence of hospital-acquired infection in a Tunisian hospital. *Journal of Hospital Infection* 2005; **59(4)**: 343–347.

Tebourski F, Ben Alaya D. Knowledge and attitudes of high school students regarding HIV/AIDS in Tunisia: does more knowledge lead to more positive attitudes? *Journal of Adolescent Health* 2004; **34(3)**: 161.

Yount KM, Agree EM, Rebellon C. Gender and use of health care among older adults in Egypt and Tunisia. *Social Science and Medicine* 2004; **59(12)**: 2479–2497.

Index

3H International Rotary Grant (USA) 204
Abbot Pharmaceuticals 388
Abinaitwe, R. 209–10, 219
Abira, R. 115
ACA (Congo, Republic of the (Congo-Brazzaville))
    271, 272
advocacy 83–5
Afiyie, K. 440
African Association of Palliative Care 178
African Comprehensive HIV/AIDS
    Partnerships (ACHAP) 262, 264
African Medical Trust 438
African Palliative Care Association 10, 11, 22, 24
    Cameroon 410
    Cote d'Ivoire 418, 419
    Lesotho 450, 453
    Malawi 291
    Nigeria 310, 312, 313
    Rwanda 473
    South Africa 150
African Union 5
AIDS Alliance 387
AIDS Control Programme (Tanzania) 373
AIDS Healthcare Foundation 9
AIDS Relief Consortium (Tanzania) 353
Akankwasa, E. 210
Alabama University (USA) 386
Algeria 403–6
    current services 403–4
    education and training 404
    epidemiology 404–5
    health care system 405
    opioid availability and
        consumption 404
    political economy 405–6
    population 404
Ali, Z. 29, 62, 73, 102, 106, 118–19, 122
Allbrook, D. 106, 115, 117–18
Aloyce, M. 358
Andrew Mitchell Christian Charitable Trust 204
Anglican Children's Project (Zambia) 387
Anglican Church (UK) 264
Anglican United Society for the Propagation of the
    Gospel (Tanzania) 350
Appleton, J. 111, 118
APSO 30, 204
Aristotle: formal theory of justice 217
Arusha conference 150
Ash, M. 72–3, 353–4, 366–7
Asia 9, 52
Association Azur Developpement 272
Association Congolese Accompagner, L' 25
Association François-Xavier Bagnoud (Uganda):
    current services 203–4
    education and training 211

history and development of
    hospice–palliative care 214–15
palliative care coverage 207
Atkins, D. 218
autonomy, ideology of 216, 217–18
awareness, raised 60–2

Backeberg, M. 169, 170–1
Bagnoud, F.-X. 215
Bakari, B. 359
Bamalete Lutheran Hospital (Botswana) 263
Barnard, A. 74–5, 171
Barnard, C. 166, 188
Basemera, B. 439–40
Bates, J. 289
Beautiful Gate Ministries (Lesotho) 447–8
Beit Trust 238
Bekezela Community Home Based Care
    (Zimbabwe) 34
    current services 235
    education and training 241
    opioid availability and
        consumption 239
    palliative care coverage 240
    palliative care workforce capacity 244
    success stories 248
beneficence 216, 218
Bill & Melinda Gates Foundation 262
Bishop, C. 80
Biya, P. 413
Blair, T. 5
Bombwa, S. 293
Bond, C. 294, 324
Bongo, O. 275
Botswana 7, 11, 13, 259–60
    current services 259–60
    education and training 262
    epidemiology 266–7
    health care system 267–8
    history and development of
        hospice–palliative care 264–5
    HIV Response Information
        Management System 267
    morphine consumption 205
    national and professional
        organizations 262
    Network of AIDS Service
        Organizations 262
    opioid availability and
        consumption 261
    palliative care coverage 262
    palliative care workforce capacity
        263–4
    political economy 268
    population 266